Immunochemistry of Proteins

Volume 1

Immunochemistry of Proteins

Volume 1

Edited by

M. Z. Atassi

Mayo Graduate School of Medicine
Rochester, Minnesota
and
University of Minnesota
Minneapolis, Minnesota

PLENUM PRESS · NEW YORK AND LONDON

Library of Congress Cataloging in Publication Data

Main entry under title:

Immunochemistry of proteins.

Includes bibliographies and index.
1. Proteins–Analysis. 2. Immunochemistry. 3. Antigens–Analysis. I. Atassi, M. Z.
QP551.I44   574.1'9245   76-2596
ISBN-13: 978-1-4613-4192-5   e-ISBN-13: 978-1-4613-4190-1
DOI: 10.1007/978-1-4613-4190-1

© 1977 Plenum Press, New York
Softcover reprint of the hardcover 1st edition 1977
A Division of Plenum Publishing Corporation
227 West 17th Street, New York, N.Y. 10011

Contributors

M. Z. Atassi · Department of Immunology, Mayo Graduate School of Medicine, Rochester, Minnesota, and Department of Biochemistry, University of Minnesota, Minneapolis, Minnesota

Håkan Bergstrand · Tornblad Institute, University of Lund, and Research Laboratory, AB Draco, Lund, Sweden

Walter B. Dandliker · Department of Biochemistry, Scripps Clinic and Research Foundation, La Jolla, California

Vithal K. Ghanta · Department of Microbiology, University of Alabama, Birmingham, Alabama

A. F. S. A. Habeeb · Division of Clinical Immunology and Rheumatology, Department of Medicine and Departments of Microbiology and Biochemistry, University of Alabama School of Medicine, Birmingham, Alabama

Raymond N. Hiramoto · Department of Microbiology, University of Alabama, Birmingham, Alabama

Dov Michaeli · Departments of Biochemistry and Biophysics and Surgery, University of California School of Medicine, San Francisco, California

Abram B. Stavitsky · Department of Microbiology, School of Medicine, Case Western Reserve University, Cleveland, Ohio

Preface

The structural features responsible for the immunogenicity of certain parts of native protein molecules have been of interest to immunochemists and protein chemists for over three decades. Following the early work of Landsteiner in 1942, which showed that peptide fragments from silk fibroin exhibited an inhibitory activity toward the reaction of the protein with its antibodies, fragments from many other protein systems have been isolated and studied. However, no concerted effort was (or could be) devoted to the elucidation of the complete antigenic structure of a protein. In order for these endeavors to be successful and meaningful, knowledge of both the amino acid sequence and the detailed three-dimensional structure of the protein is necessary. Such information was not available for a protein until early in the 1960s. This and the fact that protein chemistry was not in fact sufficiently developed early in the 1960s to enable the successful completion of the entire antigenic structure of a protein were major contributing factors for the slow progress in this field. Determination of the antigenic structures of proteins therefore posed a chemical challenge of enormous proportions. For these reasons, many investigators diverted their attention to study of the immunochemistry of homo- or mixed amino acid polymers in the hope that the information derived from these systems might prove useful in the understanding of the immunochemistry of proteins. A great many data on these systems were accumulated that have been valuable in gaining some information on the immune mechanism. Unfortunately, it has now become clear that information from amino acid polymers is not in any way helpful in understanding the immunochemistry of proteins. Proteins represent the majority of antigens associated with many immunological disorders. Knowledge of the antigenic sites of these protein antigens lies at the basis of elucidating the mechanisms of these disorders at the molecular level. From a purely chemical perspective, the reaction of protein antigens with their antibodies remains one of the most fascinating and least understood phenomena in biochemistry.

The last decade has witnessed a great deal of activity carried out by many workers to investigate the immunochemistry of several protein antigens. Although, so far, only the antigenic structure of one native protein antigen (i.e., sperm whale myoglobin—to be reviewed in Volume 2) has been completed and that of lysozyme is almost complete (Volume 2), a great wealth of information in chemistry, immunochemistry, and technology has accumulated. It is surprising that there has been little awareness of the magnitude of the progress achieved in protein immunochemistry. Many recent immunological treatises have barely touched on this subject, while amino acid polymers, haptens, polysaccharides, etc., have been reviewed extensively. Therefore, critical review of the knowledge available in protein immunochemistry appears timely and should serve as a valuable guide for present and future undertakings.

The various chapters are written by leading and highly active workers in the field. It is now well appreciated that knowledge of protein chemistry and its proper and careful employment constitute the key approach in the elucidation of the antigenic structures of proteins. This fact was recognized much earlier by enzymologists and has contributed immeasurably to the significant advances in that field. Therefore, the work starts out with a critical review and evaluation of chemical modification and cleavage reactions of proteins. Also, the effects of conformational changes and evolutionary mutations on the immunochemistry of proteins are uniquely significant and these subjects will therefore be reviewed separately in detail. In view of the fact that methods and techniques employed in immunochemistry and immunology have been the subject of many excellent texts, the present work does not propose to duplicate these aspects. However, certain approaches (such as immunoabsorbents and fluorescence polarization) are, by the very nature of the subject, of particular relevance to immunochemical studies of proteins and will be reviewed here. Other chapters in this and the following volumes describe the immunochemistry and immunobiology of protein systems whose studies have contributed significantly to our knowledge of protein immunochemistry.

The treatise is intended to be a major reference work for those engaged in research in protein immunochemistry. One of the cruel shortcomings of review articles and books is that any work inadvertently overlooked by the reviewer may tend to be less cited and studied by others. It is my hope that the meticulous effort of the authors has minimized, if not completely avoided, this hazard.

M. Z. Atassi

Rochester, Minnesota

Contents

Chapter 1
**Chemical Modification and Cleavage of Proteins and Chemical
Strategy in Immunochemical Studies of Proteins**
   M. Z. Atassi

Chapter 2

Influence of Conformation on Immunochemical Properties of Proteins

A. F. S. A. Habeeb

Chapter 3
Investigation of Immunochemical Reactions by Fluorescence Polarization
Walter B. Dandliker

Chapter 4

In Vitro Immune Responses of Lymphoid Cell Populations to Proteins and Peptides

Abram B. Stavitsky

Chapter 5

Immunochemistry of Encephalitogenic Protein

Håkan Bergstrand

Chapter 6

Immunochemistry of Collagen

Dov Michaeli

Chapter 7

Histocompatibility Antigens
  Raymond N. Hiramoto and Vithal K. Ghanta

Contents of Volume 2

Chemical Modification and Cleavage of Proteins and Chemical Strategy in Immunochemical Studies of Proteins

M. Z. Atassi

I. Introduction

The determination of antigenic structures of proteins presents a major challenge, which is primarily chemical in nature. The chemical strategy set forth (Atassi, 1972) for our delineation of the complete antigenic structure of myoglobin (Atassi, 1975) has also proved extremely effective in substantial delineation of the antigenic structure of lysozyme. Delineation of the antigenic structures of these two proteins relied (Atassi, 1972) mainly on the following five approaches: (1) determination of the influence of conformational changes on immunochemical behavior, (2) study of the immunochemistry of specifically modified chemical derivatives of the protein, (3) study of the immunochemistry of a large number of peptide fragments with varying overlaps, (4) delineation of reactive regions on immunochemically reactive peptides by study of the immunochemistry of specific chemical derivatives of these peptides. and (5) organic synthesis of the antigenic reactive sites after they had been narrowed down by approaches (1)–(4) to a conveniently small size.

It has already been emphasized (Atassi, 1972, 1975) that none of the foregoing approaches by itself is likely to yield the antigenic structure. The extent of the role played by a given approach will depend on the protein

M. Z. Atassi · Department of Immunology, Mayo Graduate School of Medicine, Rochester, Minnesota, 55901, and Department of Biochemistry, University of Minnesota, Minneapolis, Minnesota 55455.

and on the antigenic site being delineated. The findings from one approach must be confirmed by independent findings from the others. Chapter 2 deals with the influence of conformational changes on the immunochemistry of proteins. Accordingly, this chapter will be concerned with a brief review and evaluation of chemical modification and cleavage reactions of proteins.

The chemical modification approach is useful only when certain precautions are observed. It is necessary to appreciate the effectiveness as well as the limitations of this technique. The employment of fragments in studying the immunochemistry of proteins has been in use ever since Landsteiner (1942) showed that peptides from silk fibroin inhibited the interaction of the fibroin with its antibodies. Clearly, the usefulness of this approach will depend on the availability and proper implementation of various fragmentation reactions for proteins. Fruitful immunochemical exploitation of the chemical cleavage requires not only knowledge of the chemistry and experimental design but also awareness of the power as well as the shortcomings of the approach. Therefore, this chapter is not intended to be a mere cataloguing of reactions; rather, an evaluation of the merits and disadvantages of a reaction will be discussed.

PART A: CHEMICAL MODIFICATION REACTIONS

II. Usefulness and Limitations

An organic reaction seldom achieves total completion. In protein chemistry, the reaction of a reagent (usually a small molecule) is complicated by many factors associated with the environment of the side chains and their accessibility to the reagent. The environment is of course dictated by the three-dimensional mode of folding and the contact surfaces between interacting subunits (if any) *in solution.* Accordingly, the reaction of a protein with a modifying reagent will seldom yield a product which is a single homogeneous molecular species. A reaction product from chemical modification must therefore be subjected to good purification procedures of high resolving capability in order to separate the variety of molecular species that may constitute the reaction product and also to remove any unreacted parent protein. This is extremely critical in immunochemical studies since the modification of one amino acid side chain, which actively forms a part of an antigenic reactive site, will be expected quantitatively to have a limited immunochemical effect (e.g., 15–20% when the reactivity of any one antigenic site in myoglobin is entirely abolished). Failure to purify or improper purification, often overlooked by many workers, will produce ambiguous results which may be difficult to correlate with other immunochemical information on the same protein. Having achieved purification and confirmed the purity of the protein by techniques of high resolution capabilities (e.g., disc electrophoresis, immunoelectrophoresis, and isoelectric focusing), it is then necessary to determine the nature and location(s) of the modification(s).

Frequently workers apply a reagent, previously reported to be specific for a given amino acid, for modification of their particular protein and then *assume* that the reaction has proceeded according to the "known" specificity of the reagent. It is relevant to caution here against complete reliance on the known specificity of a reagent. The type of amino acids modified by a given reagent can often vary with the protein, especially with regard to the "side reactions." Therefore, the specificity of a given reagent should be confirmed for each protein independently and the nature of the side reactions determined. A more common practice in determining the modification is to subject the derivative to methods of detection that may not be capable of monitoring side reactions. For example, amino acid analysis of HCl hydrolysates is not capable of detecting side reactions that may have involved tryptophan, or caused oxidation of methionine (to methionine sulfoxide) or its conversion to a sulfonium salt. Similarly, N-acyl, O-acyl, and esterified derivatives cannot be determined by amino acid analysis of acid or alkaline hydrolysates. Other substituents may possess limited stability and require a hydrolysis time–yield correlation in order to determine the extent of modification. Spectral methods are often used when the added substituent confers a unique spectral behavior on the derivative. These methods are extremely useful and convenient but are not capable of detecting side reactions, especially when they generate colorless derivatives with various amino acid side chains. Other methods of detection may employ titration of ionizable groups or a change in charge properties. These methods are often inaccurate and incapable of detecting side reactions involving other amino acids. It is always useful to employ, when possible, an isotopically labeled reagent. Although isotopic methods are subject to the previously mentioned limitations, their sensitivity frequently facilitates determination of the location and number of modified residues. It is apparent, therefore, that any one method for determining the modification should not be relied upon to the exclusion of other methods of detection. Unfortunately, this is a very common practice and the shortcomings of such studies must be borne in mind.

Once the nature and number of the modified residues have been determined, the location(s) of the modification(s) in the primary structure of the protein must be found. Here, it may be necessary to pay attention to the instability of certain substituents under conditions of peptide mapping or ion-exchange chromatography. These problems will be pointed out subsequently in the text as each reaction is discussed. Frequently, authors report the effect of modifying a certain number or percent of a given side chain (e.g., 20% of the amino groups) on the immunochemistry of a protein. Such approaches are of limited value if the locations of the modifications are not known.

Also, it is necessary to determine carefully any changes in conformation that may result from modification of the protein. Conformational changes may influence antigenic reactivity (Atassi, 1967d; Habeeb, 1967b; Andres and Atassi, 1970), and the immune response to native protein antigens, at least in early-course antisera, is directed against their native three-dimensional structure (Atassi and Thomas, 1969). Not every modification, of course, results in a conformational change, and no general rule can be given relating the nature of the modification to the presence of the conformational change. This will depend on the protein and the nature, extent, and location(s) of the modification. Therefore, the conformation of each protein derivative must be studied independently by a variety of physicochemical methods. Chemical methods may also be employed to monitor changes in protein conformation. This subject is handled in detail by Habeeb in Chapter 2. All possible parameters should be exhaustively studied and even then it is quite conceivable that the methods presently available for probing protein conformation, especially in solution, are incapable of determining with absolute certainty that the conformations of two proteins are identical. A minor change in the conformation of a protein often exerts an appreciable effect on its biological function. The magnitude of the conformational change that can be tolerated before a measurable effect on the antigenic reactivity becomes apparent need not be large and will vary with the protein.

III. Choice of Reaction and Evaluation of Results

In order to determine the role played by a modified residue in the immunochemistry of a protein, it is necessary to keep the extent of modification to a minimum. If several residues are modified simultaneously in a given derivative, it will not be possible to assign whatever immunochemical change that may be observed to any one of the altered side chains. Selectivity is usually a function of reaction conditions, and most modification reactions can be controlled so that the modification will not be extensive. This can be accomplished by controlling any one or more of the following: pH, temperature, concentration of reactants, excess of one reactant relative to the other, duration of reaction, change of solutes in the reaction medium, and in certain cases protection from light or oxygen. Ideally, it is desirable to prepare from each reaction a derivative of the protein modified at a single side chain. This may not always be possible. However, from the heterogeneous reaction product a number of derivatives are usually obtained which differ in the number and location(s) of the modification(s). Quite often, in fact, one can isolate a species of derivative modified only at one or two locations. This is possible because amino acid side chains of any given type (e.g., the lysines) show differences in their reactivities. The reactivities of given protein side chains will vary with their environment, their exposure to the reagent, the reagent itself, and with reaction conditions (Atassi and Habeeb, 1969). The reactivities with a reagent in solution are often at variance with their relative exposures in the crystalline three-dimensional structure (Lee *et al.*, 1975). For these reasons, reactivities cannot very well be predicted *a priori*.

The type of modification must also be carefully chosen for the particular purpose in mind. The absence of a change in a biological activity after modification of a residue does not necessarily suggest nonparticipation of this residue in the active site. In this case the nature of the modification must be considered. For example, guanidination of the amino groups in a protein will not usually (if no side reactions are present) change the biological properties of a protein. The guanidinium substituents can effectively discharge the functions previously imparted by the ammonium groups because of retention of the charge characteristics of the side chain. It is therefore necessary to determine if the modification is in fact chemically or sterically sufficient to impair the participation of the residue in the biological role in which it is normally involved (Atassi and Habeeb, 1969). It has been suggested (Atassi and Habeeb, 1969) that a good way to assess this is to modify the amino acid residue in question in more than one way. This, of course, is not always possible because of the limitation on the number of modification reactions that achieve a high degree of specificity and because (as mentioned above) availability of a given amino acid side chain to reaction might vary with the reagent (Atassi and Habeeb, 1969).

Bearing all the foregoing precautions in mind, changes in biological activity as a result of a specific chemical modification and in the absence of conformational changes will yield valuable information concerning the active site. Such a result may be considered a "positive" finding. There may be a tendency to consider the absence of change in biological behavior as a "negative" result of limited value. In fact, change in immunochemical reactivity after modification ("positive" result) should be interpreted with caution. It does not necessarily implicate the modified residue as a part of an antigenic site, because derivatives are often encountered where the conformational change is small, localized, and subtle, and not easily detectable by physical measurements on the protein in solution. In view of the aforementioned influence of conformation on immunochemistry, the assignment of an amino acid location to an antigenic reactive site is not straightforward and must be carefully confirmed by independent approaches. On the other hand, absence of change in immunochemical behavior after appropriate modification, a seemingly "negative" result, provides an unambiguous finding. The determination of the antigenic structure of a protein is a composite picture made up of numerous pieces of information and the parts of the jigsaw puzzle when assembled together must fit. Contradictory results suggest an error in deriving the information. Therefore, it is equally as critical to know where the antigenic reactive sites are as to know where they are not, and the two aspects should provide a double check on one another.

IV. Modification Reactions of Various Side Chains

In the following section, reactions for modification of various amino acid side chains will be reviewed briefly and their selectivity evaluated. For convenience, reactions for each functional side chain will be discussed separately. Some reagents may be used for modification of more than one type of side chain. In such cases the reagent will be cited under the amino acid for which it is usually applied. In other cases, where a reagent is used with similar frequency in modification of two or more types of amino acids, its reaction is briefly discussed under each of the respective amino acids with some relevant examples and a reminder to the section(s) dealing with its other reaction(s). Of course, even a nonselective reagent may be extremely useful if the amino acids which participate in "side reactions" are not present in the protein under study or if, alternatively, they could be reversibly masked by another reagent to protect them from participating in side reactions. It must be kept in mind that many of the following reagents could be varied so that they may carry radiolabel or a colored or a fluorescent group. Also, an environmentally sensitive reporter group may be introduced to enable, for example, performance of electron spin resonance or magnetic resonance experiments. When possible, brief mention of these applications will be given at the appropriate locations. Chemical modification reactions and their applications represent a vast subject. Therefore, in the following brief review emphasis will be placed on original reactions. Examples given are not exhaustive but are selected to demonstrate the suitability of the reaction and the difficulties that may be encountered.

A. Reactions for Amino Groups

The amino group in proteins is a quite reactive nucleophile, and therefore many reagents are available for its modification. Reactions of the amino group usually involve its unprotonated species and thus proceed between pH 8.0 and 9.5. However, higher pH conditions are frequently necessary. By lowering the pH of the reaction below 7 it is often possible to achieve preferential modification of the α-NH$_2$ group because it has a lower pK value than the ε-NH$_2$ group. Such possibilities when they exist with certain reagents will be pointed out. However, it must be remembered that the environment of a side chain in a protein plays a strong influence on its ionization properties and hence its reactivity. For example, it has been shown (Kokesh and Westheimer, 1971) that an essential lysine residue in acetoacetate decarboxylase has a pK value of about 6, which is considerably lower than the value for the free ε-NH$_2$ group.

1. Acylation with Acid Anhydrides

The modification of amino groups in proteins to the corresponding aminoacyl derivatives by reaction with acid anhydrides has been used extensively in protein chemistry. A number of mono- or dicarboxylic acid anhydrides have been employed. The reaction takes place rapidly at a slightly alkaline pH (8–9), and can be performed at neutral pH. Such acylation reactions are not specific for amino groups. In addition to α- and ε-NH$_2$ groups, phenolic and aliphatic hydroxyls and thiol and imidazole groups may be acylated. However, these side reactions are readily reversed, considerably minimized, or often avoided by careful control of reaction conditions (i.e., excess reagent, temperature, and pH). Esters of phenolic hydroxyls are unstable in a moderately alkaline medium (above pH 9), and can be removed at 0°C by a short exposure (10–15 min) of the derivative to this pH condition. Alternatively, deacylation of phenolic as well as aliphatic hydroxyls can be accomplished under milder conditions (around pH 7) by exposure to hydroxylamine (Hestrin, 1949). This forms the basis of various methods for determination of extent of esterification of phenolic (Riordan and Vallee, 1964) and aliphatic hydroxyls (Hestrin, 1949; Balls and Wood, 1956). The S-acyl groups can also be removed by hydroxylamine (Klotz and Elfbaum, 1964).

Reaction with *acetic anhydride* (Fraenkel-Conrat *et al.*, 1949) has been employed extensively for modification of amino groups. This substitution (—NHCOCH$_3$) results in the elimination of the positive charge of the ammonium group. Acetic anhydride is quite reactive, and complete acetylation of all the amino groups in a protein can be effected with a small excess of reagent. For example, all the amino groups of lysozyme were acetylated with a 3 molar excess of reagent per free amino group (Habeeb and Atassi, 1971a). In addition, seven aliphatic and some phenolic hydroxyls were esterified. With a ninefold molar excess per amino group, an average of 15 aliphatic hydroxyls were esterified. The two derivatives showed a decreased antigenic reactivity with antisera to lysozyme and suffered some conformational change (Habeeb and Atassi, 1971a). With cytochrome c, a twentyfold molar excess per amino group was necessary for complete acetylation of all the amino groups and some phenolic hydroxyls (Wada and Okunuki, 1968). A lower degree of acetylation was obtained with a onefold molar excess and a lower pH (6.3). From the reaction product, pure derivatives were obtained by ion-exchange chromatography that were acetylated at one, two, or three amino groups only and had no ester groups (Wada and Okunuki, 1968).

Acylation with *succinic anhydride* (Habeeb et al., 1958) introduces a carboxylate-carrying substituent ($-NH-COCH_2CH_2COO^-$) at the site of modification. Tyrosine residues were not modified by succinylation in bovine serum albumin, β-lactoglobulin (Habeeb et al., 1958), human IgM (Habeeb et al., 1970), or lysozyme (Habeeb and Atassi, 1971a; Lee et al., 1975), probably because of the lability of the O-succinyl moiety on tyrosine. Some proteins may yield homogeneous derivatives on succinylation (Habeeb et al., 1970). More often, however, succinylated derivatives are heterogeneous (Gounaris and Perlmann, 1967; Habeeb and Atassi, 1971a; Lee et al., 1975). In derivatives succinylated at all the amino groups, the heterogeneity may be attributed to nonuniform acylation of the aliphatic hydroxyl groups (Habeeb and Atassi, 1971a). Partial succinylation of the amino groups of lysozyme yielded a heterogeneous reaction product from which six homogeneous derivatives were isolated (Lee et al., 1975). Three of these derivatives did not show conformational changes and were instrumental in implicating lysine-33, -96, and -116 as part of antigenic reactive sites in lysozyme (Lee et al., 1975). Conformational changes are usually appreciable in succinylated proteins (Gounaris and Perlmann, 1967; Habeeb and Atassi, 1971a; Lee et al., 1975). On the other hand, succinylated α-chymotrypsin exhibited no conformational changes and retained almost its full esterase activity (Shiao et al., 1972). An approach for hybridization of native and succinylated oligomeric enzymes has been developed and applied to the study of the subunit structure of aldolase (Meighen and Schachman, 1970). Oligomeric proteins will be expected to dissociate upon complete succinylation. However, this is not a general rule and full succinylation of *Erwinia* asparaginase does not induce the tetramer to dissociate and does not destroy its catalytic activity (Shifrin et al., 1973).

Other anhydrides of dicarboxylic acids such as *glutaric* or *phthalic anhydrides* may also be employed for modification and reversal of the positive charge of the ammonium side chain. They are applications of the general acylation reaction and discussion of them here is not necessary.

The instability of N-acyl derivatives to conditions of protein hydrolysis, yielding back the original amino acid, precludes determination of the extent of modification by amino acid analysis. Usually, the number of unreacted amino groups is estimated by a spectrophotometric method or by use of a

$$\text{(a)} \qquad\qquad\qquad\qquad \text{(b)} \qquad (1)$$

suitably radiolabeled anhydride. Acylation with 3,3-*tetramethyleneglutaric anhydride* (Atassi, 1967c) obviates this instability problem. The *N*-acyl derivative, 3,3-tetramethyleneglutaryl-lysine (1a), will cyclize on acid hydrolysis of the protein derivative to 3,3-tetramethyleneglutarimidolysine (1b) and the latter can be determined by amino acid analysis. Complete acylation of sperm whale myoglobin by this reagent caused appreciable conformational changes and eliminated antigenic reactivity (Atassi, 1967c). Partial acylation in the presence of 10 molar excess of anhydride per mole of myoglobin (i.e., 0.5 mole per free amino group) gave a heterogeneous reaction product from which three homogeneous derivatives were isolated by CM-cellulose chromatography and their conformation and immunochemistry studied in detail (Atassi *et al.*, 1973b). These studies determined that lysine-98 is in an antigenic reactive region, whereas lysine-140 and -145 were not part of a reactive region in myoglobin.

Ethoxyformic anhydride $[(CH_3CH_2OCO)_2O]$ is another commercially available acylating agent. Like the other anhydrides, however, it can also acylate hydroxyl, imidazole, and sulfhydryl groups (Mühlard *et al.*, 1967). At pH 4, only the α-amino group of pepsin reacted, while in ribonuclease, amino as well as imidazole groups were modified, and in α-chymotrypsin, ethoxyformylation of the active-site serine resulted (Melchior and Fahrney, 1970). Reaction around neutrality does not improve specificity. At pH 7, only lysine residues were acylated in α-chymotrypsin (Melchior and Fahrney, 1970), while in bovine serum albumin, tryptophan residues were modified (Rosén and Fedorcsak, 1966). At pH 6, phospholipase A_2 was inactivated by acylation of one lysine residue per dimer (Wells, 1973). See also Section IVE3 for further discussion of this reagent.

The mixed anhydride (2a) has been used to introduce spin labels into proteins, and it labels both NH_2 and NH groups (Griffith *et al.*, 1967; Berger *et al.*, 1971). On the other hand, compound (2b), which is not an anhydride but a ketone (2,2,6,6-*tetramethyl-4-piperidone-1-oxyl*), labels NH_2 groups specifically (Wagner and Hsu, 1970). These are useful for electron spin resonance studies on proteins (Oakes and Cafe, 1973).

Certain anhydrides give labile *N*-acyl substituents that may be removed under certain conditions. These will be discussed in a later section together with other amino-group reversible blocking reagents.

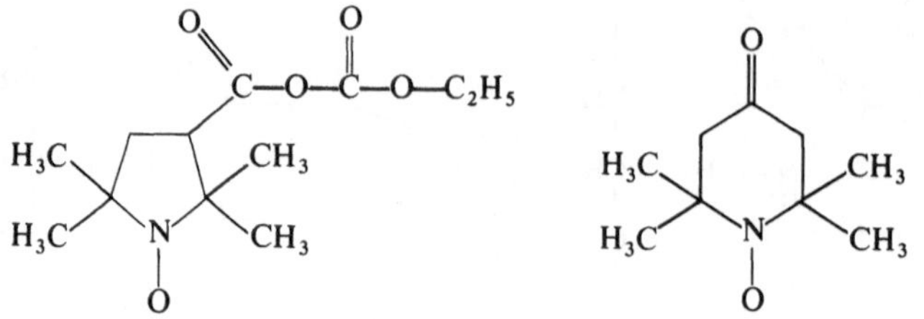

O
O
C—O—C—O—C₂H₅
H₃C
CH₃
H₃C
N
CH₃
O
O
H₃C
CH₃
H₃C
N
CH₃
O

(a) (b) (2)

2. Reaction with N-Carboxyamino Acid Anhydrides

Reaction with *N-carboxyamino acid anhydrides* is an application of the acylation reaction by acid anhydrides. However, the reaction seems to be confined to the amino and sulfhydryl groups. Reactive amino groups form an amide bond with the coupled amino acid, whose amino group will then react further so that the process continues. As a result, polypeptide chains of varying lengths polymerize onto the modified protein amino groups (Becker and Stahmann, 1953) with a free α-NH_2 group at the end of the added polymerized chain. Polymerization onto the protein can be effected in aqueous media at low temperature and neutral pH. Proline anhydride is best polymerized onto amino groups in dimethylsulfoxide (Jaton and Sela, 1968). *N*-carboxyamino acid anhydrides are relatively unstable, and the degree of polymerization cannot be entirely controlled. Polypeptidylated proteins have served as models for the study of biological and physicochemical properties of proteins (for review, see Sela and Arnon, 1972). Other than for general topical immunochemical properties, their employment for delineation of antigenic reactive sites of proteins has not been possible.

3. Thiolation

Thiol groups can be introduced into proteins by covalent modifications relying on the acid anhydride reaction described previously. This modification is useful for the introduction of heavy metal substitutions. The reaction employs either a thiolactone (3a) or an anhydride (4a). Thiolation of proteins was performed with *N-acetylhomocysteine thiolactone* (Benesch and Benesch,

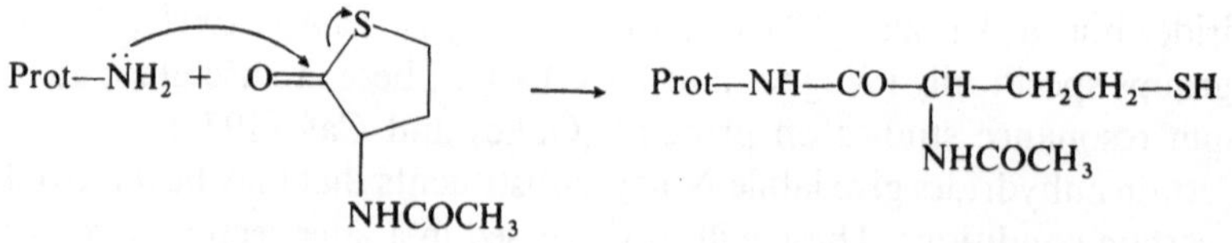

Prot—NH₂ + O
S
NHCOCH₃
Prot—NH—CO—CH—CH₂CH₂—SH
NHCOCH₃

(a) (b) (3)

1958, 1962). The reaction is catalyzed by Ag^+ (Benesch and Benesch, 1958, 1962), imidazole (Klotz and Elfbaum, 1964), or Ag^+ and imidazole together (Kendall and Barnard, 1969). Thiolations of chymotrypsinogen (Abadi and Wilcox, 1960) and ribonuclease (White and Sandoval, 1962) were possible without Ag^+, although with undesirable side reactions, including disulfide interchange in the case of ribonuclease. Thiolation in the presence of Ag^+ may be preferred because it can be performed at a lower pH (7–8) and provides an automatically protected thiol group (Kendall and Barnard, 1969). Protected thiol groups were introduced into proteins under mild conditions with *S-acetylmercaptosuccinic anhydride* (4a) (Klotz and Heiney, 1962). The *S*-acetyl group may be removed by hydroxylamine (Klotz

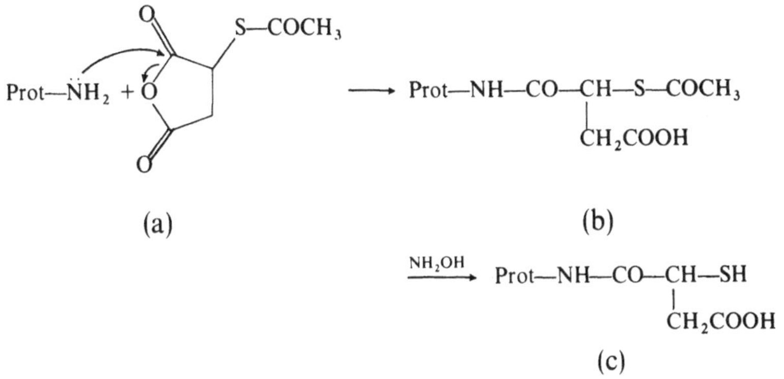

$$\text{Prot}-\overset{\cdot\cdot}{N}H_2 + \quad \xrightarrow{\quad} \quad \text{Prot}-NH-CO-\underset{\underset{CH_2COOH}{|}}{CH}-S-COCH_3$$

(a)   (b)

$$\xrightarrow{\quad NH_2OH \quad} \text{Prot}-NH-CO-\underset{\underset{CH_2COOH}{|}}{CH}-SH \qquad (4)$$

(c)

and Elfbaum, 1964). Other anhydrides designed to introduce disulfide, thioether, and protected thiol groups have been employed (Klotz *et al.*, 1965). Introduction of one or two mercaptosuccinyl groups into Taka-amylase increased its enzymatic activity considerably (Suzuki *et al.*, 1970), whereas succinylation lowered its activity. It was interesting that when the thiol groups on the mercaptosuccinyl substituent were reacted with *p*-chloromercuribenzoate or iodoacetamide, the enzyme lost its activity, suggesting an active role played in the enzymatic activity by the artificially introduced thiol groups. Thiolation by aminolysis has been reviewed (White, 1972*b*).

4. Other Acylating Agents

N-Acetylsuccinimide (Cooper *et al.*, 1970) and other *N-acylsuccinimides* (Boyd *et al.*, 1972*a*) have been shown to be effective acylating agents. These agents are soluble in water, hydrolyze relatively slowly, but are sufficiently reactive to acylate amines in aqueous solution even at low pH (Boyd *et al.*, 1972*a*). Reaction of *N*-acetylsuccinimide (5a) with ribonuclease and bovine serum albumin effected acetylation (5b) in the pH range 3–8. Acetylation was quite selective for amino groups with little or no tyrosine modifica-

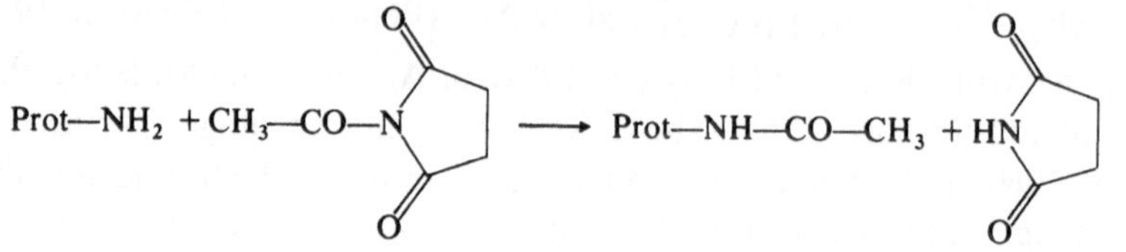

$$\text{Prot—NH}_2 + \text{CH}_3\text{—CO—N} \underset{O}{\overset{O}{\diagdown}} \longrightarrow \text{Prot—NH—CO—CH}_3 + \text{HN} \underset{O}{\overset{O}{\diagdown}} \qquad (5)$$

$$\qquad\qquad\qquad\qquad (a) \qquad\qquad\qquad\qquad\qquad\qquad\qquad (b)$$

tion. No acylation of serine, threonine, or histidine side chains was observed. Other *N*-acylsuccinimides also acylated lysine side chains selectively. These reagents should prove extremely useful for modification of amino groups. They are easy to synthesize and their high selectivity avoids many of the side reactions encountered with acid anhydrides.

The activated carcinogen *N-acetoxy-2-fluorenylacetamide* (6a) has been shown (Barry and Gutmann, 1973) to effect acetylation (6b) of some

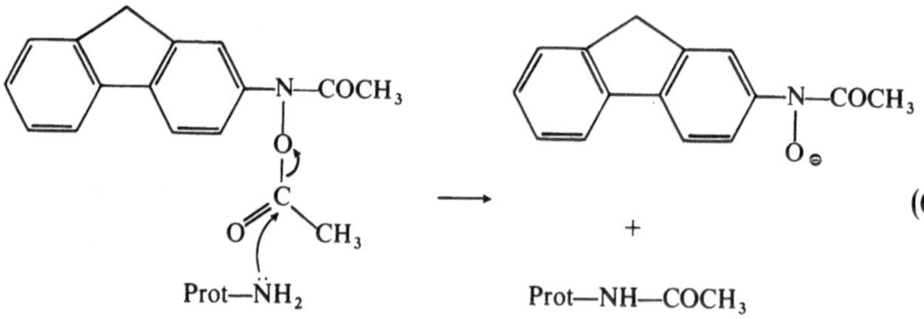

$$(6)$$

$$\qquad\qquad (a) \qquad\qquad\qquad\qquad\qquad\qquad\qquad (b)$$

lysine residues in ribonuclease. Although the reagent acted primarily as an acetyl donor, some arylamidation and other "unknown interactions" were not discounted.

An acylating agent related to the aforementioned *N*-acylsuccinimides is *N-succinimidyl 3-(4-hydroxyphenyl)propionate* (7) (Rudinger and Ruegg,

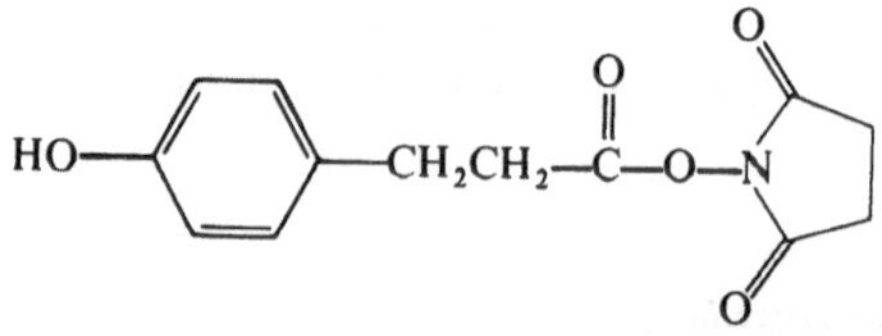

$$(7)$$

1973). This reagent, which can be readily radioiodinated, was used for labeling proteins to high radioactivities (Bolton and Hunter, 1973). Iodination of the reagent in the absence of protein followed, in a separate step, by conjugation of the labeled moiety avoids many of the problems encountered in radioiodination (see Section IVJ2). However, with this reagent the label will be on amino groups. In immunochemical studies, this may drastically affect the antigenic reactivity of many protein antigens when they have lysine residues as parts of their antigenic sites (e.g., see later chapters on myoglobin and lysozyme).

Specific N^ε-acylation of free peptides containing lysine has been obtained in good yield by reaction with *tert-butylazidoformate* (Lande, 1971). The relatively low reactivity of the reagent and the high nucleophilicity of the ε-NH_2 groups made it possible to differentiate between α- and ε-NH_2 groups. Reaction at pH 7.0 of model peptides was primarily at the N^α position. Reaction in pyridine–water–triethylamine was at the N^ε position. The two ε-NH_2 groups in β-melanotropin were specifically acylated in good yield either in pyridine–water–acetic acid or in water at pH 10.5. The reaction of model peptides with *trifluoroacetic anhydride* in trifluoroacetic acid yielded only the N^α-acyl product. The conditions for these reactions may not be well suited for protein modification. However, they may prove useful for specific modification of certain immunochemically reactive peptides at either the N^α or N^ε position.

Another acylation reaction, which may be applicable only to peptides because of the nature of the reaction medium, is trichloroacetylation by *hexachloroacetone* (Panetta and Casanova, 1970a). Trichloroacetylation of the amino group was done in simple model peptides at room temperature and under neutral conditions (8). The carboxylate group did not interfere

$$\text{Pept—NH}_2 + \text{Cl}_3\text{C—C—CCl}_3 \xrightarrow[\substack{25^\circ\text{C} \\ 12\text{-}24 \text{ hr}}]{\text{DMSO}} \text{Pept—NH—C—CCl}_3 + \text{CHCl}_3 \qquad (8)$$

with this novel reaction. The hydroxyl groups may be acylated under more basic conditions. Reaction with other functional groups was not investigated.

Trifluoroacetylation of the amino group has been accomplished using *sym-trichloro-trifluoroacetone* (9a) in dimethylsulfoxide (DMSO) (Panetta

$$\text{Pept—NH}_2 + \text{CCl}_3\text{—C—CF}_3 \xrightarrow[25^\circ\text{C, 24 hr}]{\text{DMSO}} \text{Pept—NH—C—CF}_3 + \text{CHCl}_3 \qquad (9)$$

$$\text{(a)} \qquad\qquad\qquad\qquad\qquad \text{(b)}$$

and Casanova, 1970b). The reaction conditions were mild and essentially neutral. The carboxyl and the phenolic OH groups did not react. N-Trifluoroacetylation rather than trichloroacetylation is obtained exclusively by this reagent because the trifluoromethyl group is a much poorer leaving group than is the trichloromethyl group. This reagent may prove to be more suitable for N-trifluoroacetylation of peptides than the conventional trifluoroacetic anhydride since it avoids the partial cleavage of peptide bonds encountered during trifluoroacetylation of peptides by trifluoroacetic anhydride (Weygand et al., 1966).

A transacetylation reaction has been recently reported from *aspirin* (*acetylsalicylate*) to lysine residues of hemoglobin S (Shamsuddin *et al.*, 1974). Other sites may have been acylated to a lesser extent. The transacetylation may have been catalyzed by histidine residues neighboring each of the acetylated lysines. This interesting reaction merits further investigation to determine the factors for most suitable reaction conditions and specificity. The acyl moiety on the salicylate may be altered so that a variety of acyl groups are introduced into the protein.

Acylation by active esters of *N*-substituted amino acids, especially *p-nitrophenyl* and *N-hydroxysuccinimide esters*, has been used extensively in peptide synthesis (Bodansky and Ondetti, 1966). Under appropriate conditions, there is no reason why these activated esters should not be used for modification of amino groups in proteins. Removal of the *N*-protecting group of the coupled amino acid may be accomplished by the usual procedures (see Bodansky and Ondetti, 1966). The amino groups of insulin have been coupled with *tert*-butyloxycarbonyl-*p*-nitrophenyl esters of amino acids (Levy and Carpenter, 1967).

5. Reaction with Aldehydes

Formaldehyde in acid or alkaline solution can add as methylol groups (CH_2OH) to amide groups (Fraenkel-Conrat *et al.*, 1945), arginine (Fraenkel-Conrat and Olcott, 1946), tryptophan, histidine, tyrosine, and cysteine (French and Edsall, 1945). Formaldehyde adds to the amino groups instantaneously even at neutral pH and low temperatures (Fraenkel-Conrat and Olcott, 1948). The methylol adduct can be decomposed by dilution or dialysis of the reaction mixture (French and Edsall, 1945). However, formaldehyde also irreversibly cross-links amino groups with phenol, imidazole, and indole groups (Fraenkel-Conrat and Olcott, 1948). The high, nonselective reactivity of formaldehyde makes it unsuitable for employment in immunochemical studies of proteins.

Salicylaldehyde (*o*-hydroxybenzaldehyde), a somewhat less reactive aldehyde, was used to modify the NH_2 groups in cytochrome *c* (Williams and Jacobs, 1968). In addition, it reacted with phenolic OH groups. Further work is necessary to investigate its reaction with other functional groups. The methinyl phenol groups could be removed simply by dialysis. The azomethine adduct with amino groups was reversed either at pH 3 or at pH 11 with complete restoration of enzymatic activity. Polymers of the protein were also present because of the formation of cross-links.

The dialdehyde *glutaraldehyde* [$OHC-(CH_2)_3-CHO$] has been used extensively for cross-linking purposes (see Section IVK2). It should be expected to possess broad reactivity similar to that of other aldehydes.

From the results of amino acid analysis of acid hydrolysates it has been reported to be specific for some lysine residues in carboxypeptidase A (Quoicho and Richards, 1966). However, in addition to NH_2 groups, it has been shown (Habeeb and Hiramoto, 1968) to react with thiol and phenolic OH groups, and histidine residues. It also formed cross-links in each of bovine serum albumin, ovalbumin, and human γ-globulin. It is likely that these adducts hydrolyze in acid to yield back the original amino acid and will not be detectable by amino acid analysis.

6. Reductive Alkylation

Reaction of *formaldehyde* with NH_2 groups *followed by catalytic reduction* (on Pd/charcoal) was shown to produce the $N(CH_3)_2$ derivatives (Ingram, 1950, 1953). This reaction has since been exploited under carefully controlled conditions. Reaction of proteins with an *aldehyde* or *ketone* (10a), in a small molar excess relative to the amino groups, at 0°C and pH 9.0 for a brief period (about 30 sec) was followed by reduction of the Schiff's base intermediate (10b) with $NaBH_4$ to give the corresponding *N*-alkyl derivatives (10c) (Means and Feeney, 1968). The amount of $NaBH_4$

$$\text{Prot—NH}_2 + \text{O=CHR} \underset{+H_2O}{\overset{\substack{pH\ 9.0 \\ -H_2O}}{\rightleftharpoons}} \text{Prot—N=CHR} \xrightarrow{BH_4^{\ominus}} \text{Prot—NH—CH}_2\text{R} \qquad (10)$$

(a) (b) (c)

is kept low so that disulfide bonds are not reduced. Formaldehyde gave the N^ε-$(CH_3)_2$ adduct, whereas acetaldehyde or acetone gave the N^ε-monoalkyl derivatives (Means and Feeney, 1968). The reaction was reported to be specific for amino groups. This specificity, which seems unlikely at first glance in view of the foregoing discussion on the nonselective reactivity of formaldehyde, has in fact been well established. The reaction was subsequently used for radioactive labeling of proteins with [³H]- or [¹⁴C]methyl groups by employing appropriately labeled formaldehyde (Rice and Means, 1971). Reductive alkylation of horse liver alcohol dehydrogenase with [¹⁴C]formaldehyde (Jörnvall, 1973) or unlabeled formaldehyde (Tsai et al., 1974) alkylated only lysine residues. Conformational changes accompanied the methylation of some (26 out of 60) lysine residues and the enzymatic activity increased (Tsai et al., 1974). Four lysine residues (of the 26) could be protected from methylation by NADH. Reductive methylation of ovine luteinizing hormone effected almost complete (90%) alkylation of lysine-42 and partial (50%) alkylation of lysine-20 (the derivatives were not purified), resulting in a more active luteinizing hormone (De la Llosa et al., 1974). Reductive alkylation has even recently been employed to probe the topography of ribosomal proteins (Moore and Crichton, 1974). However, in reductive alkylation the possibility of reaction of formaldehyde with thiol groups to give hemithioacetals and hemithioketals should not be overlooked.

Enzymes that carry *pyridoxal phosphate* or which have a phosphate binding site that will form specific Schiff-base complexes with pyridoxal phosphate can be reductively alkylated with $NaBH_4$ (Fischer *et al.*, 1958; for review and conditions, see Strausbauch *et al.*, 1967). The absorption maximum of the Schiff's base (about 415–425 nm) shifts (to about 325 nm) after reductive alkylation. Reduction of an NADP-specific glutamate de-hydrogenase from *Neurospora* with pyridoxal phosphate followed by reduction inactivated the enzyme, labeling it preferentially at a single lysine residue (Blumenthal and Smith, 1973). On the other hand, in the NAD-dependent enzyme from *Neurospora* which was inhibited reversibly by pyridoxal phosphate, five lysine residues per subunit were involved in the binding as determined by $NaBH_4$ reduction (Degani *et al.*, 1974) and iso-lation of the appropriate five fluorescent peptides containing ε-N-(5'-phosphopyridoxyl)lysine (Veronese *et al.*, 1974). The inactivation of fructose 1,6-diphosphatase with pyridoxal phosphate and reduction in the presence of the allosteric inhibitor AMP was shown (Colombo and Marcus, 1974) to be due to alkylation of four lysine residues per mole of enzyme. Inactiva-tion was protected by the substrate fructose 1,6-diphosphate or the inhibitor fructose 6-phosphate. Clearly, therefore, this technique will be useful for modifying ε-NH_2 groups in or near phosphate-binding sites of enzymes. Studying the immunochemistry of the derivatives thus prepared will provide information on the involvement of the modified residues in antigenic re-active sites and proximity of any of these sites to the phosphate-binding site. The reaction of pyridoxal with sulfhydryl groups should not be dis-missed.

An environmentally sensitive reporter group was introduced at the essential lysine residue in acetoacetate decarboxylase by condensation of the latter with *5-nitrosalicylaldehyde* followed by reduction of the resulting Schiff base by borohydride (Frey *et al.*, 1971). From changes in the optical absorption of the *N*-substituted 2-hydroxy-5-nitrobenzylamino reporter group, a pK value of about 6 was assigned to the essential lysine residue in the enzyme (Kokesh and Westheimer, 1971).

Finally, a novel approach for immobilization of enzymes on *aldehydic matrices* has been reported (Royer *et al.*, 1975). Supporting media containing diols were first oxidized with sodium periodate. Enzymes coupled to the oxidized supports by reduction with borohydride possessed good catalytic activities.

It is relevant to point out here that a low level of peptide bond reduction occurring as a side reaction has been observed (Paz *et al.*, 1970) when denatured collagen was treated with small amounts of tritiated sodium borodeuteride. The possibility of such a side reaction taking place on reductive alkylation of a protein should not be overlooked, even though it has not been reported with the other proteins studied so far.

7. Reaction with Aryl Halides and Aryl Sulfonyl Halides

The best-known aryl halide is 2,4-*dinitrofluorobenzene* (Sanger, 1945). Several variations of this reagent have since been utilized in protein chemistry. Some variations carried two reactive halides to introduce cross-links in proteins. Dinitrophenyl proteins have been used extensively in immunochemistry to study the immune response to the dinitrophenyl hapten and to the carrier protein. Reaction with these aryl halides proceeds by normal nucleophilic aromatic substitution, with amino, thiol, imidazole, and phenolic and, to a much lesser extent, aliphatic OH groups acting as nucleophiles. Consequently, aryl halides are not specific. However, under carefully controlled conditions it has often been possible to prepare derivatives specifically modified at amino groups. An example is the specific dinitrophenylation of ribonuclease A at certain lysine residues (Hirs and Kycia, 1965). The following (11a–c) three aryl halides (and the corresponding aryl sulfonates) which include the CF_3 group in the structure were coupled to human serum albumin (Gerig and Reinheimer, 1975). Derivatives of this

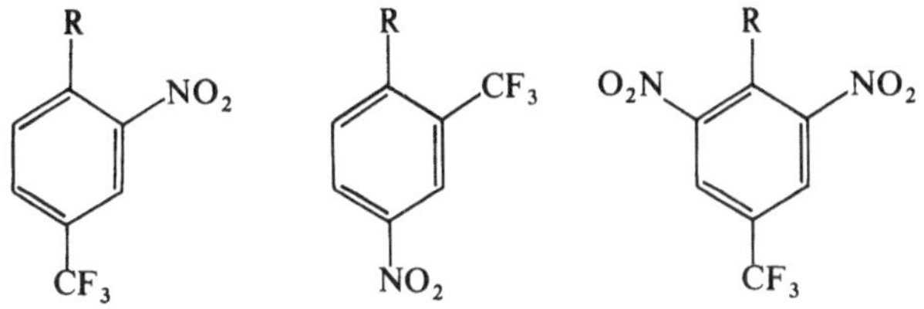

(a)   (b)   (c)   (a–c) R = F
(d)   (e)   (f)   (d–f) R = SO_3Na

(11)

type should prove useful for probing subtle changes in protein structure from the chemical shift and nuclear relaxation time data obtained from fluorine magnetic resonance experiments.

7-*Chloro-4-nitrobenzo-2-oxa-1,3-diazole* (NBD chloride), a stable non-fluorescent compound (12a), reacts with amino groups to form highly fluorescent 7-substituted derivatives (12b) (Ghosh and Whitehouse, 1968). The fluorogenic properties of NBD chloride are similar to those of dansyl chloride. However, NBD chloride has higher stability and solubility than dansyl chloride. NBD derivatives are excited by visible light (464 nm), whereas dansyl derivatives are excited at 254 or 365 nm. NBD chloride is

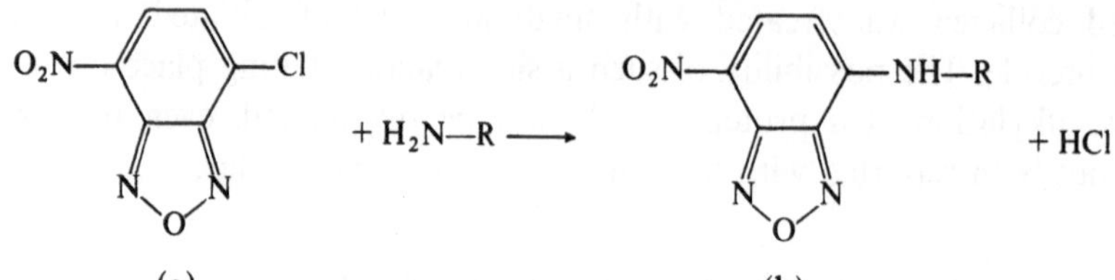

$$\text{(a)} \qquad + H_2N\text{—}R \longrightarrow \qquad \text{(b)} \qquad + HCl \quad (12)$$

not specific for amino groups and has so far been shown to react with sulf-hydryl groups (Birkett *et al.*, 1970) and with the phenolic OH groups of tyrosine (Aboderin *et al.*, 1973). Upon reaction with aryl halides, the positive charge of the ammonium group is lost.

Aryl sulfonyl halides (e.g., *p-toluenesulfonyl chloride* and *fluoride*) also possess broad reactivity. They will react with amino, thiol, imidazole, and hydroxyl (both aliphatic and phenolic) groups. Sulfonamide formation with amino groups (13) eliminates their positive charge. These will be discussed in subsequent sections in connection with modification and cleavage at sites of other functional residues.

$$\text{Prot—NH}_2 + X\text{—}\overset{\overset{\textstyle O}{\|}}{\underset{\underset{\textstyle O}{\|}}{S}}\text{—Ar} \longrightarrow \text{Prot—NH}\text{—}\overset{\overset{\textstyle O}{\|}}{\underset{\underset{\textstyle O}{\|}}{S}}\text{—Ar} + HX \qquad X = Cl, F \quad (13)$$

Dansyl chloride (1-dimethylaminonaphthalene-5-sulfonyl chloride) (14a), a nonfluorescent reagent which was first reported by Weber (1952) to give fluorescent conjugates with proteins, was subsequently studied in more detail by Hartley and Massey (1956) with amino acids, peptides and proteins. The high fluorescence of *N*-dansyl amino acids made this reagent

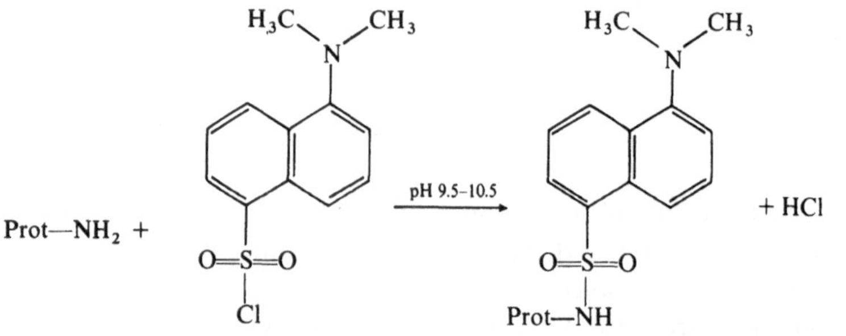

$$\text{Prot—NH}_2 + \qquad \text{(a)} \qquad \xrightarrow{\text{pH } 9.5\text{–}10.5} \qquad \text{(b)} \qquad + HCl \quad (14)$$

extremely useful in *N*-terminal determination, enabling scaling down of the operation about a hundredfold relative to fluorodinitrobenzene (for review, see Narita, 1970). Fluorescence is excited at 254 or 365 nm. The re-agent is not soluble in aqueous solvents and, in addition to amino groups (reaction 14), it reacts with sulfhydryl, phenolic OH, and imidazole groups. The broad selectivity of dansyl chloride has not precluded its employment in the specific modification of proteins. It has been possible to modify only amino groups in many proteins by this reagent. For example, lobster arginine kinase has been dansylated by reaction with a 100 M excess of reagent at pH 8.2 and 0°C for 20 min (Benyamin *et al.*, 1973). The six thiol groups modified by the reagent were regenerated quantitatively by dithio-threitol (6 mM) at pH 8.8 and 25°C for 90 min. The resulting derivative was specifically modified at amino groups (whose locations were not determined). The dansylated preparation showed no conformational changes and retained full antigenic reactivity with antibodies to native arginine kinase. A sensitive method for determination of lysyl and tyrosyl residues by [^{14}C]dansyl chloride in the presence of sodium dodecylsulfate has been reported (Casola *et al.*, 1974).

Isotopically labeled *p-iodobenzenesulfonyl (pipsyl) chloride* (with [^{131}I]) was introduced for the quantitative determination of N-terminal residues of proteins (Keston *et al.*, 1946; Udenfriend and Velick, 1951). Determination of free amino groups was performed on seven proteins with [^{35}S]-pipsyl chloride (Oratz *et al.*, 1966), giving good agreement with the expected number of free ε-NH$_2$ groups. Pipsyl chloride has also been reported to react with tyrosine residues in bovine insulin (Fletcher, 1967).

8. Reaction with Aryl Sulfonates

Aryl sulfonates give similar amino group derivatives to those of the corresponding aryl halides. Thus 2,4-*dinitrobenzene sulfonate* (Eisen *et al.*, 1953) gives the same dinitrophenyl derivative as that obtained by 2,4-dinitrofluorobenzene. However, the sulfonates are more selective for amino groups. Light dinitrophenylation of cytochrome *c* (at undetermined sites) by dinitrobenzene sulfonate enhanced its immunogenicity (Wang and Reichlin, 1974). Introduction of 2,4,6-*trinitrobenzene sulfonic acid* (TNBS, 15a) (Okuyama and Satake, 1960) has served as the basis of a very sensitive colorimetric method for amino group determination (Habeeb, 1966b). The adduct (15b) has an absorption maximum at 335 nm. This spectro-

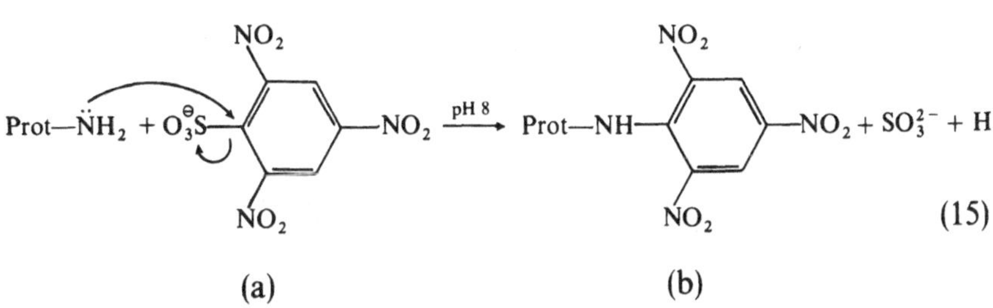

$$\text{Prot}-\overset{..}{\text{N}}\text{H}_2 + \text{O}_3^{\ominus}\text{S} \overset{\text{(a)}}{-\!\!\!\!\bigcirc\!\!\!\!-}\text{NO}_2 \xrightarrow{\text{pH 8}} \text{Prot}-\text{NH} \overset{\text{(b)}}{-\!\!\!\!\bigcirc\!\!\!\!-}\text{NO}_2 + \text{SO}_3^{2-} + \text{H}^+ \qquad (15)$$

photometric method, or some variations of it, has been used extensively and the subject has been reviewed by Fields (1972). Thiol groups will be modified by TNBS. The reagent, which was once believed to be more reactive with amino groups (Kotaki et al., 1964), has in fact been found to have a much higher reactivity with thiol groups (Friedman, 1973). In addition to its use in spectrophotometric determinations of total amino groups, TNBS can be employed for the modification of a limited number of amino groups under controlled conditions. For example, in bovine liver glutamate dehydrogenase two amino groups (lysine-428 and -425) were modified specifically by reaction with TNBS (Coffee et al., 1971). Lysine-425 became available to reaction only when lysine-428 (on a different polypeptide chain) had been trinitrophenylated. Nucleotide ligands did not protect against trinitrophenylation and the resulting loss of activity.

A group of *trifluoromethyl*-substituted *aryl sulfonates* (see structures 11d–f) have been introduced (Gerig and Reinheimer, 1975) to enable probing of protein structure by fluorine magnetic resonance.

β-Naphthoquinone-4-sulfonic acid reacts with amino groups between pH 7.5 and 9.3, and the degree of reaction can be determined by absorption at 480 nm (Matsushima et al., 1967). Also, *β-naphthoquinone-4,6- and 4,7-disulfonic acids* react with amino groups at pH 8.4–9.1, and the extent of reaction can be determined by difference spectrophotometry at 480 nm (Matsushima et al., 1968). Other aryl mono- and disulfonates have been used and possess similar selectivity.

9. Other Alkylating Agents

Alkyl halides are not selective and will react with other side chains. Thiol, imidazole, and thioether groups as well as carboxyl groups may be modified in addition to amino groups (for review, see Cohen, 1968).

Dimethylsulfate is a nonspecific base-methylating agent (Lawley and Brookes, 1964). It reacts at different rates with many amino acid side chains, including esterification of carboxyl groups. However, [^{14}C]dimethylsulfate has found use as a probe to study the organization of ribosomal proteins and RNA (Moore, 1975). It may find similar application in the study of biological membranes.

2-Methoxy-5-nitrotropone (16a) can also be used to modify amino groups (Tamaoki et al., 1967). The extent of modification can be determined

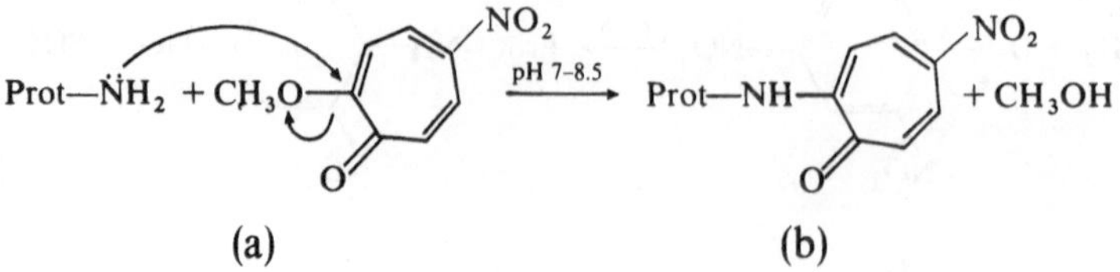

$$\text{Prot—}\dot{\text{N}}\text{H}_2 + \text{CH}_3\text{O} \text{—} \overset{\text{NO}_2}{\bigcirc} \xrightarrow{\text{pH 7-8.5}} \text{Prot—NH—} \overset{\text{NO}_2}{\bigcirc} + \text{CH}_3\text{OH} \quad (16)$$

              (a)   (b)

from the absorbance at 420 nm of the adduct (ε_m at 420 nm $= 2.07 \times 10^4$). The reagent seems to possess good specificity for amino groups. With yeast 3-phosphoglycerate kinase, modification by 2-methoxy-5-nitrotropone implicated three essential lysines and the reagent did not modify the single thiol group which was available for reaction with sulfhydryl reagents (Markland *et al.*, 1975). Up to three lysines were protected by MgITP and one lysine by 3-phosphoglycerate. Slight conformational changes were present in the nitrotroponylated enzyme (Markland *et al.*, 1975).

Compounds containing activated double bonds can react with amino groups. *Acrylonitriles* can react with ε-NH_2 groups (Riehm and Scheraga, 1966*a*), thiol groups (Weil and Seibles, 1961), and imidazole groups (Bosshard *et al.*, 1969). Cyanoethyl derivatives of these amino acids hydrolyze to the corresponding carboxyethyl amino acids, which can be determined on the amino acid analyzer. Acrylonitrile and more so *N*-ethylmaleimide are usually more employed in thiol group modification and the latter reagent is discussed in that section.

10. Guanidination

Amino groups can be guanidinated by reaction (17) with *O-methylisourea* (17a) at high pH (for review, see Kimmel, 1967). *O*-Methylisourea, believed for a long time (Hughes *et al.*, 1949) to be specific for amino groups, was found only relatively recently to *S*-methylate sulfhydryl groups below pH 10 (Banks and Shafer, 1970). More recently, it was reported to *S*-methylate the single thiol group in papain, causing its inactivation (Banks and Shafer, 1972). On the other hand, with human serum β_1-lipoprotein it has been shown (Margolis and Langdon, 1966) to modify histidine residues, in addition to lysine, under conditions normally employed in protein guanidination (i.e., pH 10.4, 0°C).

$$\text{Prot—NH}_2 + \text{CH}_3\text{O—}\overset{\overset{\displaystyle NH_2}{|}}{\underset{+}{C}}\text{=NH}_2 \xrightarrow{\text{pH 10.5}} \text{Prot—NH—}\overset{\overset{\displaystyle NH_2}{|}}{\underset{+}{C}}\text{=NH}_2 + \text{CH}_3\text{OH} \qquad (17)$$

$$\qquad\qquad\qquad\text{(a)} \qquad\qquad\qquad\qquad\qquad\qquad\qquad \text{(b)}$$

Guanidination of proteins with 1-*guanyl-3,5-dimethylpyrazole nitrate* (18a) (Habeeb, 1959, 1960) proceeds under milder conditions than those necessary for reaction with *O*-methylisourea.

1-*Nitroguanyl-3,5-dimethylpyrazole* (18b) (Habeeb, 1964) will introduce nitroguanyl substituents on amino groups. Guanidination results in retention of the positive charge of the side chain and usually of the physical and biological properties. Guanidinated bovine serum albumin retained 91% of its reactivity with antisera to the native protein (Habeeb, 1967*b*). On

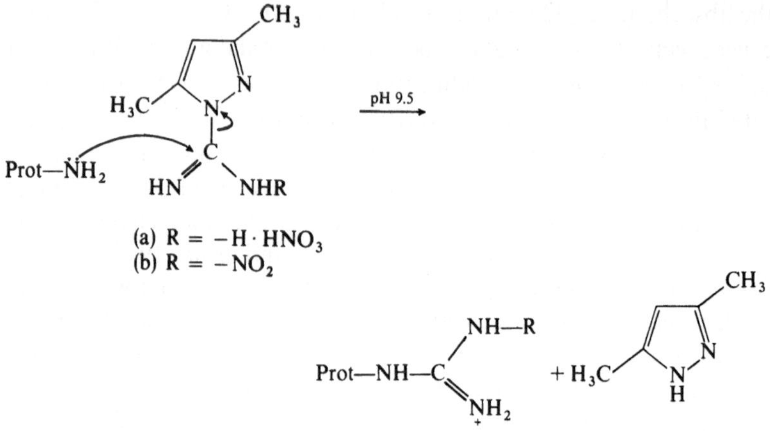

$$\text{Prot—NH}_2 \quad + \quad \underset{HN}{\overset{CH_3 \text{ pyrazole ring}}{\text{C}}}\diagdown NHR \quad \xrightarrow{\text{pH 9.5}}$$

(a) $R = -H \cdot HNO_3$
(b) $R = -NO_2$

$$\text{Prot—NH—C}\underset{\overset{+}{N}H_2}{\overset{NH-R}{\diagup}} \quad + H_3C\text{—(pyrazole-NH, CH}_3) \tag{18}$$

the other hand, with antisera to the derivative, albumin reacted only 42 % (Habeeb, 1968). It appears that new antigenic determinants are created by guanidination while simultaneously maintaining the determinants characteristic of the native protein (Habeeb, 1968). Guanidinated lysozyme retained full enzymatic activity (Habeeb and Atassi, 1971a). These reagents are quite specific for amino groups. However, the possibility of their reaction with thiol groups should be tested. The homoargine obtained on guanidination of the $\varepsilon\text{-NH}_2$ is stable to acid hydrolysis and can be determined on the amino acid analyzer. Guanidination has been reviewed by Habeeb (1972b). Another reagent for nitroguanidination is *N-methyl-N'-nitro-N-nitrosoguanidine* (McCalla and Reuvers, 1968). This reagent has been reported to react with a thiol group in enol-lactone hydrolase (Johnson and Greenbert, 1973).

11. Reaction with Imido Esters

Amidination (reaction 19), like guanidination, results in retention of the positive charge of the side chain. The reaction of *imido esters* (19a) with proteins appears to be specific for the amino groups, and side reactions involving other side chains have not been observed (Hunter and Ludwig, 1962; Wofsy and Singer, 1963). Amidination can be effected at a lower pH than is necessary for guanidination by *O*-methylisourea. Several imido esters, varying in the nature of the R side chain, have been employed (Hunter

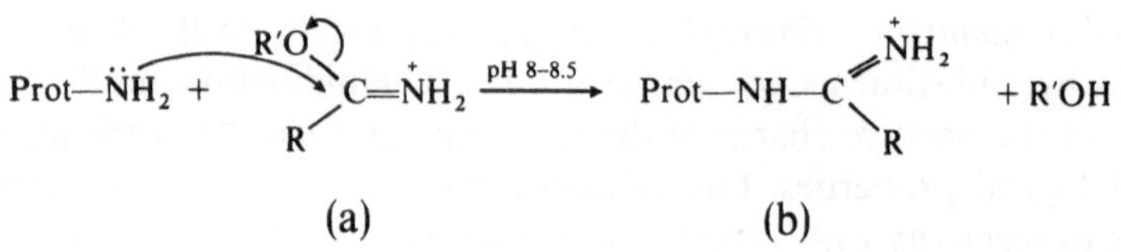

$$\text{Prot—NH}_2 \quad + \quad \underset{R}{\overset{R'O}{\diagdown}}\text{C}=\overset{+}{N}H_2 \quad \xrightarrow{\text{pH 8-8.5}} \quad \text{Prot—NH—C}\underset{R}{\overset{\overset{+}{N}H_2}{\diagup}} \quad + R'OH \tag{19}$$

(a)   (b)

and Ludwig, 1972). *Methyl acetimidate* (Hunter and Ludwig, 1962), *ethyl acetimidate* (Wofsy and Singer, 1963), and *methyl picolinimidate* (20a) (Benisek and Richards, 1968) may be mentioned. The extent of modification by methyl picolinimidate can be followed spectrally (Perham and Richards, 1968) from the increase in absorbance at 262 nm ($\varepsilon = 5700$) and it can be utilized to introduce metal-chelating groups. It is more resistant to hydrolysis in aqueous solution than aliphatic imidates (Roger and Neilson, 1961). The homologous reagent 5-*iodopyridine* 2-*carboximidate* (methyl iodopicolinimidate, 20b) has been introduced (Riley and Perham, 1973) as a possible method for preparing isomorphous heavy atom derivatives of proteins. At

$$\tag{20}$$

(a)   (b)

pH 5.0 it reacted specifically with the aromatic NH_2 group of 3-aminotyrosine without modification of aliphatic NH_2 groups (Riley and Perham, 1973). This is an attractive possibility for limiting the reaction to the very small number of aminotyrosine sites. The preparation of aminotyrosyl proteins is discussed under tyrosine modification reactions (Section IVJ6). *Mercaptopropionimidate* has been developed for introduction of additional thiol groups into proteins (Perham and Thomas, 1971). Amidination usually causes no change in physical and biological properties of the protein. Acetimidation of BSA did not change its antigenic properties (Habeeb, 1967*b*), and the immunochemical properties of antibodies were not changed by a similar modification (Wofsy and Singer, 1963). Acetimidation can be reversed at pH 11.3 with a great deal of denaturation (Reynolds, 1968) or in concentrated NH_3–glacial acetic acid (15:1 v/v) (Ludwig and Hunter, 1967). These conditions may be undesirable for most proteins. Methyl picolinimidate, by virtue of its bulky side chain, has been employed in studying the topography of tobacco mosaic virus protein (Perham and and Richards, 1968) and some mutants (Perham, 1973). Amidination of a single amino group (lysine-228) in horse liver alcohol dehydrogenase by methyl [^{14}C]acetimidate enhanced enzymatic activity thirteenfold (Dworschack *et al.*, 1975). In contrast, modification of lysine-228 by reductive alkylation with pyridoxal phosphate partially inactivated the enzyme (Sogin and Plapp, 1975). Acetimidation of β-trypsin at the ε-NH_2 groups yielded a soluble active derivative which was stable to autohydrolysis Nureddin and Inagami, 1975).

Diimidoesters would be expected to act as bifunctional reagents and have been employed to effect cross-links between amino groups. They are discussed in the section dealing with cross-linking reagents.

12. Fluorescent Labeling

The following group of compounds will incorporate a fluorescent label into proteins. They do not necessarily react via the same mechanism. However, in view of the special interest in fluorescent labeling in immunochemistry and biology, they will be grouped together. Detection of protein in cells by ultraviolet light has been reviewed (Nairns, 1964). Of course, ever since its introduction the fluorescent antibody technique (Coon *et al.*, 1942) has been used extensively in immunology (see Goldman, 1968; Hijmans and Schaeffer, 1975). In protein immunochemistry, a fluorescent label can function as an environmentally sensitive reporter group for binding and for changes in conformation.

Dansyl chloride and *NBD chloride* have already been discussed. A recently introduced compound related to dansyl chloride is *5-di-n-butyl-aminonaphthalene-1-sulfonyl chloride* (Seiler *et al.*, 1973), in which the dimethylamino group of dansyl chloride (see structure 15a) is replaced by the *di-n-butylamino* group. The reagent, which should possess the same specificity, gives derivatives which exhibit the same fluorescence activation properties but their fluorescence quantum yields exceed those of the corresponding dansyl derivatives by about 15%.

The popular fluorescent label *fluorescein isothiocyanate* (21a) re-

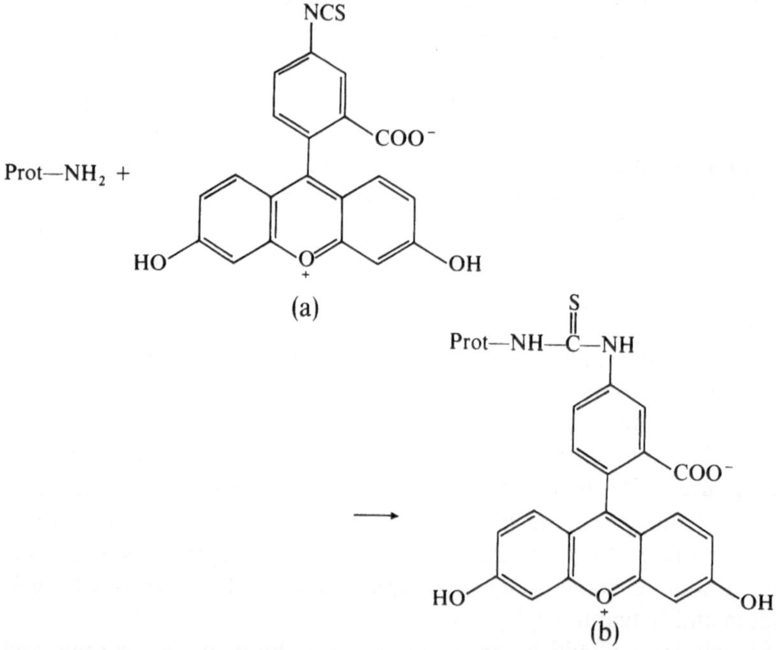

$$(21)$$

acted with insulin at ε-NH$_2$ groups (Bromer *et al.*, 1967). It was also found that fluorescein isothiocyanate will react primarily with α-NH$_2$ groups below pH 9.5 (Maeda *et al.*, 1969). At higher pH, ε-NH$_2$ groups became reactive. Noncovalent dye binding was also demonstrated with bovine serum albumin and hen lysozyme (Maeda *et al.*, 1969). Trifluoroacetic acid treatment of fluorescein-thiocarbamylated insulin released the *N*-terminal-labeled amino acids only. This label has served as a reporter group to modify a reactive lysine (residue 183) in yeast glyceraldehyde 3-phosphate dehydrogenase after reversible protection of the thiol groups (Stallcup and Koshland, 1973). The modified lysine was outside the active site, but was sufficiently close to report some environmental changes resulting from the binding and catalytic properties of the enzyme. Such approaches may be utilized to study immunochemical binding of proteins.

Fluorescamine has been developed as a new reagent for the preparation of fluorescent protein derivatives (Böhlen *et al.*, 1973) based on the ability of 2-oxysubstituted 3(2*H*)-furanones to produce highly fluorescent adducts with amines (Weigele *et al.*, 1972). The fluorophors are stable only in the pH range 8–9. In contrast *2-methoxy-2,4-diphenyl-3(2H)-furanone* (22a)

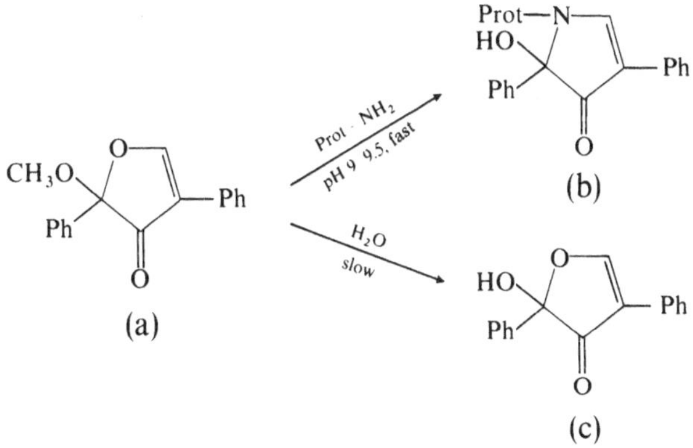

also itself nonfluorescent, reacts with amino groups to form highly stable (over a wide pH range) fluorescent (at 480 nm) *N*-substituted 3,5-diphenyl-5-hydroxy-2-pyrrolin-4-ones (22b) (Weigele *et al.*, 1973). Antibodies labeled by this reagent produced intense immunofluorescent staining.

13. Carbamylation

Cyanate ion was shown (Stark *et al.*, 1960) to react with α- and ε-NH$_2$ groups. The reaction is not specific for NH$_2$ groups and many functional groups are modified. Below pH 7.0, potassium cyanate carbamylates α-NH$_2$ groups about 100 times faster than ε-NH$_2$ groups (Stark, 1965*b*). However, at lower pH values (around pH 5) mixed anhydrides are obtained with carboxyl groups which can give rise to cross-links, but this side reaction is not encountered between pH 7 and 8 (Stark, 1965*b*). The reaction of thiol groups is rapid (Stark, 1964). However, the adduct, which is somewhat stable at pH 5, decomposes readily at pH 8 to yield the free SH group (Stark, 1964). Carbamyl derivatives of the imidazole group are unstable at neutral pH (Stark, 1965a) and the derivatives of phenolic and aliphatic OH groups are also extremely labile (Smyth, 1967; Rimon and Perlmann, 1968). The reaction can therefore be utilized for specific modification of the amino groups (23) with resultant elimination of the positive character of the side chain. Carbamylation and its application to protein modification have been

$$\text{Prot—NH}_2 + \text{NCO}^- \longrightarrow \text{Prot—NH—}\overset{\displaystyle O}{\overset{\displaystyle \|}{\text{C}}}\text{—NH}_2 \qquad (23)$$

reviewed (Stark, 1972). The reaction is also applied to the N-terminal determination of proteins and large peptides (for reviews, see Stark, 1970; Narita, 1970). Homocitrulline, which is obtained from carbamylation of ε-NH$_2$ groups, reverts to lysine on acid hydrolysis, whereas the N^α-carbamyl derivative cyclizes to the corresponding hydantoin of the terminal amino acid. In the carbamylation of pepsinogen at pH 8.8–8.85, ε-NH$_2$ groups reacted but not the α-NH$_2$ of the terminal leucine, whereas in pepsin at the same pH the α-NH$_2$ of isoleucine reacted but not the ε-NH$_2$ of the single lysine (Rimon and Perlmann, 1968). In each case, hydroxyl groups were carbamylated but were extremely labile and did not withstand isolation procedures. The proteolytic activity of carbamylated pepsin toward N-acetyl-DL-phenylalanyldiiodotyrosine increased 2.8-fold and the changes were reversed by hydroxylamine. Carbamylation of all the ε-NH$_2$ groups in a λ-type Bence Jones protein did not alter its conformation or its immunoprecipitability (Liaw et al., 1974). Cyanate has been employed as an antisickling agent (see Cerami et al., 1973, for review).

1,3-*Disubstituted* 1-*nitrosoureas* decompose at neutral pH to generate isocyanates that will react with NH$_2$ groups to yield the carbamoyl derivatives. Of these, 1,3-*bis*(2-*chloroethyl*)-1-*nitrosourea* and 1-(2-*chloroethyl*)-3-*cyclohexyl*-1-*nitrosourea* (24a) may be cited (Bowdon and Wheeler, 1971; Schmall et al., 1973). The reaction of compound (24a) with ε-NH$_2$ groups has been shown (Schmall et al., 1973) to yield the N^6-cyclohexyl-carbamoyl adduct of lysine (24b). These reagents need further study and have not been exploited in protein modification for biological activity studies.

$$\text{Prot—(CH}_2)_4\text{—NH}_2$$

$$\text{pH 7.2} \quad \text{ClCH}_2\text{CH}_2\text{—N—}\overset{\displaystyle O}{\overset{\displaystyle \|}{\text{C}}}\text{—NH—}\bigcirc \qquad (a)$$
$$\underset{\displaystyle \text{NO}}{\big|}$$

$$\text{Prot—(CH}_2)_4\text{—NH—}\overset{\displaystyle O}{\overset{\displaystyle \|}{\text{C}}}\text{—NH—}\bigcirc \qquad (b) \qquad (24)$$

14. Other Modification Reactions

2-*Diazoquinoline tetrafluoroborate* (25a) has been reported to react specifically with amino groups, unlike other diazonium compounds (discussed later) which suffer from lack of specificity. Trypsin was modified exclusively at three out of the 14 lysyl residues (Kanazawa et al., 1971). The remarkably stable reaction product with amino groups has been characterized (Kanazawa and Ishii, 1974) as 1,2,3-triazolo[4,5-c]quinoline (25b). The derivative is stable to acid hydrolysis and can be determined by amino acid analysis. It is also fluorescent when excited at 321 nm, giving emission spectra that are dependent on the protein (Kanazawa and Ishii, 1974). In addition to trypsin, the specificity of the reaction for lysyl residues has been confirmed with insulin and lysozyme (Kanazawa and Ishii, 1974).

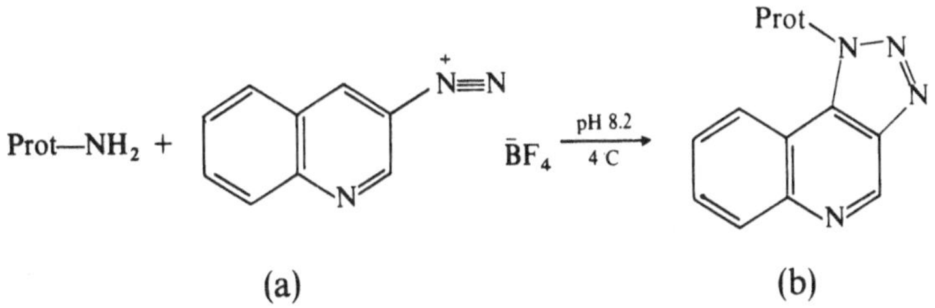

$$\text{Prot—NH}_2 + \qquad \qquad \xrightarrow[\text{4 C}]{\text{pH 8.2}} \qquad \qquad (25)$$

(a)   (b)

2,4,6-*Trimethylpyrylium perchlorate* salt (26a) or the chloroferrate salt will react with amino groups and has been shown to modify amino groups in α-chymotrypsin (O'Leary and Samberg, 1971). The chloroferrate salt is more water soluble than the perchlorate salt. The reaction product with amino groups, a pyridinium salt (26b), is stable to acid hydrolysis and has an absorption maximum at 268 nm. The reagent exhibited apparent steric selectivity.

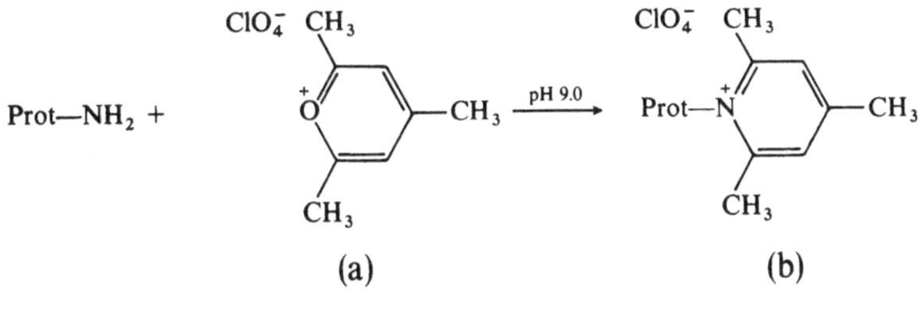

$$\text{Prot—NH}_2 + \qquad \qquad \xrightarrow{\text{pH 9.0}} \qquad \qquad (26)$$

(a)   (b)

Amino groups have been modified by α-*acetyl-β-ethoxy-N-ethoxycarbonylacrylamide* (Dewar and Shaw, 1961), which was also used for N-terminal analysis of ribonuclease and insulin. The product (a 5-acetyluracil) is stable to acid hydrolysis.

15. Deamination

Nitrous acid has been frequently employed for the deamination of amino groups in proteins. However, it is not a selective reaction. Nitrosation of tyrosine was demonstrated very early (Philpot and Small, 1938). *N*-Terminal proline residues are nitrosated at the secondary amine group (Stewart, 1969). Tryptophan residues are nitrosated at the *N*-1 position of the indole system and histidine nitrosation should be expected (Bonnett and Holleyhead, 1974). Although it has been applied successfully by some investigators, it is not a recommended procedure for modifying amino groups in proteins in view of the availability of a large number of reactions for amino groups, many of which, as discussed in the preceding sections, achieve a high degree of specificity, elegance, and controllability. For other discussions of deamination, see Cohen (1968) and Means and Feeney (1971).

16. Reversible Masking Reagents

The foregoing sections demonstrate the high reactivity of amino groups in a protein. Many reagents employed in modification of other functional groups would be reasonably selective if their reaction with amino groups could be prevented. Reversible masking of the amino groups will therefore protect them from side reactions when a more selective modification of a protein or peptide is needed. Also, such protecting groups are useful for rendering hydrolysis with trypsin specific for cleavage at arginine peptide bonds. Many such reversible masking reagents are now available. *Carbon disulfide* has been used to modify amino groups reversibly in proteins and peptides (Li and Bertsch, 1960) but does not afford complete protection. Amidination suffers from the same problem, and the conditions for its reversal are not desirable (see Section IVA11). As mentioned earlier, trifluoroacetylation by *trifluoroacetic anhydride* may cause partial cleavage of peptide bonds (Weygand *et al.*, 1966). The use of *ethyl thiotrifluoroacetate* for trifluoroacetylation (Goldberger and Anfinsen, 1962) probably overcomes this problem, but the lability of the trifluoroacetyl groups under the alkaline conditions of the reaction necessitates the use of a large excess of the reagent. The large amounts of ethanethiol liberated and the alkaline conditions will cause reduction and reshuffling of disulfide bonds (Goldberger and Anfinsen, 1962) if they are present. Furthermore, trifluoroacetylated proteins are mostly insoluble. Peptides derived from them will tend to aggregate, making it necessary to employ dissociating solvents for their chromatography and causing a decrease in yield (Harris and Perham, 1968). Reversible protection of amino groups by *2-methoxy-5-nitrotropone* (see reaction 16) was first demonstrated on Taka-amylase A (Tamaoki *et al.*, 1967). The nitrotroponyl groups could be removed with alkali (over pH 12), but the method would be drastic for most proteins. A milder procedure for denitrotropony-lation was by hydrazine (1–2 M) at pH 8.5–9, which resulted in good recovery of amylase activity and physicochemical properties of the enzyme. Other reversible modifications for amino groups in proteins are *maleylation* (Butler *et al.*, 1967, 1969), *acetoacetylation* (Marzotto *et al.*, 1968), *tetrafluorosuccinylation* (Braunitzer *et al.*, 1968), and *citraconylation* (Dixon and Perham, 1968). With this collection of reversible blocking reagents, it was most desirable to determine in a systematic study on the *same* set of proteins which would be the most suitable reagent to be employed in protein chemistry. The behavior of diketene (for acetoacetylation) and tetrafluorosuccinic, maleic, and citraconic anhydrides was studied in detail both with myoglobin (Singhal and Atassi, 1971) and with lysozyme (Habeeb and Atassi, 1970). The results have also been recently reviewed (Atassi and Habeeb, 1972), and a summary will suffice here. Complete unmasking of the amino groups was not achieved with acetoacetylated, tetrafluorosuccinylated, and maleylated derivatives. The deblocked proteins were highly heterogeneous (in disc electrophoresis), with partial recovery of enzymatic activity (for lysozyme), immunochemical properties (for both lysozyme and myoglobin), and native conformation. In contrast, the corresponding citraconyl derivatives gave, on deblocking, which proceeded readily (pH 4.2, 40°C, 3 hr), homogeneous preparations with 100% recovery of free amino groups, enzymatic activity, immunochemical properties, and native conformation. Thiol groups will react irreversibly with citraconic (Gibbons and Perham, 1970) and maleic anhydrides. Previously, the addition product of cysteine and citraconic anhydride (27b) had been shown to be a tricarboxylic acid (27c) containing a thioether bond (Black, 1966), which of course would be irreversible.

$$
\begin{array}{c}
\mathrm{NH_2} \\
| \\
\mathrm{CH\!-\!CH_2\!-\!SH} \\
| \\
\mathrm{COOH}
\end{array}
+
\text{(maleic anhydride)}
\longrightarrow
\begin{array}{c}
\mathrm{NH_2} \qquad \mathrm{CH_3} \\
| \qquad\quad | \\
\mathrm{CH\!-\!CH_2\!-\!S\!-\!C\!-\!COOH} \\
| \qquad\quad | \\
\mathrm{COOH} \quad\;\; \mathrm{CH_2\!-\!COOH}
\end{array}
\qquad (27)
$$

    (a)   (b)   (c)

Citraconic anhydride was found almost suitable for effecting specific tryptic cleavage at arginine peptide bonds. The peptides from myoglobin were isolated and deblocked, and their immunochemistry (Singhal and Atassi, 1971) as well as their conformation (Atassi and Singhal, 1970*b*) was studied. Citraconylation of disulfide-containing proteins introduced conformational changes into the protein (Habeeb and Atassi, 1970), which formed the basis for a novel approach to obtain all the tryptic peptides with intact disulfide bonds from lysozyme (Atassi et al., 1973a) and bovine serum albumin (Habeeb et al., 1974). From the respective tryptic hydrolysates, disulfide peptides were isolated and characterized, which accounted for the entire antigenic reactivity in both lysozyme (Atassi et al., 1973a) and bovine serum albumin (Habeeb et al., 1974; Atassi et al., 1976a).

It is interesting that antibodies against the succinyl substituent could distinguish it from the maleyl substituent (by partial reaction), the discriminating ability being obviously directed against the double bond (Habeeb and Atassi, 1971a). On the other hand, the citraconyl group did not react with antibodies to the succinyl substituent. More recently, conformational changes were demonstrated (Nakagawa et al., 1972) on citraconylation of human IgG, and, on deblocking, the native conformation and antigenic reactivity (qualitatively by immunodiffusion) with antisera to human IgG were recovered. Treatment of antibodies against the phthalyl group with maleic anhydride indicated that only a small percentage of these antibodies had lysine residues in their combining sites (Mayers et al., 1973), but no conformational measurements were carried out. Conformational changes have also been shown to take place on citraconylation of human IgG fragments Fab(t) and Fc(t) and Bence Jones proteins (Nakagawa et al., 1974). Restoration of native conformation was more complete on deblocking of Fab(t) than of Fc(t) and especially of the k and λ Bence Jones proteins. An interesting application of citraconylation has been in the selective release of proteins from water-extracted human erythrocyte membranes (Lundahl, 1975).

Reversible protection of amino groups in parvalbumin has been obtained by acylation with *phthalic anhydride* (at pH 8.5) to give the O-carboxybenzoyl derivative (Bertrand et al., 1974). The protecting group could be removed at pH 3.5 (50°C, 48 hr). Although comparative studies on this reagent have not been carried out, the protecting group is considerably more stable than the citraconyl moiety and may not be completely removed. Also, the higher temperature necessary for its reversal will be undesirable for many proteins.

Recently, the methylsulfonylethyloxycarbonyl protecting group was introduced onto N^{α}-(Gly-A1) and N^{ε}-(Lys-B29) positions in insulin by reaction of the latter with *methylsulfonylethyloxycarbonyl-N-hydroxysuccinimidester* (Geiger et al., 1975) in $NaHCO_3$-dimethylformamide. Deprotection was carried out in dilute NaOH (pH 11–13) at 0°C with seemingly no damage to the molecule and with full recovery of biological activity. This new reagent has not been subjected to comparative studies with other reversible reagents on the same set of proteins. However, it should be expected that the alkaline conditions necessary for deblocking will have detrimental effects on many proteins. The reagent needs further study.

B. Reactions for Aliphatic Hydroxyls

Specific modification of aliphalic hydroxyl groups in a protein is difficult to achieve even though they often participate in "side reactions" when other functional groups are being modified (see Section IVA on reactions of amino groups). Because of the low reactivity of aliphatic hydroxyl groups, not many protein derivatives have been prepared with specific modifications at these side chains. *Sulfonyl halides* as mentioned earlier (Section IVA7), react with many (NH_2, SH, phenolic OH, and imidazole) groups in proteins. However, under carefully controlled conditions it has been possible to obtain specifically modified derivatives at the essential serine of many "serine enzymes." Reaction of α-chymotrypsin with *p-toluenesulfonyl chloride* tosylated the enzyme specifically at the active-site serine and abolished its activity (Strumeyer *et al.*, 1963). Active-site serine residues in trypsin, acetylcholinesterase (Fahrney and Gold, 1963), and subtilisin (Neet and Koshland, 1966) have also been modified by sulfonyl halides. *O*-Tosyl serine derivatives (28a) will undergo β-elimination under alkaline conditions to give dehydroalanine residues (Photaki, 1963). Studies of model serine derivatives showed that *N*-carbobenzoxy derivatives formed only dehydroalanine, whereas *N-p*-nitrobenzoyl compounds can form either dehydroalanine or oxazoline products (Ginsburg and Wilson, 1964). Strong bases favored the formation of dehydroalanine, while more polar solvents favored the formation of oxazolines. It is relevant to caution here that the dehydroalanine side chain is quite reactive. Favorably placed nucleophilic groups can add to the double bond to form cross-links (Zahn, 1961; Bohak, 1964).

The β-elimination reaction was employed (Strumeyer *et al.*, 1963; Weiner *et al.*, 1966*b*) to convert the tosylated serine (28a) to an inactive dehydroalanine (anhydro) chymotrypsin (28b). Inactive sulfonylated (at serine-195) α-chymotrypsin has been desulfonylated and reactivated by hydrogen peroxide (Radomsky *et al.*, 1973) to the normal hydroxy enzyme, but methionine-192 was oxidized to the sulfoxide. Arylsulfonyl halides failed

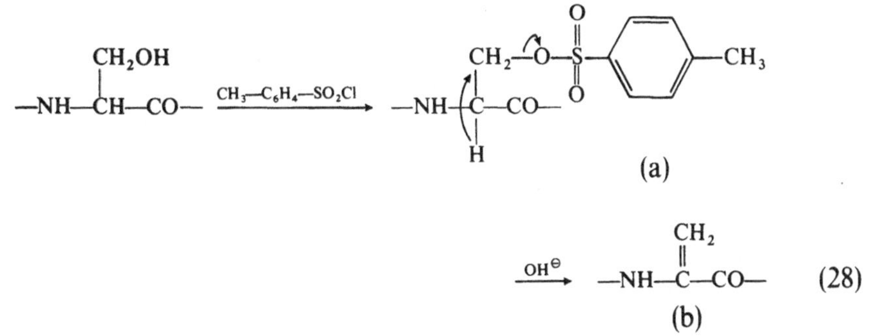

(a)

(b)

(28)

to inactivate deoxyribonuclease, but the enzyme was inactivated by *methane sulfonyl chloride* (Poulos and Price, 1974). Reaction at pH 7.0 sulfonylated eight sites on the enzyme, whereas reaction at pH 5.0 resulted mainly in a single sulfonylation at a serine residue. The sulfonylated serine on deoxyribonuclease was reacted with the nucleophile β-mercaptoethylamine to form S-aminoethylcysteine. The stability of the latter to acid hydrolysis enabled determination of the extent of modification by amino acid analysis. Reaction of thioacetate and other thiol anions with O-tosyl and O-phosphorylserine peptides in dimethylformamide or aqueous media (at pH 7) effected (reaction 29) their quantitative conversion to optically active S-acetyl-L-cysteine peptides (29b) via an S_N2 displacement mechanism (Zioudrou *et al.*, 1965). The S-acetyl group may be removed by hydroxylamine. This approach has been applied to convert the active serine in subtilisin to a cysteine residue (Neet and Koshland, 1966). Thiosubtilisin was inactive.

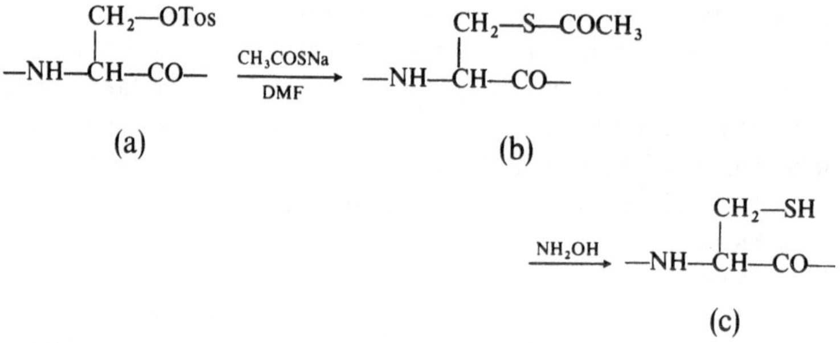

$$
\underset{\text{(a)}}{\overset{\overset{\displaystyle CH_2-OTos}{|}}{-NH-CH-CO-}} \quad \xrightarrow[\text{DMF}]{CH_3COSNa} \quad \underset{\text{(b)}}{\overset{\overset{\displaystyle CH_2-S-COCH_3}{|}}{-NH-CH-CO-}}
$$

$$
\xrightarrow{NH_2OH} \quad \underset{\text{(c)}}{\overset{\overset{\displaystyle CH_2-SH}{|}}{-NH-CH-CO-}} \qquad (29)
$$

Aryl cyanates seem to offer a promising approach since their reactivity can be controlled by varying the substituents on the aromatic ring. *p*-Nitrophenyl cyanate with α-chymotrypsin has been shown (Robillard *et al.*, 1972) to carbamylate mainly serine-195, whereas in S-chymotrypsin the reagent carbamylated both serine-195 and the N^α position.

O-Acylation of aliphatic and phenolic OH groups has been obtained by *carboxylic acid chlorides* in anhydrous trifluoroacetic acid (Previero *et al.*, 1972a). Amino groups did not react under these conditions, while thiol groups were acylated. Phenolic O-acyl and S-acyl groups could easily be removed. A more serious side reaction was the cleavage of a peptide bond next to S-acylcysteine which could occur through an $S \to N$ acyl shift (Previero *et al.*, 1972a). Also, cleavage may occur through an $N \to O$ acyl shift in anhydrous trifluoroacetic acid (see Section VIIF). However, the reaction may prove useful for the modification of certain immunochemically reactive peptides. *Benzoyl amino acid amides* have been shown to react with the OH groups of serine (Previero *et al.*, 1969a). The reaction also takes place in anhydrous trifluoroacetic acid at 50°C. However, such conditions are likely to be too drastic for most protein antigens.

C. Reactions for Arginine

Simple aldehydes such as formaldehyde have long been known to react with arginine as well as many other functional groups (Fraenkel-Conrat and Olcott, 1946) in proteins (see Section IVA5). The nonselectivity of these reagents precluded their employment in specific arginine modifications. Dicarbonyl compounds, on the other hand, have proved more suitable for selective arginine modification. *Benzil* ($C_6H_5COCOC_6H_5$) has been shown to react with the guanidinium group under strong alkaline conditions (Itano and Gottlieb, 1963). *1,2-Cyclohexanedione* (Toi *et al.*, 1965, 1967) has proved to be a more suitable reagent for arginine modification. Originally the reaction was carried out under strong alkaline conditions (0.2 N NaOH). However, this solvent is undesirable for many proteins, especially those with disulfide bonds. For example, trypsin inhibitor (Liu *et al.*, 1968) and lysozyme (Atassi *et al.*, 1972) each lost their respective activities, while myoglobin (Atassi and Thomas, 1969) was insolubilized up to 50%. However, in many cases it has been possible to prepare specifically modified derivatives for immunochemical studies, as, for example, in the case of myoglobin (Atassi and Thomas, 1969) and parvalbumin (Gosselin-Rey *et al.*, 1973). Subsequently, 0.1 M triethylamine was shown (Habeeb and Bennett, 1971) to be a very effective solvent for arginine modification by cyclohexanedione. Ten out of eleven arginine residues in lysozyme could be modified specifically by cyclohexanedione in 0.1 M triethylamine (Atassi *et al.*, 1972). Cyclohexanedione may also modify amino groups (Liu *et al.*, 1968). Reaction of a large fragment from lysozyme with cyclohexanedione in 0.1 M triethylamine resulted in the modification (in addition to arginine) of tryptophan and α- and ε-NH_2 groups (Atassi *et al.*, 1976c). Modification by cyclohexanedione has been shown to take place at pH 8–9 in borate at 25–40°C (Patthy and Smith, 1975a). A single product, N^7,N^8-(1,2-dihydroxycyclohex-1,2-ylene)-L-arginine (30b), was obtained which was stable in acid or in borate buffers (pH 8–9), forming with the latter the complex (30c). On the other hand, the product obtained (Toi *et al.*, 1967) on reaction in strong alkaline solutions is N^5-(4-oxo-1,3-diazaspiro[4.4]non-2-ylidene)-L-ornithine (30a). Arginine could be regenerated from compound (30b) by hydroxylamine at pH 7.0 and 37°C for 7–8 hr (Patthy and Smith, 1975a). This should prove extremely useful for preparation of lysine tryptic peptides which, after cleavage and deprotection of the arginines, will not have internal modifications that may complicate immunochemical studies (see Part B). Hydroxylamine converted the blocking groups in (30b) to cyclohexanedione dioxime, which gave a red complex with nickel and formulated the basis for a specific color reaction (Patthy and Smith, 1975b). All the aforementioned improvements make cyclohexanedione a highly suitable reagent for arginine modification.

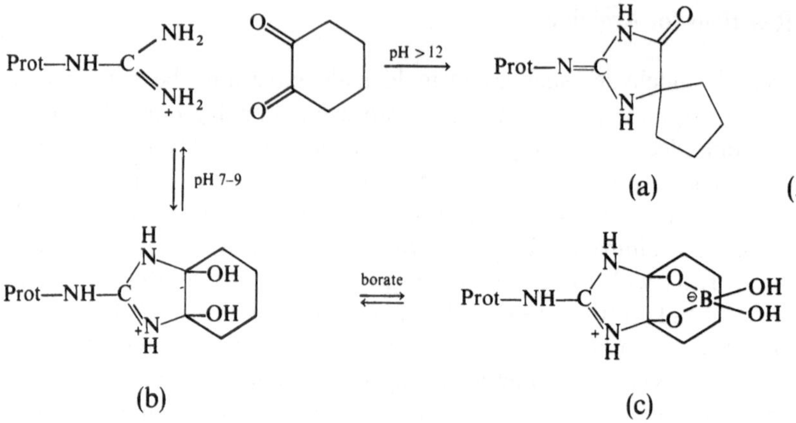

(a)   (30)

(b)   (c)

Phenylglyoxal (31a) condenses (two molecules of C_6H_5—COCOH) with the guanido group at pH 7–8 and 25°C (Takahashi, 1968). The adduct reverted slowly to arginine at neutral or alkaline pH. The α-NH_2 was deaminated and, in excess reagent, the ε-NH_2 groups were modified (Takahashi, 1968). However, specifically modified derivatives have been prepared under carefully controlled conditions. For example, lysozyme was modified specifically at one arginine (residue 61), causing small conformational changes that decreased enzymatic activity slightly but had no effect on its immunochemistry (Atassi *et al.*, 1972). Specific arginine derivatives of carboxypeptidase B (Werber and Sokolovsky, 1972), carboxypeptidase A (Ikenaga and Takahashi, 1975), and trypsin (Delarco and Liener, 1973) have been reported. In the case of trypsin, one arginine could be protected from reaction by binding the enzyme with trypsin inhibitor. In the reaction of a large peptide fragment from lysozyme, amino groups were modified and their reversible protection by citraconylation was necessary to achieve a specific arginine modification (Atassi *et al.*, 1976c).

Recently, a mechanism has been proposed independently (Werber *et al.*, 1975) for reaction of arginine residue with phenylglyoxal in the presence of borate, which resembles the mechanism described (reaction 30) for cyclohexanedione. Reaction of phenylglyoxal with the guanido group (reaction 31) was proposed to yield a *cis*-diol (31b), which will form a complex with borate (31c) and prevent further condensation of the *cis*-diol with another molecule of phenylglyoxal by which (31d) would otherwise form. The borate complex can dissociate to regenerate the reactants or to give a more stable product with incorporation of 1 mole of phenylglyoxal (31e). Compound (31e) will not dissociate to regenerate arginine and accounts for the ability to determine extent of arginine modification by amino acid analysis.

2,3-*Butanedione* reacts with the guanido group (Yankeelov *et al.*,

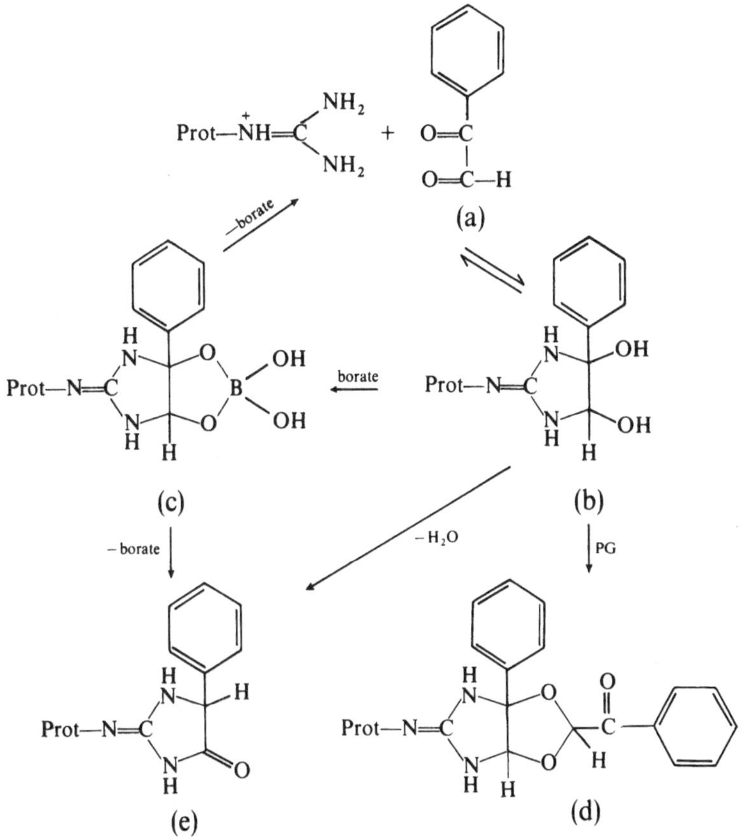

$$(31)$$

PG = phenylglyoxal

1966) after undergoing self-condensation to a dimer or trimer (Yankeelov et al., 1968; Yankeelov, 1970, 1972). The dimer and trimer show similar specificity and reactivity, each giving multiple products that will decompose back to arginine, although only very slowly at neutral pH (Yankeelov, 1970). Its reversion back to arginine on acid hydrolysis is more appreciable, but it may be possible to employ a suitable extrapolation or correction. This reagent reacts appreciably with amino groups, aliphatic hydroxyl groups, and methionine, and to a lesser extent (below 10%) with other functional groups (Yankeelov et al., 1968). Although the nature of these side reactions is unknown, acylation of amino and hydroxyl groups is one possible route which would preclude detection of such modifications by amino acid analysis of acid hydrolysates. A noncovalent interaction was proposed for methionine modification (Yankeelov et al., 1968). The elution position of the methionine adduct on the analyzer is more consistent with a sulfonium salt or a sulfoxide, both of which cannot be determined by amino acid analysis of acid hydrolysates. Reversible protection of the amino groups by citraconylation was reported to protect these, as well as other functional groups, from participating in side reactions (Yankeelov and Acree, 1971). It must be remembered in this connection that citraconic anhydride will modify thiol groups irreversibly (see Section IVA16). The possibility of reaction of butanedione with indole and thiol groups has not been considered. The reagent has been used to modify arginine residues in bovine serum albumin, ribonuclease A (Yankeelov, 1970), antibodies (Grossberg and Pressman, 1968), lysozyme (Davies and Neuberger, 1969), carboxypeptidase A (Riordan, 1973), and glyceraldehyde 3-phosphate dehydrogenase (Nagradova and Asryants, 1975). In these studies, derivatives were not purified and characterization relied on amino acid analyses of acid hydrolysates, which precluded determination of tryptophan and of hydrolyzable modifications.

Glyoxal (HCOCOH) has been shown to react with arginine as well as lysine residues, forming with the latter an adduct which, as expected, reverted to lysine on acid hydrolysis (Nakaya *et al.*, 1967). The possibility of modifying tryptophan, cysteine, histidine, and hydroxyl groups, which would be expected for a reactive aldehyde of this type (Fraenkel-Conrat and Olcott, 1946; Habeeb and Hiramoto, 1968), cannot yet be discounted. After acid hydrolysis, such adducts would be expected to give mostly the original amino acid, and the modification cannot therefore be determined by amino acid analysis. Its application to modify arginine residues in antibodies to the 3-nitro-4-hydroxy-5-iodophenylacetyl group (Joniau *et al.*, 1970) did not consider these side reactions, the purity of the derivative(s), or conformational changes therein. Glyoxal requires further study.

Malonaldehyde (OHCCH$_2$CHO) will condense with the guanido groups of arginine in 10 N HCl at 25°C (King, 1966). Such conditions preclude utility of this reagent in arginine modification and correlation with biological function. *Nitromalondialdehyde* [OHC—Č(NO$_2$)—CHO], a more reactive compound because of the electron-withdrawing nitro group, has also been shown to condense with the guanido group in 0.5 M NaOH (Signor *et al.*, 1971). This solvent may be unsuitable for most proteins (see discussion relating to cyclohexanedione), especially those containing disulfide bonds (Section IVH8). Furthermore, this reagent (like malonaldehyde) will be expected to react with both amino and thiol groups (Buttkus, 1969), at pH values from neutrality or higher.

D. Reactions for Carboxyl Groups

1. Esterification

Esterification had until recently been the most commonly used reaction for carboxyl group modification. Several procedures are available for esterification of carboxyl groups. Reaction with *alcohol* (usually methanol or ethanol) *HCl* is often used but it is not specific and can cause an $N \rightarrow O$ acyl shift (Cohen, 1968; Levy and Carpenter, 1970) and deamidation (Cohen, 1968). Acid esterification of lysozyme caused denaturation (Kravchenko *et al.*, 1968) and the methyl ester groups introduced showed appreciable instability (Chentsova and Kravchenko, 1974). In long reaction periods (50 hr or more) of lysozyme, methoxy groups were incorporated at sites other than carboxyl groups (Kramer and Rupley, 1973*b*). *Diazomethane*, which is a good methylating agent, is not specific for carboxyl groups. *Aliphatic diazo compounds* will exhibit higher specificity for carboxyl groups when a carboxyl group is present next to the diazotized carbon (Wilcox, 1972), but they will also react with thiol groups. A number of aliphatic diazo compounds have been effective as site-specific reagents (Wilcox, 1972). However, they have not been employed in general modification of protein carboxyl groups because of their instability in aqueous solution and the poor yields of derivatives, as, for example, in the reaction of diazoacetoglycine amide with ribonuclease A (Riehm and Scheraga, 1965).

Esterification of carboxyl groups can be effected in aqueous solution by *triethyloxonium fluoroborate* (Meerwein, 1937), which undergoes nucleophilic attack (32) by ionized carboxyl groups. The reaction can be

$$
\text{Prot—COO}^- \quad \begin{array}{c} \text{CH}_2\text{CH}_3 \\ | \\ ^+\text{O—CH}_2\text{CH}_3 \\ | \\ \text{CH}_2\text{CH}_3 \end{array} \xrightarrow{\text{pH 4-5}} \text{Prot—COOCH}_2\text{CH}_3 + \text{CH}_3\text{CH}_2\text{—O—CH}_2\text{CH}_3
$$

$$\text{(a)} \hspace{4cm} \text{(b)} \tag{32}$$

performed in aqueous solutions under mild conditions. Two single ester derivatives of lysozyme were prepared (Parsons *et al.*, 1969), one of which was esterified at the essential Asp-52 (Parsons and Raftery, 1969). The yield of esterified carboxyl groups in model peptides was shown to improve as the pH increased from 2 to 7 (Yonemitsu *et al.*, 1969*a*). Some nonspecificity has been reported in the formation of the ethyl sulfonium salt of methionine and quaternary imidazolium salt of histidine (Yonemitsu *et al.*, 1969*a*). Such side reactions, as well as the esterification of carboxyl groups, cannot be determined by amino acid analysis of acid or alkaline protein hydrolysates. The use of an isotopically labeled reagent is recommended. The carboxyl groups in trypsin have been esterified by this reagent (Nakayama *et al.*, 1970) at pH 4.5. More recently, the essential carboxyl groups in pepsin were studied by reaction with [^{14}C]trimethyloxonium fluoroborate at pH 5.0 (Paterson and Knowles, 1972).

2,2-*Dimethoxypropane* has been shown to give methyl esters of amino acids in high yields (80–90%) without effect on amino, phenolic OH, or thioether side chains (Rachele, 1963). This reagent may be suitable for the esterification of peptides in high yield. Its applicability to proteins requires further study.

2. Coupling with Nucleophile after Activation

Activated carboxyl groups can be coupled with nucleophiles. Activation may be effected with water-soluble *carbodiimides* (Khorana, 1953). When the modification employed only the carbodiimide, the derivatives obtained were not easily characterized (Sheehan and Hlavka, 1956; Franzblau *et al.*, 1963; Goodfriend *et al.*, 1964; Riehm and Scheraga, 1966b). *Carbodiimide activation followed by coupling with a nucleophile* (33) (Hoare and Koshland, 1966, 1967; Wilcheck *et al.*, 1967a) presented a substantial improvement in yield and ease of characterization. The reaction has now been applied to many proteins and a variety of nucleophiles have been employed. Examples

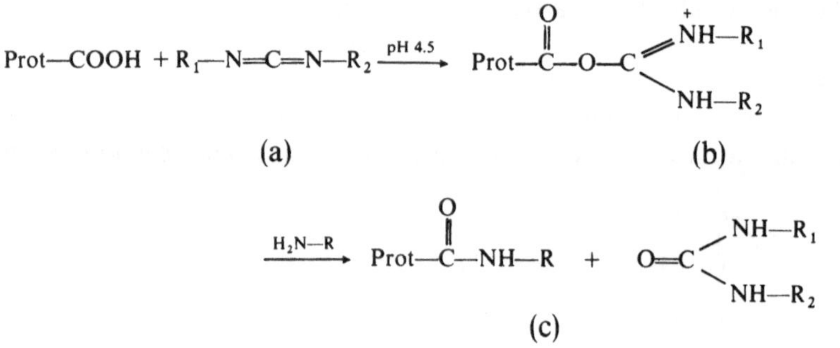

$$\text{Prot—COOH} + R_1\text{—N=C=N—}R_2 \xrightarrow{\text{pH 4.5}} \text{Prot—C(=O)—O—C} \overset{\overset{+}{N}H\text{—}R_1}{\underset{NH\text{—}R_2}{}}$$

(a)   (b)

$$\xrightarrow{H_2N\text{—}R} \text{Prot—C(=O)—NH—R} + O=C \overset{NH\text{—}R_1}{\underset{NH\text{—}R_2}{}} \qquad (33)$$

(c)

of this are its application to the study of the role in activity and/or reactivity of carboxyl groups in lysozyme by coupling with H_2N—CH_2—SO_3H, glycine methyl ester or glycinamide (Lin and Koshland, 1969), sulfanilic acid (Kramer and Rupley, 1973a), histidine methyl ester (Atassi *et al.*, 1974). Glycine esters or glycinamide have been coupled to carboxyl groups in α-chymotrypsin (Carraway *et al.*, 1969), α-lactalbumin (Lin, 1970), and insulin (Ozawa, 1970). A dipeptide (AlaGly) was coupled to ribonuclease A (Wilcheck *et al.*, 1967a). Cystamine has been coupled to carboxyl groups of tobacco mosaic virus (King and Leberman, 1973). The effects of modifying the *same* carboxyl groups (in a given protein) in two different ways on the immunochemistry and conformation of myoglobin (Atassi and Singhal,

1972*a,b*) and on the enzymatic activity, immunochemistry, and conformation of lysozyme (Atassi *et al.*, 1974; Atassi and Rosemblatt, 1974) were studied. Under carefully controlled conditions, it was possible to couple the *same* sites in a given protein to glycine methyl ester or to histidine methyl ester. By using ammonium chloride as the nucleophile, exposed carboxyl groups in five proteins were recently converted, after activation with carbodiimide, to their corresponding carboxamido groups (Lewis and Shafer, 1973). This interesting modification will convert aspartic and glutamic acid residues to asparagine and glutamine residues. A *spin-labeled carbodiimide* has been synthesized (Azzi *et al.*, 1973) and permits the performance of electron paramagnetic resonance studies on the protein derivative.

Carboxyl groups have been converted (Hoare *et al.*, 1968) to amino groups by using a procedure which employed both the esterification and the carbodiimide activation reaction (34). The carboxyl groups were first esterified and the ester groups then converted to hydroxamic acid groups (34c) by reaction with hydroxylamine. In a third step, the conversion of hydroxamic acids to amino groups is effected by reaction with carbodiimide. This proceeds through a reactive isocyanate intermediate (34e) which can cause cross-links in the protein. A method has been developed (Hargrave and Wold, 1973) for isolating glycinamide-coupled, carboxy-terminal tryptic peptides from proteins.

$$\text{Prot—COOH} \xrightarrow{\text{ROH}} \text{Prot—COOR} \xrightarrow{\text{NH}_2\text{OH}} \text{Prot—CONHOH} \xrightarrow{\text{R'—N=C=N—R''}}$$

$$\text{(a)} \qquad\qquad \text{(b)} \qquad\qquad \text{(c)} \qquad\qquad\qquad (34)$$

$$\left[\text{Prot—CO—NH—O—C}\overset{\text{NHR'}}{\underset{\overset{+}{\text{NHR''}}}{}}\right] \longrightarrow \left[\text{Prot—N=C=O}\right] \longrightarrow \text{Prot—NH}_2$$

$$\text{(d)} \qquad\qquad\qquad\qquad \text{(e)}$$

Carbodiimides have been shown to modify tyrosine residues (Carraway and Koshland, 1968). The modification, which is stable to acid hydrolysis, can be reversed by hydroxylamine. Another complication in the application of carbodiimides is their reaction with sulfhydryl groups (Carraway and Triplett, 1970), giving an irreversible, stable derivative. A carbodiimide has been shown to react with the active serine residue in α-chymotrypsin (Banks *et al.*, 1969). In addition to these problems, reaction with carbodiimides could give rise to intra- and intermolecular cross-links between activated carboxylate groups and favorably placed amino groups. Intermolecular cross-links may be minimized if reactions are performed on dilute protein solutions.

Isoxazolium salts will react with carboxyl groups at room temperature to form an enol ester (Woodward and Olofson, 1961, 1966). *N-Alkyl-5-phenylisoxazolium salts* have been used for the modification of protein carboxyl groups (Bodlaender *et al.*, 1969). The activated enol esters (which possessed sufficient stability to permit isolation) were displaced with [^{14}C]-nucleophiles. This reaction has been employed in the modification of essential carboxyl groups in trypsin (Feinstein *et al.*, 1969). An isoxazolium salt inactivated yeast phosphoglycerate kinase (which could be protected from inactivation by Mg-ATP), implicating an essential carboxyl group (Brake and Weber, 1974). Like the carbodiimide activation reaction, activation by isoxazolium salts could give rise to intra- and intermolecular cross-links.

In addition to the aforementioned complications, these modifications are not permanent to acid or alkaline hydrolysis, and therefore the modified residue cannot be identified by amino acid analysis.

3. Reduction

Specific reduction of carboxyl groups in peptides and proteins have been reported (Rosenthal and Atassi, 1967; Atassi and Rosenthal, 1969) by reaction with *diborane* in tetrahydrofuran. Specificity of the reaction was demonstrated on 20 different model peptides and six different proteins. For reduction, the carboxyl groups must be protonated. Under carefully controlled conditions the peptide bonds and carboxamido groups were not reduced. The specific reduction of a limited number of available carboxyl groups may be generally accomplished by reaction at $-10°C$ and, with some proteins, specificity was maintained when reactions were carried out at $0°C$ (Atassi and Rosenthal, 1969). Under relatively more vigorous conditions (e.g., room temperature and/or long reaction periods), side reactions may be encountered. Amino acids that suffered modification in proteins under these conditions were histidine, arginine, and proline (Atassi and Rosenthal, 1969) and in certain model peptides a hydrolytic type of reaction was observed under these vigorous conditions (Rosenthal and Atassi, 1967). In all cases, reduction at $-10°C$ was entirely specific for the carboxyl groups.

This chemical modification has the advantage of permanence, since the original carboxyl groups cannot be inadvertently regenerated by subsequent hydrolytic procedures. Reduction of aspartyl and glutamyl residues whose α-carboxyl groups are involved in peptide linkage gives rise to homoserine and 2-amino-5-hydroxyvaleric acid, respectively (Atassi and Rosenthal, 1969). Some γ- and δ-lactones are formed from these aminohydroxy acids during acid hydrolysis and drying of the hydrolysates. The decrease in aspartic and glutamic acid contents is accounted for quantitatively by the total recovery of the corresponding hydroxy acids and their respective lactones. Amino acids at the *C*-terminus are usually reduced to their corresponding amino alcohols, which appear on the analyzer with, or close to, ammonia.

The change in the size of the side chain is small on conversion of the —COOH group to —CH_2OH, and this is an extremely useful procedure when it is desired that loss of hydrophilicity or introduction of bulky side chains is to be avoided.

It is possible to control the reaction, and it has been applied to the preparation of a myoglobin derivative that had been reduced only at two carboxyl groups and whose immunochemistry and conformation were studied in detail (Atassi and Perlstein, 1972a). It has also been used to reduce certain carboxyl groups in human hemoglobin and to study subunit interaction, immunochemistry, and conformation of the homogeneous derivative (Atassi and Nakhleh, 1975). Diborane was applied in the reduction of N-terminal pyroglutamic acid residues to proline in an analogue of gastrin and bovine γ-globulin (Takahashi and Cohen, 1969). Reduction by diborane has proved extremely valuable in identifying γ-carboxyglutamic acid residues $[(HOOC)_2—CH—CH_2—CH(NH_2)—COOH]$ in bovine and rat vitamin-K-dependent proteins (Nelsestuen et al., 1974; Zytkovicz and Nelsestuen, 1975). The reduction product of γ-carboxyglutamic acid by [^{3}H]diborane was the expected 5,5'-[^{3}H]dihydroxyleucine $[(HOCH_2)_2—CH—CH_2CH(NH_2)—COOH]$, and its presence was demonstrated in hydrolysates of reduced rat prothrombin, bovine prothrombin, and bovine factor X (Zytkovicz and Nelsestuen, 1975). The stability of dihydroxyleucine permitted its identification, whereas γ-carboxyglutamic acid undergoes decarboxylation during acid hydrolysis into glutamic acid. Recently, the aforementioned specificity of diborane reduction to carboxyl groups and its ineffectiveness on carboxamido groups formulated the basis of a method (Airoldi and Doonan, 1975) to distinguish between aspartic acid and asparagine and between glutamic acid and glutamine during sequence analysis by the dansyl-Edman procedure. Reduction of two carboxyl groups in the antigenic reactive site of a large, immunochemically reactive fragment of sperm whale myoglobin abolished its reactivity (Perlstein and Atassi, 1974).

Disulfide bonds undergo reductive cleavage by diborane (Atassi and Rosenthal, 1969). However, this should not present a problem, and recently correct re-formation of disulfide bonds was demonstrated in a homogeneous lysozyme derivative in which two carboxyl groups had been reduced to their corresponding alcohols by diborane (Atassi et al., 1975b). In early studies, reduction in tetrahydrofuran yielded protein derivatives that were largely insoluble in aqueous solvents. This complication was entirely avoided by replacing tetrahydrofuran with dioxane at the end of the reduction and before drying the residue (Atassi and Perlstein, 1972a). Highly soluble derivatives of myoglobin (Atassi and Perlstein, 1972a), hemoglobin (Atassi and Nakhleh, 1975), and lysozyme (Atassi et al., 1975b) were obtained in this manner.

Recently, two alkylboranes with differing degrees of steric requirements were employed to achieve steric control of the direction of hydroboration (Atassi *et al.*, 1973c). *Disiamylborane*, a dialkylborane with large steric requirements, enabled the specific reduction of accessible glutamic acids in lysozyme and myoglobin, and unhindered end-chain carboxyl groups. On the other hand, 9-*borabicyclo*[3.3.1]-*nonane*, a bicyclic dialkylborane with appreciable hindrance, exhibited good selectivity for glutamate and un-hindered *C*-terminal carboxylate groups, with only marginal reduction of β-carboxyl groups of aspartic acid. It was suggested that, in addition to their usefulness in specific chemical modification, these reagents may prove to be valuable conformational probes (Atassi *et al.*, 1973c).

Esters have been reduced to their corresponding alcohols by $LiBH_4$ or $LiAlH_4$ in ether, and the reduction was accompanied by some peptide-bond cleavage (Crawhill and Elliott, 1955; Yonemitsu *et al.*, 1968). Peptide-bond cleavage of model peptides was avoided when their esters were reduced by $NaBH_4$ in aqueous solutions at room temperature (Yonemitsu *et al.*, 1969b). Under these conditions, reduction of the disulfide bonds should be expected and some peptide bond reduction has been reported (Kimmel and Parcells, 1960; Gillespie *et al.*, 1960; Paz *et al.*, 1970) in proteins. Reduction of esters is subject to the limitations of the esterification reaction, which have been discussed (see Section IVD1), as well as those of the reduction procedure.

Acyl-phosphate compounds have been reduced by borohydride (Degani and Boyer, 1973). The reaction has been employed to identify carboxyl groups at the site of phosphorylation of several ATP-phosphorylases (Degani and Boyer, 1973; Nishigaki *et al.*, 1974) and at the site of *Escherichia coli* acetate kinase (Todhunter and Purich, 1974).

4. Carboxamido Groups

Carboxamido groups in *internal* positions in peptides can be dehydrated by *ethylene chlorophosphite* in *triethyl phosphite* (Ressler and Kashelikar, 1966). The procedure is not recommended for modification but should be quite useful for identification of asparaginyl and glutaminyl residues in *endo* positions in peptides. Dehydration of these residues gave the cyano derivatives (i.e., $-(CH_2)_n-C\equiv N$ side chains; $n = 1$ or 2). These were subjected directly to a Birch reduction in Na in liquid ammonia to give the corresponding amines, i.e., $(CH_2)_n-CH_2NH_2$. Therefore, asparagine will give rise to 2,4-diaminobutyric acid and glutamine will give ornithine, both of which can be determined by amino acid analysis. The method has been applied only to peptides.

E. Reactions for Histidine

It is not easy to modify histidine specifically in a protein. The reagents usually employed for histidine modification also participate in many side reactions. The following reactions have been employed, and in many cases it has been possible to obtain good selectivity with certain proteins.

1. Photooxidation

Dye-sensitized photooxidation (Weil *et al.*, 1951) has been frequently used to modify amino acids in proteins. In addition to histidine, the reaction can oxidize methionine, tryptophan, tyrosine, and cysteine residues. However, the rates of oxidation of these amino acids can be controlled considerably by varying the conditions. Photooxidation is influenced by the nature of the dye, the pH, and the temperature of the reaction. Photooxidation of histidine follows sharply its titration curve and apparently only un-ionized imidazole groups are subject to oxidation, which is not appreciable below pH 6. With some dyes, tyrosine photooxidation decreases below pH 8. In general, at neutral or higher pH values all the aforementioned susceptible amino acids are oxidized, while at low pH values only tryptophan, methionine, and cysteine are photooxidized (Spikes and MacKnight, 1970; Westhead, 1972). However, in certain cases, selective histidine oxidation has been reported. For example, photooxidation of 3-phosphoglyceraldehyde dehydrogenase in the presence of rose bengal at pH 6.5 and 2°C inactivated the enzyme appreciably and effected oxidation of a single histidine residue per monomer (Bond *et al.*, 1970). Also, a single histidine residue per subunit was oxidized in glutamate dehydrogenase with a little inactivation, by employing pyridoxal-5′-phosphate as photosensitizer (Hucho *et al.*, 1973). Photooxidation of apoperoxidase at pH 9 using protoporphyrin IX as photosensitizer gave a slightly active, homogeneous derivative in which one histidine residue had been oxidized (Mauk and Girotti, 1974). Photooxidation of papain (which has no methionine) in the presence of methylene blue at pH 7.5 resulted in tryptophan, histidine, and smaller extent of tyrosine modification and effected inactivation of the enzyme (Okumura and Murachi, 1975). Covalent coupling of dye to proteins has been shown to take place on increasing dye concentration (Brandt *et al.*, 1974). This complication ought to be taken into consideration.

2. Alkylation

Alkyl halides can undergo nucleophilic substitution with amino, thiol, imidazole thioether, and phenolic OH groups. The reaction proceeds with the uncharged nucleophile and will therefore take place close to or above the pK of the functional group. Therefore, control of the result of reaction may be achieved to a certain extent by proper selection of the pH of the reaction. However, the reactivity of the thioether side chain shows little change with pH

Carboxymethylation with *iodoacetate* or *bromoacetate* or their corresponding amides has been used frequently for alkylation of histidine residues in protein. Carboxymethylation of proteins has been reviewed (Gurd, 1972, and references therein). Carboxymethylation for the purpose of modifying histidine residues is usually carried out around pH 6. At this pH the reactivity of the amino groups is appreciably suppressed but not always entirely eliminated. Alkylation of tyrosine residues in proteins by iodoacetamide has been reported in the pH range 7–10 (Cotner and Clagett, 1973). It increased rapidly above pH 8.5 but was significant at pH 7. Methionine, if unhindered, will also react. For example, in the reaction of oxidized beef cytochrome *c* with iodoacetic acid at pH 5–6 two methionines and a histidine were modified (Ando *et al.*, 1966), while in oxidized human cytochrome *c* alkylation occurred at these two residues as well as a third methionine. On the other hand, the reaction of *Pseudomonas* cytochrome *c* with bromoacetate at pH 7 resulted in the carboxymethylation of one and two methionine residues in the absence and presence of cyanide, respectively (Fanger *et al.*, 1967). Histidine was unaffected even at this pH. Other examples of the lack of reaction of histidine were reported in the carboxymethylation of pig heart isocitrate dehydrogenase by iodoacetate at pH 5.6 (Colman, 1968), and of yeast inorganic phosphatase by iodoacetamide at pH 5.5 (Yano *et al.*, 1973). In each case, only a methionine residue reacted. An unusual modification was reported on reaction of ribonuclease T_1 with iodoacetate. The latter, acting as an active site-directed reagent, esterified a glutamate residue in ribonuclease T_1 (Takahashi *et al.*, 1967). The reaction of bromoacetate at pH 6.8 with harbor seal and sperm whale myoglobins gave heterogeneous reaction products which were not fractionated. It was, however, possible to identify histidine alkylation in the heterogeneous product as well as some ε- and α-NH_2 carboxymethylation (Nigen and Gurd, 1973). Alkylation of sperm whale myoglobin with iodoacetate at pH 6 also yielded a heterogeneous product from which six homogeneous derivatives were isolated and characterized and their conformation and immunochemistry were studied (Atassi *et al.*, 1975a). Of these, four derivatives were alkylated specifically at certain histidine residues only. One derivative was alkylated at two histidines and a single lysine, while the sixth derivative was alkylated at three histidines and at the α-NH_2 group. The reaction of bovine α-lactalbumin•with iodoacetate was studied at pH 5.5, 6.5, and 7.5 (Castellino and Hill, 1970). Methionine was modified under all of these conditions. At pH 5.5 some histidine alkylation was obtained but no reaction of lysine was observed. At pH 6.5 carboxymethylation of lysine appeared and carboxymethylation of histidine was almost complete. At pH 7.5 alkylation of lysine was further increased and histidine modification was still almost complete. The reaction of human myoglobin with bromoacetate was studied at several pH intervals in the pH range 3–10 and the heterogeneous reaction products were fractionated (Harris and Hill, 1969). No alkylation of lysine was detected below pH 7.5 and it increased very sharply above pH 7.5. Histidine alkylation increased at a steady but slower rate between pH 4 and 10. No modification of methionine was detected in the pH range 5.5–9, but it was observed above and below this pH range. A novel phenomenon was reported in the reactivation, by carboxymethylation of a histidine residue, of human 17β-estradiol dehydrogenase which had been previously inhibited by covalent labeling of the same histidine with a site-specific inhibitor (Boussioux et al., 1973). The steroid inhibitor was eliminated from the active site by carboxymethylation. The carboxymethylated enzyme exhibited a threefold activation and a dramatic decrease in the apparent affinity for estradiol, suggesting that the labeled histidine was not essential for catalytic activity but was located near the substrate binding site. In porcine mitochondrial malate dehydrogenase, two histidine residues were selectively modified by iodoacetamide, causing inactivation of the enzyme. The inactivation was completely prevented in the presence of reduced NADH (Foster and Harrison, 1974).

Carboxyalkylation of histidine residues in proteins can give rise to 1-carboxyalkyl, 3-carboxyalkyl, and 1,3-dicarboxyalkyl derivatives. With lysine, ε-mono- and ε-dicarboxyalkyl derivatives can be obtained. Methionine can give rise to the carboxyalkyl sulfonium salt. The N-alkyl derivatives are stable to hydrolysis and can be determined on the amino acid analyzer. The sulfonium salts are not stable, and this will be discussed subsequently under methionine (Section IVF2). The reactivity to alkylation of the imidazole nitrogens in histidine has recently been studied (Wieghardt and Goren, 1975). However, in proteins the type of the reaction products will be dependent entirely on the reaction conditions and on the protein. It has been reported that tritium-labeled carboxymethyl derivatives of various functional groups in proteins will exchange the ^{3}H label at different rates when exposed to standard protein acid hydrolysis conditions (Chin and Wold, 1975). The differential rate of hydrogen exchange was proposed as a means for the rapid identification of the carboxymethylated side chain. This method may prove to be useful when only small quantities of protein are available.

The reaction of *bromoacetone* with trypsin has been reported to yield a derivative alkylated at a single histidine (residue 46), and it was suggested that the reagent may react specifically with "surface" histidine residues (Beeley and Neurath, 1968). This specificity may have been more a function of the protein and the reaction conditions rather than the reagent since it has been shown more recently that iodoacetamide at room temperature and pH 7.0 also specifically alkylated the same histidine residue (i.e., His-46) in trypsin (Kasai and Ishii, 1973). Bromoacetone and dibromoacetone should be expected to react with thiol groups (Husain and Lowe, 1968; Moore and Fenselau, 1972a). From the foregoing examples, it can be seen clearly that the selectivity of alkylation by haloacetyl reagents, even though it is influenced by the reaction conditions, is highly dependent on the protein. The heterogeneity of the product, the extent of modification, and the nature of the residues alkylated under a given set of conditions for a new protein cannot really be predicted and may not be assumed.

Methylation of a single histidine (residue 57) in α-chymotrypsin has been obtained by reaction at pH 8 with *methyl p-nitrobenzenesulfonate* (Nakagawa and Bender, 1970). However, this reagent also reacts extremely well with thiol groups and it will be discussed later (Section IVG6).

3. Carbethoxylation

Ethoxyformic anhydride (*diethyl pyrocarbonate*, 35a) reacts with several amino acid side chains at neutral and alkaline pH values to give the carbethoxy derivatives (Muhlard et al., 1967). This has already been discussed briefly in connection with amino group modification (Section IVA1). Its reported selectivity at pH 6 for histidine residues (Muhlard et al., 1967) is no longer valid in view of many subsequent studies which documented modification of other functional groups (see Section IVA1 for examples). The pattern of reaction cannot therefore be predicted. There have been many reports of seemingly selective histidine modification by this reagent. Histidine has been selectively modified (usually between pH 6 and 7) in bovine glutamate dehydrogenase (Wallis and Holbrook, 1973), actin (Hegyi et al., 1974), yeast pyruvate kinase (Bornmann and Hess, 1974), choline acetyltransferase and acetylcholine esterase (Roskoski, 1974), and rabbit muscle pyruvate kinase (Dann and Britton, 1974). In some, but not all, of these studies either specific histidine modification was assumed or the analytical procedures employed did not permit detection of the modification of other functional groups. Thermolysin is inactivated by ethoxyformylation of a histidine (Blumberg et al., 1973; Burstein et al., 1974), but, at the same time, several other ethoxyformyl groups are introduced into the enzyme (Burstein et al., 1974). In the case of dihydroxyfolate reductase from *E. coli*, ethoxyformic anhydride caused modification of sulfhydryl, amino, and imidazole groups (Greenfield, 1974). In K-casein, this reagent was reported to modify (at pH 6–6.5) histidine and tyrosine residues as well as amino groups (Reimerdes and Kiostermeyer, 1973). The rates of reaction of ethoxyformic anhydride with several nucleophiles were studied by Osterman-Golkar et al. (1974). Even though differences in the rates of its reaction were found, the authors concluded that reaction of ethoxyformic anhydride with proteins "is expected to occur in a random fashion with various groups." The extent of histidine carbethoxylation (35b) can be determined from the increase in absorbance at 230 nm. The carbethoxyl substituent can be removed at room temperature with 0.1 M hydroxylamine at pH 7 (Melchior and Fahrney, 1970).

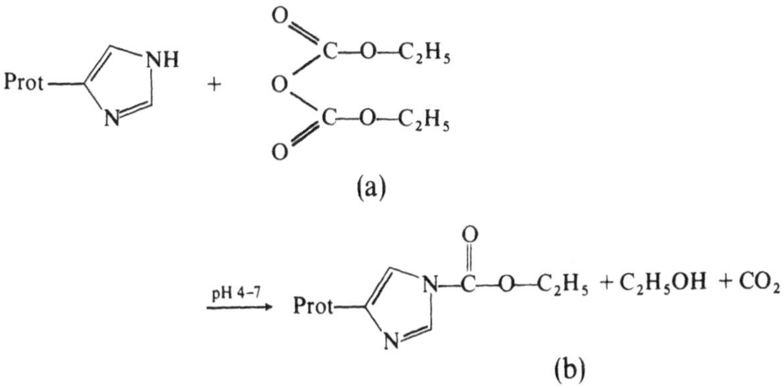

$$Prot{-}\left\langle \begin{array}{c} NH \\ N \end{array} \right\rangle + \begin{array}{c} O{=}C{-}O{-}C_2H_5 \\ O \\ O{=}C{-}O{-}C_2H_5 \end{array}$$

(a)

$$\xrightarrow{pH\ 4-7}\ Prot{-}\left\langle \begin{array}{c} N{-}\overset{O}{\overset{\|}{C}}{-}O{-}C_2H_5 \\ N \end{array} \right\rangle + C_2H_5OH + CO_2 \qquad (35)$$

(b)

4. Reaction with Diazonium Salts

Although *diazonium compounds* give colored adducts with histidine and tyrosine (Pauly, 1915), they will also react with several other functional groups in proteins to give colorless products (Cohen, 1968). *Diazonium-1H-tetrazole* was subsequently introduced (Horinishi et al., 1964) and appeared as a very promising reagent that apparently avoided the nonselectivity problems of other diazonium compounds. This reagent has been applied to differentiate free and bound histidine residues in proteins (Horinishi et al., 1964), to determine free and iron-linked histidines in some cytochromes (Horinishi et al., 1965), to study the role of tyrosine in the activity of myosin (Shimada, 1970), and to differentiate histidine residues in insulin (Suzuki et al., 1969), hemoglobin, myoglobin, and their apoproteins (Takenaka et al., 1970). The specificity of diazonium-1H-tetrazole was carefully determined with myoglobin and human serum albumin at two different pH values (i.e., pH 6.9 and 8.8) (Andres and Atassi, 1973). Studies of the electrophoretically homogeneous derivatives showed that diazonium-1H-tetrazole possessed a marked lack of specificity even under carefully controlled conditions where (for example, in myoglobin), from spectral measurements, one histidine residue was expected to have reacted. Several other amino acids were modified to significant extents as well. In addition to histidine and tyrosine, diazonium-1H-tetrazole also reacted with α- and ε-NH_2 groups, tryptophan, methionine, proline, cystine, and even phenylalanine (Andres and Atassi, 1973). Previous studies had reported its reaction with amino (Sokolovsky and Vallee, 1967; Takenaka, *et al.*, 1969) and thiol groups (Shimada, 1970). Myoglobin derivatives suffered severe conformational changes and entirely lost their antigenic reactivity with antisera to the native protein (Andres and Atassi, 1973). Diazotized human serum albumin cross-reacted strongly (82%) with antisera to diazotized myoglobin, with the added substituents acting as haptens and the nature of the carrier backbones bearing little consequence. It was concluded that diazonium-1*H*-tetrazole is completely nonspecific and totally unsatisfactory as a reagent for selective modification of proteins (Andres and Atassi, 1973). This provides an example of the inadvisability of relying on spectral measurements alone in chemical modification studies.

Aryl diazonium ions function as electrophilic reagents and can undergo diazo coupling without loss of nitrogen. Their coupling reactions with imidazole and phenol groups in proteins will yield the mono- and bisazo compounds. Monoazo coupling will most likely be obtained with other modified functional groups. Diazonium-1H tetrazole will react in a similar fashion. The two histidine adducts are shown in structures (36a) and (36b) and the two tyrosine derivatives are in (36c) and (36d). Derivatives with amino groups (36e) and with thiol groups (36f and 36g) are also shown. The chemistry of the reaction of the indole group with diazonium salts at acidic and neutral pH has been studied by Spande and Glenner (1973).

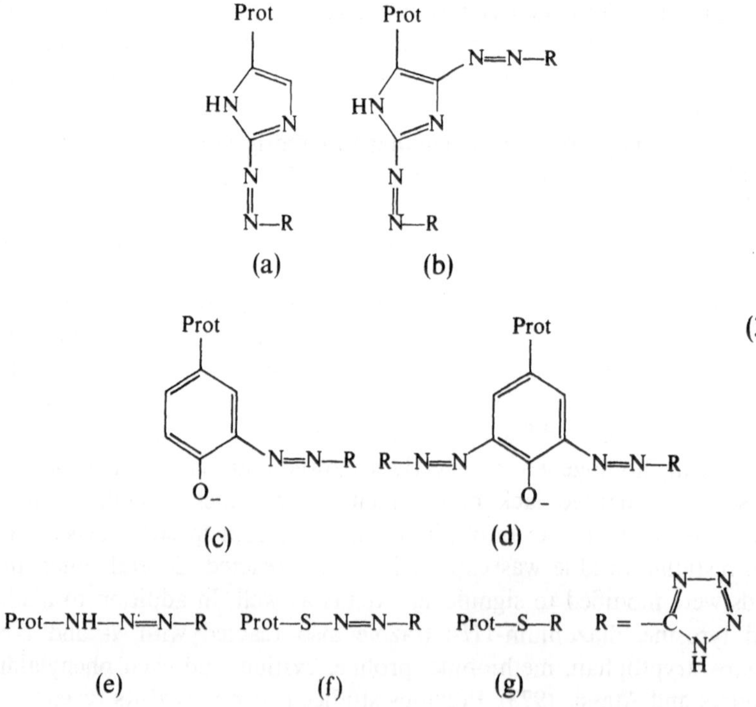

(36)

The general nonselective nature of their reactivity has led to the wide application of diazonium compounds for coupling of aryl substituents onto protein molecules. These derivatives have then been utilized to prepare antibodies with specificity directed against these small substituents (haptens) (Landsteiner, 1945; Singer, 1967; Nisonoff, 1967). Also, some diazonium compounds have been used as affinity labels and this will be discussed later (Section IVL3).

5. Other Modification Reactions

Iodination of proteins yields mono- and diiodo derivatives of histidine and tyrosine. Factors that determine the reactivity of histidine residues in proteins have been studied (Wolff and Covelli, 1969). In addition to reaction of histidine and tyrosine residues, iodine will cause oxidation of tryptophan, methionine, cysteine, and cystine as well as other covalent changes. Iodination is discussed in detail under tyrosine modification (Section IVJ2). Oxidizing agents such as *N*-bromosuccinimide and *N*-chlorosuccinimide can effect the modification, in addition to histidine, of methionine, tryptophan, cysteine, and tyrosine residues and are discussed in the relevant sections in this article.

F. Reactions for Methionine

1. Oxidation

The thioether side chain of methionine can be oxidized by any of a number of oxidizing agents. The specificity of the oxidation reaction and the nature of the oxidation product will be dependent on the oxidizing agent employed, the protein under study, and the reaction conditions.

Photooxidation has already been discussed in connection with histidine modification (Section IVE1). Photooxidation of α-chymotrypsin at pH 7.2 in the presence of methylene blue effected preferential oxidation of the three methionine residues (Schachter and Dixon, 1964). This is to be contrasted with examples of photooxidation around neutrality which resulted in histidine modification (Section IVE1). Clearly, the results are unpredictable. Selective methionine oxidation to methionine sulfoxide was reported when the reactions were performed in aqueous acetic acid in the presence of rose bengal or methylene blue as sensitizer (Jori *et al.*, 1968), or in aqueous solution (pH 2.5–6.5) employing hematoporphyrin as sensitizer (Jori *et al.*, 1969). The reaction was applied to modify methionine-12 in lysozyme. The possibility of covalent coupling of dye to protein at higher dye concentration (Brandt *et al.*, 1974) has been mentioned.

Hydrogen peroxide will oxidize methionine, cystine, cysteine, tyrosine, tryptophan, and histidine residues (Neumann, 1972). At low pH its selectivity for methionine improves and has been used to oxidize methionine residues at pH 2.5 in ribonuclease (Neumann *et al.*, 1962) and at pH 3 in α-chymotrypsin (Koshland *et al.*, 1962; Weiner *et al.*, 1966a). However, some disulfide interchange may occur during oxidation (Weiner *et al.*, 1966a) and selectivity at low pH is not always obtained. For example, action of H_2O_2 on cytochrome *c* in the pH range 2.2–13 effected oxidation of methionine, cystine, tyrosine, and histidine (O'Brien, 1967). Also, in the presence of substrate, chymotrypsin was oxidized at tryptophan and cystine as well as methionine (Schachter *et al.*, 1964).

Sodium metaperiodate can yield excellent selectivity with appropriate control of conditions. Its use to oxidize the *N*-terminal serine (Dixon, 1962) and a methionine (Knowles, 1965) in corticotropin and α-chymotrypsin, respectively, was reported. In a detailed investigation, using sperm whale myoglobin and apomyoglobin as models, the action of periodate was studied under different conditions of pH, temperature, and reagent excess (Atassi, 1967a). In the presence of a large molar (60–70) periodate excess, selectivity of the reaction increased with decrease in pH and decrease in temperature. The heme group catalyzed the reaction and was itself degraded. Selectivity was best at pH 5 and 0°C when methionine, tryptophan, and tyrosine were oxidized, with the rate of oxidation of the methionines being greater than those of the other two amino acids in the protein. Oxidation of tyrosine and tryptophan residues in apomyoglobin was eliminated, and reaction at pH 5 and 0°C was entirely specific for the two methionines when periodate was present in equimolar excess relative to the number of methionine residues in the protein (Atassi, 1967a). The apomyoglobin derivative recombined with unmodified ferriheme and showed no change in immunochemical behavior relative to native myoglobin (Atassi, 1967a). In the presence of a larger periodate excess at 32°C and pH 8.5, oxidation of the glycoprotein ovotransferrin at three tyrosines and one tryptophan was reported (Azari and Phillips, 1970) without effect on the carbohydrate moiety.

Oxidation of methionine (and other sulfides) was shown to take place rapidly and efficiently at neutral pH in the presence of Mn^{2+}, *oxygen*, and *sulfite ion* (Yang, 1970). The aerobic oxidation of sulfite was necessary for sulfoxide formation and the reaction was inhibited by superoxide dismutase. *S*-Methylcysteine was not appreciably oxidized by the Mn–*sulfite*–O_2 system but was oxidized when horseradish peroxidase, Mn^{2+}, and phenol were present (Yang, 1970). This reaction has not yet been applied to the oxidation of methionine residues in proteins.

Trichloroisocyanuric acid reacted with several amino acids at acid pH (3.5), but a remarkable narrowing down of its specificity was observed at pH 7.0 with free amino acids and proteins (Atassi, 1973). Action of the reagent on free amino acids at pH 7.0 exhibited selectivity for methionine, cystine, and tryptophan. Derivatives of lysozyme and egg albumin were prepared in which methionine and tryptophan were oxidized without change in the cystine and cysteine contents of the proteins. Methionine was oxidized to its sulfone, and tryptophan was probably converted to an oxindole derivative (Atassi, 1973). *Trichloromethanesulfonyl chloride* (CCl_3SO_2Cl) was reported to oxidize Met-192 to the sulfoxide in α-chymotrypsin at pH 3.5 in a rapid stoichiometric reaction (Taylor *et al.*, 1973). This derivative existed entirely in the active substate in the pH range 7–9. *Tetrachloroauric (III) acid* ($HAuCl_4$) was reported to effect a quantitative and stereospecific oxidation of methionine to methionine sulfoxide in free solution and in model peptides in the pH range 2–5 (Bordignon *et al.*, 1973). No traces of the sulfone were detected, and only one of the two possible diastereoisomers was obtained. This reaction has not been applied to protein modification but it may prove useful. *Chloramine T* (sodium *p*-toluenesulfonchloramide, $pCH_3C_6H_4SO_2N\ NaCl$), a reagent used in the radioiodination of proteins (Greenwood *et al.*, 1963), has been employed to oxidize methionine residues in a group of rabbit IgG allotypes and resulted in loss of the allotypic specificity (McBurnette and Mandy, 1974). The selectivity of this relatively strong oxidizing agent, which often causes undesirable denaturation, needs further study.

Azide, which has been used extensively in binding studies with hemoglobin, does not confine its effect to binding with the heme group. It has long been known (Misani *et al.*, 1951; Whitehead and Bentley, 1952) that azide will react with both methionine and its sulfoxide to form methionine sulfoximine (37d). Acid hydrolysis converts the sulfoximine into methionine. The rate of azide reaction increases with decrease in pH and has been shown to inactivate horseradish peroxidase as a result of methionine oxidation (Brill and Weinryb, 1967). Lack of agreement concerning the cooperativity of the binding process of azide with hemoglobin (for discussions, see Barksdale *et al.*, 1975) may be attributed to the covalent change in the protein part of the molecule which is either overlooked or ignored. Different degrees of oxidation may produce different binding results, especially if heterogeneous reaction products are formed. Total reliance on physical and kinetic measurements without examining any covalent and/or conformational changes may lead to erroneous conclusions.

Methionine sulfoxide in protein derivatives can be reduced by a thiol reagent to methionine (Dedman *et al.*, 1957), often with regeneration of full activity. Acid hydrolysis converts methionine sulfoxide back to methionine (Ray and Koshland, 1962), and the modification is undetectable by amino acid analysis of acid hydrolysates, but can be determined by analysis of alkaline hydrolysates. A colorimetric procedure, based on rearrangement of sulfoxide with acetic anhydride, has been introduced (Lunder, 1972) for the determination of methionine sulfoxide in the intact protein. The rearrangement product can be determined colorimetrically using chromotropic acid.

2. Alkylation

Methionine sulfonium salts have long been known to be produced from reaction at acid pH of methionine with *alkyl halides* such as *methyl iodide* or *bromide, allyl bromide, cinnamyl chloride* (Toennies, 1940; Toennies and Kolb, 1945), or mustard gas (Stein and Moore, 1946). *Methyl iodide* was later reintroduced for selective methionine alkylation at low pH (Link and Stark, 1968). Reaction of methyl iodide with bovine ribonuclease A in 8 M urea at low pH was shown to be selective for the methionine residues (Stark and Link, 1975). By chromatography of the heterogeneous reaction product and characterization of the derivatives, it was demonstrated that methylation of Met-29 or Met-79 had no effect on the enzymatic activity, while methylation of Met-13 or Met-30 resulted in conformational changes. Studies of alkylation with *iodoacetate* at low pH showed that the reaction becomes quite selective for methionine, particularly in the absence of sulfhydryl groups (Gundlach *et al.*, 1959*a*). *Carboxymethylation* has been discussed in connection with histidine modification (see Section IVE2). Unlike the *N*-alkyl derivatives of lysine and histidine and the *S*-alkyl derivatives of cysteine, the sulfonium salts of methionine are not stable to acid hydrolysis and cannot be determined by amino acid analysis of protein hydrolysates. The carboxymethylsulfonium salt of methionine (38a) gave methionine and *S*-carboxymethylhomocysteine (38c) on acid hydrolysis (Gundlach *et al.*, 1959*b*).

Alkylation of methionine residues is usually carried out at pH 2–3. There are examples of selective methionine alkylations being obtained at higher pH (see Section IVE2). Also, certain site-directed reagents have alkylated methionine residues at higher pH. For example, α-chymotrypsin was selectively alkylated at pH 5 on methionine-192 by reaction with *p*-nitrophenyl *N*-bromoacetyl-α-aminobutyrate (Lawson and Schramm, 1965). Selective alkylation of horse heart cytochrome *c* at the two methi-

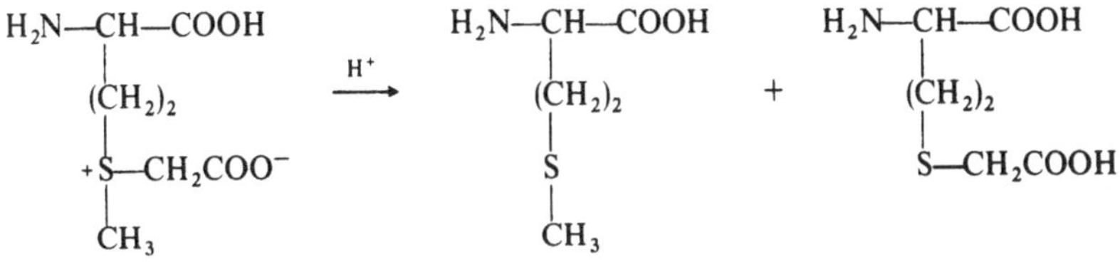

$$
\begin{array}{ccc}
\underset{\displaystyle\substack{|\\ (CH_2)_2 \\ | \\ +S-CH_2COO^- \\ | \\ CH_3}}{H_2N-CH-COOH}
&
\underset{\displaystyle\substack{|\\ (CH_2)_2 \\ | \\ S \\ | \\ CH_3}}{H_2N-CH-COOH}
&
\underset{\displaystyle\substack{|\\ (CH_2)_2 \\ | \\ S-CH_2COOH}}{H_2N-CH-COOH}
\end{array}
$$

(a) $\xrightarrow{H^+}$ (b) $+$ (c) (38)

onine residues was obtained by reaction with bromoacetate at pH 7.0 (Schejter and Aviram, 1970; Ikeda-Saito *et al.*, 1975).

β-Propiolactone (39b) was shown to alkylate methionine specifically when reaction was carried out at pH 3.0 and 0°C (Taubman and Atassi, 1968). This reagent possessed unique specificity for methionine. The reaction proceeds through a nucleophilic attack (39) by the sulfur on the β-carbon

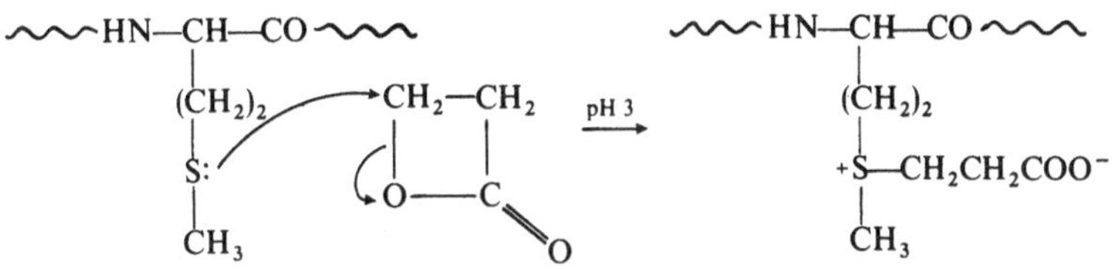

$$
\begin{array}{ccc}
\sim\!\!\sim\!\!HN-CH-CO\!\!\sim\!\!\sim & & \sim\!\!\sim\!\!HN-CH-CO\!\!\sim\!\!\sim \\
| & CH_2-CH_2 & | \\
(CH_2)_2 & | \quad\quad | & (CH_2)_2 \\
S: & O-C & +S-CH_2CH_2COO^- \\
| & \quad\quad \searrow O & | \\
CH_3 & & CH_3
\end{array}
$$

(a) (b) $\xrightarrow{pH\ 3}$ (c) (39)

of β-propiolactone, resulting in cleavage at the alkyl–oxygen bond of the lactone and the formation of the carboxyethylsulfonium salt (39c) (Taubman and Atassi, 1968). Reaction of β-propiolactone with sperm whale myoglobin gave a homogeneous derivative which was specifically carboxyethylated at the two methionine residues. The modification caused no changes in the conformation or in the immunochemical properties of the protein (Atassi, 1969a). The reagent has also been employed recently for the carboxyethylation of the two methionine residues in hen egg white lysozyme (Atassi *et al.*, 1976b). The homogeneous derivative showed no conformational changes by ORD and CD measurements, but slight changes in conformation were detected by disulfide reducibility. The enzyme lost half its lytic activity but its immunochemical reactivity remained unchanged.

Ethylenimine (aziridine) has been reported to alkylate methionine at pH 8.6, but cysteine was also aminoethylated, even at pH 2 (Schroeder *et al.*, 1967). Sulfonium salt formation from reaction of methionine with some *aziridine alkylating agents* at pH 7.4 was studied in more detail by Capps and Jones (1974). These sulfonium salts were, as expected, unstable to acid or alkaline hydrolysis, giving, in addition to methionine, several products which were identified (Capps and Jones, 1974). *2-Methoxy-5-nitrobenzyl bromide* reacts with methionine but has equal reactivity with tryptophan and thiol groups (Horton *et al.*, 1965).

Methionylsulfonium derivatives have been shown to be especially susceptible to attack by sulfur nucleophiles (Naider and Bohak, 1972). The rate of regeneration of the methionyl side chain depended on the nature of both the sulfonium salt and the nucleophile employed. Regeneration by thiols was proposed as a method to distinguish methionine alkylation from that of other functional groups in proteins (Naider and Bohak, 1972). Methionine sulfonium salts are stable to cyanogen bromide cleavage (Spande et al., 1970), to performic acid oxidation (Neumann et al., 1962), and to mild periodate oxidation (Atassi et al., 1976b). These properties can also be used for their determination and identification.

3. Other Modification Reactions

Cleavage of the thioether side chain of methionine was achieved by reaction with *boron tribromide* or *boron triiodide* (Atassi and Perlstein, 1972b). *Boron trihalides* will cleave thioethers at room temperature to give the corresponding alkyl halide side chain, either directly or through the thioxydihaloborane intermediate (40) (Atassi and Perlstein, 1972b). With

$$R\text{—}S\text{—}R + BI_3 \longrightarrow RSBI_2 + RI$$
$$3RSBI_2 \longrightarrow 3RI + BI_3 + B_2S_3$$

(40)

methionine, the thioxydihaloborane side chain could oxidize in air to give homocysteic acid. From the alkyl halide side chain, homoserine and homoserine lactone were produced on acid hydrolysis. Selectivity of the reaction for methionine was demonstrated on hemoglobin, myoglobin, and lysozyme, where, in each case, no other amino acids were modified (Atassi and Perlstein, 1972b). Unfortunately, solvents employed in the reaction (BBr_3 itself, and for BI_3 chloroform was used) subsequently rendered the protein derivative highly insoluble. This reaction should prove useful, however, in selective modification of immunochemically reactive peptides at methionine residues.

Production of ethylene from methionine occupying end-chain position in several model peptides was obtained by *FMN in light* at pH 5 (Ku and Leopold, 1970). Methionine residues in internal or *N*-terminal positions were ineffective as substrates for ethylene production. The generality and specificity of this interesting reaction have not been tested on proteins.

G. Reactions for Sulfhydryl (Thiol) Groups

The sulfhydryl group is the most reactive side chain in proteins. The reagents discussed under the modification of other functional groups will, with only a very few exceptions, modify sulfhydryl groups as well. The chemistry of the thiol groups is therefore quite extensive. Numerous and diverse modification reactions are available to the investigator, depending on the type of adduct desired (e.g., fluorescent, spin-labeled, chromophoric, reversible). It is not possible to give a comprehensive discussion of sulfhydryl group chemistry here. The chemistry and biochemistry of the sulfhydryl group have been the subject of an excellent and extensive review by Friedman (1973). The biochemistry of the SH group has also been reviewed (Jocelyn, 1972). The following section emphasizes only the main reactions and recent developments in these reactions.

1. Oxidation

Several reagents are available for the oxidation of sulfhydryl groups in proteins. Oxidation of sulfhydryl groups, previously derived from reduction of disulfide bonds, back to the disulfide bonds is discussed later (Section IVH). Oxidation of preexisting sulfhydryl groups in a protein normally does not give rise to disulfide bond formation because their proximity is precluded by their three-dimensional positioning in the protein. The reaction, therefore, will proceed to the higher oxidation states (i.e., sulfinic and sulfonic acids).

Hydrogen peroxide will oxidize sulfhydryl groups to sulfonic acid (Cecil and McPhee, 1959; Neumann, 1972). Other strong oxidizing agents such as *lipid peroxides, N-bromosuccinimide,* and *iodine* will also give the higher oxidation product (Friedman, 1973). The reaction of rabbit muscle creatine kinase with limited excess of iodine at pH 6.1 resulted in oxidation of the thiol groups to the sulfenate with inactivation (Trundle and Cunningham, 1969). Oxidation was reversed and the enzyme reactivated by a thiol reagent. However, these reagents will usually also oxidize other functional groups (any one or more of methionine, tyrosine, histidine, tryptophan, and cystine) and are discussed subsequently in detail. *Peroxyacetyl nitrate,* previously shown to oxidize sulfhydryl groups in proteins to the sulfonic acid (Mudd *et al.,* 1966) has more recently been found to cause methionine oxidation (Leh and Mudd, 1974). Peroxyacetyl nitrate is a toxic gas which is not available commercially and therefore is not likely to find extensive application. *Performic acid* oxidation (Hirs, 1967*a*) is more often used for oxidative cleavage of disulfide bonds. It is also employed for analytical purposes to convert cysteine (and cystine) residues quantitatively into cysteic acid, which can be determined with more accuracy than cysteine (or cystine) on the amino acid analyzer. Performic acid is also not specific for cysteine or cystine.

Tretranitromethane, a reagent employed for nitration of tyrosine residues in proteins (see Section IVJ6), will in fact oxidize sulfhydryl groups more rapidly than it will nitrate tyrosine residues (Riordan and Christen, 1968).

Thiol group oxidation in aldolase decreased with decreasing pH. The final products of oxidation of thiol compounds were mainly the disulfide and the sulfinic ($-SO_2^-$) acid derivatives (Sokolovsky et al., 1969) and in proteins disulfide bonds were primarily obtained. Tetranitromethane has been used to modify a thiol group in cytoplasmic aspartate aminotransferase at pH 7.5 (Birchmeier et al., 1973; Wilson et al., 1974). However, the use of tetranitromethane for modification of sulfhydryl groups is not recommended, since, at pH 7.5, tyrosine nitration will be considerable and in addition other functional groups can be modified (Section IVJ6). Ortho-iodosobenzoate will modify sulfhydryl groups (Hellerman et al., 1941) and the modification can be reversed (Rafter, 1957) by mercaptoethanol. The reagent has been applied to modify reversibly the essential sulfhydryl group in rabbit muscle glyceraldehyde phosphate dehydrogenase, but the extent of reversibility was not determined (Moore and Fenselau, 1972b). A new method for determining cysteine by this reagent using ascorbic acid and iodine has been reported (Verma and Bose, 1974). Specificity of this reagent has not been well studied and the nature of the oxidation products in proteins has not been established. Other reagents are available which are better suited for reversible modification of the thiol group (Section IVG10).

2. Acylation Reactions

Acid anhydrides, often employed in acylation of amino groups, will in addition react with thiol as well as other functional groups. These have previously been discussed in detail (Section IVA1). Choline selenol esters (41a) have been found to acylate thiol groups in slightly acidic conditions under which histidine and amino groups did not react (Makriyannis et al., 1973). The thiol esters produced (41b) and the selenol ester reagents had

$$
\text{Prot}-\text{SH} + \text{R}-\overset{\overset{\displaystyle O}{\|}}{\text{C}}-\text{SeCH}_2\text{CH}_2\overset{+}{\text{N}}(\text{CH}_3)_3 \underset{-\text{NH}_2}{\overset{\text{H}^+}{\rightleftharpoons}} \text{Prot}-\text{S}-\overset{\overset{\displaystyle O}{\|}}{\text{C}}-\text{R} + \text{HSeCH}_2\text{CH}_2\overset{+}{\text{N}}(\text{CH}_3)_3
$$

(a)   (b)

(41)

$$\text{R} = -\text{CH}_3 \text{ or } -\text{C}_6\text{H}_5$$

different ultraviolet absorption maxima, and the reaction therefore could be conveniently followed by monitoring simultaneously at different wavelengths. This reaction should prove useful in the modification of thiol groups in proteins since the reagents are very soluble in aqueous solvents and the modification, which is quite stable to experimental manipulation, can be readily reversed by the addition of free amine (Günther and Mautner, 1965). The S-acetyl group may also be removed by hydroxylamine (Klotz and Elfbaum, 1964).

3. Reaction with Mercuric Compounds

Mercuric salts or better *organic mercurials* react with thiol groups quite selectively at neutral pH. Divalent mercury can react with two SH groups to form S—Hg—S bridges. Following the introduction of *p-hydroxymercuribenzoate* (Hellerman *et al.*, 1943), which was subsequently employed in spectral determination of the extent of modification (Boyer, 1954), a variety of organic mercurials have been introduced for modification of the thiol group. Protein mercurial derivatives are of course useful in X-ray diffraction studies. A group of *chloromercurinitrophenols* were introduced as chromophoric reagents for thiol groups in proteins and were applied to modify a specific site in lobster glyceraldehyde 3-phosphate dehydrogenase (McMurray and Trentham, 1969). The reagents acted as chromophoric probes as well as "reporter groups" that could monitor environmental changes. One of these reagents, 2-chloromercuri-4-nitrophenol, has been used to modify two nonessential thiol groups in chicken creatine kinase and its complexes with substrate (Quiocho and Olson, 1974). *Fluorescein mercuric acetate* reaction with protein thiol groups (Karush *et al.*, 1964) can be followed by absorption spectroscopy or by fluorescence spectroscopy. Its action as an irreversible inhibitor of calf liver sorbitol dehydrogenase was also followed by gel filtration (Heitz, 1973). *Mercurichrome* is another recent protein thiol-group reagent which will also introduce a fluorescent label at the site of modification (Weltman *et al.*, 1972). More recently, *S-mercuric-N-dansyl cysteine* was shown to react with SH groups rapidly and stoichiometrically over a wide range of pH to form mercury-bridged mercaptides (Leavis and Lehrer, 1974). Considerable fluorescence enhancements and spectral shifts were obtained when the label was attached to tropomyosin, troponin C, and actin. A spin-labeled *p*-mercuribenzoate analogue, carrying the iminoxyl radical 2,2,6,6-tetramethyl-4-oxypiperidine-1-oxyl, has been used to label the reactive thiol group in glyceraldehyde phosphate dehydrogenase and monitor conformational changes by paramagnetic resonance studies (Elek *et al.*, 1972).

It is relevant to point out here that when thiol groups in oxidized protein derivatives are being determined by reaction with mercurials it may be necessary to take into account the finding that mercurials will react with disulfide monoxide (thiosulfinate, RSOSR) and to a lesser extent with cystine dioxide (RSO_2SR) residues that may be present (MacLaren *et al.*, 1965). Another significant finding is that the *p*-mercuribenzoate group has been reported to migrate from one protein subunit to another in glyceraldehyde phosphate dehydrogenase (Szabolcsi *et al.*, 1960; Smith and Schachman, 1971) and in human hemoglobin A (Waterman, 1974). The migration took place at neutral pH and low temperature ($4°C$).

4. Reaction with Haloacetates and Analogues

Reaction of *iodo-* and *bromoacetates*, or their amides, with proteins has already been discussed in connection with histidine (Section IVE2) and methionine (Section IVF2) modifications. The thiol group is more reactive with haloacetates than any of the other nucleophilic side chains in proteins. Usually, *S*-carboxymethylations are performed in the pH range 7–8.5. Since thiol groups react at a much faster rate, alkylation of amino groups is often avoided or greatly minimized. However, the possibility of amino group, histidine, methionine, and perhaps tyrosine modification (see Section IVE2) cannot be dismissed. In general, better selectivity is achieved with organic mercurials, but the stability of *S*-carboxymethyl-cysteine to acid hydrolysis enables its determination by amino acid analysis where it appears just before aspartic acid. For the determination of total thiol groups in proteins, carboxymethylation has to be performed in a dissociating solvent in order to achieve complete accessibility of the SH groups. It has been shown that *S*-carboxymethylcysteine (42a) can undergo intramolecular cyclization under acid conditions to yield a thiazine deriva-tive (42b). The thiazine derivative escaped detection by amino acid analysis

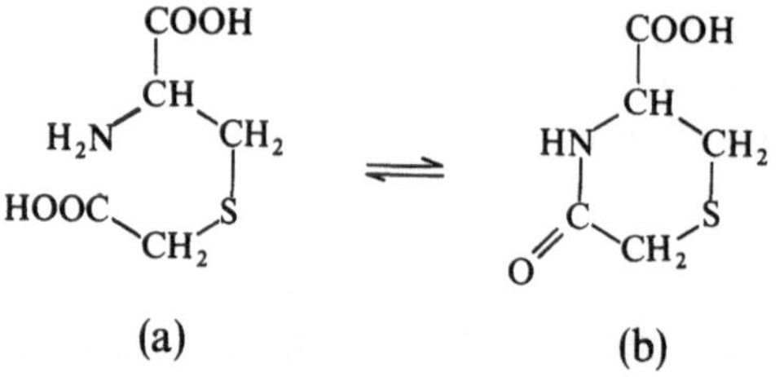

$$\tag{42}$$

(a)   (b)

because it lacks a free amino group (Bradbury and Smyth, 1973). 3-*Bromo-propionic acid* ($BrCH_2CH_2COOH$), which yields *S*-carboxyethylcysteine, avoided this complication. *S*-Carboxyethylcysteine did not cyclize and appeared on the analyzer between serine and glutamic acid (Bradbury and Smyth, 1973). Performic acid oxidation of *S*-carboxymethylcysteine, either in the free state or in proteins, yielded the sulfoxide predominantly at $-10°$ to $-20°C$, while at 37°C the product was exclusively *S*-carboxymethyl-cysteine sulfone (Takahashi, 1973). Upon acid hydrolysis, the sulfoxide decomposed mostly to cysteine. The sulfone, which also decomposed extensively, gave products that have not been identified.

A large number of derivatives of iodo- or bromoacetamide have been prepared with a variety of chromophoric, fluorescent, and other side chains. 2-*Bromoacetamide-4-nitrophenol* (Burr and Koshland, 1964) enabled the introduction of an environmentally sensitive conformational probe (re-porter group) (i.e., 2-acetamide-4-nitrophenol) at the active-site thiol group in each of the four subunits of rabbit muscle glyceraldehyde phosphate dehydrogenase (Kirtley and Koshland, 1970). *Iodoacetamide naphthylaminesulfonates* have been developed to introduce a fluorescent probe at the site of the modified thiol group (Hudson and Weber, 1973). *Spin-labeled iodoacetamide* derivatives have been valuable in protein paramagnetic resonance studies. The reagents N-(1-oxyl-2,2,5,5-tetramethyl-3-pyrrolidinyl)iodoacetamide (43a) and N-(1-oxyl-2,2,6,6-tetramethyl-4-piperidinyl)-iodoacetamide (43b) have been employed to study oxygenation-induced conformational changes in hemoglobin labeled at a sulfhydryl group (Ogawa and McConnell, 1967; Deal *et al.*, 1971). An application of reagent (43a)

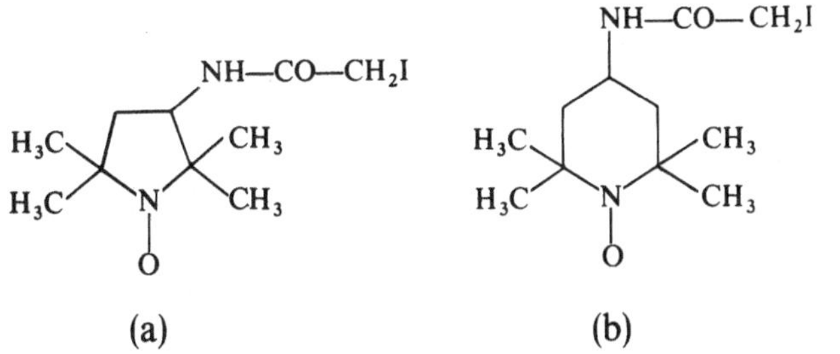

$$(43)$$

(a)   (b)

has been in monitoring small conformational changes associated with inhibitor binding in human carbonic anhydrases (Carlsson *et al.*, 1975). Iodoacetamide analogues, with a spin-label at increasing distances from the reactive halide, have been used to study the binding site of carbonic anhydrases (Chignell *et al.*, 1972) and to estimate the sulfhydryl group crevice in bovine serum albumin (Hull *et al.*, 1975). It should be noted here that the attachment of spin-labeled iodoacetamides similar to (43b) was found to induce conformational changes in glyceraldehyde 3-phosphate dehydrogenase. In contrast, when the same thiol group was modified with non-labeled iodoacetate, conformational changes were not observed (Elek *et al.*, 1972). This is most likely caused by the bulky side chain of the spin-label. Furthermore, nitroxyl radicals have been shown to oxidize sulfhydryl groups over a wide pH range (Morrisett and Drott, 1969). The oxidative effect was reduced when the label was used in a small concentration and excess reagent was removed immediately after reaction. The azo dye *4-iodoacetamido-2,3'-dicarboxyazobenzene* has been used to label the reactive SH group (β93) in human hemoglobin A (Fasold *et al.*, 1973).

5. Addition to Double Bond

Ability of the thiol group to undergo rapid nucleophilic addition to double bonds formulates the basis of a class of compounds comprising a large number of versatile and useful reagents. Maleimides (44a) are the most widely used compounds in this class. Reaction with thiol side chains

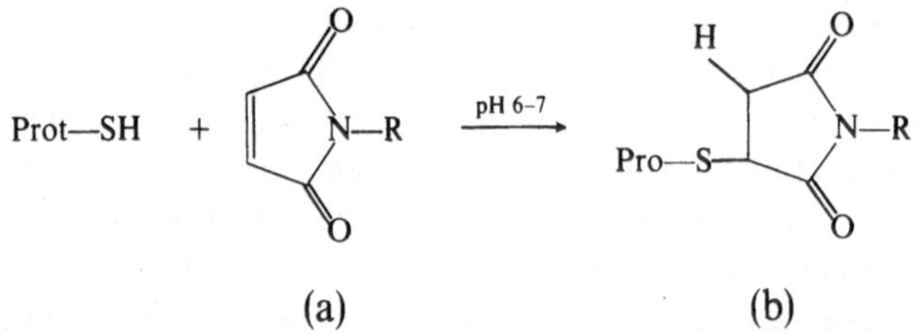

$$\text{Prot—SH} \quad + \quad \underset{(a)}{\text{(maleimide, N—R)}} \quad \xrightarrow{\text{pH 6-7}} \quad \underset{(b)}{\text{(Pro—S adduct, N—R)}} \qquad (44)$$

takes place rapidly at neutral pH. The group R in (44a) can be varied to impart a variety of desired characteristics to the reagent. *N-Ethylmaleimide* was first shown to react with thiol groups by Friedmann *et al.* (1949) and was subsequently used (Tsao and Bailey, 1953) for titration of these groups in proteins. This reaction has since been studied extensively. The reagent is most stable between pH 5 and 7 and reacts rapidly with thiol groups between pH 6 and 7 (Gregory, 1955). It also reacts with α-amino groups and with histidine residues (Smyth *et al.*, 1960). A high degree of selectivity is obtained when the reaction is carried out below neutrality and excess reagent is avoided (Smyth *et al.*, 1964). Hydrolysis of the cysteine adduct (44b) under the usual acid conditions of protein acid hydrolysis yields predominantly *S*-succinylcysteine [*S*-(1,2-dicarboxyethyl)-L-cysteine, HOOC—CH(NH$_2$)—CH$_2$—S—CH(COOH)—CH$_2$—COOH] and ethyl-amine (Smyth *et al.*, 1964). Reaction with amino groups yields the *N*-alkylamine derivative (Sharpless and Flavin, 1966), and their hydrolysis also gives ethylamine and the *N*-succinyl adduct of the modified amino acid. Recovery of *S*-succinylcysteine and ethylamine in equimolar quantities indicates the specificity of the reaction toward thiol groups. *S*-Succinyl-cysteine elutes on the amino acid analyzer before aspartic acid, and ethyl-amine appears between ammonia and arginine (Smyth *et al.*, 1964). *N*-Ethylmaleimide has been employed in the study of numerous proteins to determine the role of protein thiol groups in a given biological function. It has even been applied to determine the topography of ribosomal proteins (Bakardjieva and Crichton, 1974). However, its application in studies of this type (e.g., topography of cellular particles and membranes) may be quite unreliable (Glick and Brubacher, 1975).

The group R (44a) could be a colored label such as *N-dimethylamino-dinitrophenylmaleimide* (Witter and Tuppy, 1960). A fluorescent label could also be introduced such as in *N-(p-(2-benzimidazolyl)phenyl)maleimide* (Sekine *et al.*, 1972; Machida *et al.*, 1974) and *N-(1-anilinonaphthyl-4)-maleimide* (45a) (Kanaoka *et al.*, 1973). The long-life fluorescent reagent *N-(3-pyrene)maleimide* (45b) (Weltman *et al.*, 1973) gave protein adducts (excited at 345 nm) whose fluorescence (380 and 405 nm) lifetimes were as long as 100 nsec. Spin-labeled 2,2,5,5-*tetramethylpyrrolidine-1-oxyl-3-maleimide* (45c) has been developed for carrying out electron spin resonance

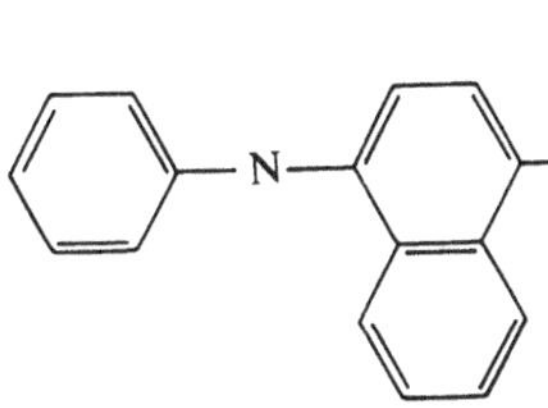

(a) 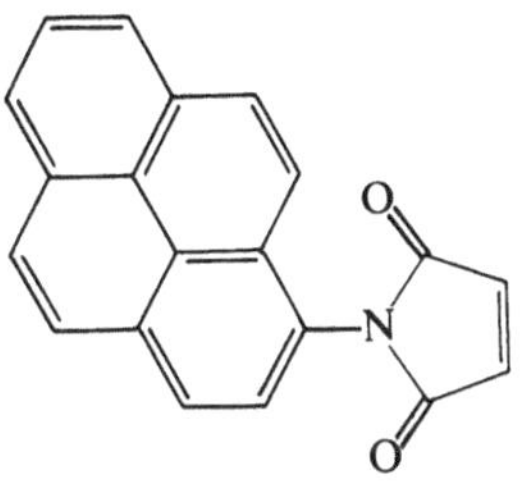   (b)

(45)

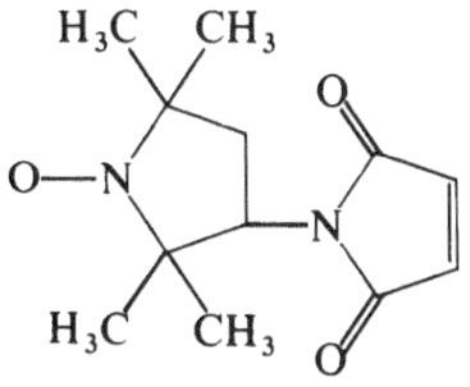

(c)

spectral studies on the protein derivatives (Barratt *et al.*, 1971). Maleimides carrying spin-labels at increasing distances from the modified thiol group have been used to estimate the depth of the thiol-group crevice in bovine serum albumin (Hull *et al.*, 1975).

Thiol groups will add rapidly to α,β-unsaturated compounds of the general formula $CH_2{=}CHR_1R_2$. The reaction usually takes place around neutrality (pH 6–8). Acrylates such as *acrolein* ($CH_2{=}CHCHO$), *acrylonitrile* ($CH_2{=}CHCN$), *acrylamide* ($CH_2{=}CHCONH_2$), and *methyl acrylate* ($CH_2{=}CHCOOCH_3$) are examples of such compounds. However, they will react with thiol (Weil and Seibles, 1961; Plummer and Hirs, 1964), amino (Plummer and Hirs, 1964; Riehm and Scheraga, 1966a), and imidazole (Bosshard *et al.*, 1969) groups. Their reaction with thiol and amino groups (see Section IVA9) was found to be a function of pH in the range 6–8, but thiol groups were modified more rapidly (Cavins and Friedman, 1968). When reagents were used in equimolar excess relative to the free thiol groups, high selectivity for these groups was obtained (Cavins and Friedman, 1968). Other useful compounds of this type are 4-*vinylpyridine* (Friedman and Krull, 1969) and 2-*vinylquinoline* (Krull *et al.*, 1971). 4-Vinylpyridine yielded *S*-pyridylethylcysteine residues which were stable to acid hydrolysis and which had an absorption maximum at 255 nm. 2-Vinylquinoline afforded a colored adduct (*S*-quinolylethylcysteine) which absorbed at 318 nm and could therefore be used for spectrophotometric determination of reactive thiol groups. *S*-Pyridylethylcysteine was reported to oxidize in performic acid to the sulfone and to cysteine sulfinic acid (Stevenson, 1973).

On acid hydrolysis, S-pyridylethylcysteine sulfone suffered partial decomposition, giving mainly cysteic acid and alanine. It is relevant to take this into account if S-pyridylethyl-protein derivatives are to be subjected to performic acid oxidation.

6. Other Alkylation Reactions

β-Bromoethylamine (Br—CH$_2$CH$_2$—NH$_2$) was introduced in order to convert cysteine residues to S-β-aminoethylcysteine residues (Prot—S—CH$_2$CH$_2$NH$_2$), which were then susceptible to tryptic hydrolysis (Lindley, 1956). However, complete alkylation of the thiol groups is not usually achieved, even though the reaction is ordinarily carried out at pH 11. In fact, at this high pH, the reaction is quite likely not specific for thiol groups. *Ethylenimine* (*aziridine*, 46a) was subsequently reported to give more quantitative S-aminoethylation (46) at a lower pH (Raftery and Cole, 1966). Methionine can be modified under these conditions (Section

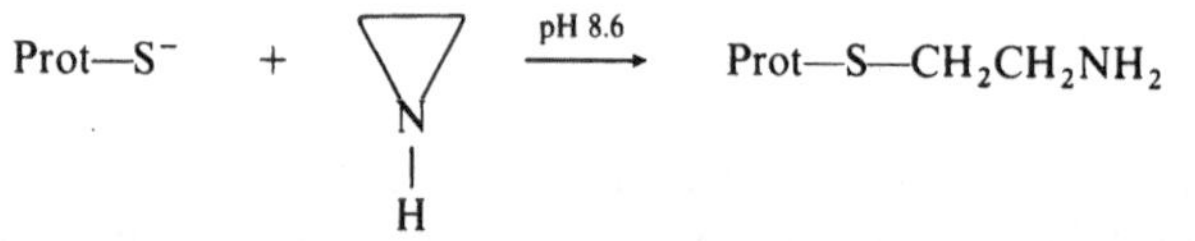

$$\text{Prot—S}^- \quad + \quad \underset{\overset{|}{\text{H}}}{\overset{\displaystyle\bigtriangledown}{\text{N}}} \quad \xrightarrow{\text{pH 8.6}} \quad \text{Prot—S—CH}_2\text{CH}_2\text{NH}_2 \qquad (46)$$

$$\text{(a)} \qquad\qquad\qquad\qquad \text{(b)}$$

IVF2). Also, histidine modifications, in addition to that of thiol groups, has been reported with an N-substituted derivative of aziridine (Shapiro *et al.*, 1969). More recently, quantitative aminoethylation of thiol groups in peptides and proteins was achieved, seemingly without side reactions, by the action of aziridine in liquid ammonia at boiling point temperature ($-33°C$) (Kuromizu and Meienhofer, 1972). This may prove to be the method of choice since the reaction proceeded rapidly and offered the advantage of rapid workup under mild conditions. S-Aminoethylcysteine is stable to acid hydrolysis and appears on the analyzer between lysine and histidine (Raftery and Cole, 1966). *N-Dansylaziridine* was recently developed to prepare fluorescent protein derivatives by reaction at pH 7.5 (Scouten *et al.*, 1974). A *spin-labeled aziridine* derivative, N-substituted with the group 2,2,6,6-tetramethyl-4-oxypiperidine-1-oxyl, introduced a spin-label at the site of modification (Shapiro *et al.*, 1969; Elek *et al.*, 1972).

3-Bromo-1,1,1-*trifluoropropanone* (BrCH$_2$COCF$_3$) has been employed at pH 7.15 to attach 3,3,3-trifluoroacetonyl groups on two reactive thiol groups (out of a total of six) in human hemoglobin and study its interaction with ligands by fluorine nuclear magnetic resonance spectroscopy (Huestis and Raftery, 1972) and its oxygenation equilibrium (Lee *et al.*, 1973). However, reaction of other functional groups cannot be excluded since modification of the thiol groups was determined only spectrophotometrically by back-reaction with 5,5′-dithiobis(2-nitrobenzoic acid) (see Section IVG9). Further study is necessary to establish the selectivity of this reagent, especially since bromoacetone and dibromoacetone also react with histidine residues (Husain and Lowe, 1968; Beeley and Neurath, 1968).

Introduction of a quaternary ammonium group was accomplished by reaction with (2-*bromoethyl*)*trimethylammonium bromide* (47a) to give the thioethyltrimethylammonium derivative (47b) (Itano and Robinson, 1972). The thioether linkage was of course stable to acid hydrolysis and the cysteine derivative (4-thialaminine) eluted between lysine and histidine on the amino acid analyzer. This reagent should prove especially useful in reduction and alkylation of the disulfide bonds since derivatives thus obtained were readily soluble in aqueous solvents (Itano and Robinson, 1972). *S*-Ethyltrimethylammonium sites were not hydrolyzable by trypsin. Imidazole groups have been introduced at modified thiol sites by alkylation with α-*bromo*-β-*(5-imidazolyl)propionic acid* (Yankeelov and Jolley, 1972).

$$Prot\!-\!SH + Br\!-\!CH_2CH_2\!-\!\overset{\overset{\displaystyle CH_3}{|}}{\underset{\underset{\displaystyle CH_3}{|}}{\overset{\oplus}{N}}}\!-\!CH_3 \longrightarrow Prot\!-\!S\!-\!CH_2CH_2\!-\!\overset{\overset{\displaystyle CH_3}{|}}{\underset{\underset{\displaystyle CH_3}{|}}{\overset{\oplus}{N}}}\!-\!CH_3 \qquad (47)$$

(a)   (b)

Iodoalkanesulfonates were used to modify the thiol groups, after reduction of the disulfides, in human serum albumin (Jermyn, 1966). 2-*Bromoethanesulfonate* has been introduced for complete alkylation of thiol groups under mild conditions (Niketic *et al.*, 1974). This procedure should prove extremely useful since *S*-sulfoethylated proteins were comparable in solubility and charge properties to *S*-sulfonated or performic acid oxidized derivatives. Furthermore, *S*-sulfoethylcysteine [$H_2NCH(COOH)CH_2\!-\!S\!-\!CH_2CH_2SO_3H$] was stable to standard conditions of protein acid hydrolysis and eluted on the analyzer almost at the position of cysteic acid (Niketic *et al.*, 1974). Another useful method for attaching sulfonate groups at cysteine sites is the reaction (48) with 1,3-*propane sultone* (3-*hydroxypropanesulfonic acid γ-sultone*, 48a) under mild conditions (Ruegg and Rudinger, 1974). *S*-3-Sulfopropylcysteine (48b) was stable to acid hydrolysis and eluted on the analyzer also before aspartic acid.

$$Prot\!-\!S^- \diagdown\!\!\!\diagup\!\!\!\diagup_{SO_2} \overset{pH\ 8.3}{\longrightarrow} Prot\!-\!S\!-\!CH_2\!-\!CH_2\!-\!CH_2\!-\!SO_3^- \qquad (48)$$

(a)   (b)

Methylation of thiol groups by *O-methylisourea* which also guanidinates amino groups has already been mentioned (Section IVA10). *S*-Methylation by *methyl iodide* has problems of selectivity, extensive losses of methyl-cysteine and methionine (Rochat *et al.*, 1970a), and a tendency of CH_3I to decompose, yielding free iodine. *S*-Dinitrophenyl groups (49b) can undergo β-elimination at high alkaline pH (Patchornik and Sokolovsky, 1964a; Cremona *et al.*, 1965) to give reactive dehydroalanine residues (49c). Reaction of dehydroalanine side chains with methylmercaptan yielded *S*-methyl-cysteine (49d) (Gross and Morell, 1967). This route for *S*-methylation suffers

$$-HN-CH-CO- \xrightarrow[\text{pH 5-6}]{\text{FDNB}} -HN-CH-CO- \xrightarrow{\text{pH} > 10.5} -HN-C-CO-$$
$$\quad\quad | \quad\quad\quad\quad\quad\quad\quad\quad\quad\quad | \quad\quad\quad\quad\quad\quad\quad\quad\quad\quad ||$$
$$\quad CH_2-SH \quad\quad\quad\quad\quad\quad\quad CH_2-SDNP \quad\quad\quad\quad\quad\quad CH_2$$

(a)   (b)   (c)

$$\xrightarrow{CH_3SH} -HN-CH-CO- \quad\quad (49)$$
$$\quad\quad\quad\quad\quad\quad\quad | $$
$$\quad\quad\quad\quad\quad\quad CH_2-S-CH_3$$
(d)

from the problem that dehydroalanine residues are quite reactive and may couple with a favorably situated nucleophilic group in the protein. Also, the alkaline conditions necessary for β-elimination are detrimental for most proteins. *Methyl p-nitrobenzenesulfonate* is the most selective reagent for quantitative *S*-methylation under mild conditions (Heinrikson, 1970 and 1971). *S*-Methylcysteine was stable to acid hydrolysis and suffered no more than 10% decomposition (probably by oxidation to the sulfone). It eluted on the analyzer on the descending side of the proline peak (Heinrikson, 1971). One useful application of the $-SCH_3$ derivatives of proteins and peptides is the possibility of cleavage at these sites by cyanogen bromide (Gross and Morell, 1967). After reduction of the four disulfide bonds in hen egg white lysozyme, the resultant thiol groups were quantitatively *S*-methylated by methyl *p*-nitrobenzenesulfonate (Lee and Atassi, 1973). The homogeneous derivative possessed, unlike the *S*-carboxymethyl ana-logue, considerable antigenic reactivity with antisera to native lysozyme.

Reaction of 4,4′-*bis-dimethylaminodiphenylcarbinol* (45a) has been intro-duced for the selective modification, as well as the quantitative colorimetric determination, of thiol groups in proteins (Rohrbach *et al.*, 1973; Humphries and Harrison, 1974). The reagent, under slightly acidic conditions, dissoci-ates to give three species (50a), of which the monocation is presumably the one that reacts with the thiol group. The resonance-stabilized carbonium-immonium ion exhibits an absorption maximum around 606 nm ($\varepsilon_{max} =$

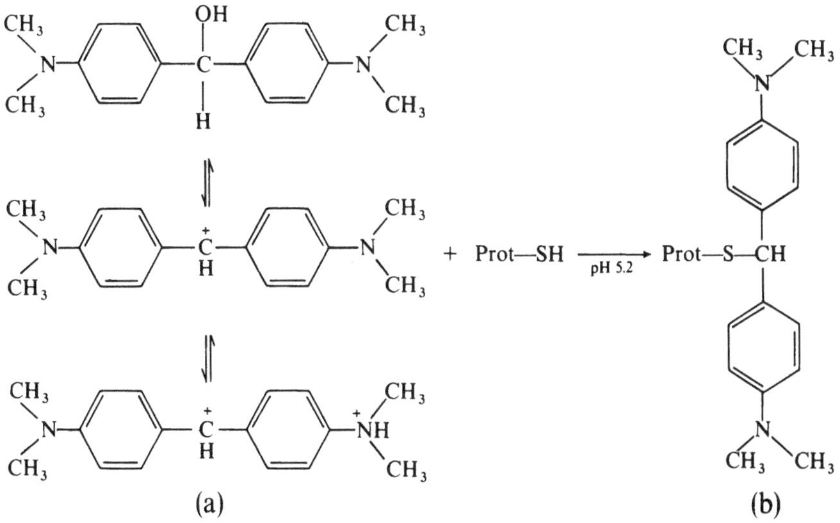

(50)

$128,000 \pm 4000$ M^{-1} cm^{-1}). Its reaction with thiol groups formed the stable S-(4,4'-bis-dimethylaminodiphenylmethyl-) adduct (50b), with an accompanying quantitative loss in absorbance. Utility of the reagent has been demonstrated on five proteins (Rohrbach *et al.*, 1973) and has been used to modify an essential thiol group in porcine heart malate dehydrogenase (Humphries and Harrison, 1974).

7. Thioaryl Derivatives

The reaction of aryl halides with proteins has been discussed in connection with amino group modification (Section IVA7). S-Dinitrophenyl derivatives are discussed later (Section IVG10). *7-Chloro-4-nitrobenzo-2-oxa-1,3-diazole (NBD chloride)* has been employed as a thiol fluorescent label (Allen and Low, 1973). The reaction of NBD chloride with amino and phenolic OH groups has been mentioned (Section IVA7). *Diazotized 3-aminopyridine adenine dinucleotide* has been used to inactivate yeast alcohol dehydrogenase by the modification of four thiol groups, giving S-(3-pyridyl)-cysteine residues (Chan and Anderson, 1975). As expected, other amino acid residues were modified. Although the reaction of aryldiazonium salts with thiol groups has been known for over seven decades (Friedmann, 1903), such compounds are not selective for any given side chain (see Section IVE4). Addition of thiol groups at low pH to *ortho-quinones* such as *aminochrome* (Powell and Heacock, 1972) and *adrenochrome* (Powell and Heacock, 1973) needs further study to determine its selectivity in protein modification.

8. Desulfurization

Desulfurization of cysteine with Raney nickel was shown to take place very rapidly (a few minutes) at pH 7.0 and 22°C (Perlstein *et al.*, 1971). The reaction exhibited a high degree of specificity since all other amino acids, including methionine, were unchanged even after reaction for 10 h. The six cysteine residues of globin (from adult human hemoglobin) were almost completely desulfurized without effect on the other amino acids. On the other hand, the cystine residues in hen egg white lysozyme and bovine α-lactalbumin were only partially desulfurized as a result of their inaccessibility to the reagent. Desulfurization was appreciably increased (but not complete) after reduction of the disulfide bonds. Desulfurization of cysteine or cystine gave rise to alanine (Perlstein *et al.*, 1971).

Other desulfurization reactions (for review, see Friedman, 1973) may not be suitable for application to proteins because of the undesirable or drastic conditions necessary for the reaction.

9. Thiol–Disulfide Interchange Reactions

Interchange reactions between thiol groups and disulfides in simple compounds have long been known (Parker and Kharasch, 1959) and proceed through a reversible nucleophilic attack by the —S^- on the S—S bond (51). A mixed disulfide is formed as shown in (51a). In the presence of an excess of disulfide, reaction (51a) predominates and the modification of thiol groups in the protein goes essentially to completion. Reaction (51b), which can also take place, is not usually favored in proteins because of steric

$$\text{Prot—}S^- + \text{RSSR} \xrightarrow{\text{pH} > 7.5} \text{Prot—SSR} + \text{RS}^- \qquad \text{(a)}$$

$$\qquad\qquad\qquad\qquad\qquad\qquad\qquad\qquad\qquad\qquad (51)$$

$$\text{Prot—SSR} + \text{Prot—}S^- \longrightarrow \text{Prot—SS—Prot} + \text{RS}^- \qquad \text{(b)}$$

inaccessibility that precludes formation of such disulfide bond derivatives. An exception, of course, is when the thiol groups have been derived by previous reduction of disulfide bonds. However, intra- and intermolecular protein disulfide bond formation is sometimes possible (Habeeb, 1972*a*). The reaction is quite specific for thiol groups, especially if the pH of the reaction is not high enough to effect disulfide bond cleavage.

The best known compound in this class of reagents is 5,5'-*dithiobis*-(2-*nitrobenzoic acid*) (52a), which, on reaction with thiol groups, liberates an equimolar quantity of 3-carboxyl-4-nitro-thiophenolate anion (Ellman, 1959). The yellow color of the thionitrobenzoate anion (see structure 55b) has enabled the employment of this reaction in the spectrophotometric

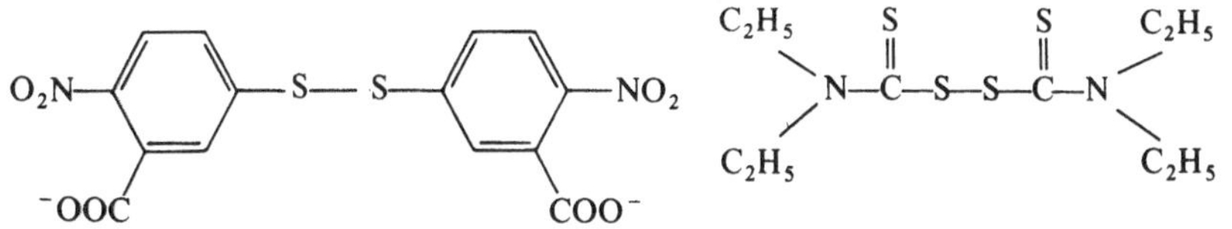

$$\text{(a)} \qquad\qquad\qquad \text{(b)} \qquad\qquad (52)$$

determination (ε at 412 nm = 13,600 M^{-1} cm^{-1}) of free thiol groups and has been applied extensively for this purpose (for review, see Habeeb, 1972a). The only reported interference is the reaction of this disulfide reagent with thiosulfate and sulfite ions (Man and Bryant, 1974) and an appreciable instability of the reagent above pH 9.5 (Danehy *et al.*, 1971). A reported attack by thionitrobenzoate on protein disulfide bonds (Robyt *et al.*, 1971), which was proposed as a method for quantitative determination of disulfide bonds, has not been substantiated by subsequent work (Brocklehurst *et al.*, 1972; Ando and Steiner, 1973; Telegdi and Straub, 1973; Weitzman, 1975). Examples of recent applications are its employment to modify the thiol groups in *E. coli* succinic thiokinase and to study the effect on enzymatic activity and immunochemistry (Nishimura *et al.*, 1973). However, conformational changes and dissociation into subunits were inferred but not investigated. More recently, the reagent was used to demonstrate a substantial increase in reactivity of a thiol group in mitochondrial aspartate aminotransferase, from chicken and pig heart, when covalent enzyme–substrate intermediates were formed (Gehring and Christen, 1975). The increased reactivity of the thiol group resulted from the conformational adjustments of the enzyme–coenzyme–substrate compound. A potentially useful application has been the attachment of the reagent (through its carboxylate groups) to agarose 1,6-diaminohexane by carbodiimide (see Section IVD2) (Lin and Foster, 1975). The affinity columns were useful in covalently attaching sulfhydryl-containing proteins and thus enabled their separation from thiol-lacking proteins. The attached proteins could be released by a thiol reagent.

This group of disulfide reagents can obviously offer a great deal of versatility in the type of the side chain to be attached to the site of modification and only some examples will be given here. *Tetraethylthiuram disulfide* (52b) with ^{35}S label has been employed to determine thiol groups and to modify such groups in amino acid oxidase and hemoglobin (Neims *et al.*, 1966a,b). 2,2′-*Dithiopyridine* and 4,4′-*dithiopyridine* (53a) have been developed for the spectrophotometric determination of thiol groups (Grassetti and Murray, 1967), based on the absorption maxima of 2-thiopyridone (343 nm) and 4-thiopyridone (53b) (324 nm). The ultraviolet spectral characteristics of these compounds over a wide range of pH have been determined

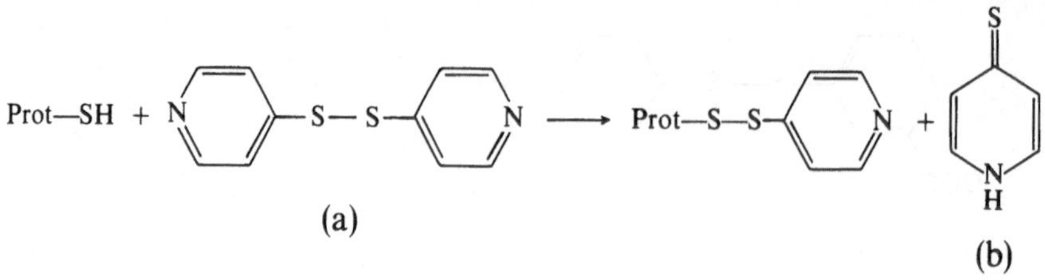

(a)

(b)

(53)

and employed for the modification of an essential thiol group in papain (Brocklehurst and Little, 1973). *Di-dansylcystine* has been introduced to enable attachment of a fluorescent substituent at the site of the modified thiol group (Cheung *et al.*, 1971; Wu and Stryer, 1972). The reagent has enabled the modification of thiol groups, probably situated within a nonpolar environment, in rat liver cystathionase and caused great inactivation (Oh and Churchich, 1974). *6,6'-Dithiobis-(inosinyl imidodiphosphate)*, a purine disulfide analogue of ATP, has been used to form mixed disulfides, most likely near or at the ATP regulatory sites of myosin (Wagner and Yount, 1975).

10. Reversible Reactions

An obvious reversible method for protection of protein thiol groups is modification by *disulfide interchange* (51a). Protein-bound mixed disulfides are stable to air oxidation (Smithies, 1965). They can be isolated, and the label is removable by a thiol reagent via the backward reaction (51a). Any of the mixed disulfide reagents described in Section IVG9 may be employed for this purpose.

2,4-Dinitrofluorobenzene reacts with several functional groups in proteins (see Section IVA7). However, the thiol group because of its strong nucleophilic character is the most reactive. Therefore, dinitrophenylation of the sulfhydryl group can be carried out even below neutrality (pH 5–6). Under these conditions, amino groups will not usually react and histidine modification can mostly be avoided if the reaction is carried out for brief periods. The advantage of this reaction is that dinitrophenyl groups (on cysteine, histidine, and tyrosine) can be removed under mild conditions by thiolation with mercaptoethanol (Shaltiel, 1967). On the other hand, the stability of the label to other experimental manipulation permits identification of the labeled site in the protein. The method has been used, for example, for labeling a single thiol group in rabbit muscle glyceraldehyde 3-phosphate dehydrogenase, which was identified, and the dinitrophenyl group was subsequently removed by thiolation (Shaltiel and Tauber-Finkelstein, 1970). Thiolysis of dinitrophenylated rabbit muscle phosphorylase *b* removed all except one S-dinitrophenyl group, presumably because it was buried in the AMP binding site and thus was inaccessible to attack by mercaptoethanol (Baumert et al., 1973).

The oxidation of thiol groups in papain by *peroxyacetyl nitrate* could be reversed by thiol compounds (Leh and Mudd, 1974). However, this reaction in general is not very selective and it is not the most convenient to use. *Sodium tetrathionate* will oxidize cysteine into S-sulfocysteine [HOOC—CH · (NH_2)—CH_2—SSO_3^-] residues (Phil and Lange, 1962). S-Sulfonated proteins are stable in neutral and acidic solutions but deprotection can be effected by thiolysis. Another method has been described for complete S-sulfonation of protein thiol groups by *sodium sulfite* and catalytic amounts of cysteine in the presence of oxygen and 8 M urea in the pH range 7.0–8.5 (Chan, 1968). Aldolase was completely sulfonated (and inactivated) within 1 hr. Treatment with mercaptoethanol regenerated the thiol groups, and the enzymatic activity was fully recovered (Chan, 1968). Sulfonation of rabbit muscle glyceraldehyde 3-phosphate dehydrogenase by tetrathionate modified a single thiol group, and the modification was reversed by mercaptoethanol or dithioerythritol with the recovery of 80–90% of the enzymatic activity (Moore and Fenselau, 1972b).

Thiol esters, formed by reaction with *choline selenol esters* (see Section IVG2), provide excellent protecting groups (Makriyannis et al., 1973) because of the high selectivity of the reagent, stability of the group to normal experimental conditions, and ease of removal by aminolysis (Günther and Mautner, 1965).

Modification of the sulfhydryl group by *mercurials*, even though it gives strongly bound adducts, can be reversed readily by adding an excess of a low molecular weight thiol. Reversibility has been achieved with organic mercurials carrying a variety of side chains of different size and charge character.

Azobenzene-2-sulfenyl bromide has been shown to react selectively with thiol groups, in contrast with other aryl sulfenyl halides which react with tryptophan as well (Fontana et al., 1968b). The reagent, which is highly soluble in water because of its saltlike structure, reacted selectively and stoichiometrically with cysteine residues around pH 5. The adduct, being a mixed disulfide, was stable in neutral and acid pH but the modification was easily reversed by mercaptoethanol, thioglycolic acid, or sodium borohydride.

Cyanate reacts rapidly with thiol groups to give thiocarbamyl derivatives (—$SCONH_2$). The stability of the adduct at pH 5 and its instability at pH 8 or higher permit the use of this reaction in the reversible modification of thiol groups. Carbamylation and the nature of other reactive functional groups have been discussed earlier (see Section IVA13). Reversible reaction of cyanate with a reactive thiol group at the glutamine-binding site in the light chain of carbamyl phosphate synthetase from *E. coli* has been reported

(Anderson and Carlson, 1975). The thiol group was protected from reaction by glutamine or its analogues. Reversibility was not influenced by pH in the range 6–10, but was greatly increased by bicarbonate and ATP. *Methoxymethylisocyanate* (54a) has been developed for the selective carbamylation of thiol groups in proteins (Tschesche and Jering, 1973). Reaction proceeded

$$\text{Prot—SH} + \text{O}{=}\text{C}{=}\text{N—CH}_2\text{—O—CH}_3 \underset{\text{pH} > 6}{\overset{\text{pH 4-5}}{\rightleftharpoons}} \text{Prot—S—CO—NH—CH}_2\text{—O—CH}_3$$

$$\text{(a)} \hspace{5cm} \text{(b)} \hspace{3cm} \text{(54)}$$

at pH 4–5, and under these conditions α- and ε-amino groups did not react. The modification was readily reversed at pH values above neutrality. Reversibility of the reaction was demonstrated on papain and on trypsin inhibitor with a reduced disulfide bond.

Selective cyanylation of the thiol group has been obtained under mild conditions by *2-nitro-5-thiocyanobenzoic acid* (55a), resulting in the conversion of cysteine residues into β-thiocyanoalanine residues (Degani *et al.*, 1970). The thionitrobenzoate formed (55b) can be determined spectro-

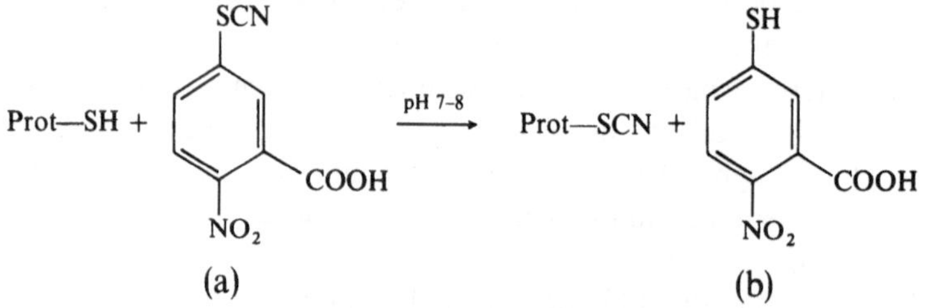

photometrically at 412 nm (cf. Ellman's reagent, 53a, Section IVG9). This modification could also be reversed by treatment with excess thiol.

H. Reactions for Disulfide Bonds

1. Oxidation

Performic acid oxidation is the most widely used procedure for oxidative cleavage of disulfide bonds in proteins and peptides. Oxidation of a disulfide bond yields two residues of cysteic acid. The latter is stable to acid hydrolysis and elutes very rapidly on the amino acid analyzer, considerably before aspartic acid. The reaction is useful, therefore, for determination of the total half-cystine residues by amino acid analysis, but is not specific for cystine and as mentioned earlier thiol groups will also oxidize to cysteic acid. In addition, methionine and tryptophan are normally oxidized and quite often tyrosine and histidine are modified. For a detailed discussion of performic acid oxidation, see Hirs (1967a).

2. Reduction

The reduction of disulfide bonds by a low molecular weight thiol compound is by far the most selective procedure for cleavage of the disulfide bond. In the presence of a considerable excess of thiol, the reduction will reach completion. 2-*Mercaptoethanol* has been applied extensively for this purpose (Hirs, 1967*b*).

Upon removal of the reducing agent, the thiol groups readily reoxidize in air to reform the disulfide bonds. This can be prevented by the modification of the thiol groups thus generated by a suitable method as described in Section IVG. Alkylation by iodoacetate is the most frequently used procedure because of the stability of S-carboxymethylcysteine to acid hydrolysis and the convenience of its determination by amino acid analysis. However, the method employed should obviously be chosen to suit the particular purpose of the investigation. For example, it may be desirable to have a reversible protecting group, or a highly soluble derivative, or ability to cleave subsequently by trypsin at the cysteine sites, then the appropriate modification reaction (from Section IVG) may be employed.

Dithiothreitol and *dithioerythritol*, the threo and erythro isomers of 2,3-dihydroxy-1,4-dithiolbutane, have been found to reduce disulfide bonds completely within several minutes at pH 8 (Cleland, 1964). The mixed disulfide produced in reaction (56a) can undergo an intramolecular displacement reaction to form the sterically favored cyclic disulfide (56b). This effectively displaces the equilibrium to the right, especially in dilute

$$R—S—S—R + HS—CH_2(CHOH)_2CH_2—SH$$

$$\underset{pH\ 8}{\rightleftharpoons} RSH + R—S—S—CH_2(CHOH)_2CH_2—SH \quad (a)$$

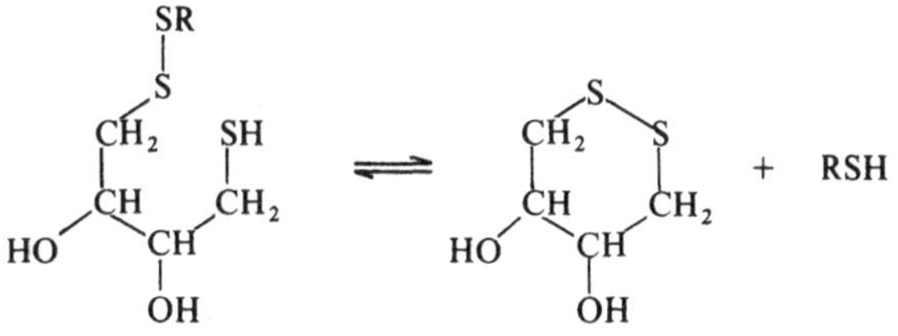

$$+ \quad RSH \quad (b) \quad (56)$$

solutions. A lower reagent excess is therefore needed. The thiol groups produced are maintained in the reduced state by the reagent. In addition, these two reagents have little thiol odor and are water soluble, in both the oxidized and the reduced forms. The reduced forms are quite stable to air oxidation. The two isomers have similar properties. These two compounds have been used extensively for reduction of disulfide bonds and as protective reagents for protein thiol groups. The thiol groups thus generated can also be protected by a suitable thiol reagent (Section IVG). Disulfide bonds in peptides and proteins can be readily reduced by dithiothreitol in liquid ammonia (Meienhofer *et al.*, 1972). This finding proved useful because addition of aziridine to the liquid ammonia solution enabled complete reduction and concurrent *S*-aminoethylation of the cystine residues (Kuromizu and Meienhofer, 1972). The procedure yielded homogeneous derivatives in high yield from insulin (hexa-*S*-aminoethyl), basic trypsin inhibitor (hexa-*S*-aminoethyl), neocarzinostatin (tetra-*S*-aminoethyl), and lysozyme (octa-*S*-aminoethyl), and no side reactions with other amino acids were observed. This procedure should be extremely useful in future studies.

Trialkyl phosphines have been shown to effect reduction of disulfide bonds (MacLaren and Sweetman, 1966). Alkylation of the resultant thiol groups can be performed in the presence of the reducing agent. Water-soluble trialkyl phosphines, such as *tris-hydroxymethyl phosphine* and *tris-carboxyethylphosphine*, enabled reduction of the disulfide bonds in IgG in aqueous solution and in the presence of an alkylating agent (Levison *et al.*, 1969). The reduction of disulfide bonds by *sodium borohydride* has been studied and compared to the reduction with 2-mercaptoethanol (Crestfield *et al.*, 1963). The latter compound was a more satisfactory reducing agent. In some cases, borohydride caused peptide-bond cleavage.

Diborane, which reduces carboxyl groups selectively to their corresponding alcohols (see Section IVD3) also effects the reduction of disulfide bonds (Atassi and Rosenthal, 1969; Atassi *et al.*, 1975*b*). Since carboxyl groups are not reduced unless they are previously protonated, it has been shown (Atassi and Rosenthal, 1969) that diborane may be employed to achieve disulfide bond reduction in nonprotonated proteins without effect on the carboxyl groups.

Electroreduction of disulfide bonds by use of a dropping mercury electrode has been known for over four decades (Brdicka, 1933) and has been studied by several workers. Cecil and Weitzman (1964) showed that electroreduction can be employed to yield complete reduction of the disulfide bonds in insulin, ribonuclease, chymotrypsin, trypsin, and bovine serum albumin. The reduction could be carried out under acid conditions to minimize thiol–disulfide interchange and was seemingly selective for disulfide bonds. Reducing agents or dissociating solvents were not necessary. The disulfide bonds in insulin were also reduced electrolytically by Markus (1964). It was later reported (Leach *et al.*, 1965) that electrolytic reduction of the disulfide bonds in bovine serum albumin, lysozyme, wool keratin. ribonuclease, and insulin required the addition of a small amount of a thiol compound. These workers also obtained a high but incomplete extent of reduction without the use of denaturing agents. One-electron reduction of simple disulfides in aqueous solution has been studied using the fast reaction technique of pulse radiolysis and kinetic absorption spectrophotometry (Hoffman and Hayon, 1972; Schafferman, 1972). The disulfide radical anions (RSSR$^-$), produced by reaction with e_{aq}^-, decayed over a wide pH range to produce thiyl RS$^.$ radicals and RSH. Thiyl radicals were also produced by the reaction of H atoms with disulfide (Hoffman and Hayon, 1972). In view of the complex reactions involved, electroreduction of disulfide bonds should be expected to possess considerable nonselectivity. If reductive cleavage is desired, thiol compounds are more highly recommended.

3. Disulfide Bond Re-formation

When thiol groups, previously obtained from reduction of disulfide bonds in ribonuclease, were allowed to reoxidize in air, the disulfide bonds re-formed in the correct manner with partial recovery of enzymatic activity (Sela et al., 1957; Anfinsen, 1961; Anfinsen and Haber, 1961; White, 1961). This formulated the basis for the hypothesis that the amino acid sequence protein carries the information that determines its three-dimensional structure. Subsequent to these observations, similar results were obtained by other workers with a variety of disulfide proteins (for review, see White, 1972a). A lysozyme derivative which had been reduced by diborane at the four disulfides, as well as two carboxyl groups, was found to regenerate the correct pairing of the disulfide bonds by chemical, conformational, and immunochemical studies (Atassi et al., 1975b). On the other hand, the introduction of a previously nonexistent disulfide bond into pig lipoamide dehydrogenase was demonstrated (Mathews and Williams, 1974; Thorpe and Williams, 1975) by treatment with cupric ions, which were known to inactivate the enzyme (Veeger and Massey, 1962). Conformational and immunochemical studies on reduced S-methylated or S-carboxymethylated lysozyme derivatives showed that long-range interactions exerted a considerable driving force for reorganizing the molecule into its native conformation (Lee and Atassi, 1973). In S-carboxymethyl lysozyme this directive effect could not give rise to a structure that resembled the native protein because of steric effects and the like–like charge electrostatic repulsion between the carboxymethyl anions as they approach one another. By contrast, in S-methyl lysozyme, the smaller size of the S-methyl groups and their ability to participate in hydrophobic interactions induced stabilization of the conformation of the derivative, or at least certain regions of it.

4. Extension of the Disulfide Bond

The ability of a mercuric ion to react with two sulfhydryl groups to give S—Hg—S bridges has been exploited to lengthen the disulfide bonds in some protein derivatives. This should give information on the length of the disulfide bond required for proper maintenance of conformation and biological function. Reduction of the disulfide bonds followed by reaction with mercuric chloride enabled the introduction of Hg cross-links in papain (Arnon and Shapira, 1969), ribonuclease (Sperling et al., 1969; Sperling and Steinberg, 1971), and Fab and Fc fragments from a myeloma protein (Steiner and Blumberg, 1971). Minimal conformational changes were detected in each case. *Mercurous acetate* has been reported to effect simultaneous reduction and mercuration (57) of disulfide bonds (David et al., 1974). Reaction of monovalent mercury with ribonuclease for 2 days resulted in the introduction of about three mercury atoms per mole of protein and a partial retention of enzymatic activity. The determination of mercury bridges is difficult because of the reversibility of the binding. Its identification has been achieved by eliminating the mercury with EDTA in the presence of $[^{14}C]$iodoacetate, which enabled simultaneous S-carboxymethylation (Burstein and Sperling, 1970).

$$\text{R—S—S—R} + \text{Hg}_2^{2+} \rightleftharpoons \begin{bmatrix} 2(\text{R—SHg}^+) \\ \Updownarrow \\ \text{R—S—Hg—S—R} + \text{Hg}^{2+} \end{bmatrix} \quad (57)$$

Reaction of *selenious acid* with mercaptoethanol-reduced ribonuclease A and resulted in the introduction of some selenium bridges (—S—Se—S—) into the protein (Ganther and Corcoran, 1969). The incorporation of selenium was higher at pH 2 than at pH 7. However, at pH 7, little or no selenium was released from the reaction product. Also, partial incorporation (one bridge) of selenium was obtained by an exchange reaction between reduced ribonuclease and the selenium trisulfide derivative of 2-mercaptoethanol $[(\text{HOCH}_2\text{CH}_2\text{S})_2\text{Se}]$ at pH 2–7. These derivatives showed conformational changes and had little residual enzymatic activity.

5. Disulfide Interchange and Mixed Disulfides

Disulfide bonds in proteins have been shown to undergo an interchange reaction when treated with an excess of a low molecular weight disulfide reagent in the presence of catalytic amounts of thiol (Smithies, 1965). The reaction (58) resulted in cleavage of the disulfide bonds as a result of the formation of mixed disulfides. The extent of cleavage was readily controlled

$$\text{Prot—S—S—Prot}' + \text{R—S—S—R} \overset{\text{RS}^-}{\rightleftharpoons} \text{Prot—S—S—R} + \text{R—S—S—Prot}' \quad (58)$$

by the pH of the reaction, the temperature, and the addition of urea. Exposure of mixed disulfide derivatives to catalytic amounts of thiol resulted in correct re-formation of the original disulfide. The method could also be used for protection of thiol groups in native proteins.

During chemical modification reactions, disulfide interchange may be encountered. Incubation of the protein with cystamine ($\beta\beta'$-diaminodiethyl disulfide) under the conditions of the reaction was shown to serve as a control for detection of any possible interchange (Koshland and Mozersky, 1964). After removal of excess cystamine, followed by performic acid oxidation, liberated taurine ($H_2N—CH_2CH_2SO_3H$) was determined by amino acid analysis. Disulfide interchange reactions between cystine and di-dinitrophenyl-cystine have been found to be catalyzed, in concentrated HCl solutions, by selenium and tellurium oxy acids (Lawrence, 1969). Because of the strongly acidic conditions necessary for the catalysis, this finding cannot be exploited in protein modification.

Phosphorothioate (59a) gives a mixed disulfide on reaction with disulfides in proteins (Neumann et al., 1967a,b). Nucleophilic attack by the reagent (59a) on the disulfide bond gives the mixed disulfide (59b) and the protein thiolate anion (59c). The latter reoxidizes to the disulfide, which

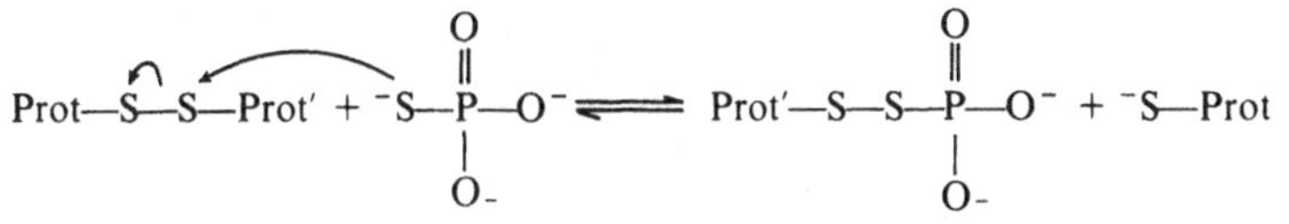

$$
\text{Prot—S—S—Prot'} + {}^-\text{S—P—O}^- \rightleftharpoons \text{Prot'—S—S—P—O}^- + {}^-\text{S—Prot} \qquad (59)
$$

(a)   (b)   (c)

is further attacked by phosphorothioate until all the product is in the mixed disulfide form (59b). This mixed disulfide, like other mixed disulfides, can be reduced by excess thiol reagent and the original disulfide can be regenerated. This reaction has been demonstrated with lysozyme, ribonuclease, papain, and ficin.

6. Reaction with Cyanide

Cyanide anion has long been known to react with cystine (Mauthner, 1912; Fraenkel-Conrat, 1941). The kinetics of the reaction were shown to be bimolecular and the rate depended on pH (Gawron and Fernando, 1961). In the pH range 7.5–12.5, the rate constant increased markedly with protonation of cystine, which suggested intramolecular catalysis by hydrogen ion (Gawron et al., 1964). The action of cyanide on proteins was shown to produce lanthionine (Nicolet, 1931). Lanthionine can be produced either via dehydroalanine (60b and 60c) or by direct displacement of thiocyanate by a thiolate anion (60d) (Catsimpoolas and Wood, 1964). It is relevant to mention here that in alkaline solutions, without cyanide, lanthionine can be formed by β-elimination of cystine followed by addition of a sulfhydryl group to the double bond of dehydroalanine (Horn et al., 1941; Zahn, 1961). The reaction of bovine serum albumin with cyanide has been studied

$$\begin{array}{c}\diagdown\!\!\!\!\!\!\!\text{CH}\!-\!\text{CH}_2\!-\!\text{S}\!-\!\text{S}\!-\!\text{CH}_2\!-\!\text{CH}\diagup +\text{CN}^-\longrightarrow\diagdown\!\!\!\!\text{CH}\!-\!\text{CH}_2\!-\!\text{S}^- +\underset{\underset{\displaystyle\text{CN}}{|}}{\text{S}}\!-\!\text{CH}_2\!-\!\text{CH}\diagdown\quad\text{(a)}\end{array}$$

$$\diagdown\!\!\!\!\!\text{CH}\!-\!\text{CH}_2\!-\!\text{S}\!-\!\text{CN}\xrightarrow{\ \text{OH}^-\ }\diagdown\!\!\!\!\text{C}\!=\!\text{CH}_2 +\text{SCN}^-\qquad\qquad\qquad\text{(b)}$$

$$\diagdown\!\!\!\!\!\text{C}\!=\!\text{CH}_2 +{}^-\text{S}\!-\!\text{CH}_2\!-\!\text{CH}\diagup\longrightarrow\diagdown\!\!\!\!\text{CH}\!-\!\text{CH}_2\!-\!\text{S}\!-\!\text{CH}_2\!-\!\text{CH}\diagup\qquad\text{(c)}$$

$$\diagdown\!\!\!\!\!\underset{\underset{\displaystyle\text{CN}}{|}}{\text{CH}}\!-\!\text{CH}_2\!-\!\text{S}^- +\text{S}\!-\!\text{CH}_2\!-\!\text{CH}\diagup\longrightarrow\diagdown\!\!\!\!\text{CH}\!-\!\text{CH}_2\!-\!\text{S}\!-\!\text{CH}_2\!-\!\text{CH}\diagup +\text{SCN}^-\quad\text{(d)}$$

$$\text{(60)}$$

(Catsimpoolas and Wood, 1964, 1966). Thiocyanate was produced only in reactions with cyanide at pH 8 and above. Alkaline degradation of the protein accompanied the reaction due to the high pH conditions. Thiocyanate production resulted from cyanolysis of the persulfide (RSSSR) produced (mechanism not shown here) in the alkaline degradation of the protein and from β-elimination of the thiocyanoalanine moiety (60b). At pH 7, four disulfide bonds were cleaved in bovine serum albumin with the formation of iminothiazolidine groups instead of thiocyanoalanine. Formation of the iminothiazolidine ring was accompanied by cleavage of a peptide bond at the cystine amino group.

The employment of cyanide to obtain disulfide bond cleavage is not a desirable approach because of the complexity of the reactions involved, both in reaction with cyanide and in alkaline degradation.

7. Reaction with Sulfite

Cleavage of disulfide bonds with sulfite has been studied extensively and is known to proceed stoichiometrically at a slightly alkaline pH, forming soluble S-sulfonated derivatives (Cecil, 1963). Sulfite is more S-nucleophilic than cyanide toward cystine derivatives (Gawron et al., 1964). The reaction has been carried out on lysozyme at pH 4.7 and pH 9.0 in 8 M urea with equal effectiveness (Azari, 1966). Cleavage of the disulfide bond yields (61) the S-sulfonyl derivative and thiolate anions. The latter

$$\text{Prot}\!-\!\text{S}\!-\!\text{S}\!-\!\text{Prot}' +\text{SO}_3^{2-}\rightleftharpoons\text{Prot}'\!-\!\text{SSO}_3^- +\text{Prot}\!-\!\text{S}^-\qquad\text{(61)}$$

will re-form into disulfide bonds which are attacked again by sulfite and the cycle of reactions continues until conversion of the disulfides into S-sulfonates is complete. Cupric ion will facilitate the formation of disulfides from the thiolate anions formed in (61). In sulfitolysis of unsymmetrical disulfides, it has been found that steric hindrance to the approach of the entering group exerted a predominating influence on the substitution at a given sulfur atom and that the electron displacement effect was of less importance (van Rensburg and Swanepoel, 1967). Also, the influence of pH in the range 5–9.5 was not significant. A procedure for complete S-sulfonation of proteins containing cysteine or cystine residues (Chan, 1968) has been discussed previously (Section IVG10). S-Sulfonyl groups can be used for reversible protection of the thiol groups (see Section IVG10).

8. Alkaline Hydrolysis of Disulfide Bonds

Instability of the disulfide bond in alkaline solutions has been studied extensively (for review, see Danehy, 1966) following the early observations (Nicolet, 1931) of cleavage of disulfide bonds by alkali. The mechanism of cleavage is rather complex and proceeds through α- and β-elimination reactions followed by cleavage of the S—S bond or a carbon–sulfur bond. Alkaline cleavage via the β-elimination mechanism (Nicolet, 1931; Tarbell and Harnish, 1951) is shown below (62). Also, the hydroxide ion can partic-

$$
\underset{(a)}{\text{H}-\overset{|}{\underset{|}{\text{C}}}-\text{CH}_2-\text{S}-\text{S}-\text{CH}_2-\overset{|}{\underset{|}{\text{C}}}-\text{H}} \xrightarrow{\text{OH}^{\ominus}} \underset{(b)}{\text{H}-\overset{|}{\underset{|}{\text{C}}}-\text{CH}_2-\text{S}-\overset{\frown}{\text{S}}\text{CH}_2-\overset{|}{\underset{|}{\text{C}}}{}^{\ominus}} \longrightarrow \underset{(c)}{\overset{|}{\underset{|}{\text{C}}}=\text{CH}_2}
$$

$$+ \qquad (62)$$

$$
\underset{(e)}{\overset{|}{\underset{|}{\text{HC}}}-\text{CH}_2-\text{S}^{\ominus}+\text{S}} \longleftarrow \underset{(d)}{\overset{|}{\underset{|}{\text{HC}}}-\text{CH}_2-\text{S}-\overset{\frown}{\text{S}}{}^{\ominus}}
$$

ipate in a direct nucleophilic attack on a sulfur atom. It has been proposed that, in the presence of an amine, decomposition of a cystine residue in intact proteins will yield 2 moles of dehydroalanine (Asquith and Carthew, 1972). In other words, the thiol group in (62e) will undergo further decomposition in alkali to give one residue of dehydroalanine and hydrogen sulfide. Dehydroalanine is a reactive side chain and can react further with a suitably placed nucleophilic side chain (—NH$_2$ and SH groups). Its reaction with ε-NH$_2$ groups has been observed with alkali-treated lysozyme, ribonuclease, chymotrypsin, papain, and bovine serum albumin (Bohak, 1964). Lysinoalanine has also been found after alkaline treatment of ovomucoid (Donovan and White, 1971). Alkaline treatment of keratin in the presence of alkyl amines gave large amounts of new β-N-alkyl amino acid residues (Asquith and Carthew, 1972). The reaction of dehydroalanine with thiol groups has already been mentioned (Section IVG6; reaction 49).

It should be cautioned here that modification reactions carried out on disulfide proteins under alkaline conditions (e.g., some arginine modification reactions, Section IVC) can lead to the aforementioned complications. Alkaline decomposition of disulfides is appreciable above pH 9.5 and proceeds extremely rapidly around pH 10.5 (Andersson and Berg, 1969; Danehy et al., 1971). The decomposition of disulfides is even faster in proteins (Bohak, 1964).

9. Reactivity of Disulfide Bonds and Its Utility as a Conformational Monitor

The reactivities of disulfide bonds differ with the protein and, within the same protein, disulfide bonds exhibit various degrees of reactivity. Other functional groups, of course, show differences in their reactivities. However, the disulfide bonds, because of their importance in covalent stabilization of protein structure, merit a brief discussion. There are many reports in the literature of preferential cleavage of one (or more) disulfide bonds within a given protein. For example, preferential cleavage of the inter-heavy-chain disulfide bond in rabbit γG-globulin was achieved by reduction with 2-mercaptoethanol or 2-mercaptoethylamine with minimal cleavage of disulfide bonds linking light and heavy chains (Palmer et al., 1963; Hong and Nisonoff, 1965). Human immunoglobulin M was reduced by mercaptoethylamine to give 7 S subunits and release the J chain (Tomasi, 1973). Immunoglobulin A was reduced to a 10 S dimer and 7 S monomer, leaving intact the disulfide bonds linking heavy chains together, heavy and light chains, or heavy and J chains (Hauptman and Tomasi, 1975). Cleavage of some disulfide bonds in a protein often does not lead to a major change in activity, indicating that not all the disulfide bonds in a protein are always required for proper maintenance of the native conformation. Examples of this were demonstrated in antibodies where mixing of previously isolated heavy and light chains recovered almost full antigen-binding capacity in antitoxin antibodies (Franek and Nezlin, 1963) and in antibodies to bacteriophages f(1) and f(2) (Edelman et al., 1963). Other workers subsequently recorded similar observations with a variety of antibodies. A partial cleavage of disulfide bonds in bovine pancreatic ribonuclease (Neumann et al., 1967a), bovine trypsin inhibitor (Kress and Laskowski, 1967), and trypsin (Light and Sinha, 1967) had little effect on their respective biological activities. The homogeneous ribonuclease derivative in which disulfides 3–8 and 4–5 had been cleaved (by phosphorothioate at pH 9.0, in the absence of urea) retained fully, in addition to enzymatic activity toward RNA, its immunochemical reaction with antiserum to ribonuclease (Neumann et al., 1967a). On the other hand, cleavage of one disulfide bond in hen egg white lysozyme (Caputo and Zito, 1961) and in bovine milk α-lactalbumin (Shechter et al., 1973) was detrimental to their activities. By contrast, the activity of trypsinogen with one cleaved disulfide enhanced its affinity for an active-site reagent (Knights and Light, 1974). Clearly, the effect of partial disulfide bond cleavage will depend on the protein and on the location of the bond cleaved within a given protein. Proteins in which all the disulfide bonds are broken usually lose their biological activity and are immunochemically unrelated to the native protein such as in performic acid oxidized ribonuclease (Brown, 1962) and reduced-carboxymethylated lysozyme (Gerwing and Thompson, 1968; Young and Leung, 1970; Lee and Atassi, 1973). Porcine lactogenic hormone with ruptured disulfide bonds has been reported to retain some antigenic reactivity (Clarke and Li, 1974).

Conformational changes in a protein result in an increased reactivity of its disulfides to reduction or oxidation. This formulated the basis of a chemical method to evaluate conformational differences between native and modified proteins (Habeeb, 1966a). The approach has been extensively employed and has proved to be a very effective and sensitive method for monitoring small conformational changes that were undetectable even by optical rotatory dispersion and circular dichroism measurements (Atassi et al., 1972; Atassi and Rosemblatt, 1974; Lee et al., 1975). It also proved effective in demonstrating conformational differences among closely related proteins such as lysozyme and α-lactalbumin (Atassi et al., 1970; Habeeb and Atassi, 1971b). This subject is discussed in detail in Chapter 2.

10. Sulfide Bonds

In the antibiotic nisin, the two amino acids lanthionine (see structure in 60c and 60d) and β-methyllanthionine were found (Gross and Morell, 1968). These amino acids are seldom encountered in proteins and carry a sulfide bridge (i.e., a thioether linkage). Cleavage of these bridges was accomplished by desulfurization with Raney nickel at a high temperature (Gross and Morell, 1970). It must be remembered that under these conditions cysteine, if present, will desulfurize much more rapidly than thioether linkages (see Section IVG8). The sulfide bridge was also oxidized to the sulfone by performic acid (Gross and Morell, 1970). Even though these reactions are not specific, they served elegantly in the solution of the unique structure of nisin.

I. Reactions for Tryptophan

1. Oxidation Reactions

N-Bromosuccinimide has been used to modify tryptophan residues in proteins (Witkop, 1961). Oxidation of histidine, tyrosine, cysteine, and cystine was believed to proceed more slowly at low pH and became minimal when complete tryptophan oxidation was achieved. The extent of tryptophan oxidation decreased with increase in pH (Spande *et al.*, 1966). Tryptophan oxidation (to oxindole) was usually followed by decrease in optical density at 280 nm (Patchornik *et al.*, 1958). Subsequent studies showed that *N*-bromosuccinimide will react with and cleave at peptide bonds of tryptophan, histidine, and tyrosine residues (see Sections VIIE, VII I, and VIIJ). The oxidation of a single tryptophan was obtained with lysozyme (Hayashi *et al.*, 1965; Imoto *et al.*, 1974). Other workers (Kronman *et al.*, 1967) found no pH dependence of tryptophan oxidation in lysozyme. Extensive tyrosine and histidine destruction was found at pH 4 and 5.5, even when incomplete tryptophan reaction was indicated spectrally. Brief oxidation of subtilisin at pH 6 in the presence of varying molar excess of *N*-bromosuccinimide showed simultaneous modification of methionine, tyrosine, and tryptophan (Ohtsuki *et al.*, 1969). Reaction of horse heart ferricytochrome *c* with incremental amounts of reagent at pH 4.1 resulted in the oxidation of one tryptophan, two tyrosine, and both methionine residues (Myer, 1972). From the reaction product, two components have been recently isolated (O'Hern *et al.*, 1975). One component was modified at one tryptophan (residue 59) and one methionine (residue 65), and the other was modified at these two residues as well as at the second methionine (residue 80). Brief reaction of cobrotoxin (which has no methionine) at pH 4 oxidized tyrosine, histidine, and tryptophan residues (Chang and Yang, 1973). There have been recent reports of *N*-bromosuccinimide selectivity for tryptophan in various proteins, but these have relied on spectral measurements solely (Irie *et al.*, 1972; Morgan and Müller-Eberhard, 1974; Lowe and Whitworth, 1974) or together with amino acid analyses of acid hydrolysates (Ryan and Tollin, 1973; Samy *et al.*, 1974). Spectral methods have already been found to be misleading in monitoring this reaction (Kronman *et al.*, 1967), and in acid hydrolysis methionine sulfoxide reverts to methionine (see Section IVF1). Also, thiol groups are oxidized by *N*-bromosuccinimide to sulfonic acid (Friedman, 1973).

   Iodine is another strong oxidizing agent that has been employed in tryptophan modification studies (Fraenkel-Conrat, 1950). In addition to tryptophan oxidation, iodine will modify histidine, tyrosine, methionine, cysteine, and cystine residues and also effects other covalent changes (Section IVJ2). However, it has been possible to employ the reaction, for example, in the selective oxidation at pH 5.5 of a single tryptophan (residue 108) in lysozyme (Hartdegen and Rupley, 1967, 1973; Imoto and Rupley, 1973; Iomoto *et al.*, 1973).

   Performic acid and other *peroxides* are also strong oxidizing agents which exhibit no satisfactory selectivity. Invariably, methionine is oxidized to the sulfone and cystine and cysteine to the sulfonic acid. Histidine and tyrosine residues are often oxidized.

Photooxidation (already discussed in detail in Sections IVE1 and IVF1) at low pH will modify tryptophan, methionine, and cysteine. If cysteine is absent (or reversibly protected), tryptophan may be oxidized selectively since methionine sulfoxide can be reduced back to methionine by a thiol reagent (Dedman, 1957). Using proflavin as the sensitizer, the tryptophan and methionine residues in lysozyme were completely photooxidized in 100% formic acid solution (Galiazzo *et al.*, 1968). However, in this solvent, hydroxyl groups will be extensively esterified (Habeeb and Atassi, 1969). A singlet-oxygen mechanism has been proposed for photooxidation of lysozyme at pH 4 in the presence of methylene blue (Churakova *et al.*, 1973). In practice, the direction of photooxidation cannot be predicted (see Sections IVE1 and IVF1) and other reactions with better selectivity for tryptophan are preferrable.

Reaction with 2-(2-*nitrophenylsulfenyl*)-3-*methyl*-3'-*bromoindolenine* (BNPS-skatole) in 80% acetic acid was shown (Omenn *et al.*, 1970) to oxidize methionine and tryptophan residues with equal effectiveness at a low excess (up to 10 equivalents) relative to tryptophan. Thiol groups reacted much faster than tryptophan. Cystine and, to a lesser extent, tyrosine were modified in the presence of a higher reagent excess or longer reaction periods. These conditions also effected considerable cleavage of tryptophyl peptide bonds (Section VII I). *Ozone* oxidation in anhydrous acetic acid (Witkop and Graser, 1944) will oxidize tryptophan residues to *N*-formylkynurenine. However, ozonization will also oxidize methionine, cysteine, and tyrosine residues (Scoffone *et al.*, 1966b). Action of ozone on lysozyme in anhydrous formic acid resulted in the oxidation of two tryptophan residues (Previero *et al.*, 1967c). However, as mentioned above, anhydrous formic acid causes extensive esterification of hydroxyl groups. Reaction of *trichloroisocyanuric acid* with proteins at pH 7.0 (Atassi, 1973) shows comparable selectivity for methionine and tryptophan (see Section IVF1).

It is clear from the foregoing that oxidation reactions are not the most desirable for selective tryptophan modification.

2. Reaction with Arylsulfenyl Halides

Arylsulfenyl halides have been shown to react selectively with tryptophan and cysteine residues (Scoffone *et al.*, 1966a, 1968). Originally, the reaction was carried out in 99% formic acid (Scoffone *et al.*, 1966a), which is an undesirable solvent, and was subsequently found to proceed in aqueous solvents such as 30–50% acetic acid (Scoffone *et al.*, 1968). Reaction with tryptophan residues (63) resulted in the addition of the aryl substituent, through a thioether linkage, at the 2-position of the indole nucleus (63b). Thiol groups gave the mixed disulfide, which could be reversed by a thiol reagent (Fontana *et al.*, 1968a). The 2-*nitro*- and 2,4-*dinitrophenylsulfenyl*

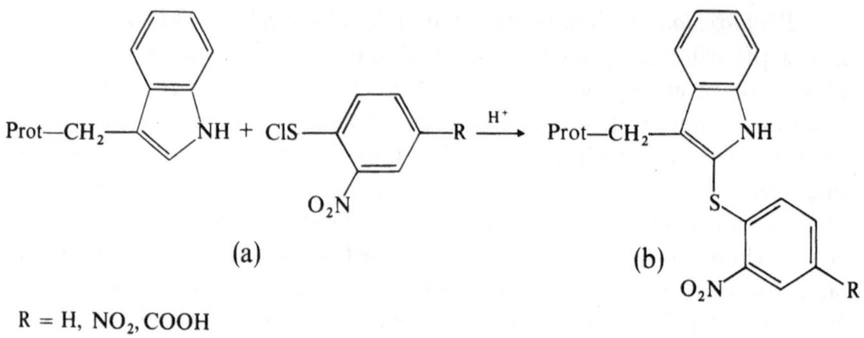

(a)   (b)

R = H, NO$_2$, COOH

(63)

chlorides (Scoffone *et al.*, 1966*a*) and *2-nitro-4-carboxyphenylsulfenyl chloride* (Veronese *et al.*, 1968) have been used. These modifications introduce a chromophoric group, which has been utilized for the determination of tryptophan and cysteine residues in proteins (Boccù *et al.*; 1970). The adduct is stable to alkaline hydrolysis and the extent of modification can be determined by amino acid analysis (Habeeb and Atassi, 1969). Sulfenylation has been applied extensively to protein modification.

The foregoing reaction conditions give extensive modification of all, or most, of the tryptophan residues in a protein. The reaction of 2-nitrophenylsulfenyl chloride with hen egg white lysozyme has been studied under various pH conditions and found to proceed at pH 3.5, effecting modification of a single tryptophan (residue 62) in the enzyme (Shechter *et al.*, 1972). The derivative had no enzymatic activity. These conditions (pH 3–4) have subsequently been used to modify a single tryptophan (residue 149) in ovine pituitary lactogenic hormone (Kawauchi *et al.*, 1973) and two residues (tryptophan-60 and -118) in bovine α-lactalbumin (Shechter *et al.*, 1974). The latter derivative retained full antigenic reactivity, but lost its activity in the lactose synthesis reaction.

Desulfenylation of tryptophan residues in peptides was recently achieved by catalytic hydrogenolysis of 2-nitrophenylsulfenyl derivatives in the presence of tritium (Marche *et al.*, 1975). The reaction permitted replacement of the thioether group by a tritium atom. This procedure has the advantage of recovering the original tryptophan residue and its simultaneous radiolabeling. Its application to proteins merits further study.

3. *Reaction with Substituted Benzyl Halides and Benzylsulfonium Salts*

2-Hydroxy-5-nitrobenzyl bromide was shown to modify tryptophan and cysteine residues in proteins (Koshland *et al.*, 1964; Horton and Koshland, 1965). The incorporation of the 2-hydroxy-5-nitrobenzyl group could be followed spectrophotometrically. The absorption spectrum of the chromophore was sensitive to changes in pH (Koshland *et al.*, 1964). The substituent also served as a sensitive probe for conformational changes in its environment and as a procedure for determination of tryptophan residues in proteins (Barman and Koshland, 1967). Alternatively, the extent of modification could be determined by amino acid analysis of alkaline hydrolysates of the protein derivative (Koshland *et al.*, 1964). The addition of the reagent to tryptophan has been shown to involve a complex set of reactions (Spande *et al.*, 1968; Loudon and Koshland, 1970). Its reaction with N-acetyltryptophan methyl ester yielded three derivatives, with the disubstituted adduct predominating (Spande *et al.*, 1968). In the formation of monosubstituted adducts, addition was initially at position 3 of the indole ring to give two indolinine diastereoisomers (64a) (Loudon and Koshland, 1970). Compound (64a) could cyclize to (64b) and (64c) or undergo

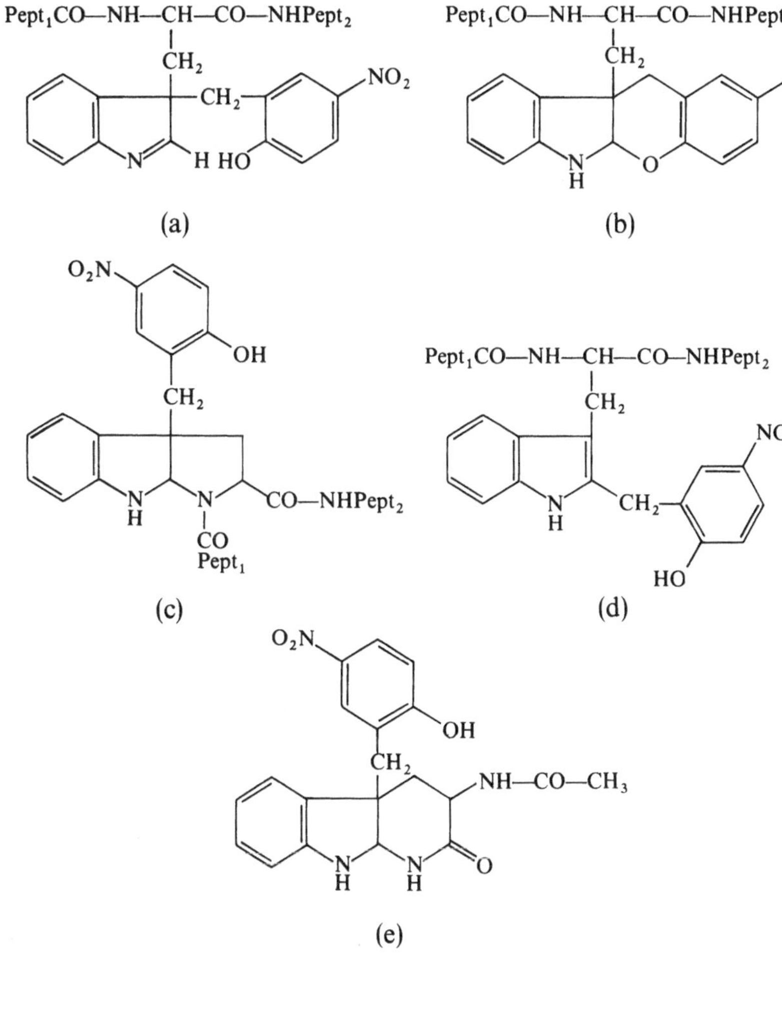

(a)

(b)

(c)

(d)

(64)

(e)

acid-catalyzed rearrangement to compound (64d). Because of these various reaction routes, heterogeneous reaction products with proteins may be formed. To prevent the reaction of thiol groups, they can be reversibly protected (Section IVG10). The analogue, 2-*acetoxy-5-nitrobenzyl chloride*, was developed to introduce the *p*-nitrophenyl group near the active site of enzymes which possess *p*-nitrophenylesterase activity, thereby generating the reactive 2-hydroxy-5-nitrobenzyl bromide (Horton and Young, 1969). 2-*Methoxy-5-nitrobenzyl bromide* reacts with tryptophan, but it will also modify methionine and cysteine residues (Horton et al., 1965).

The three aforementioned reagents suffer from insolubility in water, which necessitates the use of a solution of the reagent in water-miscible organic solvents. Such solvents have frequently effected appreciable denaturation of the protein being modified. Also, the nonpolar nature of the alkylating substituent will often render the modified peptide or protein insoluble. The problem of reagent insolubility in water has been overcome by the use of dimethyl(2-*hydroxy-5-nitrobenzyl*)*sulfonium* salts (Horton and Tucker, 1970). However, this reagent also reacts with thiol groups (Horton and Tucker, 1970) and the protein or peptide derivative will still suffer from insolubility problems due to the nonpolar nature of the alkylating side chain. In addition, the reagent suffers from serious instability problems and quantitative tryptophan recoveries are not possible. Furthermore, it has been suggested (Heinrich et al., 1973) that methylation reactions may have to be taken into account. Alkylations by this reagent are also complex and have been shown (Heinrich et al., 1973) to give at least ten different reaction products with N-acetyl-L-tryptophan amide. Two products had structures similar to (64b) and (64c). The major and most stable product had the structure (64e). At pH 6, each of 2-hydroxy-5-nitrobenzyl bromide and dimethyl-(2-hydroxy-5-nitrobenzyl)sulfonium bromide was less specific (than at pH 2.7) on reaction with α-lactalbumin (Barman, 1972), resulting in each case in the modification of a histidine residue in addition to three tryptophans. Reaction of 2-hydroxy-5-nitrobenzyl bromide with bovine carboxypeptidase A at pH 7 has been reported to result in N^{α}-alkylation of the amino-terminal residues (Bradshaw et al., 1969a). On the other hand, reaction of the enzyme with dimethyl(2-hydroxy-5-nitrobenzyl)sulfonium chloride at pH 7.5 was shown to effect only tryptophan modification and gave no N^{α}-alkylation (Naik and Horton, 1971). Yet another complication with this reaction has been reported with a hen egg white lysozyme derivative which had been modified at a single tryptophan (residue 62) by reaction with 2-hydroxy-5-nitrobenzyl bromide. The derivative has been found to be unstable in acidic and neutral solutions at room temperature. It yielded the native enzyme and liberated 2-hydroxy-5-nitrobenzyl alcohol (Reiss and Lukton, 1975).

In spite of these complications, the reagents have been employed successfully in protein modification. 2-Hydroxyl-5-nitrobenzyl bromide was instrumental in determining the role of tryptophan residues in the conformation and their noninvolvement in the antigenic reactivity of sperm whale myoglobin (Atassi and Caruso, 1968). This reagent has also been employed to modify the single tryptophan residue in each of human chorionic somatomammotropin (Neri *et al.*, 1973), Taiwan cobra toxin (Chang and Yang, 1973), and Indian cobra toxin (Ohta and Hayashi, 1974*b*) and to study its role in the immunochemistry of the respective proteins. Tryptophan modification in rabbit IgG or its Fc fragment has been studied with regard to its effect on anticomplementary activity (Allan and Isliker, 1974), and it was concluded that at least one tryptophan was involved in complement fixation by IgG. Other studies have included the effects of tryptophan modification on the encephalitogenic properties of the basic myelin protein (Chao and Einstein, 1970), on the association–dissociation equilibrium and regulatory properties of bovine liver glutamate dehydrogenase (Witzemann *et al.*, 1974), and on retinol-binding ability of prealbumin (Horwitz and Heller, 1974).

Applications of dimethyl(2-hydroxy-5-nitrobenzyl)sulfonium bromide have included the modification of three tryptophan residues in bovine α-lactalbumin (Barman, 1972), causing small conformational changes and loss of specific protein activity (Barman and Bagshaw, 1972). Tryptophan modification in yeast apotransketolase could be protected (and loss of enzymatic activity prevented) by the coenzyme thiamine pyrophosphate (Heinrich *et al.*, 1972). The modification of two tryptophans (residues 7 and 14) in a sperm whale myoglobin fragment (sequence 1–31) did not change its antigenic reactivity (Perlstein and Atassi, 1974). One tryptophan (residue 193) modified in glyceraldehyde 3-phosphate dehydrogenase caused the loss of enzymatic activity but no conformational change (Heilmann and Pfleiderer, 1975).

4. Acylation Reactions

N-Formylation of tryptophan residues in peptides and proteins was reported to take place in anhydrous formic acid saturated with HCl gas at room temperature (Previero *et al.*, 1967*b*). The reaction proceeded with apparent selectivity for tryptophan and the adduct was stable at neutral or acid pH but was completely reversed at pH 9.5 or higher, yielding back tryptophan. The modification caused a shift in the ultraviolet absorption maximum to 298 nm, which was employed to estimate the extent of tryptophan reaction. The reaction was proposed for reversible modification of tryptophan residues in proteins (Previero *et al.*, 1967*b*). However, the severe conditions of the reaction may prove detrimental to many proteins. Also, the high pH conditions often employed in the deformylation step (Aviram and Schejter, 1971) preclude its application in many proteins, especially those containing disulfide bonds. These complications are evidenced in the incomplete recovery of esterase and proteolytic activity of trypsin even when full (100%) deformylation of tryptophan had been obtained (Colletti-Previero et al., 1969). Deformylation of E. coli thioredoxin under various conditions recovered only between 15 and 38% of its activity, while the recovery of activity in one preparation approximated 50% (Holmgren, 1972). However, high recoveries (85–100%) of activities have been reported upon deformylation of horse heart cytochrome c (Aviram and Schejter, 1971). Despite its shortcomings, the reaction provides the only reversible tryptophan modification so far available.

Carboxylic acid halides or anhydrides in anhydrous trifluoroacetic acid have been reported to effect C-acylation of tryptophan residues mostly to the 2-acyl and in part to the 5-acyl and 1-acyl indole derivatives (Previero et al., 1972b). Rapid condensation of the carbonyl group with the α-NH_2 group in free 2-acyltryptophan gave 1-alkyl-3,4-dihydro-β-carboline-3-carboxylic acid. This cyclization did not take place in proteins and peptides but was obtained on acid hydrolysis of the derivative. C-Acylated tryptophan peptides and proteins absorbed at 305 and 315 nm, and the stability of the β-carboline system to acid hydrolysis enabled its determination by amino acid analysis. Aliphatic and aromatic hydroxyl groups were also acylated. This reaction needs further study. The conditions of the reaction may not be suitable for most proteins, but they could find application in tryptophan modification of certain immunochemically reactive peptides.

5. 2,3-Dioxo-5-indolinesulfonic Acid

2,3-Dioxo-5-indolinesulfonic acid has been introduced as a new highly specific reagent for modification of tryptophan residues in peptides and proteins (Atassi and Zablocki, 1975). Its reaction with free amino acids in aqueous solution (0.1 M acetic acid, pH 2.9) at room temperature modified tryptophan rapidly, and no other amino acid was modified. In the presence of high reagent excess and on long reaction periods, the modification of proline was appreciable and cysteine modification became detectable (12 hr, 7%). Proline engaged in peptide linkage did not react in the presence of high molar excess and long reaction periods. No modification of proline was obtained, even when it occupied the N-terminal position (Atassi and Zablocki, unpublished work). The mechanism of reaction with tryptophan has not yet been determined. Reaction of egg albumin with the reagent was entirely specific for tryptophan and showed no modification of proline or cysteine residues (Atassi and Zablocki, 1975). A single tryptophan (residue 123) has been modified by the reagent in egg white lysozyme, and the conformation, enzymatic activity, and immunochemistry of the derivative have been studied (Atassi and Zablocki, 1976). Two tryptophans (residues

62 and 63) have been modified in an immunochemically reactive lysozyme peptide and were shown to be part of an antigenic reactive site which overlapped with the enzyme active site (Lee and Atassi, 1975). The reagent offers the advantages of stability, easy handling, high water solubility, and high specificity. It affords protein and peptide derivatives that are completely water soluble because of the polar nature of the substituent. The yellow color (λ_{max}, 367 nm) of the derivatives offers advantages of easy determination of the extent and location of the modification.

6. Other Modification Reactions

Selective *deuteration* or *tritiation* of tryptophan residues has been achieved to a considerable extent in CF_3COOD and CF_3COOT, respectively (Bak *et al.*, 1969). The labels were at positions 2, 4, 5, 6, and 7 of the indole nucleus and these exchanged slowly with the aqueous solvent. The method has been applied to glucagon. Although its application to proteins may not be satisfactory, it may prove useful in labeling tryptophan-containing, immunochemically reactive peptides and merits further study.

N-Benzoyloxy-N-methyl-4-aminobenzene (Poirier *et al.*, 1967: Lin *et al.*, 1969) and *3-acetoxyxanthine* (Stohrer *et al.*, 1973), both potent oncogens, modify tryptophan but will also react with methionine and aromatic amino acids.

J. Reactions for Tyrosine

1. Oxidation

Various oxidation reactions that may also effect tyrosine oxidation have been discussed in connection with oxidation of other functional groups (see Sections IVE1, IVF1, IVG1, and IVI1). The chemistry of the reaction of tyrosine residues with *N-bromosuccinimide* and cleavage of tryosyl peptide bonds by the reagent have been studied in detail (Wilchek *et al.*, 1967b, 1968a). Amino-terminal tyrosine residues gave the indole derivatives. The absorption maximum of the latter (λ_{max} 315 nm) was used as the basis of a spectrophotometric procedure for a rapid assay of amino-terminal tyrosine residues (Wilchek *et al.*, 1968b). For reactions and examples of N-bromosuccinimide applications, see Section IVI1). *Potassium nitrosodisulfonate* oxidized amino-terminal tyrosine to 2-carboxy-5,6-dihydroxyindole, while tyrosine in the middle or at the carboxyl end of a peptide gave 3,4-dihydroxyphenylalanine derivatives (Dukler *et al.*, 1971). This reaction would not be expected to exhibit good selectivity, but this has not been investigated.

2. Iodination

Radioiodination is extensively employed in immunochemistry and for immunoassays. Selective substitution (to mono- and diiodo derivatives) on the phenolic side chain (Hughes and Straessle, 1950) does not obtain, and the reaction has also been found to iodinate histidine (Fraenkel-Conrat, 1950; Covelli and Wolff, 1966) to the mono- and the diiodo products. Histidine iodination was relatively slower than that of tyrosine in proteins and increased with increase in pH (Wolff and Covelli, 1969). The reaction will also oxidize methionine (Lavine, 1943; Koshland et al., 1963), tryptophan (Section IVI1), cysteine (Section IVG1), and cystine (Friedman, 1973). Iodo derivatives of histidine and tyrosine are destroyed on acid hydrolysis. Alkaline hydrolysis permitted a substantial recovery of iodotyrosines, and, in amino acid analysis, monoiodotyrosine eluted before lysine while diiodotyrosine emerged just after ammonia (Sherman and Kassell, 1968). The nature and extent of the modification are usually determined from enzymatic hydrolysates or, unfortunately, often assumed.

These reactions are carried out at an alkaline pH (usually between pH 8 and 9.5) employing I_3^-, I_2, or more efficiently, ICl (McFarlane, 1958). Iodide in the presence of an oxidizing agent such as chloramine T (Greenwood et al., 1963) yields radioiodinations with higher specific activities. However, chloramine T is a strong, rather nonselective oxidizing agent. Enzymatic iodination with lactoperoxidase or horseradish peroxidase (Rombauts et al., 1967; Morrison and Bayse, 1970) was developed as a gentle procedure for selective iodination of tyrosine residues. It has been shown that the chemical as well as the enzymatic iodination procedures oxidize tryptophan very rapidly to the oxindole over the pH range 4–7.5 (Alexander, 1973, 1974). In acid pH, the oxidized derivatives suffered considerable cleavage of tryptophyl peptide bonds, but the cleavage was minimal at pH 7.5. In addition, the iodinating agents, N-iodosuccinimide (Junek et al., 1969), ICl, and chloramine T–potassium iodide can effect oxidative cleavage of diiodotyrosyl peptide bonds, whereas with I_2 and I_3^- substitution occurs but the iodinated tyrosine sites undergo no subsequent cleavage (Alexander, 1974). Clearly, therefore, selectivity of iodination for tyrosine may not be assumed with any of the iodination reactions. This assumption has often been the basis for developing methods to determine relative rates of iodination of various protein tyrosyl residues (Roholt and Pressman, 1967). Spectral measurements (320 nm) used to determine the extent of iodination will be misleading.

Iodination with KI_3 has been applied, for example, to study the active sites of several antihapten antibodies together with ICl (Grossberg et al., 1962), but the nature of the modified residues, conformational changes, and homogeneity of the derivatives were not investigated. The reaction of KI_3 with 11 proteins was studied in detail and found to modify histidine, tryptophan, and thiol groups (Wolff and Covelli, 1969). With bovine trypsin inhibitor, selective iodination of three tyrosine residues was reported (Sherman and Kassell, 1968). Its reported selectivity for two tyrosine residues in lysozyme (Hayashi *et al.*, 1968) has not been confirmed (Wolff and Covelli, 1969). Thus iodination of tyrosine residues in horse cytochrome *c* (McGowan and Stellwagen, 1970) does not exclude tryptophan and histidine iodination since they were not investigated. Investigations with ICl on antibodies (Zappacosta and Rossi, 1967; Miles and Hales, 1968) and ribosomal proteins (Miller and Sypherd, 1973) and with chloramine T–KI in radioimmunoassay (Hunter, 1970) have neglected to study selectivity of the reaction. Enzymatic iodination has been extended to study the surface of mammalian cell membranes (Phillips and Morrison, 1971; Podulso *et al.*, 1972) and relative degrees of exposure of ribosomal proteins (Miller and Sypherd, 1973). In such complex systems, the type of selectivity achieved cannot be determined. Radioiodination is, nevertheless, a very effective tool in immunochemical studies of proteins. The foregoing complications, however, should not be overlooked.

A novel approach employing an entirely different concept has been applied to radioiodination of proteins and other polyanionic macromolecules by Little *et al.* (1975). In this approach, iodine was *not* directly incorporated into the antigen. Tyramine (2-*p*-hydroxyphenylethylamine, $HOC_6H_4CH_2CH_2NH_2$) was conjugated to soluble DEAE-dextran by the cyanogen bromide activation reaction of Axén *et al.* (1967). The *tyramine-DEAE-dextran* conjugate was then radioiodinated by the chloramine T method. Mixing of the radioiodinated DEAE-dextran with a polyanionic antigen gave a soluble antigen–iododextran complex which, on interaction with appropriate specific antibodies, gave a radioactive antigen–antibody–dextran complex. This complex could then be employed in a conventional radioimmunoassay technique to determine free and antibody-bound antigen. Since in this approach the antigen suffers no covalent modification, chemical alteration of antigenic reactive sites is avoided. High specific activities of antigen–dextran complexes were achieved (Little *et al.*, 1975), which enabled detection in the nanogram range.

3. Acylation Reactions

N-Acetylimidazole was reported to effect the specific *O*-acetylation of phenolic hydroxyl groups, and selectivity was demonstrated on carboxypeptidase A (Simpson *et al.*, 1963). Subsequent studies showed the reagent to cause acylation of amino groups as well, which was, as expected, less extensive than acylation with acid anhydrides. Acylation of amino groups accompanied tyrosine acylation, for example, in horse heart cytochrome *c* (Cronin and Harbury, 1965), in hen egg white lysozyme (Parsons *et al.*,

1969; Nakae *et al.*, 1972), and quite extensively in protein A from *Staphylococcus aureus* (Sjoholm *et al.*, 1972). With trypsin, a serine was O-acetylated together with ε-NH_2 and phenolic OH groups (Houston and Walsh, 1970). Thiol groups are also acetylated by N-acetylimidazole (Riordan *et al.*, 1965). In addition to these side reactions, phenolic O-acetyl substituents are quite labile and may be inadvertently removed at pH values moderately away from neutrality or by buffer anions (Riordan and Vallee, 1972). Reaction is therefore performed at neutral pH. The extent of tyrosine O-acetylation has been evaluated spectrophotometrically from the decrease in absorption at 257 nm (Riordan and Vallee, 1972) or by removal with hydroxylamine (see Section IVA1). The reagent hydrolyzes rapidly in aqueous solution and has moderate stability in dry benzene. Amino- and thiol-group acetylations may be avoided by their respective reversible protection. Reversible amino-group protection has been employed in O-acetylation of the single tyrosine residue in bovine neurophysin II (Furth and Hope, 1970). Also, S-acyl groups can be reversed (Section IVA3).

In reaction with an N-acylimidazole (65), the acyl group may be varied to introduce substituents with certain desired properties. A pyrroline 1-oxyl

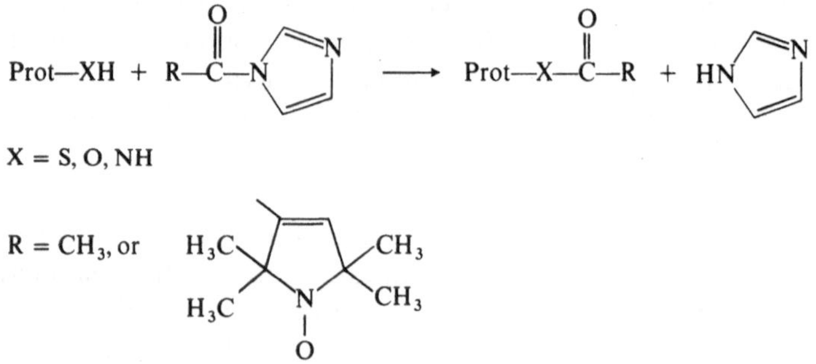

$$\text{Prot—XH} + \underset{\text{R—C—N}}{\overset{O}{\underset{\|}{}}}\text{—N} \longrightarrow \text{Prot—X—C—R} + \text{HN}$$

X = S, O, NH   (65)

R = CH_3, or   (structure)

substituent has been developed to introduce spin-labels on tyrosine residues (Barratt *et al.*, 1969). However, the reagent should not be expected to be specific for tyrosine, and its selectivity properties will be similar to those of N-acetylimidazole. Also, the labile nature of O-acyl substituents complicates the utility of this spin-label.

4. Reaction with Cyanuric Halides

Cyanuric halides, and in particular cyanuric fluoride, were introduced as selective reagents for tyrosine residues in proteins (Kurihara *et al.*, 1963). Optimum reaction proceeded between pH 10 and 12 (Gorbunoff, 1972). Since reaction of cyanuric halides is believed to proceed by nucleophilic substitution (Schaefer *et al.*, 1951), it is to be expected that at the pH range of the supposed tyrosine modification other protein nucleophilic side chains should react, especially with the highly reactive and also highly unstable cyanuric fluoride. Therefore, substitution should take place with amino, thiol, imidazole, phenolic, and (to a lesser extent) aliphatic hydroxyl groups. Also, tryptophan and methionine residues will most likely react. In addition, the alkaline conditions of the reaction will be detrimental for disulfide-containing proteins (Section IVH8). Reports of high selectivity of the reagent for tyrosine residues (Kurihara et al., 1963; Gorbunoff, 1970) were based solely on spectrophotometric titrations. Cyanuric fluoride has been applied extensively to study the "state" or "exposure" of tyrosine residues in proteins. Unfortunately, these studies shed little light on the property being investigated. The extensive modification of other protein side chains by the reagent should induce drastic conformational changes. These changes will influence both accessibility and reactivity of tyrosyl residues as well as the spectral properties employed to monitor tyrosine modification. The "state" of residues in such grossly modified proteins cannot be relevant to the situation in the native protein. Cyanuric halides and diazonium salts are probably the least suitable reagents for selective protein modification.

5. Reaction with Diazonium Salts

The nonselectivity of diazonium salts in reaction with proteins has already been discussed in connection with histidine modification (Section IVE4). An unusual selectivity has been reported in the reaction of p-azobenzene arsonate with crystals of bovine carboxypeptidase A, giving rise to diazotization of a single tyrosine (residue 248) in the protein (Johansen et al., 1972). Reaction of porcine carboxypeptidase B with the reagent in solution modified two tyrosine and three lysine residues, with only minimal histidine and tryptophan modification (Sokolovsky and Eisenbach, 1972). One tyrosine residue could be protected from modification by 3-phenylpropionate. These differing reactivity results were attributed to conformational differences between the crystalline and solution states (Johansen and Vallee, 1973). Reduction of 3-azotyrosyl residues to 3-aminotyrosyl residues by sodium hydrosulfite has been reported in model peptides and in ribonuclease A (Gorecki et al., 1971).

6. Nitration

Tetranitromethane, which was known to nitrate phenols (Schmidt and Fischer, 1920), was suggested (Herriott, 1947) as a reagent for nitration of proteins. It was subsequently reported to react specifically with tyrosine and cysteine residues (Riordan et al., 1966; Sokolovsky et al., 1966). Reaction

$$\text{Prot}-\langle\text{C}_6\text{H}_4\rangle-\text{OH} + \text{C(NO}_2)_4 \xrightarrow{\text{pH 8}} \text{Prot}-\langle\text{C}_6\text{H}_3(\text{NO}_2)\rangle-\text{O}^- + \text{C(NO}_2)_3^- + \text{H}^+$$

$$\qquad\qquad\text{(a)}\qquad\qquad\qquad\qquad\text{(b)}\qquad\qquad\text{(c)}\qquad\text{(66)}$$

of tyrosine residues with tetranitromethane (66) gave 3-nitrotyrosine (66b), which had an absorption maximum at 428 nm and nitroformate anion (66c) (λ_{max} 350 nm). In addition to spectral measurements (Riordan et al., 1967), modification could be determined by amino acid analysis of acid hydrolysates since 3-nitrotyrosine appeared on the analyzer after phenylalanine (Riordan et al., 1966). Conversion of 3-nitrotyrosine to 3-aminotyrosine was accomplished in peptides and proteins by reduction with sodium hydrosulfite (Sokolovsky et al., 1967). Subsequent to these studies, tetranitromethane was widely employed in numerous protein systems and it soon became evident that the reagent was not as selective as it was first believed to be. Its oxidation of thiol groups has already been mentioned (Section IVG1). It was found to form cross-links, first with γ-globulin and collagen (Doyle et al., 1968), and subsequently with trypsinogen and trypsin (Vincent et al., 1970), insulin (Boesel and Carpenter, 1970), ovotransferrin (Williams and Lowe, 1971), thyroid-stimulating hormone (Cheng and Pierce, 1972), and papain (Tsukamoto and Ohno, 1974). Its ability to effect intermolecular cross-links has been exploited to identify neighbor relationships among proteins in 30 S ribosomal subunits (Shih and Craven, 1973). With model phenols (Bruice et al., 1968) and tyrosine (Williams and Lowe, 1971), reaction was shown to be complex, giving several reaction products. Glycyltyrosine gave a single, quantitatively nitrated reaction product (Atassi and Habeeb, 1969; Boesel and Carpenter, 1970) in nitration at low pH but formed cross-links in reaction at pH 8 (Boesel and Carpenter, 1970). Tryptophan oxidation was observed on reaction of denatured staphylococcal nuclease with 60 molar excess (Cuatrecasas et al., 1968), and of native bovine α-lactalbumin with 10 molar excess (Atassi et al., 1970) of tetranitromethane. Under the latter conditions, tryptophan residues in hen egg white lysozyme were not modified. The reaction of tetranitromethane with tryptophan analogues and substituted indoles has been studied (Sokolovsky et al., 1970). Also, its reaction with histidine, tryptophan, and methionine peptides has been observed (Sokolovsky et al., 1969). Furthermore, the reagent has been shown to nitrate the vinyl side chains of heme (Atassi, 1969b), which makes results from direct nitrations of hemoproteins difficult to interpret. However, cross-linking, tryptophan modification, and other side reactions are not always obtained and the results will depend on the conditions, such as in human serum albumin and thyroglobulins (Malan and Edelhoch, 1970), and on the protein, as seen in α-lactalbumin and lysozyme (Atassi *et al.*, 1970).

On nitration of tyrosyl residues at the *ortho* position, the inductive effect of the nitro group on the aromatic nucleus will increase the acidity of the phenolic OH, thus promoting its ionization since the resultant anion will be stabilized by the electron-withdrawing mesomeric effect (Atassi, 1968). The increased acidity is shown by a decrease of the pK_a value from 10.1 for tyrosine to 7.2 for 3-nitrotyrosine (Sokolovsky *et al.*, 1967). The pK_a value for 3-aminotyrosine is 10.0 (Sokolovsky *et al.*, 1967). The decrease in the pK_a value has been shown to be sufficient to abolish the reactivity of an antigenic reactive site in sperm whale myoglobin (tyrosine-146 and -151; Atassi, 1968) and in lysozyme (tyrosine-20 and -23; Atassi and Habeeb, 1969). In the latter case, the antigenic reactivity lost on nitration was entirely recovered upon reduction of the nitrotyrosine residues to aminotyrosine. This was not attempted in myoglobin. The results with lysozyme showed that, by modifying the same amino acid residues in more than one way, the nature of the modification determines its effect on biological activity (Atassi and Habeeb, 1969) and on conformation (Atassi *et al.*, 1971). A large number of proteins have been subjected to nitration, often with useful results. In addition to the above, other examples include its employment to study the immunochemistry of tetanus toxin (Bizzini *et al.*, 1973) and Indian cobra toxin (Ohta and Hayashi, 1974a). Its effects on the enzymatic activity of aspartate transcarbamylase (Polyanovsky *et al.*, 1972), on the conformation and activity of its catalytic subunit (Kirschner and Schachman, 1973), and on the iron-binding capacity of ovotransferrin (Tsao *et al.*, 1974) have been studied.

7. Other Modification Reactions

Diisopropylfluorophosphate (67a) inhibits many hydrolases, such as trypsin, chymotrypsin, and acetylcholinesterase, through alkylphosphorylation of a single serine residue at the active site of the enzyme. The reagent has been reported to react with stem bromelain at *tyrosine* residues (Murachi and Yasui, 1965) without causing loss in activity (Murachi *et al.*, 1965). Similar results have been obtained with papain (Chaiken and Smith, 1969). In lysozyme, two tyrosines (residues 20 and 23) were partially modified by the reagent (Kato and Murachi, 1971). The extent of tyrosine modification increased with increase in pH from 9.5 to 10.7. The reaction most likely

Prot—X—O—H F—P(O—CH(CH₃)₂)₂ →(pH 9.5) Prot—X—O—P(O—CH(CH₃)₂)₂

(a)   (b)   (67)

X = Ser, Tyr

proceeds by nucleophilic substitution (67), with a reactive hydroxyl resulting in alkylphosphorylation (67b) of the protein. No reports of reaction with NH_2 or SH groups have appeared, although some results suggest modification at sites other than tyrosine (Murachi *et al.*, 1970).

α-*Nitroso-β-naphthol* was shown to react with tyrosine to give colored adducts in the presence of an oxidizing agent (Gerngross *et al.*, 1933). The reaction is not selective, but only tyrosine gives a colored derivative. Although it is not useful in selective modification studies, many spectrophotometric methods for tyrosine determination in peptides and proteins are based on this reaction (Uehara *et al.*, 1970). Also, tyrosine residues in peptides have been detected fluorometrically because of the intense fluorescence of the condensation product (Håkanson *et al.*, 1973). The reaction is very useful in detection of tyrosine peptides in peptide maps (Block *et al.*, 1958).

K. Cross-Linking Reagents

Compounds carrying more than one reactive group will effect cross-links between the modified amino acid side chains. Cross-linking reagents are being applied increasingly in several kinds of studies. In immunochemistry, cross-linking of peptides or poorly immunogenic proteins to a high molecular weight polypeptide or a protein carrier enables the preparation of antibodies with specificity against the coupled peptide or protein. With proper choice of carrier, antibody synthesis against the carrier may be avoided. Cross-linking of protein antigens to erythrocyte cell wall is employed extensively in hemagglutination tests.

Other applications of cross-linking have been mostly in deriving information about the distance or spacing in the three-dimensional structure of the side chains that had been cross-linked. The distance derived from such studies will be approximate because the amino acid side chains can move to accommodate to the length of the cross-linking reagent, which is unlikely to match the preexisting distance in the native protein. Such studies, of course, presume that after coupling of the first functional group conformational changes remain minimal until the second functional group finds the amino acid side chain with which it will react. Alternatively, both reactive groups have to possess the unlikely capability of coupling simultaneously with two respective amino acid side chains, thus "trapping" the protein molecule in its original conformation. Even though it appears that many factors complicate these studies and interpretation of their conformational implications, some useful and interesting results have been obtained. In some cases, the links could be made only by some (Hartman and Wold, 1966) or appreciable (Moore and Day, 1968) distortion of the crystalline three-dimensional structure. These reagents have also been employed to effect cross-links between, or close to, contact surfaces of subunits in oligomeric proteins which can also undergo conformational changes as a result of the cross-linking (Hanschumacher and Gaumond, 1972). Intermolecular cross-links have been employed in nearest-neighbor analysis to gain information on the geometrical arrangement or topography of proteins in membranes and in ribosomal particles.

The cross-linking reagents incorporate reactive groups similar to those previously described for the monofunctional reagents. Their selectivity properties will follow closely the properties of the respective monofunctional reagents already described in Sections IVA to IVJ. Therefore, selectivity will not be discussed here in detail and the preceding sections should be consulted. Also, cross-linking to insoluble nonprotein supports will not be reviewed.

1. Aryl and Alkyl Halides and Sulfonyl Halides

4,4'-Difluoro-3,3'-dinitrodiphenyl sulfone (68a) was first introduced by Zahn and Zuber (1953) and has since been used to introduce intramolecular cross-links in bovine serum albumin (Wold, 1961) and lysozyme (Stevens and Long, 1969). It has been employed to prepare several mixed protein conjugates (Ram, 1963), including those of horseradish peroxidase–IgG (Nakane and Pierce, 1967; Modesto and Pesce, 1971), and to enrich proteins with amino acid residues (Brazil and Ram, 1965). Dinitrodifluorobenzene was used for the introduction of cross-links between an α-NH$_2$ and an

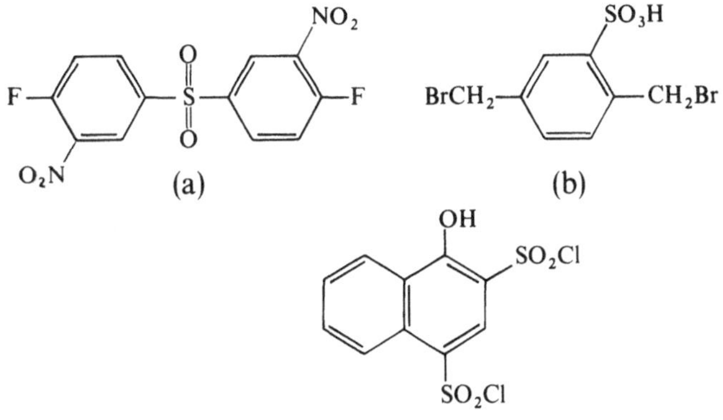

(a)   (b)   (68)

(c)

ε-NH$_2$ group in insulin (Zahn and Meienhofer, 1958). The reagent has subsequently found wide application. The selectivity of the two reagents will be similar to that of the monofunctional fluorodinitrobenzene (Section IVA7). α,α'-Dibromo-p-xylenesulfonic acid (68b), a soluble bifunctional reagent, was used for effecting cross-links between two ε-NH$_2$ groups in lysozyme (Hiremath and Day, 1964). 1-*Naphthol-2,4-disulfonyl chloride* (68c) (Zahn and Meienhofer, 1958) and *phenol-2,4-disulfonyl chloride* (Moore and Day, 1968) have been used for effecting cross-links between amino groups. The links in both cases are identical in length, and therefore the smaller phenol reagent may be preferable.

2. Aldehydes

Formaldehyde was shown (Fraenkel-Conrat and Olcott, 1948) to effect irreversible cross-links with several protein functional groups (Section IVA5) and to yield intermolecularly linked protein oligomers (Fraenkel-Conrat and Mecham, 1949). It has since been applied extensively, most recently in the cross-linking histones in chromatin to learn about their spatial relationships (Hyde and Walker, 1975). *Glutaraldehyde* gave inter-molecular cross-links on reaction with crystals of carboxypeptidase A (Quiocho and Richards, 1964) to produce insoluble preparations with substantial enzymatic activity. It has been used to polymerize trypsin into an enzymatically active insoluble preparation (Habeeb, 1967a) and subsequently many other proteins, and to prepare enzyme–cellophane membranes (Broun *et al.*, 1969). It has been applied to demonstrate extensive interactions of the proteins (and not the glycoproteins) in beef ghost erythrocyte membrane (Capaldi, 1973). The shorter dialdehyde *malonaldehyde* has been shown to inactivate and intermolecularly cross-link ribonuclease and other enzymes, giving fluorescent derivatives (Chio and Tappel, 1969). *o-Hydroxybenzaldehyde* (*salicylaldehyde*) was shown to produce cytochrome *c* polymers (Williams and Jacobs, 1968). (For selectivity information on aldehydic reagents, see Section IVA5).

3. Diimido Esters

Diimido esters (69) with increasing length of the alkyl chain have been employed in cross-linking studies. *Dimethyladipimidate* ($n = 4$), first to be introduced in this series, was used to effect intramolecular cross-links in bovine ribonuclease A and to obtain a dimer and higher oligomers, all with enzymatic activity (Hartman and Wold, 1966, 1967). *Diethylmalonimidate* (69, $n = 1$) was employed to conjugate ferritin and bovine serum albumin to human IgG (Dutton *et al.*, 1966). The derivatives of bovine serum albumin and human IgG suffered little change in antigenic reactivities.

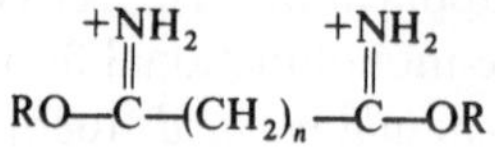

$$\underset{\text{RO—C—(CH}_2)_n\text{—C—OR}}{\overset{\overset{+NH_2}{\|}\qquad\quad\overset{+NH_2}{\|}}{}} \qquad (69)$$

Dimethylsuberimidate ($n = 6$) was shown to produce cross-links which, under appropriate conditions, were mostly intramolecular such as in ribonuclease (Davies and Stark, 1970). With five different oligomeric proteins intermolecular links among the subunits were formed. The adipimidate, the suberimidate and the *pimerlinidate* ($n = 5$) have been used to investigate the quaternary structure of beef liver glutamate dehydrogenase (Hucho and Janda, 1974). Dimethylsuberimidate was employed in the cross-linking of the subunits of L-asparaginase from *E. coli* (Handschumacher and Gaumond, 1972). The cross-linking resulted in over 70% loss of enzymatic activity, presumably due to conformational changes since lysine modification by itself did not affect the activity. This reagent was used to cross-link 30 S and 50 S subunits of *E. coli* (Slobin, 1972) and in the identification of neighboring proteins in the 30 S subunit (Barritault *et al.*, 1975). The mechanism of action of chain initiation factor 3 was studied with 70 S *E. coli* ribosomes which had been cross-linked with dimethylsuberimidate (Hawley *et al.*, 1974). The factor was also cross-linked with 50 S and 30 S ribosomal subunits. The reagent has been employed in the cross-linking of the initiation factor IF-2 to the same subunit (Bollen *et al.*, 1975). The proteins S 5 and S 8 in the 30 S subunit were cross-linked by dimethyladipimidate and the reagent was used to cross-link the glycoproteins in human erythrocyte membranes (Ji, 1974).

Because of the good selectivity of imido esters for amino groups (see Section IVA11) and their ability to react under mild conditions, affording protein derivatives that suffer no change in net charge, they present an extremely useful class of reagents for cross-linking studies. Amidination can be reversed, although the conditions necessary for its reversal are too drastic for most proteins (see Section IVA11). Some removal of the cross-links by ammonolysis was reported in two of the foregoing studies (Ji, 1974; Barritault *et al.*, 1975).

Cross-linking reagents containing disulfide bonds were first described by Traut *et al.* (1973) by oxidation of *methyl-4-mercaptobutyrimidate* derivatives to the disulfides. The presence of the disulfide enables a facile cleavage of the cross-link. Other bifunctional reagents with disulfide bonds have been reported (Wang and Richards, 1974a). Of these reagents, the diimido ester *dimethyl dithiobispropionimidate** was employed in nearest-neighbor analysis of proteins of human erythrocyte membrane (Wang and Richards, 1974b). The same reagent has been used to introduce cross-links in aldolase, concanavalin A, and intact human erythrocytes (Ruoho *et al.*, 1975). Cross-links in the last case did not prevent the reversible oxygenation of hemoglobin, and reduction of the disulfides in the links caused lysing of the cells.

$$*(-SCH_2CH_2\overset{\overset{+NH_2}{\|}}{C}-OCH_3)_2.$$

Recently, an artifactual staining was observed with the suberimidate cross-linking reaction in sodium dodecylsulfate (SDS) polyacrylamide gel electrophoresis (Burke and Reeves, 1975). The artifact had an apparent molecular weight (in SDS gels) of about 40,000. This is noteworthy since SDS gel electrophoresis is routinely used in investigating the molecular weights of cross-linked protein oligomers.

4. Reagents with Activated Carboxyl Groups

Carboxyl groups may be converted to certain derivatives such as the *p*-nitrophenyl ester or azide derivatives, which will readily couple with amino groups through an amide linkage (Schröder and Lübke, 1965). This fact has been exploited in the design of some bifunctional reagents.

Di(p-nitrophenyl)sebacate (70a) has been used to cross-link ε-NH$_2$ groups in wool (Zahn *et al.*, 1965), and the structure of the cross-linked product with lysine has been determined (Caldwell *et al.*, 1971). *Carbonyl-bis(L-methionine p-nitrophenyl ester)* (70b) is an interesting new reagent which has been introduced for reversible cross-linking (Busse and Carpenter, 1974). The reagent was used to effect intramolecular cross-linking in bovine

$$
R\text{—OOC—(CH}_2)_8\text{—COO—R}
$$

(a)

$$
R = p\text{-C}_6\text{H}_4\text{NO}_2
$$

$$
\begin{array}{c}
\qquad\qquad\qquad\quad \overset{\textstyle O}{\overset{\textstyle \|}{\quad}} \\
ROOC\text{—CH—NH—C—NH—CH—COOR} \\
\quad\ \ | \qquad\qquad\qquad\quad | \\
\ \ (CH_2)_2 \qquad\qquad\ (CH_2)_2 \\
\quad\ \ | \qquad\qquad\qquad\quad | \\
\quad\ \ S \qquad\qquad\qquad\quad S \\
\quad\ \ | \qquad\qquad\qquad\quad | \\
\ \ CH_3 \qquad\qquad\quad CH_3
\end{array}
$$

(b)

(70)

insulin between residue Al (α-NH$_2$) and residue B29 (ε-NH$_2$). The cross-link could be removed by cleavage with cyanogen bromide (see Section VIIG) in 70–75% yield to give a product which was identical with native insulin electrophoretically, spectrally, and immunochemically (Busse and Carpenter, 1974). On reduction and reoxidation of cross-linked insulin the disulfides reformed in the correct manner in about 80% yield by physical and immuno-chemical criteria (Busse *et al.*, 1974). *Diazide tartarate* derivatives (71a–c) offer another new series of cross-linking reagents of varying chain length which carry vicinal hydroxyl groups (Lutter *et al.*, 1974). This latter feature permitted cleavage of the cross-links by periodate oxidation. The method has been applied to effect protein cross-links in *E. coli* 30 S ribosomal sub-unit (Lutter *et al.*, 1974). *Trimesyl-tris-β-alanylazide* (71d) was recently introduced as a *trifunctional* reagent and was used to effect inter- and intra-subunit cross-links in hemoglobin (Wetz *et al.*, 1974).

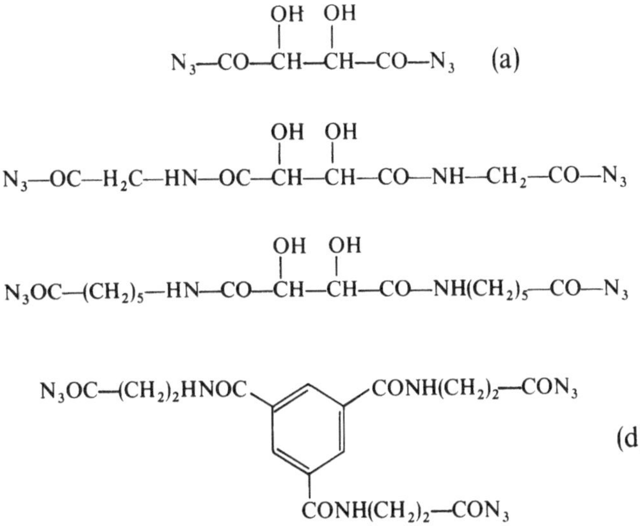

$$\underset{\text{(a)}}{N_3-CO-\underset{\overset{|}{OH}}{CH}-\underset{\overset{|}{OH}}{CH}-CO-N_3}$$

$$\underset{\text{(b)}}{N_3-OC-H_2C-HN-OC-\underset{\overset{|}{OH}}{CH}-\underset{\overset{|}{OH}}{CH}-CO-NH-CH_2-CO-N_3}$$

(71)

$$\underset{\text{(c)}}{N_3OC-(CH_2)_5-HN-CO-\underset{\overset{|}{OH}}{CH}-\underset{\overset{|}{OH}}{CH}-CO-NH(CH_2)_5-CO-N_3}$$

$$N_3OC-(CH_2)_2HNOC \diagdown \text{(ring)} \diagup CONH(CH_2)_2-CON_3$$

(d)

$$CONH(CH_2)_2-CON_3$$

5. Carboxyl-Group Activating Reagents

In cross-linking by carboxyl-group activating reagents, unlike the approach in the preceding section, derivatives with activated carboxyl groups are not isolated. The activated carboxyl groups are usually on the protein and not on a reagent. The carboxyl-group activation and the cross-linking are carried out in a single-step reaction. Carboxyl-group activation by water-soluble *carbodiimides* and *isoxazolium* salts has already been discussed in detail (Section IVD2). The reaction can introduce intramolecular cross-links between an activated carboxyl and a favorably placed amino group. Reaction on concentrated protein solutions will introduce intermolecular cross-links.

6. Isocyanates and Isothiocyanates

Diisocyanates, such as *toluene-2,4-diisocyanate* (72a), *m-xylelene diisocyanate* (72b), and *3-methoxydiphenylmethane-4,4'-diisocyanate* (72c) have been used to conjugate ferritin or bovine serum albumin to antibody (Schick and Singer, 1961; Singer and Schick, 1961). The coupling with reagent (72a) can be carried out in two steps since the —NCO group in position 4 is more reactive than the group in position 2. The reagent has been employed in the preparation of antigen–erythrocyte conjugates for passive hemagglutination tests (Gyenes and Sehon, 1965). Other reagents in this class of compounds include *azophenyldiisocyanate* and *azophenyldiisothiocyanate* derivatives (73a and 73b) and others with longer aromatic

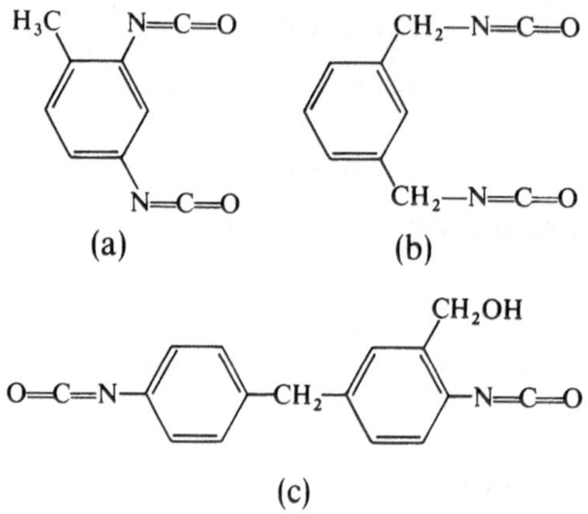

$$(72)$$

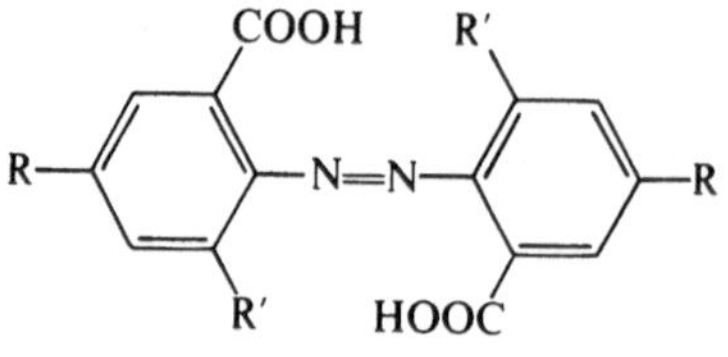

(a)   (b)

(c)

(a) R = —N=C=O or —N=C=S

R′ = H (73)

(b) R = H; R′ = —N=C=O

spacings between the reactive groups (Fasold *et al.*, 1971). The selectivity features of cyanates have been discussed (Section IVA13). Isothiocyanates, although known primarily as NH_2 group reagents, can also modify thiol, imidazole, and aliphatic and phenolic hydroxyl groups.

7. Cross-Linking by Thiol-Selective Reagents

It has already been mentioned that *divalent mercury* can form S—Hg—S bridges (Section IVG3). *Organic dimercurials* can be utilized for formation of cross-links through thiol groups. The most suitable procedures for cross-link formation through thiol groups have been compounds with two maleimide groups. *N,N′-o-Phenylenedimaleimide, N,N′-p-phenylenedimaleimide* (74a), and *N,N′-m-phenylenedimaleimide* (Moor and Ward, 1956) have been used extensively. Some examples of recent applications include the cross-linking of ribosomal proteins (Chang and Flaks, 1972), of the essential sulfhydryl groups in myosin (Reisler *et al.*, 1974), and of the subunits

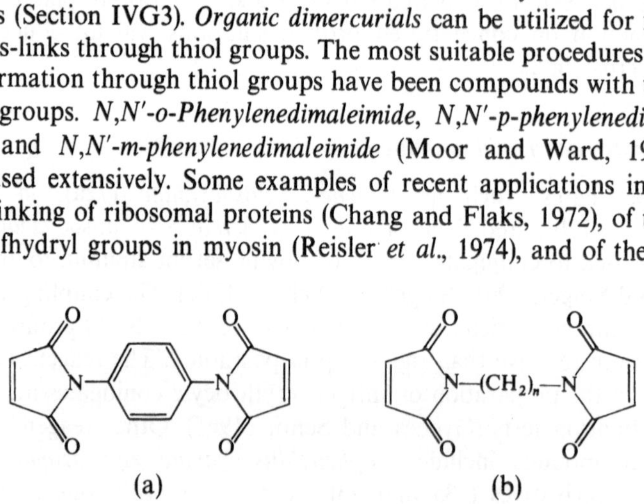

$$(74)$$

(a)   (b)

of *E. coli* succinic thiokinase (Teherani and Nishimura, 1975). *Alkyl dimaleimides* of varying chain lengths (74b) have also been employed in cross-linking studies (Fasold *et al.*, 1971; Wold, 1972). Selectivity properties of maleimides have already been discussed in detail (see Section IVG5). *Dihaloacetyl* compounds have also been used as cross-linking alkylating agents. The azodihaloacetamide benzene derivatives (75a) (Fasold *et al.*, 1964) have been used to cross-link hemoglobin subunits through both thiol and amino groups (Fasold *et al.*, 1971). The *diiodoacetamide compounds* (75b) have been used to effect cross-links, mostly between thiol groups, in rabbit muscle aldolase (Ozawa, 1967).

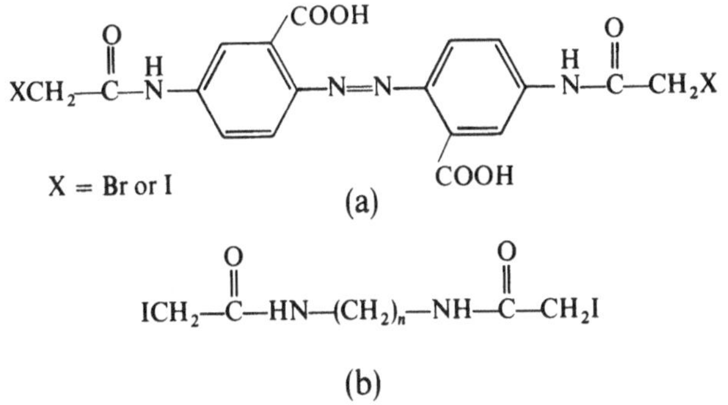

$$XCH_2-\overset{\overset{O}{\|}}{C}-\overset{H}{N}-\text{(benzene ring, COOH)}-N=N-\text{(benzene ring, COOH)}-\overset{H}{N}-\overset{\overset{O}{\|}}{C}-CH_2X$$

X = Br or I

(a)

(75)

$$ICH_2-\overset{\overset{O}{\|}}{C}-HN-(CH_2)_n-NH-\overset{\overset{O}{\|}}{C}-CH_2I$$

(b)

The bifunctional reagent *dibromoacetone* has been employed to study neighbor relationships of some thiol and imidazole groups in several plant proteases (Husain and Lowe, 1968). With glyceraldehyde 3-phosphate dehydrogenase, dibromoacetone acted mainly as a monofunctional alkylating agent for the essential thiol groups (Moore and Fenselau, 1972a). Selectivity properties of haloacetyl compounds have been discussed (Section IVG4).

8. Other Cross-Linking Reagents

2,4-*Dinitro*-1,5-*phenyldisulfenyl chloride* has been developed to introduce intertryptophan cross-links, and it will also cross-link thiol groups (Veronese *et al.*, 1970). With glucagon, it gave a dimer in which the molecules were linked through the single tryptophan residue. The dicarboxaldehyde 2-*nor*-2-*formylpyridoxal* 5'-*phosphate* has been developed for exploring the spatial relationships of amino acid side chains at the pyridoxal 5'-phosphate site in glycogen phosphorylase and other enzymes (Pocker, 1973). A series of *bisbiotinyl diamines* with varying chain lengths were designed to cross-link subunits of avidin *noncovalently* through their binding sites (Green, 1967; Green *et al.*, 1971). *Benzoquinone*, which has been used for covalent attachment of proteins to polysaccharide (Brandt *et al.*, 1975), can probably be applied for the purpose of cross-linking proteins because of its ability to

$$\text{Seph—OH} \xrightarrow{\text{CNBr}} \text{Seph—O—C} \equiv \text{N} \xrightarrow{\text{Prot}_1\text{—NH}_2} \text{Seph—O} \overset{\overset{\displaystyle +\text{NH}_2}{\|}}{\text{C}} \text{—NH—Prot}_1$$

(a)

$$\xrightarrow{\text{Prot}_2\text{—NH}_2} \text{Seph—OH} + \text{Prot}_2\text{—NH} \overset{\overset{\displaystyle \text{HN}}{\|}}{\text{C}} \text{—NH—Prot}_1 \qquad (76)$$

(b)

undergo a 2,5-disubstitution. The reaction will involve NH_2, SH, and phenolic OH groups (Morrison et al., 1969). A novel cross-linking reaction (76) has been reported in which bovine serum albumin released insulin from Sepharose-linked insulin (76a). As a result, insulin and albumin were, most likely, cross-linked (76b) through an N_1,N_2-disubstituted guanidine (Wilchek et al., 1975). Cross-linking reagents with long hydrophobic backbones tend to denature proteins. The preparation of longer reagents containing hydrophilic proline chains on an azophenyl center, and in which the carboxyl groups of the two end proline residues were activated to their azide, has been reported (Wetz et al., 1974). The cross-links could be reductively cleaved by dithionite.

L. Affinity-Labeling (Active-Site-Directed) Reagents

In the affinity-labeling approach, a protein, which binds a given molecule at a specific active site, is made to interact with an analogue of the molecule that carries a reactive functional group. The reactive functional group can then react with a contact amino acid at or near the active site. Following its introduction (Jansen et al., 1949; Schaffer et al., 1954) and revival (Baker et al., 1961; Schoellman and Shaw, 1962; Lawson and Schramm, 1962; Wofsy et al., 1962), the approach has proved to be versatile and extremely powerful for labeling protein active sites. Although the vast majority of the applications have been in chemical studies of active sites of various enzymes, it has in recent years been employed to study the combining sites of antibodies. Affinity labeling therefore is an extensive subject and its detailed analysis is not within the scope of this chapter. Several reviews on the subject (Baker, 1967; Singer, 1967; Shaw, 1970) and on site-specific reagents for serine proteases (Shaw, 1972) and for triosephosphate isomerase (Hartman, 1972) have appeared.

This section will deal briefly with the various reactive functional groups that may be employed for covalent labeling and the examples cited will demonstrate the effectiveness of the technique and the versatility of the systems that may be investigated by it. Results from the studies of antibody combining sites are obviously of direct relevance to immunochemistry of proteins. However, enzyme active-site-directed reagents are also extremely useful since they provide a route for chemical modification of a strategic location on the enzyme and determination of the effect of this, usually singular, modification on its immunochemistry.

A variety of reactive functional groups have been incorporated into analogues of different natural binding molecules. Their chemical nature is designed to meet the specificity requirements of the protein active site.

1. Alkylating and Acylating Agents

Alkyl halide functional groups may be used. For example, *β-chloro*-L-*alanine* inactivated L-aspartate β-decarboxylase and covalently labeled the enzyme (Tate *et al.*, 1969). 4-*Bromocrotonate*, acting as a substrate analogue, inactivated fumarase (Bradshaw *et al.*, 1969*b*). Other acylating and alkylating agents have been used as affinity labels. *Acetyl phosphate* and *p-nitrophenyl-acetate* acetylated a thiol group (Harris *et al.*, 1963) and an ε-NH_2 group (Mathew *et al.*, 1965) in rabbit muscle 3-phosphoglyceraldehyde dehydrogenase. At pH 8.5, *S*-acetyl group migration was observed via an S–N transfer reaction which was prevented by DPN (Mathew *et al.*, 1967). *Quinacillin* has been used to label covalently the active site of penicillinase from *S. aureus* (Virden *et al.*, 1975). Reaction of quinacillin was by the β-lactam carboxyl group and the enzyme was acylated predominantly at one or two amino groups. *Methyl p-nitrobenzenesulfonate* methylated a histidine (residue 57) in α-chymotrypsin and inactivated the enzyme (Nakagawa and Bender, 1970). Note that this reagent methylates thiol groups (Section IVG6). Firefly luciferose was inhibited slowly by the same reagent but more rapidly by a luciferin analogue, *ethyl 2-benzothiazolesulfonate*, presumably by alkylation of a histidine residue (White and Branchini, 1975).

Diisopropylfluorophosphate inhibition of a number of esterases was shown to be due to alkylphosphorylation (see reaction 67) of a unique serine residue (Schaffer *et al.*, 1954). A large number of serine esterases (e.g., chymotrypsin, trypsin, elastase, acetylcholinesterase, subtilisin) are inhibited by the reagent (Singer, 1967). The zymogens were believed to be unaffected. However, more recent work has shown that this active-site-directed reagent reacted with both trypsinogen and chymotrypsinogen and inhibited their potential enzymatic activities (Morgan *et al.*, 1972). In the case of trypsinogen, inhibition was due to alkyl-phosphorylation of a serine (residue 183) in the active site. "Side" reactions of this reagent have been discussed (Section IVJ7).

2. Haloacetyl Compounds

Haloacetyl or *halomethyl ketone* functional groups (i.e., $-COCH_2X$; X = Br or Cl) are more frequently used because of their higher reactivity. A bromoacetyl derivative of an immunochemically reactive peptide from performic acid oxidized bovine ribonuclease A was shown to link covalently with antibodies to oxidized ribonuclease at unidentified sites (Guldalian et al., 1965). A series of derivatives of the dinitrophenyl hapten, in which the bromoacetyl group was at increasing distances from the hapten, effected covalent labeling of antidinitrophenyl antibodies at tyrosine and lysine in a distribution that varied with the animal (Strausbauch et al., 1971). Subsequently, it was found that two types of antibodies were actually present, one reacting with the label exclusively through tyrosine and the other exclusively through lysine (Weinstein et al., 1973). The affinity labeling of anti-p-azobenzenearsonate antibodies with N-bromoacetylmono(p-azobenzenearsonic acid)-L-tyrosine suggested that lysine-N59 in the hypervariable region of the heavy chain may be a contact residue in the antibody combining site (Koo and Cebra, 1974). Antilactose antibodies were affinity-labeled by two bromoacetyl-lactose derivatives, also in the hypervariable region of the heavy chain (Gopalakrishnan and Karush, 1975). Reaction of a mouse myeloma protein having antidinitrophenyl activity with eight dinitrophenyl ligands, which carried bromoacetyl groups at increasing distances, showed that the site of labeling depended mainly on the length of the reagent (Givol et al., 1971). A unique tyrosine on the light chain and a unique lysine on the heavy chain were involved and could in fact be cross-linked by a bifunctional bisbromoacetyl dinitrophenyl compound of appropriate length. The labeled residues were in the hypervariable regions of the heavy chain (lysine-54) and of the light chain (tyrosine-34) (Haimovich et al., 1972).

In enzyme active-site studies, the chymotrypsin quasi-substrate p-nitrophenyl bromoacetyl-α-aminoisobutyrate formed an acylserine intermediate at the active site. The acylserine intermediate then enabled the bromoacetyl group to alkylate a methionine residue followed by hydrolysis of the ester bond, giving back serine and a partially active enzyme (Lawson and Schramm, 1962). A well-known reagent in this class of compounds is L-1-tosylamido-2-phenylethyl chloromethyl ketone, which inactivated α-chymotrypsin (Schoellman and Shaw, 1962) due to alkylation of a histidine (residue 57) at the active site (Ong et al., 1965). More recent work suggests that, in addition to histidine-57, other residues in the enzyme may react with the reagent (Blair et al., 1972). Another reagent, 1,4-dibromo-2-phenylacetoin, was shown to inhibit and alkylate α-chymotrypsin at histidine-57 (Schramm, 1967). The halomethyl ketone (1-chloro-3-tosylamido-7-amino-2-heptanone), which fulfills the specificity requirements of trypsin, inactivated the enzyme (Shaw et al., 1965) and alkylated a histidine (residue 46) in the active site (Shaw and Springhorn, 1967). Benzyloxycarbonyl-phenylalanine chloromethyl ketone met the specificity requirements of subtilisin and inactivated the enzyme, also by alkylation of a histidine residue (Shaw and

Ruscia, 1968). Similarly, carbobenzoxyphenylalanine bromomethyl ketone inactivated aspergillopeptidase B by alkylation of a histidine residue (Dworschack *et al.*, 1973). Peptide chloromethyl ketones have been developed as active-site-specific inhibitors of elastase (Powers and Tuhy, 1972; Thompson and Blout, 1973). Peptides terminating with *C*-terminal lysine chloromethyl ketone have been developed for affinity labeling of proteinases with tryptic specificity, such as subtilisin, thrombin, and plasma kallikrein (Coggins *et al.*, 1974). The structural analogues of NAD$^+$ and NADH, [3-(3-bromoacetylpyridinopropyl)]adenosine pyrophosphate and nicotinamide-[5-(bromoacetyl)-4-methylimidazole]dinucleotide have been shown to inhibit alcohol dehydrogenase (Woenckhaus *et al.*, 1970) through *S*-alkylation in both the yeast (Cys-43) and horse (Cys-174) enzymes (Jörnvall *et al.*, 1975). Carbamyl phosphate synthetase was shown to have a reactive cysteine residue at the glutamine binding site by affinity labeling with L-2-amino-4-oxo-5-chloropentanoic acid (Pinkus and Meister, 1972). 3-Bromo-2-butanone 1,4-biphosphate has been developed as an affinity label for ribulosebiphosphate carboxylase (Hartman *et al.*, 1973). Aspartate aminotransferase was inactivated and alkylated at a thiol group by bromopyruvate (Okamoto and Morino, 1973). Chloropyruvate inactivated *N*-acetylneuraminate lyase through alkylation of an active-site thiol group (Barnett and Kolisis, 1974). Triosephosphate isomerase was affinity-labeled by 3-chloroacetolphosphate (Davis *et al.*, 1973).

Examples of *N*-substituted α-bromoacetamides are found in the affinity labeling of α-chymotrypsin (Schramm and Lawson, 1963; Bittner and Gerig, 1970). *N*-Bromoacetylethanolamine phosphate labeled a histidine residue in rabbit muscle aldolase (Hartman and Welch, 1974). *N*-Bromoacetylacetazolamide caused histidine modification in human and bovine carbonic anhydrase (Wong *et al.*, 1972; Cybulsky *et al.*, 1973). *N*-Bromoacetyl-β-D-galactosylamine reversibly alkylated a methionine residue in β-glactosidase (Naider *et al.*, 1972). Carboxypeptidase B was modified at a glutamic acid (residue 270) by *N*-bromoacetyl-*N*-methyl-L-phenylalanine (Hass *et al.*, 1972) or by *N*-bromoacetyl-D-arginine (Kimmel and Plummer, 1972). On the other hand, bromoacetyl-*p*-aminobenzylsuccinic acid was shown to label a methionine residue (Zisapel and Sokolovsky, 1974). Deoxyribonucleic acid dependent RNA polymerase from *E. coli* was affinity-labeled by the pseudosubstrate, 6-methyl-thioinosinedicarboxyaldehyde, at ε-amino groups (Nixon *et al.*, 1972). An analogue of the antibiotic rifamycin (which binds to RNA polymerase and inhibits bacterial RNA synthesis), 3-(2-bromo[1-^{14}C]acetamidoethyl)-thio-rifamycin SV, was shown to label covalently DNA-dependent RNA polymerase (Stender *et al.*, 1975). The site of label has not been identified. An *N*-bromoacetyl analogue of puromycin has been used to identify components of *E. coli* ribosomes situated in the active site for the peptidyl transferase function of the ribosome (Greenwell *et al.*, 1974). One of the early affinity labels, 4-iodoacetamido-salicylate, was devised as an active-site-directed reagent for glutamate dehydrogenase (Baker *et al.*, 1961) and the inactivation has been attributed to a lysine modification (Holbrook *et al.*, 1973), a cysteine modification (Malcolm and Radda, 1970), or more convincingly a methionine modification (Rosen *et al.*, 1973).

3. Diazonium Salts

Diazonium functional groups have been employed in the design of a variety of affinity labels. Early experiments with *p*-(arsonic acid)benzene-diazonium fluoroborate and antibenzenearsonic acid antibodies demon-strated the presence of tyrosine residues in the active site of the antibody (Wofsy *et al.*, 1962), and these residues were located on both heavy and light chains (Metzger *et al.*, 1964). It was subsequently shown that the extent of labeling and the nature of the modified residues in rabbit anti-bodies varied with the preparation (Koyama *et al.*, 1968). Significantly, one antibody population was able to bind the label but was not modified by it. Affinity labeling of rabbit and mouse antidinitrophenyl antibodies with *m*-nitrobenzenediazonium fluoroborate again effected tyrosine modi-fication in the variable region and implicated both heavy and light chains (Thorpe and Singer, 1969). In porcine antibodies of similar specificity, the reagent also labeled tyrosine residues on light and heavy chains and the modified tyrosines in the heavy chains were identified at positions 33 and 93 (Franek, 1971), which situates them in the hypervariable region. Also, in guinea pig antibodies of this specificity, the affinity label modified tyrosine residues in the hypervariable region of the heavy chain (Ray and Cebra, 1972). *m*-Nitrobenzenediazonium fluoroborate labeled a mouse myeloma IgA with nitrophenyl binding activity at a tyrosine residue in the variable region of the light chain (Goetzl and Metzger, 1970). Another mouse my-eloma IgA which had a phosphorylcholine-binding activity was affinity-labeled with *p*-diazonium phenylphosphorylcholine (Chesebro and Metzger, 1972) at a tyrosine residue in the light chain. The azotyrosines in the two affinity-labeled myeloma proteins were reduced by dithionite to 3-amino-tyrosine, which were cross-linked to other amino acids by difluorodinitro-benzene (Hadler and Metzger, 1973).

Diazonium salts have also been employed as affinity labels in enzyme studies such as diazotized 5'-(4-aminophenyl-phosphoryl)uridine 2'(3')-phosphate for modifying ribonuclease A (at tyrosine-73) (Gorecki *et al.*, 1971). α-Chymotrypsin was inhibited by active-site-directed diazonium compounds and *p*-diazo-*N*-acetyl-L-phenylalanine labeled a tyrosine (resi-due 146) in the enzyme (Yoshida *et al.*, 1973).

4. Epoxy Compounds

Epoxy groups have been incorporated in active-site-directed reagents. A series of irreversible inhibitors were first designed for lysozyme (Thomas *et al.*, 1969). These were the *2',3'-epoxypropyl β-glycosides* of N-acetylglucosamine or its $\beta(1 \to 4)$-linked dimers and trimers. In reaction with lysozyme, they were linked by an ester linkage to aspartic acid-52 in the enzyme (Moult *et al.*, 1973; Eshdat *et al.*, 1973). Borohydride reduction converted the ester bond to homoserine, yielding a catalytically inactive enzyme which was nevertheless still capable of binding saccharide inhibitors of the enzyme (Eshdat *et al.*, 1974). This was a convincing chemical demonstration of the catalytic role of aspartic acid-52. Epoxide affinity labels have been used to inactivate pepsin (Tang, 1971) and penicillopepsin (Mains and Hofmann, 1974) and in each case the reagent was esterified to an aspartic acid side chain.

5. Reagents with Other Functional Groups

Alkyl isocynates were proposed as general active-site-directed reagents because of their broad reactivity and the fact that many enzymes act on substrates containing aliphatic chains (Twu and Wold, 1973). Butyl isocyanate inactivated yeast alcohol dehydrogenase by *S*-butylcarbamoylation of three cysteine residues in the enzyme (Twu and Wold, 1973). The reagent also inactivated α-chymotrypsin and elastase, effecting *O*-butylcarbamoylation of a serine residue in each enzyme (Brown and Wold, 1973). *Cyanoalkyl* derivatives have also been used as substrate analogues. An example is the modification of the tryptophan synthetase tetramer or its β_2 subunits by α-cyanoglycine (Miles, 1975).

Mixed disulfide formation has been used as a basis for covalent labeling by active-site reagents. A purine disulfide analogue of ATP, 6,6'-dithiobis-(inosinyl imidodiphosphate), removed the ATPase activity of myosin and formed mixed disulfides with two cysteine residues per head (Wagner and Yount, 1975).

N-Bromosuccinimide, a compound which reacts with many protein functional groups (Sections IVI1, VIIE, VIII, and VIIJ) has been used as an analogue for the intermediate of L-asparaginase from *E. coli* (Menge and Jaenicke, 1974). Inactivation was attributed to the modification of two tyrosines and one histidine, and the modification was detected spectrophotometrically and fluorophotometrically. The nonselectivity of the reagent, the methods employed in detection of the modification, and the accompanying conformational changes make conclusions concerning active-site residues uncertain.

3-Amino-1:2:4-triazole inactivated catalase (Agrawal *et al.*, 1970) and bovine lactoperoxidase (Chang and Schroeder, 1973) when they were in the enzyme–H_2O_2 form. In catalase, only a histidine (residue 74) was modified (Agrawal et al., 1970; Chang and Schroeder, 1972), while in lactoperoxidase two histidine residues and four or five tyrosine residues were lost (Chang and Schroeder, 1973).

p-Nitrophenylcarbamyl-methionyl-tRNA (formylatable, methionine specific) was reported to act as an affinity label in binding to E. coli ribosomes (Hauptmann et al., 1974). It was shown to label primarily protein L27 in the 50 S ribosomal subunit.

6. Reactive Species Generated at the Active Site

In the generation of reactive species at the active site, the reagent carries a functional group whose reactivity is generated at the active site by enzymatic action of the enzyme on the reagent. Alternatively, the reagent, having been situated in the enzyme (or protein) active site, is then subjected to a mild activating step which converts a previously nonreactive group to a very reactive species. The latter procedure is therefore suitable for probing active sites not only of enzymes but also of other proteins with binding activity (e.g., antibodies, antigens, and hormones). Also, the broad reactivity of the species enables it to label any contact group. On the other hand, in the preceding reagents labeling is determined by the type of reactions in which the functional group is potentially able to participate and the label therefore will be attached only if an appropriate residue is within binding distance. Generation of the reactive group in situ avoids side reactions that may be encountered with reagents carrying an already reactive functional group. Furthermore, this highly specific labeling technique can, at least in principle, be employed to effect selective labeling of the desired protein in impure systems.

The generation of a reactive species by the action of the enzyme on the reagent has been exploited in the action of α-chymotrypsin on 2-acetoxy-5-nitrobenzyl chloride; it hydrolyzed the nitrophenyl ester and released the tryptophan-modifying reagent, 2-hydroxy-5-nitrobenzyl chloride (see Section IV I3), which then modified tryptophan residues in the vicinity of the active site (Horton and Young, 1969). The reagent showed no reaction with chymotrypsinogen, diisopropylphosphoryl chymotrypsin, or serum albumin. 2-Chloromethyl-4-nitrophenyl(N-carbobenzoxy)glycinate was developed to label the active site of papain (Mole and Horton, 1973a). A single tryptophan was modified and the enzyme showed enhanced catalytic efficiency (Mole and Horton, 1973b). The p-nitrophenolic label also served as an environmentally sensitive conformational probe near the active site. Inhibition of β-hydroxydecanoyl thioester dehydrase by 3-decynoyl-N-acetylcysteamine proceeded through isomerization by the enzyme of the acetylene to an allene, which then alkylated a histidine residue in the active site (Bloch, 1969). Monoamine oxidase induced conversion of the chemically unreactive 3-bromoallylamine to a highly reactive intermediate which was generated at the active site, and the compound inhibited the enzyme irreversibly (Rando, 1973).

Diazoacetyl ($-CO-CHN_2$) derivatives, incorporated into the active site, when followed by photolysis yield the highly reactive carbene ($-CO-\ddot{C}H$), which could then insert into *any* contact groups (Singh *et al.*, 1962). Several amino acids (including alanine) in the active site have been modified by photolyzation of diazoacetyl and diazomalonyl chymotrypsin, trypsin (Shafer *et al.*, 1966; Hexter and Westheimer, 1971), and more recently diazoacetyl subtilisin (Stefanovsky and Westheimer, 1973). It is relevant here to mention that diazoketones (Fry *et al.*, 1968) and diazoacetyl amino acid derivatives (Delpierre and Fruton, 1966) inactivated pepsin by esterification of a β-carboxyl group in the enzyme (Fry *et al.*, 1968; Bayliss and Knowles, 1968; Bayliss *et al.*, 1969). The reaction was greatly facilitated by Cu(II) or Ag(I), probably because of the formation of a metal-complexed carbene ($-CO-CH=Cu^{2+}$) intermediate (Lundblad and Stein, 1969). Other *N*-diazoacetyl compounds have been shown to inactivate pepsin (Stepanov *et al.*, 1968) and acid proteases (Kovaleva *et al.*, 1972; Liu and Hatano, 1974) through Cu(II)-catalyzed esterification of the β-carboxyl group of a unique aspartic acid residue. In these studies, the diazoacetyl compounds were not used as photogenerated reagents.

Aryl azides ($Ar-N_3$) have been devised as nonreactive precursors from which, after binding of the reagent in the active site, photolysis (300 nm) of the conjugate generated a highly reactive aryl nitrene ($Ar-\ddot{N}$) at the active site (Fleet *et al.*, 1969). These reagents, as originally proposed (Fleet *et al.*, 1969), should prove extremely useful in the study of antibody combining sites to aryl azide haptens since the potential reactive group (i.e., $-N_3$) would be included in the determinant to which antibody specificity is directed. This avoids complications inherent in the studies which employed haloacetyl or diazonium compounds where the reactive group was not part of the determinant in the hapten. Rabbit antibodies to the hapten ε-4-azido-2-nitrophenyl L-lysine were affinity-labeled by photolysis of the antibody–hapten complex (Press *et al.*, 1971). The label (mostly in the heavy chain) was located in the hypervariable region, possibly on cystine-97 and alanine-98. A mouse IgA myeloma protein, with binding activity toward the 2,4-dinitrophenyl group, was labeled (after photolysis) with 2,4-dinitrophenylalanyl diazoketone predominantly in the light chain on the ε-NH_2 of lysine-54 (Hew *et al.*, 1973). On the other hand, 2,4-dinitrophenyl azide, which labeled mostly the heavy chain and the small amount of label in the light chain, was identified at many sites within the hypervariable regions (Hew *et al.*, 1973).

Aryl azides have also been employed in enzyme studies. The active site of glutamate dehydrogenase was labeled by the competitive inhibitors 2-azidoisophthalic acid and 5-azidoisophthalic acid by photolysis of the enzyme–inhibitor complex (White and Yielding, 1973). The aromatic-binding site of α-chymotrypsin was labeled by photolysis of acyl chymotrypsin from reaction with the p-nitrophenyl ester of p-azidocinnamate (Bridges and Knowles, 1974). In order to investigate the ribosomal binding site of chloramphenicol, an analogue of the latter, 4-denitro-4-azido-chloramphenicol, has been prepared (Seela and Cramer, 1975).

7. Bifunctional Reagents

In principle, a bifunctional reagent would be quite valuable for cross-linking residues within, or near, the active site. In the design of the reagent, the active-site-directed part carries two reactive groups which may be identical or they may differ. Only a few bifunctional reagents have been used successfully. For example, 1,3-dibromoacetone was used to cross-link the catalytic histidine and cysteine residues at the active sites of bromelin, papain, and ficin (Husain and Lowe, 1968, 1970). Two bifunctional reagents were designed to study the active site of pepsin (Husain et al., 1971). One bisdiazoketone reagent which carried two identical reactive groups, 1,1-bis(diazoacetyl)-2-phenylethane, inactivated pepsin stoichiometrically and was more efficient than the dl-1-bromo-1-diazoacetyl-2-phenylethane analogue. A mouse IgA myeloma protein with anti-2,4-dinitrophenyl activity was cross-linked in the vicinity of its binding site by a bisbromoacetyl derivative of the 2,4-dinitrophenyl ligand between a tyrosine on the light chain and a lysine on the heavy chain (Givol et al., 1971). There is evidence that 1,5-difluoro-2,4-dinitrobenzene may also act in part as a bifunctional affinity-labeling reagent for the same myeloma protein (Hadler and Metzger, 1973).

8. Concluding Remarks

Selectivity of site-directed reagents carrying a reactive group increases with decrease in dissociation constant. However, its ability to effect a covalent modification is determined by the type of reactions in which the reactive moiety is able to participate, and also by the presence of a suitable amino acid side chain in the vicinity of the binding site within bonded distance. If these conditions do not obtain, labeling cannot take place. An example of this was provided in the finding that a population of antibenzene-arsonic antibodies was able to bind the label p-(arsonic acid)benzene-diazonium fluoroborate, but underwent no covalent modification (Koyama *et al.*, 1968). When labeling takes place, the chemical properties of the reactive moiety on the reagent restrict the versatility of the approach and yield limited information. For example, diazonium affinity labels have labeled almost exclusively at tyrosine residues in antibodies, myeloma proteins, and enzymes (see Section IVL3). Bromoacetyl compounds have shown a little better versatility and have labeled antibodies and myeloma proteins at tyrosine or lysine residues. With enzymes, these reagents labeled mostly at histidine and in fewer cases at cysteine and methionine residues (see Section IVL2). The findings that either a tyrosine or a lysine is labeled in antibodies of different specificities clearly indicates that these residues may not be involved in the antigen-binding specificity of the antibody. They are, however, close to the binding site but not implicated in the binding process. This is a critical distinction when one aspires to understand antibody specificity and the amino acid residues expressing this specificity. The results nevertheless are useful for the evaluation of the total environment around the binding site, but underscore the limitations of the technique.

Of course, it should be mentioned here that when a reagent can act as an affinity label for more than one enzyme, it need not react covalently with the same type of amino acid side chain in the various enzymes. An example may be found in *p*-bromophenacyl bromide. The reagent was reported to alkylate a methionine in α-chymotrypsin (Schramm and Lawson, 1963), esterify the β-COOH group of an aspartic acid in pepsin (Erlanger *et al.*, 1966; Gross and Morell, 1966), and alkylate a histidine residue in the active site of phospholipase A_2 (Volwerk *et al.*, 1974). Such results are reassuring because they indicate that the modification is indeed determined by the type of contact amino acids and the environment of the active site where the reactive analogue is bound.

In this approach, therefore, it is desirable that the reactive moiety should have little or no selectivity and it should be highly reactive so that it can modify *any* contact amino acid. This obviously will introduce complications of possible nonselective modifications outside the active site. The photogenerated reagents (diazoacetates and aryl azides) provide perhaps the best available solution to this problem since the highly reactive species is generated mildly by photolysis *after* the reagent is bound in the active site (Section IVL6). The reactive species has the ability even to insert in a C—H bond and alanine modifications have been reported. Further applications of these labels, either as monofunctional or as bifunctional reagents, should provide important information on antibody and enzyme active sites. Identification of the labeled site should be made easier by the approach developed by Givol *et al.* (1970) in which the labeled peptide can be isolated by exploiting the natural affinity of the native protein to the ligand on the peptide. As methodology improves and reactive species gain in versatility, valuable and critical information should be derived from active-site-directed reagents. A good way to probe the active site of a given protein is to design several reagents directed toward the *same* active site but carrying *different* reactive moieties.

PART B: CHEMICAL CLEAVAGE REACTIONS

V. Usefulness, Limitations, and Evaluation of the Results

The antigenic structure of a protein cannot be completely elucidated through chemical modification studies alone. An advantage in the study of protein antigens (which cannot be obtained in the study of active sites of enzymes) is that if an antigenic reactive site can be isolated as part of a peptide fragment, the latter *may* interact with antibodies to the native protein. Therefore, the isolation and characterization of immunochemically reactive peptides should make a substantial contribution to the enormous task of delineation of the antigenic reactive sites of a protein. Unfortunately, this approach is not without its shortcomings. These limitations have previously been outlined (Atassi, 1975) and will be mentioned here for the sake of completion.

1. Purity of the peptide is of critical importance in immunochemical studies. A minor component may be immunochemically more potent than the major component. In many cases, a fragment may give an immune precipitate (e.g., see Atassi and Saplin, 1968) while a smaller overlapping fragment may inhibit (Atassi and Singhal, 1970a). The presence of the two fragments in a mixture will only complicate the investigations. Other serious situations can be envisaged. The peptide should be carefully purified and subjected to all the criteria of purity. This precaution should really never be compromised.

2. An isolated peptide will not exist appreciably in the conformation it had in the native protein (Atassi and Saplin, 1968; Singhal and Atassi, 1970; Atassi and Singhal, 1970b). The immune response to native protein antigens is directed against their native three-dimensional structure (Atassi and Thomas, 1969). For proper binding with antibody, an antigenic reactive site must achieve its native mode of folding (Atassi, 1967d, 1970; Atassi and Saplin, 1968; Habeeb and Atassi, 1971b). This question is discussed in detail in Chapter 2. As previously pointed out (Atassi, 1975), it is often possible for antibody to induce in a peptide the appropriate conformation necessary for binding with the antibody combining site. Another complication, which we observed during the course of our delineation

of the antigenic structure of myoglobin, is that attachment of bulky amino acids which occur in the natural sequence to the appropriate end of synthetic antigenic reactive sites frequently exerted some steric obstruction and reduced the binding considerably (Koketsu and Atassi, 1974a,b; Atassi and Pai, 1975). As a result the *longer* peptide in those cases *inhibited less* than the *shorter* peptide, contrary to the "normal" phenomenon. This situation may inadvertently obtain in fragmentation, and conceivably a peptide with low inhibitory ability may erroneously be dismissed as insignificant.

3. Cleavage of a protein may take place *within* a reactive region (Atassi, 1972), effecting dissection of the reactive region into two (or more) parts carried on different peptides. This will cause the loss of most (or all) of the immunochemical reactivity by one (or both) of the two dissected parts of the region (Atassi, 1972). This is an extremely serious limitation which is invariably ignored. Before subjecting the protein to cleavage at a given site (or sites), it is critical to ensure that this site (or sites) is not part of an antigenic reactive site in the protein (Atassi and Saplin, 1968; Singhal and Atassi, 1971). This should be done by prior immunochemical studies of appropriate derivatives of the intact native protein that had been modified at these sites (Atassi and Saplin, 1968; Atassi, 1972, 1975). Clearly, indiscriminate enzymatic cleavage at multiple sites (e.g., by chymotrypsin or trypsin) will yield only limited information which may even be confusing.

4. When positive results are obtained with a given peptide, the results are useful. As a general rule (which may have some exceptions; see 1 above), further delineation of reactive sites in a peptide should not be attempted by shortening the peptide, as is often done by many investigators. It has already been shown (Atassi and Saplin, 1968) that shortening a reactive peptide may lead to erroneous conclusions because of the inherent limitations of the technique. The shortened peptide may not be able to assume the necessary mode of folding for binding with antibody, even though the segment removed may not be part of a reactive region (Atassi and Saplin, 1968).

5. Although peptides in general are more unfolded than the native protein, it is often desirable to study the conformation of the resultant peptides. When this is done, the results could be quite helpful in interpretation of the immunochemical findings (Singhal and Atassi, 1970; Atassi and Singhal, 1970b).

The foregoing complications and limitations make it necessary, in order to achieve the correct conclusions, that a reactive region be isolated as part of several different overlapping peptides (Atassi, 1972). Because of the complexity of the task and the limitations of each approach, it is absolutely necessary to delineate accurately the nonreactive regions as well as the reactive regions.

VI. Choice of Reaction

For selective cleavage at a given amino acid location, many reactions
are often available and the proper choice of reaction is critical. The following
criteria ought to be taken into account in chemical cleavage.

1. The cleavage reaction should not have side reactions that cause
internal modifications in the resultant peptide. The presence of internal
modifications, often ignored, will render the immunochemical studies
difficult to interpret or even meaningless. Conditions of the cleavage reaction may often lead to undesirable complications. For example, strong
alkali conditions necessary for certain cleavage reactions will result in
alkaline hydrolysis of disulfide bonds (Section IVH8) and can often lead
to indiscriminate cleavage of peptide bonds. Certain reaction conditions
give poor yields because of insolubility of the resultant peptides, especially
when these fragments are considerable in size.

2. Optimum conditions for maximum cleavage by a given reaction
will usually vary with the protein. They are influenced by the unique structure of each protein and the availability of the potential sites of cleavage
to reaction. The nature and extent of side reactions that may cause internal
modification or undesirable cleavage are also dependent on the protein.
Therefore, a general procedure cannot usually be adopted for a given
reaction. For the best results in most of these reactions, each protein will
have to be studied independently in order to determine the most suitable
conditions for its cleavage. Often, the conditions will be a compromise
between maximum cleavage and minimum side reactions.

3. To achieve complete cleavage at given amino acid residues, it is
often necessary to resort to conditions that will increase the occurrence
of side reactions. This is in fact unnecessary, since partial cleavage at a
given location will give the respective overlapping peptides which are extremely useful for immunochemical studies.

4. Occasionally, the selection of a cleavage reaction will give one (or
more) peptide which is insoluble due to its particular composition and
structure. In order to obtain immunochemical information about that
insoluble region, it is necessary to isolate it as part of other peptides by
employing reactions which will cleave at other locations.

VII. Cleavage Reactions

Of the reactions that are now available for chemical cleavage of proteins, only a few achieve a high degree of selectivity. Nonselective modifications or cleavages that accompany the other reactions vary in extensiveness.

Many of the reactions are so drastic that they are not in fact useful for selective protein cleavage and have been demonstrated only on carefully selected model peptides. In the following section, emphasis will be placed on reactions which in the author's experience have been more useful in immunochemical studies. A comprehensive and excellent review that included all types of chemical cleavage reactions has appeared (Spande *et al.*, 1970). Many cleavage reactions are further extensions of modification reactions already discussed in the first half of the chapter. Reference to those reactions will be made at the appropriate places.

A. *N*-Terminal Removal

In immunochemical studies of proteins, it may occasionally be useful to remove an *N*-terminal residue with, preferably, no internal modification. Several procedures are available for removal of the *N*-terminal. This subject has been reviewed frequently (Start, 1970; Narita, 1970; Dixon and Fields, 1972). Only a brief mention of some of the procedures will be given here.

Transamination using glyoxylate in the presence of metal ion (Cu^{2+}, Co^{2+}, Ni^{2+}) has been shown (Dixon, 1964a,b) to effect removal of the *N*-terminal residue (for review, see Dixon and Fields, 1972). The removal of the *N*-terminal amino acid may also be accomplished (Collman and Buckingham, 1963) under mild conditions by *cis-hydroxoaquotriethylene-tetraminecobalt(III)*. However, side chains with ability to coordinate with cobalt may complicate the reaction (Buckingham *et al.*, 1967a). *Cyanate* and *phenylisothiocyanate* may be employed with some peptides that do not carry reactive side chains.

A different approach is the hydrolytic cleavage of *N*-terminal peptide bonds after reduction of 3,5-dinitropyridyl derivatives with sodium borohydride (Signor and Bordignon, 1968). Reaction with *2-chloro-3,5-dinitropyridine*, followed by reduction with borohydride under mild conditions that were not expected to reduce amide or disulfide bonds, yielded the tetrahydropyridyl derivatives. Quantitative, and seemingly exclusive, cleavage of the *N*-terminal peptide bond was obtained at pH 5–6. Aliphatic and phenolic OH groups were not modified. The reaction merits further investigation.

Other approaches to *N*-terminal cleavage have applied intramolecular aminolysis by reaction of the peptide (at pH 8–9) with *2-fluoro-3,5-dinitroaniline* (Kirk and Cohen, 1969). Cyclization of the aniline nucleophile with the carbonyl group of the first amino acid proceeded readily with concomitant scission of the first peptide bond. Cleavage of the *N*-terminal through lactam formation from a series of *o-aminophenoxy* groups on the amino end has also been investigated (Kirk and Cohen, 1972).

B. Cleavage at Carboxyl and Carboxamide Groups

Cleavage at *aspartyl* and *glutamyl* peptide bonds was reported via esterification of the carboxyl groups by methanol-HCl, reduction of the ester groups by $LiBH_4$ in tetrahydrofuran to the corresponding hydroxyl groups, followed by acidification to pH 1–2 (Burstein *et al.*, 1967). Cleavage was proposed to take place as a result of γ- and δ-lactone formation (77) from the newly formed hydroxyamino acid residues. Cleavage of the bonds Asp–Phe, Asp–Gly, and Glu–Phe was obtained in 16–43% yield in model peptides carrying only glycine or phenylalanine in addition to either aspartic acid or glutamic acid. Qualitative cleavage of aspartyl and glutamyl peptide bonds was detected in oxidized ribonuclease.

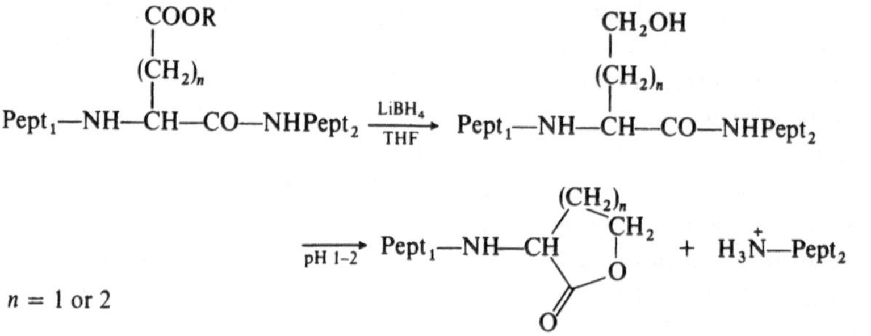

$$
\begin{array}{ccc}
\text{COOR} & & \text{CH}_2\text{OH}\\
| & & |\\
(\text{CH}_2)_n & & (\text{CH}_2)_n\\
| & \xrightarrow[\text{THF}]{\text{LiBH}_4} & |\\
\text{Pept}_1\text{—NH—CH—CO—NHPept}_2 & & \text{Pept}_1\text{—NH—CH—CO—NHPept}_2
\end{array}
$$

$$
\xrightarrow{\text{pH 1-2}} \quad \text{Pept}_1\text{—NH—CH} \overset{(\text{CH}_2)_n}{\underset{O}{\overset{\text{CH}_2}{\diagdown\diagup}}} \quad + \quad H_3\overset{+}{N}\text{—Pept}_2 \qquad (77)
$$

$n = 1$ or 2

This procedure suffers from all the shortcomings of the methanol-HCl reaction (Section IVD1) as well as those of the reduction by $LiBH_4$ (Section IVD3). It is best to perform the carboxyl group reduction directly in one step by diborane (Section IVD3). When myoglobin and lysozyme, which had been reduced at several carboxyl group sites by diborane, were subjected to pH 1–2 under a variety of conditions, no significant selective cleavage was obtained at the reduced carboxyl group sites (Rosemblatt and Atassi, unpublished results).

Asparagine peptide bonds were cleaved at the α-amino end by the Hofmann rearrangement followed by an alkaline treatment (Shiba *et al.*, 1968). In this reaction, asparagine residues were converted to imidazolidine derivatives by treatment with *sodium hypobromite* (Br_2/3NaOH) at 60°C. Following this cyclization, treatment of the product with an aqueous methanolic NaOH solution at room temperature gave cleavage in good yield of the Ala–Asn bond in the model peptide N-benzyloxycarbonyl-L-alanyl-L-asparagine. The corresponding glutamine peptide did not cyclize and therefore did not cleave. The reaction is interesting, but it is obvious that proteins cannot withstand the foregoing drastic treatment. Numerous modification and cleavage "side" reactions would take place.

Asparagine peptide bonds have been cleaved at the carboxyl end in reduced, S-carboxymethylated bovine ribonuclease with 2 M *hydroxyl-amine* at pH 9.0 (Bornstein and Balian, 1970). Cleavage was at the Asn-67–Gly-68 bond and to a minor extent at the Asn-34–Leu-35 bond. The reaction was proposed to proceed through cyclization of the asparagine to a cyclic imide derivative which was susceptible to nucleophilic attack by hydroxylamine. However, the mechanism and the general utility of the reaction are yet to be established.

Aspartic acid and asparagine peptide bonds are more susceptible to cleavage under conditions of partial acid hydrolysis (e.g., 0.25 M acetic acid or 0.03 M HCl, 105°C, few hours). Cleavage can take place at either side of aspartic acid or asparagine (for reviews, see Hill, 1965; Schultz, 1967).

C. Cleavage at Cysteine Peptide Bonds

Cleavage at the C^α–N^α bond of cysteine residues, followed by their oxidative removal at the carbonyl end, was effected by conversion of the cysteine residue to dehydroalanine and subsequent cleavage of the de-hydroalanine residue (Sokolovsky and Patchornik, 1963). Conversion of cysteine to dehydroalanine by β-elimination at alkaline pH of S-dinitro-phenyl derivatives has been described (see reaction 49, Section IVG6). Formation of dehydroalanine from S-dimethylsulfonium derivatives was found to proceed at a lower pH (8.5–9) than for the dinitrophenyl deriva-tive (0.1–0.5 N NaOH) (Sokolovsky et al., 1964). Cleavage at the dehydro-alanine sites was effected by oxidation with performic acid followed by oxidation with alkaline hydrogen peroxide (78a and 78c) (Sokolovsky and Patchornik, 1963).

$$\text{Pept}_1\text{—CONH—C—CONH—Pept}_2$$
$$\overset{\|}{\underset{\text{CH}_2}{}}$$

$$\xrightarrow[\text{(2) 0.1 N NaOH}]{\text{(1) HCO}_3\text{H}} \quad \text{Pept}_1\text{—CONH}_2 + \text{HOCH}_2\text{COCONH—Pept}_2 \quad \text{(a)}$$

$$\text{Pept}_1\text{—CONH—C—CONH—Pept}_2 \xrightarrow[\text{pH} < 7]{\text{Br}_2} \left[\text{Pept}_1\text{—CONH—}\overset{\text{Br}}{\underset{\text{CH}_2\text{Br}}{\text{C}}}\text{—CONH—Pept}_2 \right]$$

$$\xrightarrow{\text{pH} > 10} \left[\text{Pept}_1\text{—CONH—}\overset{\text{OH}}{\underset{\text{CH}_2\text{OH}}{\text{C}}}\text{—CONH—Pept}_2 \right] + 2\text{Br}^-$$

$$\longrightarrow \quad \text{Pept}_1\text{—CONH}_2 + \text{HOCH}_2\text{COCONH—Pept}_2 \quad \text{(b)}$$

$$\text{HOCH}_2\text{COCONH—Pept}_2 \xrightarrow[\text{0.1 N NaOH}]{\text{H}_2\text{O}_2} \text{H}_2\text{N—Pept}_2 + \text{CO}_2 + \text{HOCH}_2\text{COOH} \quad \text{(c)}$$

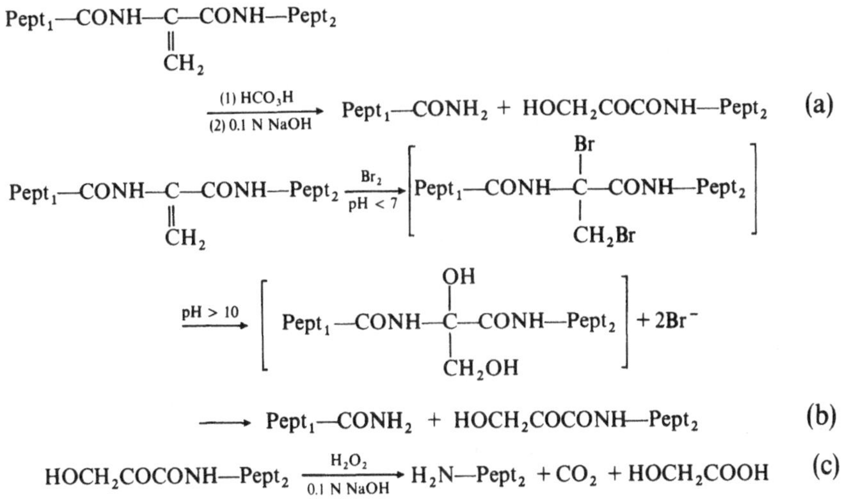

$$(78)$$

Alternatively, cleavage could be performed by oxidation with bromine (78b) followed by oxidation (78c) with alkaline hydrogen peroxide (Patchornik and Sokolovsky, 1964a) to remove the N-hydroxypyruvyl groups. The latter groups have also been removed by o,o'-diaminodiphenylamine at pH 3–6 (Degani and Patchornik, 1967). The approach was applied for cleavage of the Cys–Tyr and Cys–Pro bonds in oxytocin (Sokolovsky et al., 1964).

This cleavage procedure suffers from many problems. Side reactions of dehydroalanine with nucleophilic residues on the protein present a serious complication. The reaction of dehydroalanine with the ε-amino groups of lysine has been shown (Patchornik and Sokolovsky, 1964b) to give DL-α-amino-β(-ε-N-L-lysine)propionic acid, which eluted on the short column of the amino acid analyzer before lysine. For cleavage of ribonuclease, acetylation was necessary to avoid side reactions with amino groups (Sokolovsky and Patchornik, 1964). Permanent modification, such as the case with acetylation, precludes in most cases the usefulness of the peptides for subsequent immunochemical studies. Reversible protecting groups will not be stable under the alkaline conditions of the β-elimination and cleavage. In addition, hydrogen peroxide treatment at alkaline pH will oxidize many amino acid residues (Sections IVF1 and IVG1), giving peptides with extensive internal modification. Finally, the conditions of alkaline treatment in various steps of the reaction could give rise to indiscriminate peptide bond cleavage and disulfide bond hydrolysis (Section IVH8).

Chloroformate or *chlorothioformate* has been employed for the scission at the amino end of cysteine (Degani et al., 1966). Reaction of the two reagents with thiol groups around neutrality gave the aryloxycarbonyl or the arylthiocarbonyl derivatives, respectively. The latter formed (pH 8, 50°C) 3-acylthiazolidinone derivatives, which spontaneously hydrolyzed, resulting in an overall cleavage of the peptide bond involving the amino group of cysteine. This cleavage procedure is accompanied by extensive side reactions involving amino, hydroxyl, and carboxyl groups as well as formation of inter- and intramolecular cross-links. The procedure is not suitable for proteins if subsequent immunochemical studies of the fragments are intended.

Cyanogen bromide was utilized for cleavage at cysteine sites after methylation of the thiol groups (Gross and Morell, 1967). Methylation was originally accomplished by β-elimination of S-dinitrophenyl derivatives followed by reaction of the resultant dehydroalanine residues with methylmercaptan (see reaction 49, Section IVG6). However, methylation by methyl p-nitrobenzenesulfonate (Heinrikson, 1970, 1971) avoids the side reactions due to dehydroalanine formation and is therefore preferable. Reaction with cyanogen bromide is carried out at acid pH. The cleavage can be carried out at low temperature over several days of reaction via the oxazolinium bromide derivative, which hydrolyzes to give a serine peptide. Alternatively, it can be achieved more rapidly (about 1 hr) and with better yields at high (100°C) temperature, presumably through dehydro-alanine formation by β-elimination. The dehydroalanine site undergoes cleavage, giving a pyruvyl group at the N-terminal of the amino acid original-ly following cysteine (Gross *et al.*, 1967). The first route of cleavage is too slow and the yield is low, while the second route of cleavage will be ac-companied by side reactions due to dehydroalanine formation.

The method of choice for cleavage of cysteine peptide bonds is by *cyanylation* of the thiol group to β-thiocyanoalanine residues. Direct and selective S-cyanylation can be achieved by reaction with 2-*nitro-5-thio-cyanobenzoic acid* (Degani *et al.*, 1970) (see reaction 55, Section IVG10). The cleavage reaction was first envisaged by Degani *et al.* (1970) as a suit-able approach for cleavage at cysteine sites in the presence of cystine residues in the protein or peptide. Subsequently, cleavage has been shown to occur at the N-acyl bond of cyanylated cysteine residues by exposure to 6 M guanidine hydrochloride in 0.1 M sodium borate at pH 9.0 and 37°C for 12 hr (Jacobson *et al.*, 1973) or at pH 8 and 37–50°C (Degani and Patchor-nik, 1974). The cleavage reaction (79) resulted in the formation of 2-imino-thiazolidine-4-carboxyl peptides (79c) and it occurred by OH⁻ catalysis

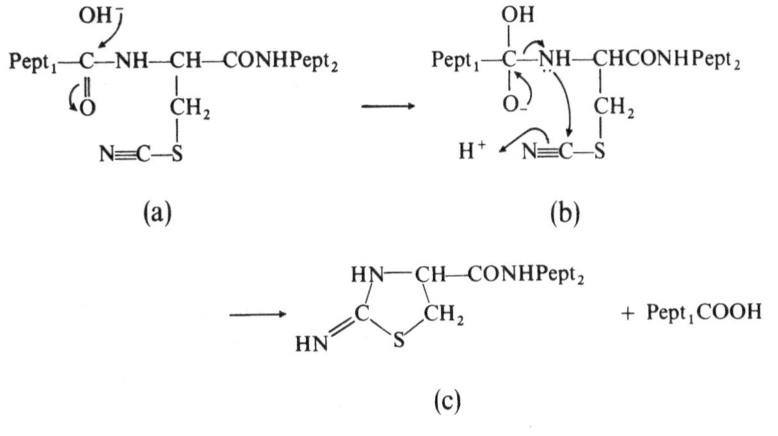

(a)   (b)

(c)

$+ \text{Pept}_1\text{COOH}$ (79)

either concerted with or subsequent to cyclization. This cyclization of thiocyano derivatives had previously been reported (Schöberl *et al.*, 1951). Cleavage was obtained in high yield and the mild alkaline condition avoided side reactions almost entirely. With increase in pH, the cleavage was more rapid, but then β-elimination of the thiocyanate group (79a) interfered. Also, cleavage was found to decrease at high concentrations of reactants (Degani and Patchornik, 1974). Cysteine peptide bonds could be selectively cleaved in the presence of cystine residues. This cleavage was demonstrated with high yields on carboxypeptidase A, ϕX174 spike protein (cistron G), and the catalytic and regulatory subunits of *E. coli* aspartate transcar-

bamylase (Jacobson *et al.*, 1973). The reaction has more recently been applied
for cleavage of human hemoglobin α-chain at cysteine-104 (Casey and Lang,
1975).

D. Cleavage at Cystine Peptide Bonds

Peptide bonds involving cystine can obviously be cleaved after reduction of the disulfide and then following this by a suitable method for cleavage
at the resultant cysteine sites. *Direct* cleavage at cystine peptide bonds,
without prior reduction of the disulfides, can be achieved to a limited extent
by reaction with *cyanide*. Reaction of disulfide bonds with cyanide has
already been discussed in detail (see reaction 60 and Section IVH6). The
first step of the reaction (60a) results in cleavage of the disulfide bond to
give a thiol and a thiocyanate group. Cleavage at the S-cyanylated cysteine
residues can then proceed according to reaction (79). The overall reaction
therefore will result in the cleavage of the peptide bond originally involving
the amino group of cystine and the release of an amino-terminal fragment
and a C-terminal fragment carrying a 2-iminothiazolidine-4-carboxylic
acid. The reaction gave some cleavage with oxytocin (at pH 7, 55°C for 72 hr)
and with bovine ribonuclease (at pH 8.0, 37°C for 48 hr) (Catsimpoolas and
Wood, 1966). Also, with bovine serum albumin thiocyanate groups were
formed at pH 8 or higher. At pH 7, thiocyanate groups were not formed,
but iminothiazolidine formation was observed with cleavage at the amino
end of some cystine peptide bonds (Catsimpoolas and Wood, 1964).
However, the reaction of disulfide bonds with cyanide is quite complex
and is accompanied by many side reactions (Section IVH6). Application
of cyanide for the preparative and "clean" cleavage at cystine peptide bonds
does not offer a suitable or a practical procedure.

Alkaline hydrolysis of disulfides and formation of dehydroalanine
residues under these conditions have been described (Section IVH8).
Cleavage at the dehydroalanine sites can be effected, at least in principle,
as described under cysteine. However, this is not a suitable route for cleavage,
because of the complex action of alkali and the reactivity of dehydroalanine,
and the reaction has not been applied in selective protein cleavage.

E. Cleavage at Histidine Peptide Bonds

N-Bromosuccinimide was employed for the oxidative cleavage of histidyl
peptide bonds (Shaltiel and Patchornik, 1963). The method relied on previously reported analogous cleavage of tryptophan (Patchornik *et al.*, 1960)
and tyrosyl (Schmir *et al.*, 1959) peptide bonds by the reagent. Histidine
carries a double bond in the imidazole ring situated in the γ-δ position,

which is an analogous position to the double bond present in tyrosyl, tryptophan, and phenylalanine residues. The last residue is nonreactive. Oxidation with N-bromosuccinimide was in pyridine acetate buffers (pH 3–4) at room temperature and cleavage was effected, after destruction of excess N-bromosuccinimide (with imidazole), by heating the reaction mixture for 1 hr at 100°C (Shaltiel and Patchornik, 1963). Model oligopeptides were cleaved in 30–55% yield at histidine sites and sperm whale myoglobin was cleaved at the His-119–Pro-120 bond in 53% yield. Cleavage of histidine, like that of tryptophan and tyrosine, was proposed to proceed (80) via the formation of a five-membered iminolactone ring (80c) which hydrolyzed readily under acidic conditions. An alternative pathway was proposed to proceed via α-ketoaldehyde and hydrated glyoxylic acid intermediates (Patchornik and Shaltiel, 1966). Differentiation between tyrosine and tryptophan peptide bonds on the one hand and histidine bonds on the other could be achieved by carrying out the reaction with N-bromosuccinimide at room temperature in pyridine-acetate (pH 3.3), where cleavage of tyrosine and tryptophan peptide bonds occurred. Under those conditions, histidine residues were oxidized but not cleaved (Shaltiel and Patchornik, 1963).

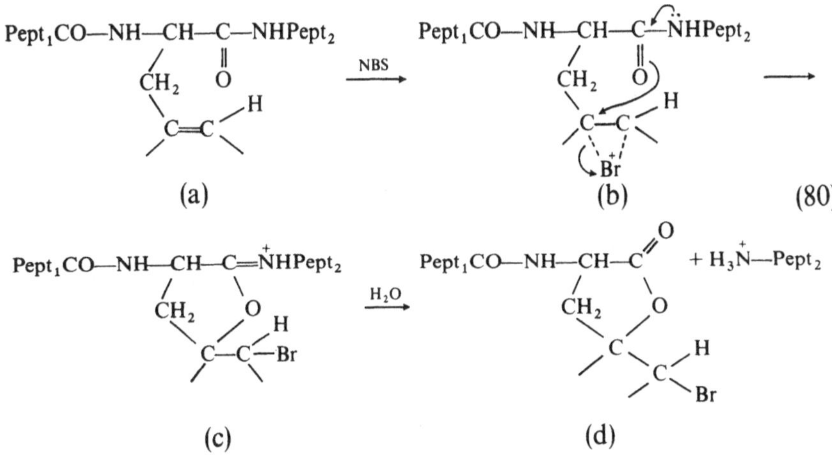

(a)   (b)   (80)

(c)   (d)

After destruction of excess N-bromosuccinimide, heating the reaction mixture effected cleavage of histidyl bonds and increased the cleavage yields of the other two linkages. Cleavage at tyrosyl peptide bonds could be prevented by O-carbobenzyloxylation or O-acetylation of the phenolic group (Shaltiel and Patchornik, 1963). Tryptophan residues could be protected from cleavage by alkylation with 2-hydroxy-5-nitrobenzyl bromide (Wilchek and Witkop, 1967) or by ozonization into N'-formylkynurenine derivatives (Previero et al., 1967a).

The nonselectivity of N-bromosuccinimide as a modifying reagent has already been discussed (Section IV I1). The strong oxidizing agent modifies (in addition to tyrosine, tryptophan, and histidine modification and cleavage) cysteine, cystine, and methionine. If used, therefore, for chemical cleavage purposes, it will produce internally modified peptides. Protection of tyrosine and tryptophan residues (by the aforementioned methods with their own particular nonselectivity problems) during histidine modification predetermines the production of internally modified peptides at those sites. Whereas such peptides may be useful for sequence studies, they will usually be of little or no utility in immunochemical studies. In cases of peptides with unique structures and amino acid compositions, the procedure may find application.

Another method for cleavage at histidyl residues utilized Bamberger's degradation of the imidazole ring by *benzoyl chloride* or *carbobenzyloxy chloride* (Sakiyama *et al.*, 1966). Mild acid hydrolysis of the resultant γ-benzamino group to a γ-oxoornithyl group, and finally elimination of the γ-oxoacyl group by tetrahydropyridazone formation with hydrazine at low pH (3.6) and high temperature (100°C, 2 hr), resulted in cleavage at the C-peptide bond of the original histidine residue. The procedure also caused tryptophan as well as nonspecific cleavage and has been applicable only to selected model peptides (Morishita *et al.*, 1967b). Most likely, it will not be useful in selective cleavage of proteins for immunochemical studies.

F. Cleavage at Aliphatic Hydroxyl Groups

Cleavage at serine residues has been obtained by *conversion of the serine to dehydroalanine*, followed by scission of the dehydroalanine sites as described under cysteine cleavage (see reaction 78) (Patchornik and Sokolovsky, 1964a). Tosylation of serine and its conversion to dehydroalanine by β-elimination have been described (reaction 28, see Section IVB). β-Elimination of O-phosphoryl groups can also be employed (Patchornik and Sokolovsky, 1964a). In glycoproteins, β-elimination of the glycosidic linkage to serine or threonine can be used for cleavage at these sites (Anderson et al., 1964). The shortcomings of cleavage reactions via dehydroalanine have been discussed (Section VIIC).

Solvolytic cleavage of O-mesyl derivative of O-methyldihydrorufomycin A proceeded in two steps (Iwasaki and Witkop, 1964). In the first step, concerted intramolecular displacement in 10% water–methyl ethyl ketone (reflux, 13 hr) gave an iminolactone which upon subsequent hydrolysis in aqueous acid (20°C, 10 hr) gave 53% cleavage at the C-δ-hydroxyleucyl peptide bond.

Anhydrous *hydrogen fluoride* induced $N \rightarrow O$ *acyl shift* has been used for cleavage at the serine and threonine sites (Lenard and Hess, 1964). The ester bonds (81c) resulting from $N \rightarrow O$ acyl shift (81) were hydrolyzed in

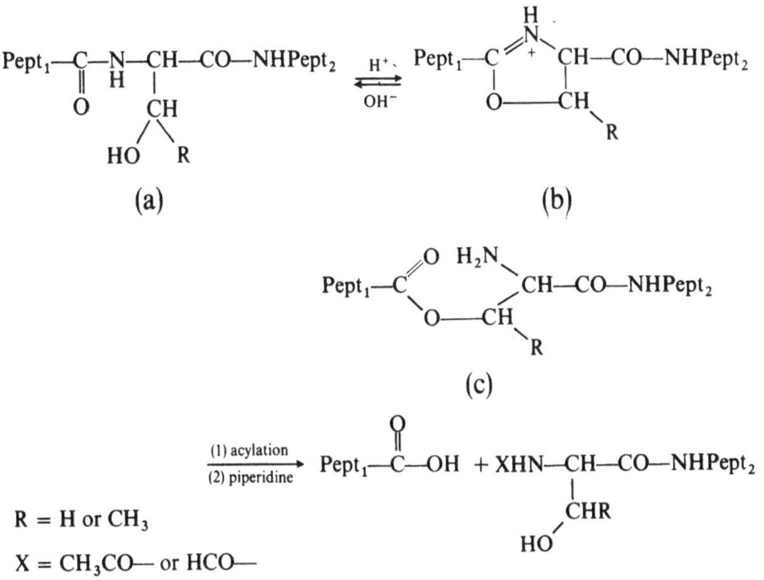

$$\text{Pept}_1\text{—C—N—CH—CO—NHPept}_2 \quad \underset{\text{OH}^-}{\overset{\text{H}^+}{\rightleftharpoons}} \quad \text{Pept}_1\text{—C} \overset{\text{N}}{\underset{\text{O—CH}}{\diagdown}} \text{CH—CO—NHPept}_2$$

(a) (b)

$$\text{Pept}_1\text{—C} \overset{\diagup\text{O}}{\underset{\text{O—CH}}{\diagdown}} \overset{\text{H}_2\text{N}}{\underset{\text{R}}{\diagdown}} \text{CH—CO—NHPept}_2$$

(c)

$$\xrightarrow[\text{(2) piperidine}]{\text{(1) acylation}} \quad \text{Pept}_1\text{—}\overset{\text{O}}{\overset{\|}{\text{C}}}\text{—OH} + \text{XHN—CH—CO—NHPept}_2 \qquad (81)$$

R = H or CH$_3$

X = CH$_3$CO— or HCO—

aqueous piperidine, after protection of the amino groups by acetylation or formylation. Protection of the amino groups was necessary to prevent the reverse shift and thus improve yield. Addition of methanol to the reaction mixture during HF treatment prevented the tendency of serine and threonine to esterify any available carboxyl groups. Cleavages of insulin A and B chains and α-melanocyte-stimulating hormone were obtained in 80–91% yield. Methionine bonds were also cleaved by HF, but this was prevented by prior oxidation of the methionine residues. Tryptophan residues were appreciably destroyed, and since acylation of the amino groups and oxidation of the methionine residues were necessary (with their own particular side reactions) in this otherwise effective method of cleavage, the peptides produced were internally modified. This limits their utility in immunochemical studies.

A two-step fragmentation of threonine-containing peptides was obtained by oxidation of threonine to α-ketoacid residues followed by cleavage of the C-peptide bond of the oxidized threonine (D'Angeli et al., 1966). Oxidation of threonine was performed by *dimethylsulfoxide-dicyclohexyl-carbodiimide-phosphoric acid* and the cleavage step was performed with *phenylhydrazine* (40–70°C, 20–30 min) to yield an N-terminal fragment ending with pyrazolone moiety and a C-terminal peptide with a free α-NH$_2$ group. The procedure has been applicable only to model peptides. Conditions of the reaction, especially those of the oxidation in phosphoric acid-carbodiimide will be expected to cause other modifications (Section IVD2).

Phosgene has been employed for cleavage of serine (Kaneko et al., 1968a) and threonine (Kaneko et al., 1968b) peptides. In this procedure, serine and threonine residues were converted to oxazolidone derivatives via O-chloro-carbonyl derivatives by treatment with phosgene and dimethylaniline followed by refluxing in xylene until evolution of HCl ceased (1 hr). Treatment of the oxazolidone peptide with alkali (1 N KOH) at room temperature resulted in cleavage at the amino end of threonine to give an N-terminal peptide with a free carboxyl end and a 5-methyl-2-oxo-oxazolidine-4-carbonyl derivative. The method has been applicable only to carefully selected model peptides and it is expected to be too drastic for proteins.

G. Cleavage of Methionine Peptide Bonds

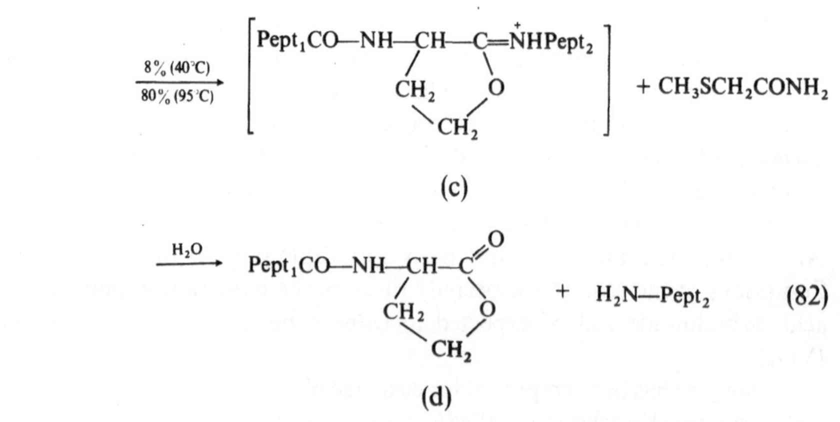

Sulfonium derivatives of methionine peptides have been shown to undergo intramolecular displacement (82) with elimination of the sulfur function (82c) and cleavage of the C-peptide bond (82d) of methionine (Lawson *et al.*, 1961). Reaction of the thioether side chain of methionine with alkyl halides at low pH has been discussed (Section IVF2). Several alkylating agents were compared and iodoacetamide was the most effective in the cleavage reaction (Lawson *et al.*, 1961). Following alkylation and removal of excess alkylating agent (ether extraction), only 8% peptide cleavage was obtained at 40°C, while brief heating at 95°C increased cleavage yields to 54–85%. Aminoethylated apocatalase (with aminoethyl sulfonium salt) was shown (Schroeder *et al.*, 1967) to give homoserine lactone at pH 2 without prior treatment with cyanogen bromide, probably due to a cleavage reaction by a pathway similar to (82).

Cyanosulfonium salts, from the reaction of a methionyl peptide with *cyanogen bromide*, are more unstable and were shown to undergo a *C*-peptide bond cleavage at acidic pH and room temperature to give a homoserine lactone derivative, methyl thiocyanate, and a *C*-terminal fragment with a free amino group (Gross and Witkop, 1961). The mechanism of cleavage is similar to pathway (82). However, since this reaction is widely applied, it is shown in (83). Peptide bonds of methionine sulfoxide or the sulfone are not cleaved by cyanogen bromide (Gross, 1967). Following its first application in the cleavage of the four methionine peptide bonds in bovine ribonuclease A (Gross and Witkop, 1961, 1962), the reaction has since become one of the most widely applied in protein chemistry. Such numerous applications cannot be discussed here and earlier work has been reviewed (Gross, 1967). Discussion will be limited here to studies and applications that bear on the conditions and specificity of the reaction. It has now become clear that the reaction is not free of complications as originally believed.

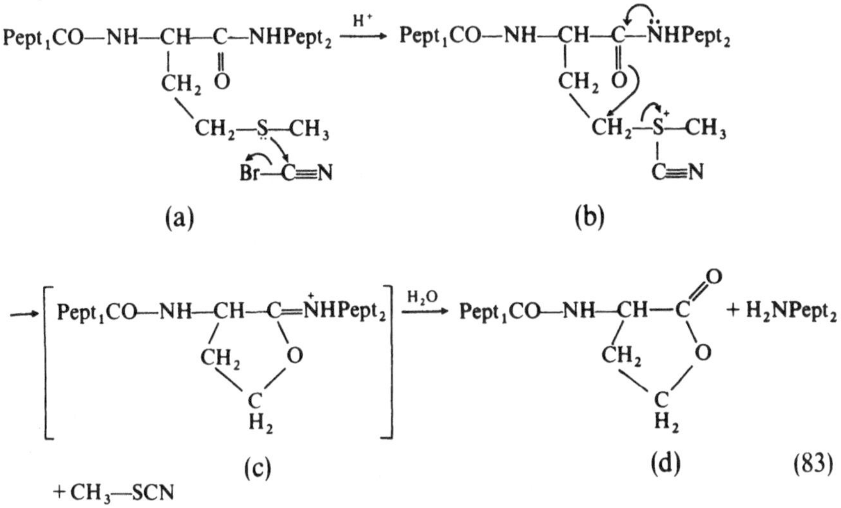

(83)

The reaction was originally carried out in 0.1 N HCl (Gross and Witkop, 1961). Subsequently, better results were obtained in 75% trifluoroacetic acid (Bargetzi *et al.*, 1964) or in 70% formic acid (Steers *et al.*, 1965). Poor cleavage often encountered with Met–Ser or Met–Thr bonds was avoided by carrying out the cleavage in 70% trifluoroacetic acid rather than in 70% formic acid (Schroeder *et al.*, 1969). It was also shown that complete conversion of methionine to homoserine was not indicative of quantitative cleavage. Higher reaction rates were obtained by increasing the concentration of the reactants. The poor cleavage of Met–Ser or Met–Thr bonds was

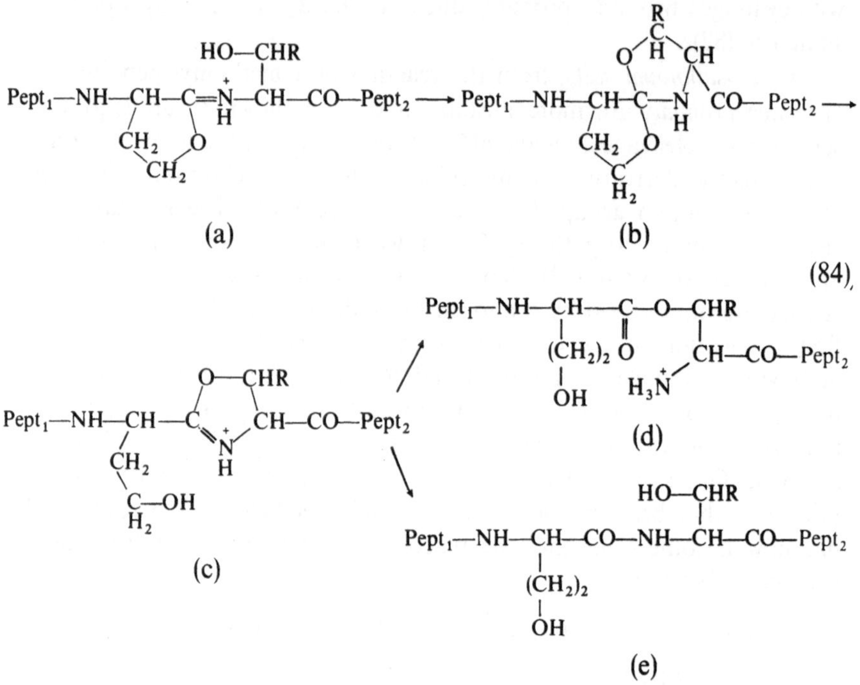

HO—CHR
Pept$_1$—NH—CH—C=N—CH—CO—Pept$_2$ $\longrightarrow$ Pept$_1$—NH—CH—C—N CO—Pept$_2$ $\longrightarrow$
       CH$_2$ O   CH$_2$ O
         CH$_2$ C
                   H$_2$

(a)   (b)

(84)

Pept$_1$—NH—CH—C—O—CHR
         (CH$_2$)$_2$ O   CH—CO—Pept$_2$
           OH   H$_3$N$^+$

(d)

O—CHR
Pept$_1$—NH—CH—C   CH—CO—Pept$_2$
       CH$_2$ N$^+$
          H
       C—OH
       H$_2$

(c)

HO—CHR
Pept$_1$—NH—CH—CO—NH—CH—CO—Pept$_2$
         (CH$_2$)$_2$
          OH

(e)

attributed to an intramolecular reaction of the hydroxyl group with the iminolactone (84a). The bicyclic structure (84b) released a homoserine side chain (84c) and the second ring opening gave either an ester linkage (84d) or a peptide linkage with the original serine or threonine hydroxyl being free (84e). Trifluoroacetic acid increased the protonation of the hydroxyl and the iminolactone groups and prevented the conversion of (84a) to (84b). Clearly reaction (84) converts methionine to homoserine without cleaving the peptide bond.

It has been shown that mixing of two fragments, previously isolated from cyanogen bromide cleavage of horse heart cytochrome c, in aqueous solution resulted in their rejoining slowly through restoration of the peptide bond originally cleaved (Corradin and Harbury, 1974).

Other examples of low yields cannot be explained by the presence of Met–Ser and Met–Thr bonds. It has been demonstrated that a reverse reaction to that shown in (83) can take place through a six-membered ring which competes with the forward reaction (Carpenter and Shiigi, 1974). The reverse reaction (85) yielded homoserine in ester linkage (85c) without an equivalent amount of peptide bond cleavage. The degree of reaction by pathway (83) or by the reverse cyclization (85) was proposed to vary with the nature of the two amino acids located on both sides of the methionine (Carpenter and Shiigi, 1974).

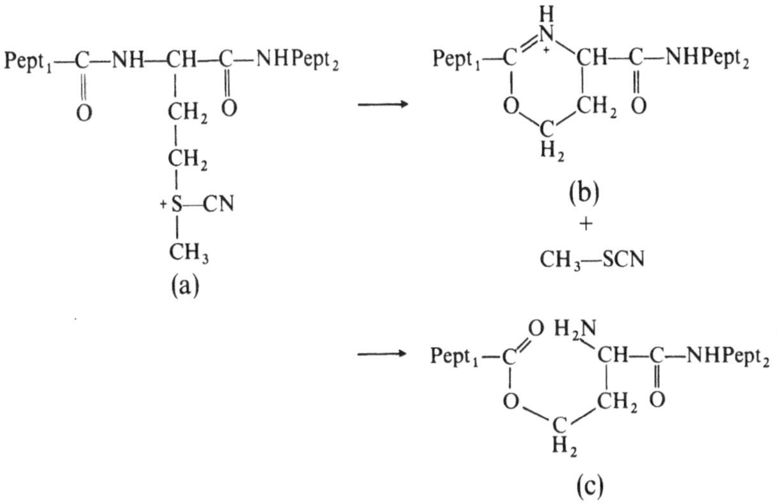

$$
\begin{array}{ccc}
\text{Pept}_1\!-\!\underset{\substack{\| \\ O}}{C}\!-\!NH\!-\!CH\!-\!\underset{\substack{\| \\ O}}{C}\!-\!NHPept_2 & \longrightarrow & \text{(figure b)} \\
\quad\quad\quad\quad | & & \\
\quad\quad\quad CH_2 & & \\
\quad\quad\quad\quad | & & \\
\quad\quad\quad CH_2 & & \\
\quad\quad\quad\quad | & & \\
\quad\quad\quad +S\!-\!CN & & \\
\quad\quad\quad\quad | & & \\
\quad\quad\quad CH_3 & & \\
\end{array}
$$

(a)   (b)
                                        +
                                 $CH_3\!-\!SCN$

$\longrightarrow$ (c)   (85)

Accordingly, quantitation of homoserine (Gross, 1967) or of methyl thiocyanate (Inglis and Edman, 1970) during cyanogen bromide cleavage may give erroneous results concerning the degree of cleavage.

Cyanogen bromide was proposed to oxidize thiol groups slowly to cysteic acid (Gross, 1967). This could be prevented by S-carboxymethylation of the protein before the reaction. It has been shown that cyanogen bromide will form disulfides from thiol compounds (Foye *et al.*, 1967). It has also been reported that cyanogen bromide acted as a thiol-oxidizing agent, forming mixed disulfides in excellent yields (Abe *et al.*, 1974). Investigators have often subjected thiol-containing proteins to cyanogen bromide cleavage without prior protection of the thiol groups. In these cases, such as myosin (Weeds and Hartley, 1968; Young *et al.*, 1968), human serum albumin (McMenamy *et al.*, 1971), and hemoglobin of the bloodworm (Imamura *et al.*, 1972), aggregation was encountered. Cyanogen bromide mediated disulfide formation (Abe *et al.*, 1974) could play a part in the aggregation. Protection of the thiol groups before reaction with cyanogen bromide should not be ignored.

Hydrogen fluoride was shown to effect cleavage of the *C*-peptide bond of methionine (Lenard *et al.*, 1964). Methionine sulfone bonds were not cleaved. Cleavage of model peptides was in high (over 95%) yields and α-melanocyte-stimulating hormone was cleaved in 45% yield. It has already been mentioned (Section VIIF) that this reaction also cleaved *N*-seryl and *N*-threonyl peptide bonds via an $N \to O$ acyl shift (see reaction 81). To prevent this during methionine cleavage, the $N \to O$ acyl shift was reversed (after removal of hydrogen fluoride) in basic aqueous solution (Lenard *et al.*, 1964). This complication has probably contributed to the fact that the reaction has not been widely applied.

An unusual rearrangement was observed in methionine model compounds upon alkylation (Jendrek *et al.*, 1967). The reaction seemed to involve cleavage of the peptide bonds, *expulsion of the methionine*, and reformation of a peptidelike bond under conditions that normally do not cause either cleavage or formation of amide bonds. Reaction was observed upon alkylation with a variety of simple alkylating agents, which included *t*-butyl iodide (or bromide), *i*-butyl bromide, ethyl bromide, and *i*-propyl bromide (or iodide). It proceeded at room temperature (48 hr) in acetic acid, methanol, ethanol, or a variety of other alcohols with erratic yields. The mechanism of the reaction is not understood, but it would imply ability to remove methionine residues from internal peptide positions leaving the peptide chain intact. The reaction needs further investigation.

H. Cleavage of Proline Peptide Bonds

Sodium in liquid ammonia was first observed to cleave the N-peptide bond of proline during removal of the p-toluenesulfonyl protecting group in synthetic α-melanocyte-stimulating hormone (Hofman and Yajima, 1961). This is similar to the Birch reduction (Birch *et al.*, 1955) of tertiary amides by the same reagent and in a similar manner required a proton donor (Guttmann, 1963). Reductive cleavage of the N-prolyl peptide bond (86) converted the amino acid preceding proline to its aldehyde or alcohol (86b) and liberated a peptide with a free proline N-terminus (86c) (Wilchek *et al.*, 1965). Reduction in the presence of methanol as proton donor cleaved the Lys–Pro bond in bovine ribonuclease (Sarid and Patchornik, 1963) in about 40% yield. Better yields (some essentially quantitative) were obtained in model peptides, in the Thr–Pro bond of insulin, and in the liberation of the C-

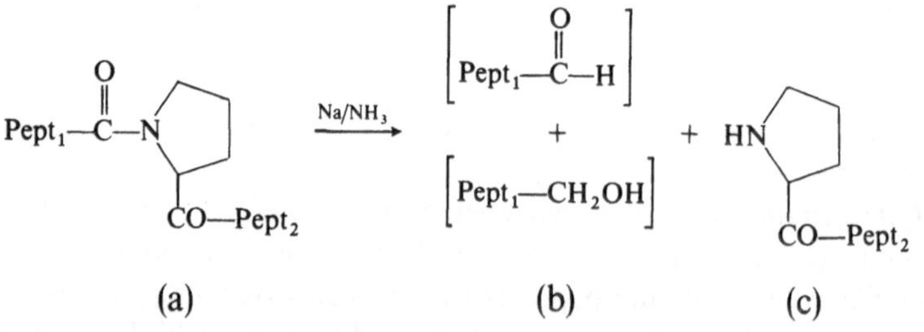

$$\text{(a)} \qquad\qquad\qquad \text{(b)} \qquad\qquad\qquad \text{(c)}$$

terminal proline in ovalbumin (Wilchek *et al.*, 1965). Other workers (Benisek and Cole, 1965; Benisek *et al.*, 1967) found the presence of proton donors unnecessary. The specificity of cleavage at proline peptide bonds and the presence of side reactions depended on the amount of sodium excess used in the reaction and on the temperature and duration of the reaction (Benisek *et al.*, 1967). Appreciable (55%) destruction of phenylalanine was observed on reductive cleavage of insulin B chain under vigorous conditions and was avoided in insulin B chain and in apoferrodoxin under milder conditions. High excess of sodium (700–1400 atoms excess), higher temperature ($-33°C$), and longer reaction periods (15 min) caused nonspecific cleavage as well as appreciable cleavage at the peptide bond formed by the N-terminal amino acid. The reaction conditions for cleavage at proline peptide bonds in sperm whale apomyoglobin, without the presence of a proton donor, were exhaustively studied (Atassi and Singhal, 1970a) at various temperatures ($-78°C$ and $-33°C$), time intervals (60, 160, and 210 sec), and sodium metal excess (200, 600, or 800 sodium atoms per mole of apomyoglobin). Best results were obtained at 600 atoms excess, $-33°C$, and 210 sec, and the peptides were isolated and their immunochemistry was studied. Milder reaction conditions gave incomplete cleavage and poor yield, while more vigorous conditions were accompanied by nonspecific cleavage. Under the optimum conditions mentioned, no side reactions were observed, as determined by the amino acid analysis of the purified peptides. Studies with apomyoglobin made it clear that the optimum conditions of cleavage will have to be determined for each protein independently. Immunochemical studies of proline peptides from apomyoglobin were critical for the delineation of the antigenic structure of sperm whale myoglobin (Atassi and Singhal, 1970a). Also, since they formed intact whole helices, their conformational analysis (Singhal and Atassi, 1970) was extremely revealing (see Chapter 2). Other than the aforementioned studies with myoglobin, this reaction has not been employed in the cleavage, isolation, and biological studies of proline peptides from other proteins.

With model compounds, opening of the proline ring was reported (Ramachandran, 1965). Also, it has been reported that Na/NH_3 caused reductive cleavage of the thioether side chains of S-carboxymethylcysteine and methionine to give cysteine and homocysteine, respectively, as the predominant reaction products (Crewther and Nicholls, 1969). Cysteine oxidized rapidly to cystine and cysteic acid and homocysteine to homocystine and homocysteic acid. Traces of other reaction products were observed. These results were obtained with very vigorous reduction conditions (30 min). Under milder conditions, no opening of the proline ring (Benisek et al., 1967; Atassi and Singhal, 1970a) or reduction of methionine (Atassi and Singhal, 1970a) has been observed.

Sodium hydrazide in hydrazine-ether at $0°C$ (45–60 min) cleaved model peptides and insulin B chain in 70–100% yields (Kauffmann and Sobel, 1963, 1966). However, several amino acids (leucine, lysine, phenylalanine, serine, threonine, and tryptophan) were modified partially (5–10%), while modifications of methionine (to homocysteine) and cystine (disulfide bond reduction) were quantitative (Kauffmann and Sobel, 1966). *Lithium in methylamine* was also shown to effect cleavage at $-70°C$ (1 hr) of N-peptide bonds of proline and hydroxyproline in model peptides (Patchornik *et al.*, 1964). The method has not been applied to proteins. Cleavage by Na/NH$_3$ is preferable because it gives higher yields and much lower nonspecific cleavage and modification side reactions. *Lithium aluminum hydride* in anhydrous tetrahydrofuran has also been used to cleave *N*-prolyl bonds in some model peptides and in the cyclic peptides gramicidin S and tyrocidine C (Ruttenberg *et al.*, 1964, 1965). The reaction reduced *C*-terminal amino acids to their corresponding alcohols and amide groups to the amines. Also, LiAlH$_4$ causes nonselective peptide bond cleavage (Yonemitsu *et al.*, 1968). In the last two reactions (i.e., Li—CH$_3$NH$_2$ and LiAlH$_4$), cleavage resulted in reduction of the amino acid preceding proline to its aldehyde. Aldehydic groups are of course quite reactive (Section IVA5). This was overcome by Ruttenberg *et al.* (1965) through reduction of the aldehyde to the corresponding alcohol by borohydride. For borohydride side reactions, see Section IVD3).

I. Cleavage of Tryptophan Peptide Bonds

N-Bromosuccinimide has been discussed in detail as a modification reagent for proteins (see Section IVI1). At acid pH, the reagent has been shown to cleave *C*-tryptophyl peptide bonds (Patchornik *et al.*, 1960). *N*-Iodoacetamide effected similar cleavage. The reaction mechanism is similar to that described for the cleavage of histidine by this reagent (reaction 80, Section VIIE). Peptide bonds of tyrosine (Corey and Haefele, 1959; Schmir *et al.*, 1959) and histidine (Section VIIE) also undergo cleavage by *N*-bromosuccinimide. Histidine cleaved preferentially at 100°C in pyridine–acetic acid–water, and tyrosine cleavage was prevented by its *O*-acylation (Shaltiel and Patchornik, 1963). The latter modification is undesirable since it gives internally modified peptides (Section VIID). An alternative approach has been proposed, to obtain selective cleavage of *C*-tryptophyl bonds in peptides containing tyrosine, by the addition of excess mercuric acetate during *N*-bromosuccinimide oxidation (Ramachandran and Witkop, 1964). This has not been tested on proteins. Selectivity of *N*-bromosuccinimide is unsatisfactory both as a modification (Section IVI1) and as a cleavage (Section VIIE) reagent.

Ozone oxidation of tryptophan residues to *N*-formylkynurenine has been described (Section IVI1). Ozonization followed by heating (100°C) in alkaline media for 1–4 hr has been used to cleave *C*-tryptophyl bonds in model peptides (Previero *et al.*, 1966a). This procedure, especially the alkaline hydrolytic step, will be too drastic for proteins. Cleavage of kynurenine peptides was also obtained, after their reduction with NaBH$_4$, by heating

(100°C) at pH 7 for 2 hr (Previero *et al.*, 1966*b*). Side reactions of borohydride reduction have been discussed (Section IVD3), and heating even at pH 7 will have a denaturing effect and possibly cause nonselective cleavage. Another approach for cleavage of kynurenine peptides employed hydrazine-acetate (pH 3.6) at 100°C for 2 hr (Morishita *et al.*, 1967*a*). This also will be too drastic for proteins and has been applied only to selected model peptides. Subsequently, hydrazine acetate was employed at 25–30°C for 24–48 hr for model peptide cleavage (Sakiyama and Sakai, 1971). At any rate, ozonization oxidizes several amino acids and the solvents during ozonization caused esterification of hydroxyl groups (Section IV I1).

Reaction of tryptophan with *BNPS-skatole* has been discussed (Section IV I1). In the presence of a large excess of the reagent (10 equivalents or greater) under acidic conditions (50% acetic acid) and room temperature (about 24 hr), cleavage of *C*-tryptophyl peptide bonds was obtained in model peptides and in staphylococcal nuclease, the latter being in 15% yield (Omenn *et al.*, 1970). Bovine encephalitogenic protein was cleaved by the reagent (10 equivalents, 50% acetic acid, 37°C, 24 hr) at the single tryptophan residue in 60% yield (Bergstrand, 1971). The basic protein A1 from bovine and human brain was cleaved at the single tryptophan, at 20°C but otherwise similar conditions, in 40% yield (Burnett and Eylar, 1971). The fragments in the foregoing two studies were isolated and their immunochemistry was studied. Modification side reactions of *BNPS*-skatole have been discussed (Section IV I1).

Periodate has been used for the oxidative cleavage of *C*-tryptophyl bonds (Atassi, 1967*b*). The first step involved oxidation of the tryptophan residues in the protein at 0°C and pH 5.0. This was followed by mild acid (0.1 N HCl) hydrolysis at room temperature (24 hr). With this procedure, cleavage of sperm whale apomyoglobin was obtained in 92–94% yield at tryptophan-7 and in 17–22% yield at tryptophan-14 (Atassi, 1967*b*). The cleavage yield was a function of the accessibility of the tryptophan residues to periodate in the oxidation step (Atassi, 1967*a*). No cleavage was obtained without the acid hydrolytic step which makes it possible to stop the reaction at the oxidation step. Oxidation gave an oxindole derivative which, upon acid treatment, suffered cleavage of the *C*-tryptophyl peptide bonds and resulted in the formation of a spirolactone (see structure 87e) (Atassi, 1967*b*). Periodate oxidized methionine very rapidly and tyrosine very slowly (Atassi, 1967*a*), but cleavage at these sites was not obtained. Methionine oxidation can be reversed by a thiol reagent (Section IVF1).

2,4,6-*Tribromo-4-methylcyclohexadienone*, a milder brominating agent than *N*-bromosuccinimide, has been used for the selective cleavage of *C*-tryptophyl peptide bonds (Burstein and Patchornik, 1972). Optimal conditions for the cleavage reaction were in the presence of 3 equivalents of reagent at room temperature and pH 3 (5–15 min). Several tryptophan model peptides were cleaved (40–60%) as well as hen egg white lysozyme (5–60%) and glucagon (30% yield). Bovine ribonuclease (which contains no tryptophan) did not undergo any cleavage. The optimum pH and the yields of cleavage obtained by this reagent were very similar to those of N-bromosuccinimide, which suggested a similar mechanism of cleavage (87). The reagent oxidized but did not cleave other amino acids. Cleavage at tryptophan could not be obtained without oxidation of cysteine and methionine (Burstein and Patchornik, 1972). In addition, cystine was oxidized in several steps to cysteic acid, histidine was brominated, and tyrosine residues gave the 2,6-dibromotyrosyl derivative. The last three side reactions could be minimized if a large excess of the reagent is not used.

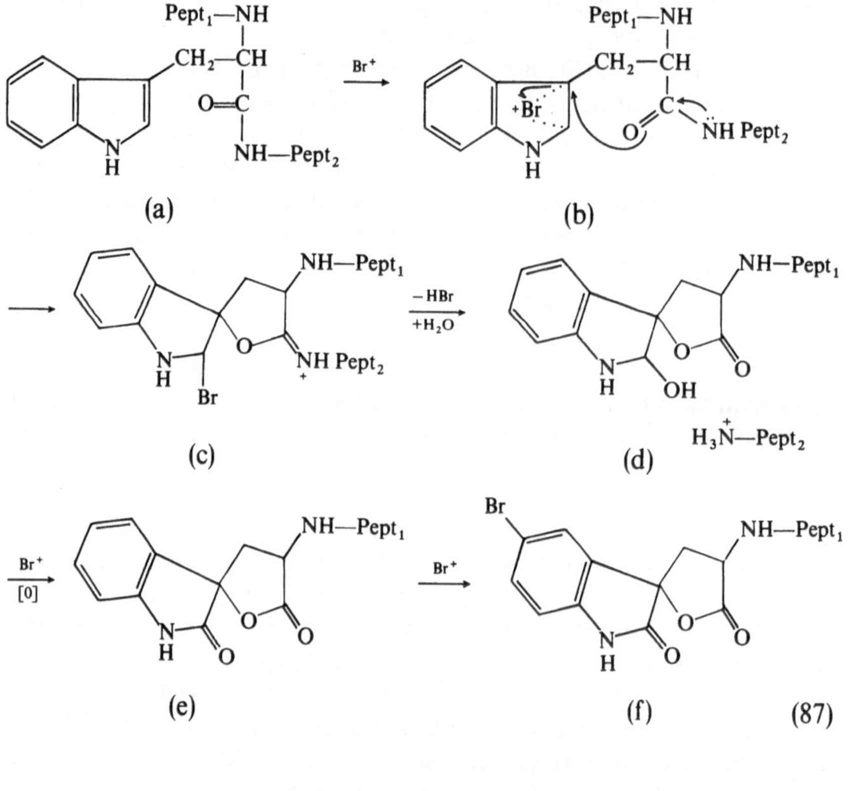

(87)

J. Cleavage at Tyrosine Peptide Bonds

N-Bromosuccinimide cleavage of the C-peptide bonds of tryptophan, histidine, and tyrosyl residues has been discussed, together with modification reactions for prevention of cleavage at tryptophan or at tyrosyl peptide bonds (Sections VII E and VII I). Other brominating agents may effect cleavage of these bonds (see Section VIIK). Bromine had been employed in the cleavage of the single tyrosyl bond in each of oxytocin and vasopressin, following prior performic acid cleavage of the disulfide (Mueller *et al.*, 1953). However, these two peptide hormones do not have histidine or tryptophan residues These reactions take place at room temperature under acidic (usually 50% acetic acid) conditions (Schmir and Cohen, 1961; Wilson and Cohen, 1963*a*) and 3–12 equivalents of *N*-bromosuccinimide has been employed with model peptides (Wilson and Cohen, 1963*a*), whereas with bovine ribonuclease 50 equivalents was necessary (Wilson and Cohen, 1963*b*). *N*-*Iodosuccinimide* has been shown to effect, in addition to diiodination of the phenolic ring, oxidative cleavage of simple tyrosyl dipeptides (Junek *et al.*, 1969). Its reactions (at pH 4.5) resulted in cleavage yields of 57–95%. On the other hand, iodine caused only ring halogenation and no cleavage was obtained, indicating that cleavage of tyrosyl peptide bonds during iodination of proteins will not pose a serious problem (Junek *et al.*, 1969). Oxidative cleavage of *C*-tyrosyl bonds by bromine, *N*-bromosuccinimide, or *N*-iodosuccinimide is probably by the same mechanism (88). Cyclization (88e) can

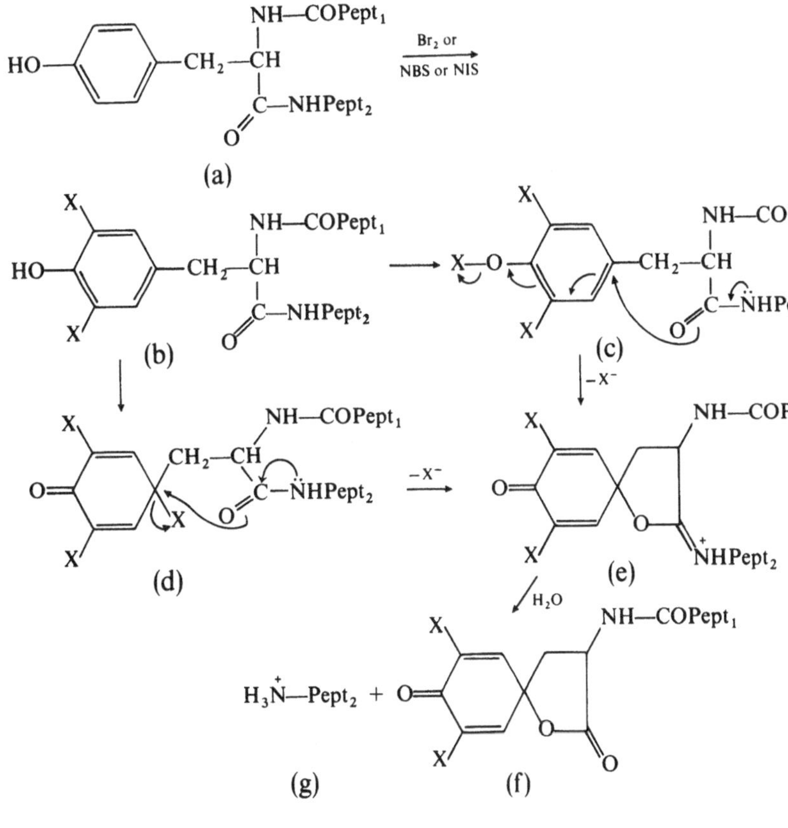

(88)

X = Br or I

proceed via the trihalogenated derivatives (88c) or (88d). The iminolactone ring in (88e) is readily hydrolyzed under the acidic conditions of the reaction to give a dienone lactone peptide (88f) and a peptide fragment with a free amino end. The oxidative action of bromine or N-bromosuccinimide is not selective either in modification (Section IV I1) or in cleavage (Sections VII E and VIII).

Mild *electrolytic oxidation* at a platinum anode and in low voltage was shown to effect cleavage at C-tyrosyl peptide bonds and, in contrast to N-bromosuccinimide, it was not accompanied by cleavage at tryptophan and histidine peptide bonds (Iwasaki et al., 1963; Iwasaki and Witkop, 1964). Destruction of the amino-terminal residue, which was found to take place at the anode during electrolysis (Iwasaki et al., 1963; Davies et al., 1964), could be essentially prevented at low pH (2–3) and lowest possible voltage (6–8V) (Farber and Cohen, 1966). Following anodic oxidation, cleavage (of phlorethylglycine) could be improved by boiling the reaction mixture at pH 3 (Farber and Cohen, 1966). This will be undesirable for proteins. Anodic oxidative cleavage (89) took place either by direct participation of the peptide bond, giving the iminolactone (89b) in 24–45% yield, while conversion to the hydroxydienone (89c) accounted for the remainder (Isoe and Cohen, 1968). Heating the hydroxydienone (89c) at pH 3 (reflux, 3 hr) effected cleavage by intramolecular participation and increased yield (to 50–65%). A continuous-flow electrolytic cell has been described for oxida-

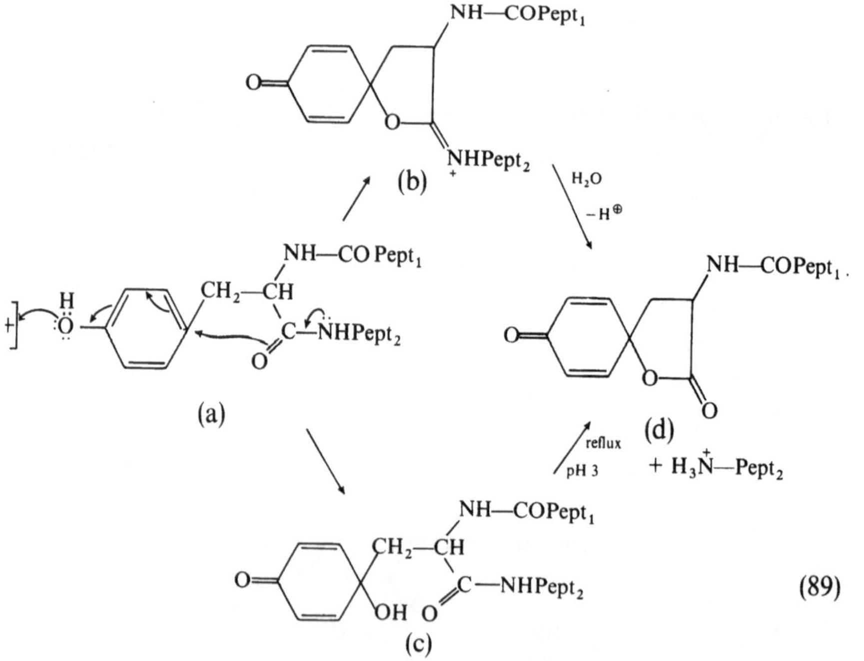

(89)

tion at low (2–3 V) potential (Isoe and Cohen, 1968). Angiotensin and insulin were cleaved at C-tyrosyl bond (except a Tyr–Gln bond in insulin) in undetermined yields (Farber and Cohen, 1966) and specific cleavage in varying yields was obtained at all six tyrosyl peptide bonds in bovine ribonuclease A. It is relevant to mention that other amino acids are oxidized (but not cleaved) by electrolysis. These include amino, imidazole, and thioether groups as well as disulfide bonds (Farber and Cohen, 1966). Some arginine modification was also observed in stationary electrolysis (Isoe and Cohen, 1968) and was avoided in the continuous-flow apparatus.

K. Miscellaneous Addition and Cleavage Reactions

N-Terminal addition of glycine to amino acid and peptide esters using triethylenetetramine-cobalt chelate $[Co(en)_2^{3+}]$ as an N-terminal protecting group and as an activating reagent has been reported (Buckingham *et al.*, 1967*b*). Treatment of $[Co(en)_2 (Gly\ O\ CH_3)]\ (ClO_4)_3$ (structure 90b) with amino acid or peptide esters in anhydrous sulfolane, dimethylsulfoxide, or acetone solutions gave quantitatively the $[Co(en)_2\ peptide\text{-}OR]^{3+}$ (structure 90c), which is an addition of the complexed glycine carbonyl group to the amino end of the peptide. This addition reaction has been demonstrated on amino acid esters and selected model peptides. Its general applicability requires further investigation.

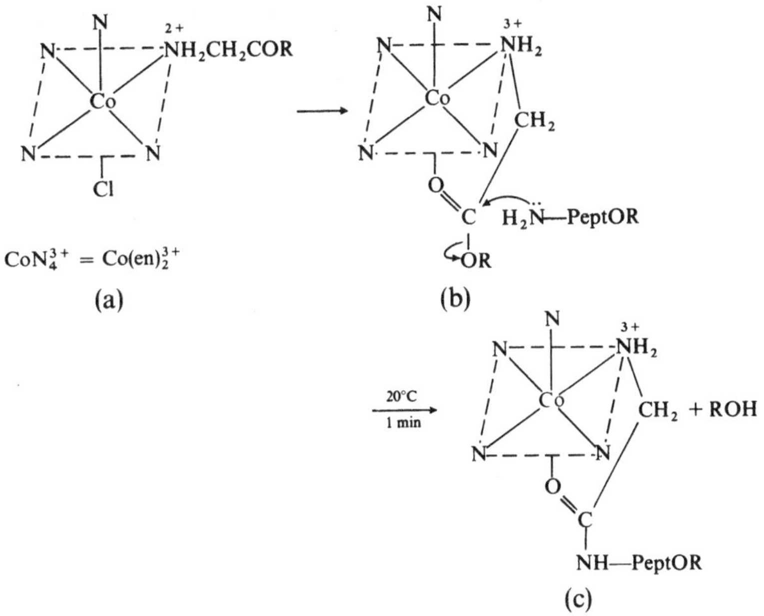

$$CoN_4^{3+} = Co(en)_2^{3+}$$

(a)   (b)

(90)

(c)

Amino acid insertion in peptides has been demonstrated (Davies *et al.*, 1971, 1973) by silylation of the amide bonds with chloro(trimethyl)silane and acylation of the product with the chloride of benzyloxycarbonyl glycine (or β-alanine) in an inert solvent. Deprotection of the *N*-acyl group by hydrogenolysis resulted in a spontaneous rearrangement in good (85%) yield, with incorporation of the aminoacyl residue (without racemization) into the peptide chain. This is an interesting reaction but it may find only limited application.

Cleavage of the *thioether bond* linking the heme to the polypeptide chain in horse heart cytochrome *c* was reported (Lederer and Tarin, 1971) by iodination of the hemoprotein with low iodine excess (6–8 molar excess of I_2 in KI) at pH 8.6 in 8 M urea (0°C, 40 min) followed by cyanogen bromide cleavage. An oxidative mechanism was proposed in which the thioether was oxidized to the sulfoxide, which then participated in cleavage by cyanogen bromide. This is unusual because methionine was not oxidized under these conditions and because cyanogen bromide is known not to react with sulfoxides (Gross, 1967; Schroeder *et al.*, 1969).

L. Modified Enzymatic Cleavage

The sites of cleavage by proteolytic enzymes can be altered by introducing into the protein substituents which will prevent enzymatic cleavage at the modified location. Alternatively, substituents may be introduced which will render the previously unsusceptible modified sites hydrolyzable by the enzyme. The enzyme most suitable for these cleavage reactions is trypsin because it possesses a very well-defined narrow specificity. Other approaches to limit enzymatic hydrolysis have been by varying the conditions of cleavage.

1. Cleavage at Cysteine Peptide Bonds

The reactions for conversion of thiol groups in proteins to *S*-β-aminoethylcysteine residues have been discussed in detail (see Section IVG6). The *S*-aminoethylcysteine peptide bond (91b) was found to be susceptible to tryptic hydrolysis (Lindley, 1956) in the same manner as lysyl peptide bonds (91) (Raftery and Cole, 1963, 1966). Of course, cleavage at cystine peptide bonds may also be achieved after reduction and aminoethylation. Cleavage may be rendered specific for aminoethylcysteine peptide bonds by the modification of lysine and arginine residues prior to tryptic hydrolysis. For example, cleavage of heavy and light chains from human and mouse immunoglobulins was achieved specifically at the cystine sites by (1) succinylation

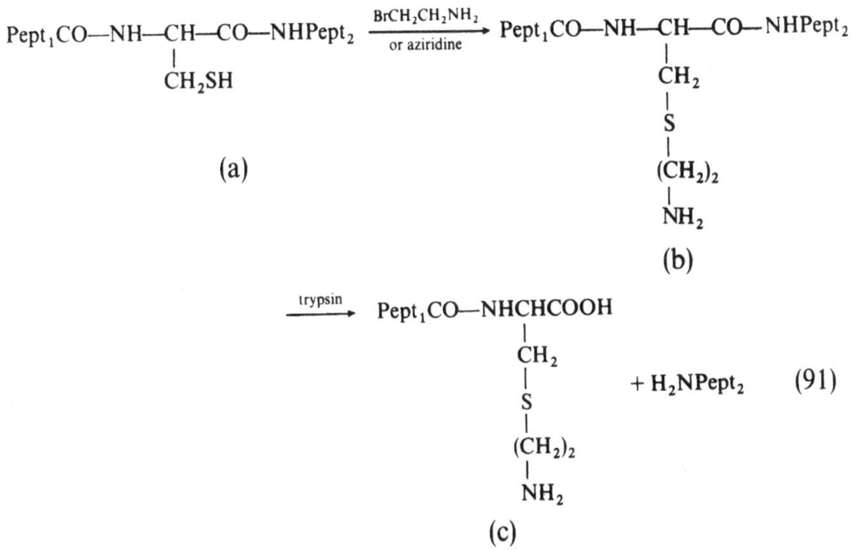

$$Pept_1CO-NH-CH-CO-NHPept_2 \xrightarrow[\text{or aziridine}]{BrCH_2CH_2NH_2} Pept_1CO-NH-CH-CO-NHPept_2$$

$$\underset{CH_2SH}{|}$$

(a)

$$\begin{array}{c} | \\ CH_2 \\ | \\ S \\ | \\ (CH_2)_2 \\ | \\ NH_2 \end{array}$$

(b)

$$\xrightarrow{trypsin} Pept_1CO-NHCHCOOH$$

$$\begin{array}{c} | \\ CH_2 \\ | \\ S \\ | \\ (CH_2)_2 \\ | \\ NH_2 \end{array} \quad + H_2NPept_2 \quad (91)$$

(c)

of the amino groups, (2) reduction of the disulfides with dithiothreitol, (3) aminoethylation of the thiol groups by reaction with aziridine, (4) modification of the arginine residues by cyclohexanedione, and finally (5) tryptic hydrolysis (Slobin and Singer, 1968). It is to be noted that this approach will give fragments which are internally modified at numerous locations. Such fragments will be useful for sequence studies but will have limited use in immunochemical studies. For the specific cleavage at cysteine sites, it would be best to protect lysine and arginine residues by reversible masking groups (see Sections IVA16 and IVC). Tryptic hydrolysis of S-aminoethylated proteins has been applied to a large number of proteins.

Carboxamidomethylation of cysteine residues (by reaction with iodoacetamide) has been reported to render them susceptible to tryptic hydrolysis (Gorecki and Shalitin, 1967). The selectivity of thiol-group modification by haloacetates has been discussed (Section IVG4). Aminoethylation by aziridine (ethylenimine) will usually be more selective and is most likely a more suitable approach for cleavage.

It is relevant to indicate here that cleavage at cysteine by reaction (91), if employed in conjunction with suitable reversible protection of lysyl and arginyl residues, will be a more specific method of cleavage and will give higher yields than the chemical cleavage reactions discussed in Sections VIIC and VIID).

Cysteine, cystine, cysteic acid, or S-carboxymethylcysteine in the carboxyterminal position is released very slowly by the action of carboxypeptidase A. However, S-β-aminoethylcysteine can be removed rapidly by carboxypeptidase B (Tietze et al., 1957), while carboxypeptidase A will rapidly remove *S*-methylcysteine (Rochat *et al.*, 1970*b*). *S*-Methylation of thiol groups has been described (Section IVG6).

2. Cleavage of Serine Peptide Bonds

Conversion of serine residues to their *O*-sulfonyl- (*p*-toluenesulfonyl, tosyl, or methanesulfonyl, mesyl) derivatives (Section IVB) can serve as the beginning for subsequent appropriate modification and cleavage at seryl peptide bonds. One approach is to convert *O*-tosylserine to cysteine residues, which has already been described in reaction (29) (Section IVB). The resultant thiol groups can then be aminoethylated and hydrolyzed by trypsin, as shown in reaction (91). An alternative approach was by direct reaction (92) of *O*-tosyl- or *O*-mesylserine peptides with β-mercaptoethyl-amine, in the presence of sodium methoxide in anhydrous dimethylform-

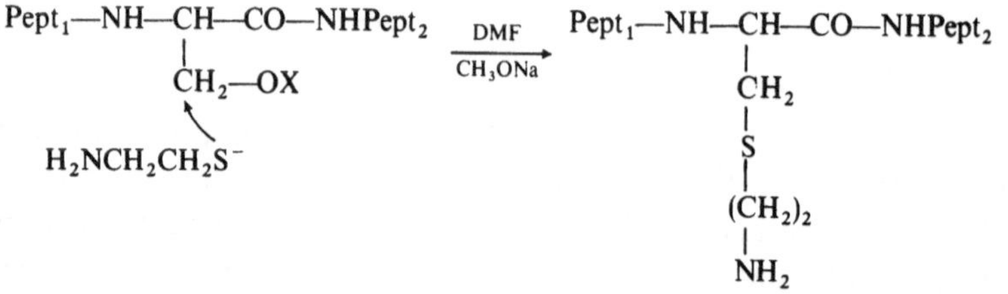

$$
\begin{array}{ccc}
\text{Pept}_1\text{—NH—CH—CO—NHPept}_2 & \xrightarrow[\text{CH}_3\text{ONa}]{\text{DMF}} & \text{Pept}_1\text{—NH—CH—CO—NHPept}_2 \\
\quad\quad\quad | & & \quad\quad\quad | \\
\quad\quad\text{CH}_2\text{—OX} & & \quad\quad\text{CH}_2 \\
\quad\quad\quad\nwarrow & & \quad\quad\quad | \\
\text{H}_2\text{NCH}_2\text{CH}_2\text{S}^- & & \quad\quad\quad\text{S} \\
& & \quad\quad\quad | \\
& & \quad\quad(\text{CH}_2)_2 \\
& & \quad\quad\quad | \\
& & \quad\quad\text{NH}_2 \\
\\
\quad\quad\text{(a)} & & \quad\quad\quad\text{(b)}
\end{array}
\tag{92}
$$

$$X = CH_3C_6H_4SO_2 \text{ or } CH_3SO_2$$

amide at room temperature (Patchornik *et al.*, 1969), to give the *S*-β-aminoethylcysteine peptides (92b). The latter can then be hydrolyzed by trypsin. Reaction (92) has been demonstrated only on model peptides.

3. Prevention of Tryptic Cleavage at Lysine or at Arginine Peptide Bonds

Cleavage by trypsin at lysyl peptide bonds has been prevented by utilizing a variety of amino group modification reactions. The most frequently employed modifications have been acetylation and succinylation, which, of course, inflict permanent modifications on the amino groups. Reversible citraconylation (Section IVA16) was shown to enable specific cleavage at arginyl peptide bonds and to yield fragments which, after deprotection, were entirely free of internal modifications (Singhal and Atassi, 1971). Cleavage of sperm whale myoglobin by this procedure aided enormously in the delineation of the antigenic structure of the protein (Singhal and Atassi, 1971). This approach has now been applied to many proteins.

Cleavage at arginyl residues may be prevented by modification of the arginine residues as described in section IVC. However, to obtain peptides free of internal modifications, the most suitable approaches are the reversible modification reactions with cyclohexanedione (reaction 30; Patthy and Smith, 1975a) or with phenylglyoxal (reaction 31; Werber *et al.*, 1975).

4. *Alteration of Tryptic Hydrolysis by Varying the Conditions*

Unlike IgG, it has been difficult to obtain Fab and Fc fragments from IgM by limited enzymatic cleavage. Hydrolysis of IgM with trypsin at high temperature (60°C) was shown to yield these fragments in high yield (Plaut and Tomasi, 1970). It was suggested that the accessibility to trypsin was made possible by relaxation of the folding in the middle part of the molecule as a result of the temperature-induced conformational change. Similar loosening up of the structure was obtained in the presence of denaturing agents such as urea (Shimizu *et al.*, 1974). Tryptic hydrolysis of human IgM in the presence of 4–5 M urea at 25°C in fact yielded Fab and Fc fragments (Shimizu *et al.*, 1974). The high-temperature tryptic cleavage method has been applied to prepare an Fc-like fragment in high yield from a human IgD myeloma protein (Wolcott *et al.*, 1975).

It is relevant to mention at this stage that in tryptic (and chymotryptic) hydrolysis of the sequence A—B—Asn—C (C = Gly preferably), cleavage of the A—B bond has been shown to result in some diketopiperazine formation due to cyclization involving aspartyl α-carboxyl groups liberated during β-aspartyl shifts (Jörnvall, 1974). This explains the presence of amino-terminal-blocked peptides sometimes obtained.

5. *Cleavage of "Tight" Proteins*

Delineation of the antigenic structures of "tight" proteins (i.e., disulfide-containing, proteolytically inaccessible proteins) has, until recently, eluded investigation because it has not been possible to prepare from these proteins a variety of long and overlapping peptides without rupturing the disulfide bonds. Scission of the disulfide bonds yielded unfolded proteins, which have been found by numerous investigators to bear no immunochemical relationship whatsoever to the native protein. These unfolded proteins were therefore totally unsatisfactory as immunochemical models for the parent native protein. This deadlock has been broken by the introduction of a novel approach for complete tryptic hydrolysis of disulfide-containing proteins (Atassi *et al.*, 1973a). Masking of the amino groups by citraconylation introduced conformational changes in the protein (Habeeb and Atassi, 1970) that rendered it completely accessible to tryptic hydrolysis at the arginyl peptide bonds. After unmasking of the amino groups, cleavage at the lysyl residues can be achieved, if desired, thus yielding the tryptic peptides with intact disulfide bonds (Atassi *et al.*, 1973*a*). Alternatively, hydrolysis can be stopped (with trypsin inhibitor) after cleavage of the arginyl peptide bonds. This approach has been applied to lysozyme, yielding fragments which accounted for almost all (90%) of the reaction of lysozyme with its antibodies (Atassi *et al.*, 1973*a*). Fragments have also been obtained from cleavage of bovine serum albumin at arginyl peptide bonds only, which accounted for all (97%) of the antigenic reactivity of the native protein (Habeeb *et al.*, 1974; Atassi *et al.*, 1976*a*). Its application to bovine ribonuclease A has also yielded fragments which reacted with antibodies to the native protein (Habeeb and Atassi, unpublished results). The ability to prepare all the tryptic peptides of a protein without rupturing the disulfide bonds was also introduced (Atassi *et al.*, 1973*a*) as a useful procedure by which the correct disulfide pairing may be determined.

Acknowledgments

I would like to thank L. Kazim, W. Zablocki, M. Litowich, and M. Odegaard for their valuable assistance in proofreading and in the tedious task of doublechecking the numerous references cited in the text. The work was supported by Grants AM 13389, AM 18920, and AI 13181 from the National Institutes of Health, U.S. Public Health Service.

VIII. References

Abadi, D. M., and Wilcox, P. E., 1960, *J. Biol. Chem.* **235**:396.
Abe, O., Lukacovic, M. F., and Ressler, C., 1974, *J. Org. Chem.* **39**:253.
Aboderin, A. A., Boedefeld, E., and Luisi, P. L., 1973, *Biochim. Biophys. Acta* **328**:20.
Agrawal, B. B. L., Margoliash, E., Levenberg, M. I., Egan, R. S., and Studier, M. H., 1970, *Fed. Proc.* **29**:732.
Airoldi, L. P. da S., and Doonan, S., 1975, *FEBS Lett.* **50**:155.
Alexander, N. M., 1973, *Biochem. Biophys. Res. Commun.* **54**:614.
Alexander, N. M., 1974, *J. Biol. Chem.* **249**:1946.
Allan, R., and Isliker, H., 1974, *Immunochemistry* **11**:175.
Allen, G., and Lowe, G., 1973, *Biochem. J.* **133**:679.
Anderson, B., Seno, N., Sampson, P., Riley, J. G., Hoffman, P, and Meyer, K., 1964, *J. Biol. Chem.* **239**:PC2716.
Andersson, L.-O., and Berg, G., 1969, *Biochim. Biophys. Acta* **192**:534.
Anderson, P. M., and Carlson, J. D., 1975, *Biochemistry* **14**:3688.
Ando, K., Matsubara, H., and Okunuki, K., 1966, *Biochim. Biophys. Acta* **118**:256.
Ando, Y., and Steiner, M., 1973, *Biochim. Biophys. Acta* **311**:38.
Andres, S. F., and Atassi, M. Z., 1970, *Biochemistry* **9**:2268.
Andres, S. F., and Atassi, M. Z., 1973, *Biochemistry* **12**:942.
Anfinsen, C. B., 1961, *J. Polym. Sci.* **49**:31.
Anfinsen, C. B., and Haber, E., 1961, *J. Biol. Chem.* **236**:1361.
Arnon, R., and Shapira, E., 1969, *J. Biol. Chem.* **244**:1033.

Asquith, R. S., and Carthew, P., 1972, *Biochim. Biophys. Acta* **278**:8.

Atassi, M. Z., 1967a, *Biochem. J.* **102**:478.

Atassi, M. Z., 1967b, *Arch. Biochem. Biophys.* **120**:56.

Atassi, M. Z., 1967c, *Biochem. J.* **102**:488.

Atassi, M. Z., 1967d, *Biochem. J.* **103**:29.

Atassi, M. Z., 1968, *Biochemistry* **7**:3078.

Atassi, M. Z., 1969a, *Immunochemistry* **6**:801.

Atassi, M. Z., 1969b, *Biochim. Biophys. Acta* **177**:663.

Atassi, M. Z., 1970, *Biochim. Biophys. Acta* **221**:612.

Atassi, M. Z., 1972, Specific receptors of antibodies, antigens and cells, in: *Third International Convocation on Immunology,* 118 pp., Karger, Basel.

Atassi, M. Z., 1973, *Tetrahedron Lett.* **1973**:4893.

Atassi, M. Z., 1975, *Immunochemistry* **12**:423.

Atassi, M. Z., and Caruso, D. R., 1968, *Biochemistry* **7**:699.

Atassi, M. Z., and Habeeb, A. F. S. A., 1969, *Biochemistry* **8**:1385.

Atassi, M. Z., and Habeeb, A. F. S. A., 1972, *Methods Enzmol.* **25(B)**:546.

Atassi, M. Z., and Nakhleh, E. T., 1975, *Biochim. Biophys. Acta* **379**:1.

Atassi, M. Z., and Pai, R.-C., 1975, *Immunochemistry* **12**:735.

Atassi, M. Z., and Perlstein, M. T., 1972a, *Biochemistry* **11**:3984.

Atassi, M. Z., and Perlstein, M. T., 1972b, *Tetrahedron Lett.* **1972**:1861.

Atassi, M. Z., and Rosemblatt, M. C., 1974, *J. Biol. Chem.* **249**:482.

Atassi, M. Z., and Rosenthal, A. F., 1969, *Biochem. J.* **111**:593.

Atassi, M. Z., and Saplin, B. J., 1968, *Biochemistry* **7**:688.

Atassi, M. Z., and Singhal, R. P., 1970a, *Biochemistry* **9**:3854.

Atassi, M. Z., and Singhal, R. P., 1970b, *J. Biol. Chem.* **245**:5122.

Atassi, M. Z., and Singhal, R. P., 1972a, *Immunochemistry* **9**:1057.

Atassi, M. Z., and Singhal, R. P., 1972b, *J. Biol. Chem.* **247**:5980.

Atassi, M. Z., and Thomas, A. V., 1969, *Biochemistry* **8**:3385.

Atassi, M. Z., and Zablocki, W., 1975, *Biochim. Biophys. Acta* **386**:233.

Atassi, M. Z., and Zablocki, W., 1976, *J. Biol. Chem.* **251**:1653.

Atassi, M. Z., Habeeb, A. F. S. A., and Rydstedt, L., 1970, *Biochim. Biophys. Acta* **200**:184.

Atassi, M. Z., Perlstein, M. T., and Habeeb, A. F. S. A., 1971, *J. Biol. Chem.* **246**:4291.

Atassi, M. Z., Suliman, A. M., and Habeeb, A. F. S. A., 1972, *Immunochemistry* **9**:907.

Atassi, M. Z., Habeeb, A. F. S. A., and Ando, K., 1973a, *Biochim. Biophys. Acta* **303**:203.

Atassi, M. Z., Perlstein, M. T., and Staub, D. J., 1973b, *Biochim. Biophys. Acta* **328**:278.

Atassi, M. Z., Rosenthal, A. F., and Vargas, L., 1973c, *Biochim. Biophys. Acta* **303**:379.

Atassi, M. Z., Rosemblatt, M. C., and Habeeb, A. F. S. A., 1974, *Immunochemistry* **11**:495.

Atassi, M. Z., Litowich, M. T., and Andres, S. F., 1975a, *Immunochemistry* **12**:727.

Atassi, M. Z., Suliman, A. M., and Habeeb, A. F. S. A., 1975b, *Biochim. Biophys. Acta* **405**:452.

Atassi, M. Z., Habeeb, A. F. S. A., and Lee, C.-L., 1976a, *Immunochemistry* **13**:547.

Atassi, M. Z., Koketsu, J., and Habeeb, A. F. S. A., 1976b, *Biochim. Biophys. Acta* **420**:358.

Atassi, M. Z., Lee, C.-L., and Habeeb, A. F. S. A., 1976c, *Immunochemistry* **13**:7.

Aviram, I., and Schejter, A., 1971, *Biochim. Biophys. Acta* **229**:113.

Axén, R., Porath, J., and Ernback, S., 1967, *Nature (London)* **214**:1302.

Azari, P., 1966, *Arch. Biochem. Biophys.* **115**:230.

Azari, P., and Phillips, J. L., 1970, *Arch. Biochem. Biophys.* **138**:32.

Azzi, A., Bragadin, M. A., Neri, G., Farnia, G., and Tamburro, A. M., 1973, *FEBS Lett.* **30**:249.

Bak, B., Led, J. J., and Pedersen, E. J., 1969, *Acta Chem. Scand.* **23**:3051.

Bakardjieva, A., and Crichton, R. R., 1974, *Biochem. J.* **143**:599.

Baker, B. R., 1967, *Design of Active-Site-Directed Irreversible Enzyme Inhibitors,* Wiley, New York.

Baker, B. R., Lee, W. W., Tong, E., and Ross, L. O., 1961, *J. Am. Chem. Soc.* **83**:3713.

Balls, A. K., and Wood, H. N., 1956, *J. Biol. Chem.* **219**:245.

Banks, T. E., and Shafer, J. A., 1970, *Biochemistry* **9**:3343.

Banks, T. E., and Shafer, J. A., 1972, *Biochemistry* **11**:110.

Banks, T. E., Blossey, B. K., and Shafer, J. A., 1969, *J. Biol. Chem.* **244**:6323.

Bargetzi, J. P., Thompson, E. O. P., Sampath Kumar, K. S. V., Walsh, K. A., and Neurath, H., 1964, *J. Biol. Chem.* **239**:3767.

Barksdale, A. D., Hedlund, B. E., Hallaway, B. E., Benson, E. S., and Rosenberg, A., 1975, *Biochemistry* **14**:2695.

Barman, T. E., 1972, *Biochim. Biophys. Acta* **258**:297.

Barman, T. E., and Bagshaw, W., 1972, *Biochim. Biophys. Acta* **278**:491.

Barman, T. E., and Koshland, D. E., Jr., 1967, *J. Biol. Chem.* **242**:5771.

Barnett, J. E. G., and Kolisis, F., 1974, *Biochem. J.* **143**:487.

Barratt, M. D., Dodd, G. H., and Chapman, D., 1969, *Biochim. Biophys. Acta* **194**:600.

Barratt, M. D., Davies, A. P., and Evans, M. T. A., 1971, *Eur. J. Biochem.* **24**:280.

Barritault, D., Expert-Bezangon, A., Milet, M., and Hayes, D. H., 1975, *FEBS Lett.* **50**:114.

Barry, E. J., and Gutmann, H. R., 1973, *J. Biol. Chem.* **248**:2730.

Baumert, H. G., Fasold, H., Keller, F., Halbach, M., and Ortanderl, F., 1973, *FEBS Lett.* **31**:23.

Bayliss, R. S., and Knowles, J. R., 1968, *Chem. Commun.* **1968**:196.

Bayliss, R. S., Knowles, J. R., and Wybrandt, G. B., 1969, *Biochem. J.* **113**:377.

Becker, R. R., and Stahmann, M. A., 1953, *J. Biol. Chem.* **204**:745.

Beeley, J. G., and Neurath, H., 1968, *Biochemistry* **7**:1239.

Benesch, R., and Benesch, R. E., 1958, *Proc. Natl. Acad. Sci. U.S.A.* **44**:848.

Benesch, R., and Benesch, R. E., 1962, *Biochim. Biophys. Acta* **63**:166.

Benisek, W. F., and Cole, R. D., 1965, *Biochem. Biophys. Res. Commun.* **20**:655.

Benisek, W. F., and Richards, F. M., 1968, *J. Biol. Chem.* **243**:4267.

Benisek, W. F., Raftery, M. A., and Cole, R. D., 1967, *Biochemistry* **6**:3780.

Benyamin, Y., Robin, Y., and van Thoai, N., 1973, *Eur. J. Biochem.* **37**:459.

Berger, K. U., Barratt, M. D., and Kamat, V. B., 1971, *Chem. Phys. Lipids* **6**:351.

Bergstrand, H., 1971, *Eur. J. Biochem.* **21**:116.

Bertrand, R., Pautel, P., and Pechere, J. F., 1974, *Biochimie* **56**:515.

Birch, A. J., Cymerman-Craig, J., and Slaytor, M., 1955, *Aust. J. Chem.* **8**:512.

Birchmeier, W., Wilson, K. J., and Christen, P., 1973, *J. Biol. Chem.* **248**:1751.

Birkett, D. J., Price, N. C., Radda, G. K., and Salmon, A. G., 1970, *FEBS Lett.* **6**:346.

Bittner, E. W., and Gerig, J. T., 1970, *J. Am. Chem. Soc.* **92**:2114.

Bizzini, B., Turpin, A., and Raynaud, M., 1973, *Eur. J. Biochem.* **39**:171.

Black, D. H., 1966, *J. Chem. Soc.* (*C*) **1123**:1708.

Blair, T. T., Marini, M. A., and Martin, C. J., 1972, *FEBS Lett.* **20**:41.

Bloch, K., 1969, *Accounts Chem. Res.* **2**:193.

Block, R. J., Durrum, E. I., and Zweig, G., 1958, *A Manual of Paper Chromatography and Paper Electrophoresis,* 2nd ed., p. 110, Academic Press, New York.

Blumberg, S., Holmquist, B., and Vallee, B. L., 1973, *Biochem. Biophys. Res. Commun.* **51**:987.

Blumenthal, K. M., and Smith, E. L., 1973, *J. Biol. Chem.* **248**:6002.

Boccù, E., Veronese, F. M., Fontana, A., and Benassi, C. A., 1970, *Eur. J. Biochem.* **13**:188.

Bodansky, M., and Ondetti, M. A., 1966, *Peptide Synthesis,* p. 98, Interscience, New York.

Bodlaender, P., Feinstein, G., and Shaw, E., 1969, *Biochemistry* **8**:4941.

Boesel, R. W., and Carpenter, F. H., 1970, *Biochem. Biophys. Res. Commun.* **38**:678.

Bohak, Z., 1964, *J. Biol. Chem.* **239**:2878.

Böhlen, P., Stein, S., Dairman, W., and Udenfriend, S., 1973, *Arch. Biochem. Biophys.* **155**:213.

Bollen, A., Heimark, R. L., Cozzone, A., Traut, R. R., Hershey, J. W. B., and Kahan, L., 1975, *J. Biol. Chem.* **250**:4310.

Bolton, A. E., and Hunter, W. M., 1973, *Biochem. J.* **133**:529.

Bond, J. S., Francis, S. H., and Park, J. H., 1970, *J. Biol. Chem.* **245**:1041.

Bonnett, R., and Holleyhead, R., 1974, *J. Chem. Soc. Perkin Trans. I* **1974**:962.

Bordignon, E., Cattalini, L., Natile, G., and Scatturin, A., 1973, *J. Chem. Soc. Chem. Commun. Part 2* **1973**:878.

Bornmann, L., and Hess. B., 1974, *Hoppe-Seyler's Z. Physiol. Chem.* **355**:1073.

Bornstein, P., and Balain, G., 1970, *J. Biol. Chem.* **245**:4854.

Bosshard, H. R., Jorgensen, K. H., and Humbel, R. E., 1969, *Eur. J. Biochem.* **9**:353.

Boussioux, A. M., Pons, M., Nicolas, J. C., Descomps, B., and Crastes de Paulet, A., 1973, *FEBS Lett.* **36**:27.

Bowden, B. J., and Wheeler, G. P., 1971, *Proc. Am. Assoc. Cancer Res.* **12**:67.

Boyd, H., Calder, I. C., Leach, S. J., and Milligan, B., 1972a, *Int. J. Peptide Protein Res.* **4**:109.

Boyd, H., Leach, S. J., and Milligan, B., 1972b, *Int. J. Peptide Protein Res.* **4**:117.

Boyer, P. D., 1954, *J. Am. Chem. Soc.* **76**:4331.

Bradbury, A. F., and Smyth, D. G., 1973, *Biochem. J.* **131**:637.

Bradshaw, R. A., Ericsson, L. H., Walsh, K. A., and Neurath, H., 1969a, *Proc. Natl. Acad. Sci. U.S.A.* **63**:1389.

Bradshaw, R. A., Robinson, G. W., Hass, G. M., and Hill, R. L., 1969b, *J. Biol. Chem.* **244**:1755.

Brake, A. J., and Weber, B. H., 1974, *J. Biol. Chem.* **249**:5452.

Brandt, J., Fredriksson, M., and Andersson, L. -O., 1974, *Biochemistry* **13**:4758.

Brandt, J., Andersson, L. -O., and Porath, J., 1975, *Biochim. Biophys. Acta* **386**:196.

Braunitzer, V. G., Beyreuther, K., Fujiki, H., and Schrank, B., 1968, *Hoppe-Seyler's Z. Physiol. Chem.* **349**:265.

Brazil, H., and Ram, J. S., 1965, *Arch. Biochem. Biophys.* **110**:205.

Brdicka, R., 1933, *Coll. Trav. Chim. Tchecosl.* **5**:148.

Bridges, A. J., and Knowles, J. R., 1974, *Biochem. J.* **143**:663.

Brill, A. S., and Weinryb, I., 1967, *Biochemistry* **6**:3528.

Brocklehurst, K., and Little, G., 1973, *Biochem. J.* **133**:67.

Brocklehurst, K., Kierstan, M., and Little, G., 1972, *Biochem. J.* **128**:811.

Bromer, W. W., Sheehan, S. K., Berns, A. W., and Arguilla, E. R., 1967, *Biochemistry* **6**:2378.

Broun, G., Selegny, E., Avrameas, S., and Thomas, D., 1969, *Biochim. Biophys. Acta* **185**:260.

Brown, R. K., 1962, *J. Biol. Chem.* **238**:1162.

Brown, W. E., and Wold, F., 1973, *Biochemistry* **12**:835.

Bruice, T. C., Gregory, M. J., and Walters, S. L., 1968, *J. Am. Chem. Soc.* **90**:1612.

Buckingham, D. A., Collman, J. P., Happer, D. A. R., and Marzilli, L. G., 1967a, *J. Am. Chem. Soc.* **89**:1082.

Buckingham, D. A., Marzilli, L. G., and Sargeson, A. M., 1967b, *J. Am. Chem. Soc.* **89**:4539.

Burke, W. F., and Reeves, H. C., 1975, *Anal. Biochem.* **63**:267.

Burnett, P. R., and Eylar, E. H., 1971, *J. Biol. Chem.* **246**:3425.

Burr, M., and Koshland, D. E., Jr., 1964, *Proc. Natl. Acad. Sci. U.S.A.* **52**:1017.

Burstein, Y., and Patchornik, A., 1972, *Biochemistry* **11**:4641.

Burstein, Y., and Sperling, R., 1970, *Biochim. Biophys. Acta* **221**:410.

Burstein, Y., Fridkin, M., and Patchornik, A., 1967, *Isr. J. Chem.* **5**:64.

Burstein, Y., Walsh, K. A., and Neurath, H., 1974, *Biochemistry* **13**:205.

Busse, W. D., and Carpenter, F. H., 1974, *J. Am. Chem. Soc.* **96**:5947.

Busse, W. D., Hansen, S. R., and Carpenter, F. H., 1974, *J. Am. Chem. Soc.* **96**:5949.

Butler, P. J. G., Harris, J. I., Hartley, B. S., and Leberman, R., 1967, *Biochem. J.* **103**:78.

Butler, P. J. G., Harris, J. I., Hartley, B. S., and Leberman, R., 1969, *Biochem. J.* **112**:679.

Buttkus, H., 1969, *J. Am. Oil Chem. Soc.* **46**:88.

Caldwell, J. B., Holt, L. A., and Milligan, B., 1971, *Aust. J. Chem.* **24**:435.

Capaldi, R. A., 1973, *Biochem. Biophys. Res. Commun.* **50**:656.

Capps, P. A., and Jones, A. R., 1974, *J. Chem. Soc. Chem. Commun.* **9**:320.

Caputo, A., and Zito, R., 1961, *Second Symp. Lysozyme Milan* 1:29.

Carlsson, U., Aasa, R., Henderson, L. E., Jonsson, B. -H., and Lindskog, S., 1975, *Eur. J. Biochem.* 52:25.

Carpenter, F. H., and Shiigi, S. M., 1974, *Biochemistry* 13:5159.

Carraway, K. L., and Koshland, D. E., Jr., 1968, *Biochim. Biophys. Acta* 160:272.

Carraway, K. L., and Triplett, R. B., 1970, *Biochim. Biophys. Acta* 200:564.

Carraway, K. L., Spoerl, P., and Koshland, D. E., Jr., 1969, *J. Mol. Biol.* 42:133.

Casey, R., and Lang, A., 1975, *Biochem. J.* 145:251.

Casola, L., Di Matteo, G., Di Prisco, G., and Cervone, F., 1974, *Anal. Biochem.* 57:38.

Castellino, F. J., and Hill, R. L., 1970, *J. Biol. Chem.* 245:417.

Catsimpoolas, N., and Wood, J. L., 1964, *J. Biol. Chem.* 239:4132.

Catsimpoolas, N., and Wood, J. L., 1966, *J. Biol. Chem.* 241:1790.

Cavins, J. F., and Friedman, M., 1968, *J. Biol. Chem.* 243:3357.

Cecil, R., 1963, *The Proteins,* Vol. 1, 2nd ed. (H. Neurath, ed.), p. 380, Academic Press, New York.

Cecil, R., and McPhee, J. R., 1959, *Adv. Protein Chem.* 14:255.

Cecil, R., and Weitzman, P. D. J., 1964, *Biochem. J.* 93:1.

Cerami, A., Manning, J. M., Gillette, P. N., De Furia, F., Miller, D., Graziano, J. H., and Peterson, C. M., 1973, *Fed. Proc.* 32:1668.

Chaiken, I. M., and Smith, E. L., 1969, *J. Biol. Chem.* 244:4247.

Chan, J. K., and Anderson, B. M., 1975, *J. Biol. Chem.* 250:67.

Chan, W. W.-C., 1968, *Biochemistry* 7:4247.

Chang, C. C., and Yang, C. C., 1973, *Biochim. Biophys. Acta* 295:595.

Chang, F. N., and Flaks, J. G., 1972, *J. Mol. Biol.* 68:177.

Chang, J. Y., and Schroeder, W. A., 1972, *Arch. Biochem. Biophys.* 148:505.

Chang, J. Y., and Schroeder, W. A., 1973, *Arch. Biochem. Biophys.* 156:475.

Chao, L.-P., and Einstein, E. R., 1970, *J. Biol. Chem.* 245:6397.

Cheng, K.-W., and Pierce, J. G., 1972, *J. Biol. Chem.* 247:7163.

Chentsova, T. V., and Kravchenko, N. A., 1974, *Biokhimiya* 39:491.

Chesebro, B., and Metzger, H., 1972, *Biochemistry* 11:766.

Cheung, H. C., Cooke, R., and Smith, L., 1971, *Arch. Biochem. Biophys.* 142:333.

Chignell, C. F., Starkweather, D. K., and Erlich, R. H., 1972, *Biochim. Biophys. Acta* 271:6.

Chin, C. C. Q., and Wold, F., 1975, *Arch. Biochem. Biophys.* 167:448.

Chio, K. S., and Tappel, A. L., 1969, *Biochemistry* 8:2827.

Churakova, N. I., Kravchenko, N. A., Serebryakov, E. P., Lavrov, I. A., and Kaversneva, E. D., 1973, *Photochem. Photobiol.* 18:201.

Clarke, W. C., and Li, C. H., 1974, *Arch. Biochem. Biophys.* 161:313.

Cleland, W. W., 1964, *Biochemistry* 3:480.

Coffee, C. J., Bradshaw, R. A., Goldin, B. R., and Frieden, C., 1971, *Biochemistry* 10:3516.

Coggins, J. R., Kray, W., and Shaw, E., 1974, *Biochem. J.* 138:579.

Cohen, L. A., 1968, *Annu. Rev. Biochem.* 37:695.

Colletti-Previero, M. A., Previero, A., and Zuckerkandl, E., 1969, *J. Mol. Biol.* 39:493.

Collman, J. P., and Buckingham, D. A., 1963, *J. Am. Chem. Soc.* 85:3039.

Colman, R. F., 1968, *J. Biol. Chem.* 243:2454.

Colombo, G., and Marcus, F., 1974, *Biochemistry* 13:3085.

Coons, A. H., Creech, H. J., Jones, R. N., and Berliner, E., 1942, *J. Immunol.* 45:159.

Cooper, H., Leach, S. J., and Milligan, B. M., 1970, *Proc. Aust. Biochem. Soc.* 3:35.

Corey, E. J., and Haefele, L. F., 1959, *J. Am. Chem. Soc.* 81:2225.

Corradin, G., and Harbury, H. A., 1974, *Biochem. Biophys. Res. Commun.* 61:1400.

Cotner, R. C., and Clagett, C. O., 1973, *Anal. Biochem.* 54:170.

Covelli, I., and Wolff, J., 1966, *J. Biol. Chem.* 241:4444.

Crawhill, J. C., and Elliott, D. F., 1955, *Biochem. J.* 61:264.

Cremona, T., Kowal, J., and Horeker, B. L., 1965, *Proc. Natl. Acad. Sci. U.S.A.* **53**:1395.

Crestfield, A. M., Moore, S., and Stein, W. H., 1963, *J. Biol. Chem.* **238**:622.

Crewther, W. G., and Nicholls, P. W., 1969, *Biochim. Biophys. Acta* **194**:606.

Cronin, J. R., and Harbury, H. A., 1965, *Biochem. Biophys. Res. Commun.* **20**:503.

Cuatrecasas, P., Fuchs, S., and Anfinsen, C. B., 1968, *J. Biol. Chem.* **243**:4787.

Cybulsky, D. L., Kandel, S. I., Kandel, M., and Gornall, A. G., 1973, *J. Biol. Chem.* **248**:3411.

Danehy, J. P., 1966, *The Chemistry of Organic Sulfur Compounds,* Vol. 2 (N. Kharasch and C. Y. Meyers, eds.), Chap. 13, Pergamon Press, Oxford.

Danehy, J. P., Elia, V. J., and Lavelle, C. J., 1971, *J. Org. Chem.* **36**:1003.

D'Angeli, F., Scoffone, E., Filira, F., and Giormani, V., 1966, *Tetrahedron Lett.* **1966**:2745.

Dann, L. G., and Britton, H. G., 1974, *Biochem. J.* **137**:405.

David, M. M., Sperling, R., and Steinberg, I. Z., 1974, *Biochim. Biophys. Acta* **359**:101.

Davies, G. E., and Stark, G. R., 1970, *Proc. Natl. Acad. Sci. U.S.A.* **66**:651.

Davies, J. S., Hassall, C. H., and Schofield, J. A., 1964, *Chem. Ind.* **1964**:1804.

Davies, J. S., Hassall, C. H., and Hopkins, K. H., 1971, *Chem. Commun.* **1971**:1118.

Davies, J. S., Hassall, C. H., and Hopkins, K. H., 1973, *J. Chem. Soc. Perkin Trans. I* **1973**:2614.

Davies, R. C., and Neuberger, A., 1969, *Biochim. Biophys. Acta* **178**:306.

Davis, R. H., Jr., Delaney, P., and Furfine, C. S., 1973, *Arch. Biochem. Biophys.* **159**:11.

Deal, W. J., Mohlman, S. G., and Sprang, M. L., 1971, *Science* **171**:1147.

Dedman, M. L., Farmer, T. H., and Morris, C. J. O. R., 1957, *Biochem. J.* **66**:166.

Degani, C., and Boyer, P. D., 1973, *J. Biol. Chem.* **248**:8222.

Degani, Y., and Patchornik, A., 1967, in: *Proceedings of the Seventh International Congress of Biochemistry (Tokyo),* Vol. 2, Abst. A-99, p. 603.

Degani, Y., and Patchornik, A., 1974, *Biochemistry* **13**:1.

Degani, Y., Patchornik, A., and Maclaren, J. A., 1966, *J. Am. Chem. Soc.* **88**:3460.

Degani, Y., Neumann, H., and Patchornik, A., 1970, *J. Am. Chem. Soc.* **92**:6969.

Degani, Y., Veronese, F. M., and Smith, E. L., 1974, *J. Biol. Chem.* **249**:7929.

De la Llosa, P., Durosay, M., Tetrin-Clary, C., and Jutisz, M., 1974, *Biochim. Biophys. Acta* **342**:97.

Delarco, J. E., and Liener, I. E., 1973, *Biochim. Biophys. Acta* **303**:274.

Delpierre, G. R., and Fruton, J. S., 1966, *Proc. Natl. Acad. Sci. U.S.A.* **56**:1817.

Dewar, J. H., and Shaw, G., 1961, *J. Chem. Soc.* **1961**:3254.

Dixon, H. B. F., 1962, *Biochem. J.* **83**:91.

Dixon, H. B. F., 1964a, *Biochem. J.* **90**:2c.

Dixon, H. B. F., 1964b, *Biochem. J.* **92**:661.

Dixon, H. B. F., and Fields, R., 1972, *Methods Enzymol.* **25B**:409.

Dixon, H. B. F., and Perham, R. N., 1968, *Biochem. J.* **109**:312.

Donovan, J. W., and White, T. M., 1971, *Biochemistry* **10**:32.

Doyle, R. J., Bello, J., and Rohom, O. A., 1968, *Biochim. Biophys. Acta* **160**:274.

Dukler, S., Wilchek, M., and Lavie, D., 1971, *Tetrahedron* **27**:607.

Dutton, A., Adams, M., and Singer, S. J., 1966, *Biochem. Biophys. Res. Commun.* **23**:730.

Dworschack, R. T., Wyborny, L. E., and Kalnitsky, G., 1973, *Arch. Biochem. Biophys.* **159**:463.

Dworschack, R., Tarr, G., and Plapp, B. V., 1975, *Biochemistry* **14**:200.

Edelman, G. M., Olins, D. E., Gally, J. A., and Zinder, N. D., 1963, *Proc. Natl. Acad. Sci. U.S.A.* **50**:753.

Eisen, H. M., Belman, S., and Carsten, M. E., 1953, *J. Am. Chem. Soc.* **75**:4583.

Elek, G., Sajgo, M., Grigorian, G. L., Chibrikin, V. M., and Keleti, T., 1972, *Acta Biochim. Biophys. Acad. Sci. Hung.* **7**:119.

Ellman, G. L., 1959, *Arch. Biochem. Biophys.* **82**:70.

Erlanger, B. F., Vratsanos, S. M., Wassermann, N., and Cooper, A. G., 1966, *Biochem Biophys. Res. Commun.* **23**:243.

Eshdat, Y., McKelvy, J. F., and Sharon, N., 1973, *J. Biol. Chem.* **248**:5892.

Eshdat, Y., Dunn, A., and Sharon, N., 1974, *Proc. Natl. Acad. Sci. U.S.A.* **71**:1658.

Fahrney, D. E., and Gold, A. M., 1963, *J. Am. Chem. Soc.* **85**:997.

Fanger, M. W., Hettinger, T. P., and Harbury, H. A., 1967, *Biochemistry* **6**:713.

Farber, L., and Cohen, L. A., 1966, *Biochemistry* **5**:1027.

Fasold, H., Gröschel-Stewart, U., and Turba, F., 1964, *Biochem. Z.* **339**:487.

Fasold, H., Klappenberger, J., Meyer, C., and Remold, H., 1971, *Angew. Chem. Int. Ed.* **10**:795.

Fasold, H., Meyer, C., and Steinkopff, Gudrun, 1973, *Eur. J. Biochem.* **32**:63.

Feinstein, G., Bodlaender, P., and Shaw, E., 1969, *Biochemistry* **8**:4949.

Fields, R., 1972, *Methods Enzymol.* **25B**:464.

Fischer, E. H., Kent, A. B., Snyder, E. R., and Krebs, E. G., 1958, *J. Am. Chem. Soc.* **80**:2906.

Fleet, G. W. J., Porter, R. R., and Knowles, J. R., 1969, *Nature (London)* **224**:511.

Fletcher, J. C., 1967, *Biochem. J.* **102**:815.

Fontana, A., 1972, *Methods Enzymol.* **25B**:419.

Fontana, A., Scoffone, E., and Benassi, C. A., 1968a, *Biochemistry* **7**:980.

Fontana, A., Veronese, F. M., and Scoffone, E., 1968b, *Biochemistry* **7**:3901.

Foster, M., and Harrison, J. H., 1974, *Biochim. Biophys. Acta* **351**:295.

Foye, W. O., Hebb, A. M., and Mickles, J., 1967, *J. Pharm. Sci.* **56**:292.

Fraenkel-Conrat, H., 1941, *J. Am. Chem. Soc.* **63**:2533.

Fraenkel-Conrat, H., 1950, *Arch. Biochem.* **27**:109.

Fraenkel-Conrat, H., and Mecham, D. K., 1949, *J. Biol. Chem.* **177**:477.

Fraenkel-Conrat, H., and Olcott, H. S., 1946, *J. Am. Chem. Soc.* **68**:34.

Fraenkel-Conrat, H., and Olcott, H. S., 1948, *J. Biol. Chem.* **174**:827.

Fraenkel-Conrat, H., Cooper, M., and Olcott, H. S., 1945, *J. Am. Chem. Soc.* **67**:950.

Fraenkel-Conrat, H., Bean, R. C., and Lineweaver, H., 1949, *J. Biol. Chem.* **177**:365.

Franek, F., 1971, *Eur. J. Biochem.* **19**:176.

Franek, F., and Nezlin, R. S., 1963, *Fol. Microbiol.* **8**:197.

Franzblau, C., Gallop, P. M., and Seifter, S., 1963, *Biopolymers* **1**:79.

French, D., and Edsall, J. T., 1945, *Adv. Protein Chem.* **2**:277.

Frey, P. A., Kokesh, F. C., and Westheimer, F. H., 1971, *J. Am. Chem. Soc.* **93**:7266.

Friedman, M., 1973, *The Chemistry and Biochemistry of the Sulfhydryl Group in Amino Acids, Peptides and Proteins,* 485 pp., Pergamon Press, Elmsford, N.Y.

Friedman, M., and Krull, L. H., 1969, *Biochem. Biophys. Res. Commun.* **37**:630.

Friedmann, E., 1903, *Beitr. Chem. Physiol. Pathol.* **4**:486.

Friedmann, E., Marrian, D. H., and Simon-Reuss, I., 1949, *Br. J. Pharmacol.* **4**:105.

Fry, K. T., Kim, O.-K., Spona, J., and Hamilton, G. A., 1968, *Biochem. Biophys. Res. Commun.* **30**:489.

Furth, A. J., and Hope, D. B., 1970, *Biochem. J.* **116**:545.

Galiazzo, G., Jori, G., and Scoffone, E., 1968, *Biochem. Biophys. Res. Commun.* **31**:158.

Ganther, H. E., and Corcoran, C., 1969, *Biochemistry* **8**:2557.

Gawron, O., and Fernando, J., 1961, *J. Am. Chem. Soc.* **83**:2906.

Gawron, O., Mahboob, S., and Fernando, J., 1964, *J. Am. Chem. Soc.* **86**:2283.

Gehring, H., and Christen, P., 1975, *Biochem. Biophys. Res. Commun.* **63**:441.

Geiger, R., Obermeier, R., and Tesser, G. I., 1975, *Chem. Ber.* **108**:2758.

Gerig, J. T., and Reinheimer, J. D., 1975, *J. Am. Chem. Soc.* **97**:168.

Gerngross, O., Voss, K., and Herfeld, T., 1933, *Chem. Ber.* **66**:435.

Gerwing, J., and Thompson, K., 1968, *Biochemistry* **7**:3888.

Ghosh, P. B., and Whitehouse, M. W., 1968, *Biochem. J.* **108**:155.

Gibbons, I., and Perham, R. N., 1970, *Biochem. J.* **116**:843.

Gillespie, J. M., O'Donnell, I. J., Thompson, E. O. P., and Woods, E. F., 1960, *J. Text. Inst.* **51**:T703.

Ginsburg, S., and Wilson, I. B., 1964, *J. Am. Chem. Soc.* **86**:4716.

Givol, D., Weinstein, Y., Gorecki, M., and Wilchek, M., 1970, *Biochem. Biophys. Res. Commun.* **38**:825.

Givol, D., Strausbauch, P. H., Hurwitz, E., Wilchek, M., Haimovich, J., and Eisen, H. N., 1971, *Biochemistry* **10**:3461.

Glick, B. R., and Brubacher, L. J., 1975, *J. Mol. Biol.* **93**:319.

Goetzl, E. J., and Metzger, H., 1970, *Biochemistry* **9**:1267.

Goldberger, R. F., and Anfinsen, C. B., 1962, *Biochemistry* **1**:401.

Goldman, M., 1968, *Fluorescent Antibody Methods,* Academic Press, New York.

Goodfriend, T. L., Levine, L., and Fasman, G. D., 1964, *Science* **144**:1344.

Gopalakrishnan, P. V., and Karush, F., 1975, *Immunochemistry* **12**:449.

Gorbunoff, M. J., 1970, *Arch. Biochem. Biophys.* **138**:684.

Gorbunoff, M. J., 1972, *Biopolymers* **11**:2233.

Gorecki, M., and Shalitin, Y., 1967, *Biochem. Biophys. Res. Commun.* **29**:189.

Gorecki, M., Wilchek, M., and Patchornik, A., 1971, *Biochim. Biophys. Acta* **229**:590.

Gosselin-Rey, C., Bernard, N., and Gerday, C., 1973, *Biochim. Biophys. Acta* **303**:90.

Gounaris, A. D., and Perlmann, G. E., 1967, *J. Biol. Chem.* **242**:2739.

Grassetti, D. R., and Murray, J. F., Jr., 1967, *Arch. Biochem. Biophys.* **119**:41.

Green, N. M., 1967, *Biochem. J.* **104**:64.

Green, N. M., Konieczny, L., Toms, E. J., and Valentine, R. C., 1971, *Biochem. J.* **125**:781.

Greenfield, N. J., 1974, *Biochemistry* **13**:4494.

Greenwell, P., Harris, R. J., and Symons, R. H., 1974, *Eur. J. Biochem.* **49**:539.

Greenwood, H. C., Hunter, W. M., and Glover, J. S., 1963, *Biochem. J.* **89**:114.

Gregory, J. D., 1955, *J. Am. Chem. Soc.* **77**:3922.

Griffith, O. H., Keana, J. F. W., Noall, D. L., and Ivey, J. L., 1967, *Biochem. Biophys. Acta* **148**:583.

Gross, E., 1967, *Meth. Enzymol.* **11**:238.

Gross, E., and Morell, J. L., 1966, *J. Biol. Chem.* **241**:3638.

Gross, E., and Morell, J. L., 1967, *J. Am. Chem. Soc.* **89**:2791.

Gross, E., and Morell, J. L., 1968, *FEBS Lett.* **2**:61.

Gross, E., and Morell, J. L., 1970, *J. Am. Chem. Soc.* **92**:2919.

Gross, E., and Witkop, B., 1961, *J. Am. Chem. Soc.* **83**:1510.

Gross, E., and Witkop, B., 1962, *J. Biol. Chem.* **237**:1856.

Gross, E., Morell, J. L., and Lee, P. Q., 1967, *Proceedings of the Seventh International Congress of Biochemistry (Tokyo),* Part XI, Abst. p. 535.

Grossberg, A. L., and Pressman, D., 1968, *Biochemistry* **7**:272.

Grossberg, A. L., Radzimski, G., and Pressman, D., 1962, *Biochemistry* **1**:391.

Guldalian, J., Jr., Lawson, W. B., and Brown, R. K., 1965, *J. Biol. Chem.* **240**:2757.

Gundlach, H. G., Stein, W. H., and Moore, S., 1959a, *J. Biol. Chem.* **234**:1754.

Gundlach, H. G., Moore, S., and Stein, W. H., 1959b, *J. Biol. Chem.* **234**:1761.

Günther, W. H. H., and Mautner, H. G., 1965, *J. Am. Chem. Soc.* **87**:2708.

Gurd, F. R. N., 1972, *Methods Enzymol.* **25(B)**:424.

Guttmann, S. T., 1963, *Peptides, Fifth European Peptide Symposium* (G. T. Young, ed.), p. 41, Pergamon Press, New York.

Gyenes, L., and Sehon, A. H., 1965, *Immunochemistry* **1**:43.

Habeeb, A. F. S. A., 1959, *Biochim. Biophys. Acta* **34**:294.

Habeeb, A. F. S. A., 1960, *Can. J. Biochem. Physiol.* **38**:493.

Habeeb, A. F. S. A., 1964, *Biochim. Biophys. Acta* **93**:533.

Habeeb, A. F. S. A., 1966a, *Biochim. Biophys. Acta* **115**:440.

Habeeb, A. F. S. A., 1966b, *Anal. Biochem.* **14**:328.

Habeeb, A. F. S. A., 1967a, *Arch. Biochem. Biophys.* **119**:264.

Habeeb, A. F. S. A., 1967b, *J. Immunol.* **99**:1264.

Habeeb, A. F. S. A., 1968, *J. Immunol.* **101**:505.
Habeeb, A. F. S. A., 1972a, *Methods Enzymol.* **25B**:457.
Habeeb, A. F. S. A., 1972b, *Methods Enzymol.* **25B**:558.
Habeeb, A. F. S. A., and Atassi, M. Z., 1969, *Immunochemistry* **6**:555.
Habeeb, A. F. S. A., and Atassi, M. Z., 1970, *Biochemistry* **9**:4939.
Habeeb, A. F. S. A., and Atassi, M. Z., 1971a, *Immunochemistry* **8**:1047.
Habeeb, A. F. S. A., and Atassi, M. Z., 1971b, *Biochim. Biophys. Acta* **236**:131.
Habeeb, A. F. S. A., and Bennett, J. C., 1971, *Biochim. Biophys. Acta* **251**:181.
Habeeb, A. F. S. A., and Hiramoto, R. N., 1968, *Arch. Biochem. Biophys.* **126**:16.
Habeeb, A. F. S. A., Cassidy, H. G., and Singer, S. J., 1958, *Biochem. Biophys. Acta* **29**:587.
Habeeb, A. F. S. A., Schrohenloher, R. E., and Bennett, J. C., 1970, *J. Immunol.* **105**:846.
Habeeb, A. F. S. A., Atassi, M. Z., and Lee, C.-L., 1974, *Biochim. Biophys. Acta* **342**:389.
Hadler, N., and Metzger, H., 1973, *Immunochemistry* **10**:455.
Haimovich, J., Eisen, H. N., Hurwitz, E., and Givol, D., 1972, *Biochemistry* **11**:2389.
Håkanson, R., Rönnberg, A. L., and Sjölund, K., 1973, *Anal. Biochem.* **51**:523.
Handschumacher, R. E., and Gaumond, C., 1972, *Mol. Pharmacol.* **8**:59.
Hargrave, P. A., and Wold, F., 1973, *Int. J. Peptide Protein Res.* **5**:85.
Harris, C. M., and Hill, R. L., 1969, *J. Biol. Chem.* **244**:2195.
Harris, J. I., and Perham, R. N., 1968, *Nature (London)* **219**:1025.
Harris, J. I., Meriwether, B. P., and Park, J. H., 1963, *Nature (London)* **198**:154.
Hartdegen, F. J., and Rupley, J. A., 1967, *J. Am. Chem. Soc.* **89**:1743.
Hartdegen, F. J., and Rupley, J. A., 1973, *J. Mol. Biol.* **80**:649.
Hartley, B. S., and Massey, V., 1956, *Biochim. Biophys. Acta* **21**:58.
Hartman, F. C., 1972, *Methods Enzymol.* **25B**:661.
Hartman, F. C., and Welch, M. H., 1974, *Biochem. Biophys. Res. Commun.* **57**:85.
Hartman, F. C., and Wold, F., 1966, *J. Am. Chem. Soc.* **88**:3890.
Hartman, F. C., and Wold, F., 1967, *Biochemistry* **6**:2439.
Hartman, F. C., Welch, M. H., and Norton, I. L., 1973, *Proc. Natl. Acad. Sci. U.S.A.* **70**:3721.
Hass, G. M., Govier, M. A., Girahn, D. T., and Neurath, H., 1972, *Biochemistry* **11**:3787.
Hauptmann, R., Czernilofsky, A. P., Voorma, H. O., Stoffler, G., and Kuechler, E., 1974, *Biochem. Biophys. Res. Commun.* **56**:331.
Hauptman, S. P., and Tomasi, T. B., Jr., 1975, *J. Biol. Chem.* **250**:3891.
Hawley, D. A., Miller, M. J., Slobin, L. I., and Wahba, A. J., 1974, *Biochem. Biophys. Res. Commun.* **61**:329.
Hayashi, J., Imoto, T., Funatsu, G., and Funatsu, M., 1965, *J. Biochem. (Tokyo)* **58**:227.
Hayashi, K., Shimoda, T., Imoto, T., and Funatsu, M., 1968, *J. Biochem.* **64**:365.
Hegyi, G., Premecz, G., Sain, B., and Muhlrad, A., 1974, *Eur. J. Biochem.* **44**:7.
Heilmann, H. D., and Pfleiderer, G., 1975, *Biochim. Biophys. Acta* **384**:331.
Heinrich, C. P., Noack, K., and Wiss, O., 1972, *Biochem. Biophys. Res. Commun.* **49**:1427.
Heinrich, C. P., Adams, S., and Arnold, W., 1973, *FEBS Lett.* **33**:181.
Heinrikson, R. L., 1970, *Biochem. Biophys. Res. Commun.* **41**:967.
Heinrikson, R. L., 1971, *J. Biol. Chem.* **246**:4090.
Heitz, J. R., 1973, *J. Biol. Chem.* **248**:5790.
Hellerman, L., Chinard, F. P., and Ramsdell, P. A., 1941, *J. Am. Chem. Soc.* **63**:2551.
Hellerman, L., Chinard, F. P., and Deitz, V. R., 1943, *J. Biol. Chem.* **147**:443.
Herriott, R. M., 1947, *Adv. Prot. Chem.* **3**:170.
Hestrin, S., 1949, *J. Biol. Chem.* **180**:249.
Hexter, C. S., and Westheimer, F. H., 1971, *J. Biol. Chem.* **246**:3934.
Hew, C.-L., Lifter, J., Yoshioka, M., Richards, F. F., and Konigsberg, W. H., 1973, *Biochemistry* **12**:4685.
Hijmans, W., and Schaeffer, M., eds., 1975, *Fifth International Conference on Immunofluorescence and Related Staining Techniques, Ann. N.Y. Acad. Sci.* **254**: 627 pp.

Hill, R. L., 1965, *Adv. Protein Chem.* **20**:37.

Hiremath, C. B., and Day, R. A., 1964, *J. Am. Chem. Soc.* **86**:5027.

Hirs, C. H. W., 1967a, *Methods Enzymol.* **11**:197.

Hirs, C. H. W., 1967b, *Methods Enzymol.* **11**:199.

Hirs, C. H. W., and Kycia, J. H., 1965, *Arch. Biochem. Biophys.* **111**:223.

Hoare, D. G., and Koshland, D. E., Jr., 1966, *J. Am. Chem. Soc.* **88**:2057.

Hoare, D. G., and Koshland, D. E., Jr., 1967, *J. Biol. Chem.* **242**:2447.

Hoare, D. G., Olson, A., and Koshland, D. E., Jr., 1968, *J. Am. Chem. Soc.* **90**:1638.

Hoffman, M. Z., and Hayon, E., 1972, *J. Am. Chem. Soc.* **94**:7950.

Hofmann, K., and Yajima, H., 1961, *J. Am. Chem. Soc.* **83**:2289.

Holbrook, J. J., Roberts, P. A., and Wallis, R. B., 1973, *Biochem. J.* **133**:165.

Holmgren, A., 1972, *Eur. J. Biochem.* **26**:528.

Hong, R., and Nisonoff, A., 1965, *J. Biol. Chem.* **240**:3883.

Horinishi, H., Hachimori, Y., Kurihara, K., and Shibata, K., 1964, *Biochim. Biophys. Acta* **86**:477.

Horinishi, H., Kurihara, K., and Shibata, K., 1965, *Arch. Biochem. Biophys.* **111**:520.

Horn, M. J., Jones, D. B., and Ringel, S. J., 1941, *J. Biol. Chem.* **138**:141.

Horton, H. R., and Koshland, D. E., Jr., 1965, *J. Am. Chem. Soc.* **87**:1126.

Horton, H. R., and Tucker, W. P., 1970, *J. Biol. Chem.* **245**:3397.

Horton, H. R., and Young, G., 1969, *Biochim. Biophys. Acta* **194**:272.

Horton, H. R., Kelly, H., and Koshland, D. E., Jr.; 1965, *J. Biol. Chem.* **240**:722.

Horwitz, J., and Heller, J., 1974, *J. Biol. Chem.* **249**:7181.

Houston, L. L., and Walsh, K. A., 1970, *Biochemistry* **9**:156.

Hucho, F., and Janda, M., 1974, *Biochem. Biophys. Res. Commun.* **57**:1080.

Hucho, F., Markau, U., and Sund, H., 1973, *Eur. J. Biochem.* **32**:69.

Hudson, E., and Weber, G., 1973, *Biochemistry* **12**:4154.

Huestis, W. H., and Raftery, M. A., 1972, *Biochemistry* **11**:1648.

Hughes, W. L., and Straessle, R., 1950, *J. Am. Chem. Soc.* **72**:452.

Hughes, W. L., Jr., Saroff, H. A., and Carney, A. L., 1949, *J. Am. Chem. Soc.* **71**:2476.

Hull, H. H., Chang, R., and Kaplan, L. J., 1975, *Biochim. Biophys. Acta* **400**:132.

Humphries, B. A., and Harrison, J. H., 1974, *J. Biol. Chem.* **249**:3574.

Hunter, M. J., and Ludwig, M. L., 1962, *J. Am. Chem. Soc.* **84**:3491.

Hunter, M. J., and Ludwig, M. L., 1972, *Methods Enzymol.* **25B**:585.

Hunter, W. M., 1970, *Radioimmunoassay Methods* (K. E. Kirkham and W. M. Hunter, eds.), p. 3, Williams and Wilkins, Baltimore.

Husain, H., and Lowe, G., 1968, *Chem. Commun.* **1968**:310.

Husain, S. S., and Lowe, G., 1970, *Biochem. J.* **117**:333.

Husain, S. S., Ferguson, J. B., and Fruton, J. S., 1971, *Proc. Natl. Acad. Sci. U.S.A.* **68**:2765.

Hyde, J. E., and Walker, I. O., 1975, *FEBS Lett.* **50**:150.

Ikeda-Saito, M., Kitagawa, T., Iizuka, T., and Kyogoku, Y., 1975, *FEBS Lett.* **50**:233.

Ikenaga, H., and Takahashi, K., 1975, *J. Biochem.* **75**:455.

Imamura, T., Baldwin, T. O., and Riggs, A., 1972, *J. Biol. Chem.* **247**:2785.

Imoto, T., and Rupley, J. A., 1973, *J. Mol. Biol.* **80**:657.

Imoto, T., Hartdegen, F. J., and Rupley, J. A., 1973, *J. Mol. Biol.* **80**:637.

Imoto, T., Fujimoto, M., and Yagishita, K., 1974, *J. Biochem.* (*Tokyo*) **76**:745.

Inglis, A. S., and Edman, P., 1970, *Anal. Biochem.* **37**:73.

Ingram, V. M., 1950, *Nature* (*London*) **166**:1038.

Ingram, V. M., 1953, *J. Biol. Chem.* **202**:193.

Irie, M., Harada, M., and Sawada, F., 1972, *J. Biochem.* (*Tokyo*) **72**:1351.

Isoe, S., and Cohen, L. A., 1968, *Arch. Biochem. Biophys.* **127**:522.

Itano, H. A., and Gottlieb, A. J., 1963, *Biochem. Biophys. Res. Commun.* **12**:405.

Itano, H. A., and Robinson, E. A., 1972, *J. Biol. Chem.* **247**:4819.

Iwasaki, H., and Witkop, B., 1964, *J. Am. Chem. Soc.* **86**:4698.
Iwasaki, H., Cohen, L. A., and Witkop, B., 1963, *J. Am. Chem. Soc.* **85**:3701.
Jacobson, G. R., Schaffer, M. H., Stark, G. R., and Vanaman, T. C., 1973, *J. Biol. Chem.* **248**:6583.
Jansen, E. F., Nutting, M.-D. F., Jang, R., and Balls, A. K., 1949, *J. Biol. Chem.* **179**:189.
Jaton, J.-C., and Sela, M., 1968, *J. Biol. Chem.* **243**:5616.
Jendrek, J. P., Barker, R. H., and Altschul, A. M., 1967, *Biochim. Biophys. Acta* **136**:409.
Jermyn, M. A., 1966, *Aust. J. Chem.* **19**:1293.
Ji, T. H., 1974, *Proc. Natl. Acad. Sci. U.S.A.* **71**:93.
Jocelyn, P. C., 1972, *Biochemistry of the SH Group,* Academic Press, New York.
Johansen, J. T., and Vallee, B. L., 1973, *Proc. Natl. Acad. Sci. U.S.A.* **70**:2006.
Johansen, J. T., Livingstone, D. M., and Vallee, B. L., 1972, *Biochemistry* **11**:2584.
Johnson, B. F., and Greenberg, J., 1973, *Chem.-Biol. Interactions* **7**:17.
Joniau, M., Grossberg, A. L., and Pressman, D., 1970, *Immunochemistry* **7**:755.
Jori, G., Galiazzo, G., Marzotto, A., and Scoffone, E., 1968, *Biochim. Biophys. Acta* **154**:1.
Jori, G., Galiazzo, G., and Scoffone, E., 1969, *Biochemistry* **8**:2868.
Jörnvall, H., 1973, *Biochem. Biophys. Res. Commun.* **51**:1069.
Jörnvall, H., 1974, *FEBS Lett.* **38**:329.
Jörnvall, H., Woenckhaus, C., and Johnscher, G., 1975, *Eur. J. Biochem.* **53**:71.
Junek, H., Kirk, K. L., and Cohen, L. A., 1969, *Biochemistry* **8**:1844.
Kanaoka, Y., Machida, M., Machida, M., and Sekine, T., 1973, *Biochim. Biophys. Acta* **317**:563.
Kanazawa, M., and Ishii, S.-I., 1974, *Biochim. Biophys. Acta* **342**:155.
Kanazawa, M., Yoshida, N., and Ishii, S., 1971, *Biochim. Biophys. Acta* **250**:372.
Kaneko, T., Takeuchi, I., and Inui, T., 1968a, *Bull. Chem. Soc. Jpn.* **41**:974.
Kaneko, T., Kusumoto, S., Inui, T., and Shiba, T., 1968b, *Bull. Chem. Soc. Jpn.* **41**:2155.
Karush, F., Klinman, N. R., and Marks, R., 1964, *Anal. Biochem.* **9**:100.
Kasai, K., and Ishii, S., 1973, *J. Biochem. (Tokyo)* **74**:631.
Kato, K., and Murachi, T., 1971, *J. Biochem. (Tokyo)* **69**:725.
Kauffmann, T., and Sobel, J., 1963, *Angew. Chem.* **75**:1177.
Kauffmann, T., and Sobel, J., 1966, *Justus Liebigs Ann. Chem.* **698**:235.
Kawauchi, H., Bewley, T. A., and Li, C. H., 1973, *Biochemistry* **12**:2124.
Kendall, P. A., and Barnard, E. A., 1969, *Biochim. Biophys. Acta* **188**:10.
Keston, A. S., Udenfriend, S., and Cannan, R. K., 1946, *J. Am. Chem. Soc.* **68**:1390.
Khorana, H. G., 1953, *Chem. Rev.* **53**:145.
Kimmel, J. R., 1967, *Methods Enzymol.* **11**:584.
Kimmel, J. R., and Parcells, A. J., 1960, *Fed. Proc.* **19**:341.
Kimmel, M. T., and Plummer, T. H., Jr., 1972, *J. Biol. Chem.* **247**:7864.
King, L., and Leberman, R., 1973, *Biochim. Biophys. Acta* **322**:279.
King, T. P., 1966, *Biochemistry* **5**:3454.
Kirk, K. L., and Cohen, L. A., 1969, *J. Org. Chem.* **34**:395.
Kirk, K. L., and Cohen, L. A., 1972, *J. Am. Chem. Soc.* **94**:8142.
Kirschner, M. W., and Schachman, H. K., 1973, *Biochemistry* **12**:2987.
Kirtley, M. E., and Koshland, D. E., Jr., 1970, *J. Biol. Chem.* **245**:276.
Klotz, I. M., and Elfbaum, S. G., 1964, *Biochim. Biophys. Acta* **86**:100.
Klotz, I. M., and Heiney, R. E., 1962, *Arch. Biochem. Biophys.* **96**:605.
Klotz, I. M., Martin, Y. C., and McConaughy, B. L., 1965, *Biochim. Biophys. Acta* **100**:104.
Knights, R. J., and Light, A., 1974, *Biochem. Biophys. Res. Commun.* **61**:1161.
Knowles, J. R., 1965, *Biochem. J.* **95**:180.
Kokesh, F. C., and Westheimer, F. H., 1971, *J. Am. Chem. Soc.* **93**:7270.
Koketsu, J., and Atassi, M. Z., 1974a, *Immunochemistry* **11**:1.
Koketsu, J., and Atassi, M. Z., 1974b, *Biochim. Biophys. Acta* **342**:21.

Koo, P. H., and Cebra, J. J., 1974, *Biochemistry* **13**:184.

Koshland, D. E., Jr., and Mozersky, S. M., 1964, *Fed. Proc.* **23**:609.

Koshland, D. E., Jr., Strumeyer, D. H., and Ray, W. J., Jr., 1962, *Brookhaven Symp. Biol.* **15**:101.

Koshland, D. E., Jr., Karkhanis, Y. D., and Latham, H. G., 1964, *J. Am. Chem. Soc.* **86**:1448.

Koshland, M. E., Englberger, F. M., and Gaddone, S. M., 1963, *J. Biol. Chem.* **238**:1349.

Kotaki, A., Harada, M., and Yagi, K., 1964, *J. Biochem.* **55**:553.

Kovaleva, G. G., Shimanskaya, M. P., and Stepanov, V. M., 1972, *Biochem. Biophys. Res. Commun.* **49**:1075.

Koyama, J., Grossberg, A. L., and Pressman, D., 1968, *Biochemistry* **7**:1935.

Kramer, K. J., and Rupley, J. A., 1973a, *Arch. Biochem. Biophys.* **156**:414.

Kramer, K. J., and Rupley, J. A., 1973b, *Arch. Biochem. Biophys.* **158**:566.

Kravchenko, N. A., Chentsova, T. V., and Kaverzneva, E. D., 1968, *Biokhimiya* **33**:355.

Kress, L. F., and Laskowski, M., Sr., 1967, *J. Biol. Chem.* **242**:4925.

Kronman, M. J., Robbins, F. M., and Andreotti, R. E., 1967, *Biochim. Biophys. Acta* **143**:462.

Krull, L. H., Gibbs, D. E., and Friedman, M., 1971, *Anal. Biochem.* **40**:80.

Ku, H. S., and Leopold, A. C., 1970, *Biochem. Biophys. Res. Commun.* **41**:1155.

Kurihara, K., Horinishi, H., and Shibata, K., 1963, *Biochim. Biophys. Acta* **74**:678.

Kuromizu, K., and Meienhofer, J., 1972, *J. Biol. Chem.* **247**:5646.

Lande, S., 1971, *J. Org. Chem.* **36**:1267.

Landsteiner, K., 1942, *J. Exp. Med.* **75**:269.

Landsteiner, K., 1945, *The Specificity of Serological Reactions,* rev. ed., Harvard University Press, Cambridge, Mass.

Lavine, T. F., 1943, *J. Biol. Chem.* **151**:281.

Lawley, P. D., and Brookes, P., 1964, *Biochem. J.* **92**:19c.

Lawrence, P. J., 1969, *Biochemistry* **8**:1271.

Lawson, W. B., and Schramm, H. J., 1962, *J. Am. Chem. Soc.* **84**:2017.

Lawson, W. B., and Schramm, H. J., 1965, *Biochemistry* **4**:377.

Lawson, W. B., Gross, E., Foltz, C. M., and Witkop, B., 1961, *J. Am. Chem. Soc.* **83**:1509.

Leach, S. J., Meschers, A., and Swanepoel, O. A., 1965, *Biochemistry* **4**:23.

Leavis, P. C., and Lehrer, S. S., 1974, *Biochemistry* **13**:3042.

Lederer, F., and Tarin, J., 1971, *Eur. J. Biochem.* **20**:482.

Lee, C.-L., and Atassi, M. Z., 1973, *Biochemistry* **12**:2690.

Lee, C.-L., and Atassi, M. Z., 1975, *Biochim. Biophys. Acta* **405**:464.

Lee, C.-L., Atassi, M. Z., and Habeeb, A. F. S. A., 1975, *Biochim. Biophys. Acta* **400**:423.

Lee, T.-T., Huestis, W. H., and Raftery, M. A., 1973, *Biochemistry* **12**:2535.

Leh, F., and Mudd, J. B., 1974, *Arch. Biochem. Biophys.* **161**:216.

Lenard, J., and Hess, G. P., 1964, *J. Biol. Chem.* **239**:3275.

Lenard, J., Schally, A. V., and Hess, G. P., 1964, *Biochem. Biophys. Res. Commun.* **14**:498.

Lewis, S. D., and Shafer, J. A., 1973, *Biochim. Biophys. Acta* **303**:284.

Levison, M. E., Josephson, A. S., and Kirschenbaum, D. M., 1969, *Experientia* **25**:126.

Levy, D., and Carpenter, F. H., 1967, *Biochemistry* **6**:3559.

Levy, D., and Carpenter, F. H., 1970, *Biochemistry* **9**:3215.

Li, C. H., and Bertsch, L., 1960, *J. Biol. Chem.* **235**:2638.

Liaw, W.-Y. V., Nakagawa, Y., and Jirgensons, B., 1974, *Makromol. Chem.* **175**:2837.

Light, A., and Sinha, N. K., 1967, *J. Biol. Chem.* **242**:1358.

Lin, J.-K., Miller, J. A., and Miller, E. C., 1969, *Biochemistry* **8**:1573.

Lin, L. J., and Foster, J. F., 1975, *Anal. Biochem.* **63**:485.

Lin, T.-Y., 1970, *Biochemistry* **9**:984.

Lin, T.-Y., and Koshland, D. E., Jr., 1969, *J. Biol. Chem.* **244**:505.

Lindley, H., 1956, *Nature (London)* **178**:647.

Link, T. P., and Stark, G. R., 1968, *J. Biol. Chem.* **243**:1082.

Little, J. R., Blanka, T. J., and Little, K. D., 1975, *Eur. J. Immunol.* **5**:373.

Liu, C. L., and Hatano, H., 1974, *FEBS Lett.* **42**:352.

Liu, W. H., Feinstein, G., Osuga, D. T., Haynes, R., and Feeney, R., 1968, *Biochemistry* **7**:2886.

Loudon, G. M., and Koshland, D. E., Jr., 1970, *J. Biol. Chem.* **245**:2247.

Lowe, G., and Whitworth, A. S., 1974, *Biochem. J.* **141**:503.

Ludwig, M. L., and Hunter, M. J., 1967, *Methods Enzymol.* **11**:595.

Lundahl, P., 1975, *Biochim. Biophys. Acta* **379**:304.

Lundblad, R. L., and Stein, W. H., 1969, *J. Biol. Chem.* **244**:154.

Lunder, T. L., 1972, *Anal. Biochem.* **49**:585.

Lutter, L. C., Ortanderl, F., and Fasold, H., 1974, *FEBS Lett.* **48**:288.

Machida, M., Sekine, T., and Kanaoka, Y., 1974, *Chem. Pharm. Bull.* **22**:2642.

MacLaren, J. A., and Sweetman, B. J., 1966, *Aust. J. Chem.* **19**:2355.

MacLaren, J. A., Savige, W. E., and Sweetman, B. J., 1965, *Aust. J. Chem.* **18**:1655.

Maeda, H., Ishida, N., Kawauchi, H., and Tuzimura, K., 1969, *J. Biochem.* **65**:777.

Mains, G., and Hofmann, T., 1974, *Can. J. Biochem.* **52**:1018.

Makriyannis, A., Gunther, W. H. H., and Mautner, H. G., 1973, *J. Am. Chem. Soc.* **95**:8403.

Malan, P. G., and Edelhoch, H., 1970, *Biochemistry* **9**:3205.

Malcolm, A. D. B., and Radda, G. K., 1970, *Eur. J. Biochem.* **15**:555.

Man, M., and Bryant, R. G., 1974, *Anal. Biochem.* **57**:429.

Marche, P., Girma, J. P., Morgat, J. L., Fromageot, P., Ghelis, C., Dubrasquet, M., and Bonfils, S., 1975, *Eur. J. Biochem.* **50**:375.

Margolis, S., and Langdon, R. G., 1966, *J. Biol. Chem.* **241**:477.

Markland, F. S., Bacharach, A. D. E., Weber, B. H., O'Grady, T. C., Saunders, G. C., and Umemura, M., 1975, *J. Biol. Chem.* **250**:1301.

Markus, G., 1964, *J. Biol. Chem.* **239**:4163.

Marzotto, A., Pajetta, P., Galzigna, L., and Scoffone, E., 1968, *Biochim. Biophys. Acta* **154**:450.

Mathew, E., Agnello, C. F., and Park, J. H., 1965, *J. Biol. Chem.* **240**:3232.

Mathew, E., Meriwether, B. P., and Park, J. H., 1967, *J. Biol. Chem.* **242**:5024.

Mathews, R. G., and Williams, C. H., 1974, *Biochim. Biophys. Acta* **370**:39.

Matsushima, A., Hachimori, Y., Inada, Y., and Shibata, K., 1967, *J. Biochem.* **63**:328.

Matsushima, A., Sakurai, K., Nomoto, M., Inada, Y., and Shibata, K., 1968, *J. Biochem.* **64**:507.

Mauk, M. R., and Girotti, A. W., 1974, *Biochemistry* **13**:1757.

Mauthner, J., 1912, *Hoppe-Seysler's Z. Physiol. Chem.* **78**:28.

Mayers, G. L., Grossberg, A. L., and Pressman, D., 1973, *Immunochemistry* **10**:37.

McBurnette, S. K., and Mandy, W. J., 1974, *Immunochemistry* **11**:255.

McCalla, D. R., and Reuvers, A., 1968, *Can. J. Biochem.* **46**:1411.

McFarlane, A. S., 1958, *Nature (London)* **182**:53.

McGowan, E. B., and Stellwagen, E., 1970, *Biochemistry* **9**:3047.

McMenamy, R. H., Dintzis, H. M., and Watson, F., 1971, *J. Biol. Chem.* **246**:4744.

McMurray, C. H., and Trentham, D. R., 1969, *Biochem. J.* **115**:913.

Means, G. E., and Feeney, R. E., 1968, *Biochemistry* **7**:2192.

Means, G. E., and Feeney, R. E., 1971, *Chemical Modification of Proteins*, pp. 254, Holden-Day, San Francisco.

Meerwein H., 1937, *J. Prakt. Chem.* **147**:257.

Meienhofer, J., Maeda, H., Glaser, C. B., and Czombos, J., 1972, *Progress in Peptide Research* (S. Lande, ed.), 295 pp., Gordon and Breach, New York.

Meighen, E. A., and Schachman, H. K., 1970, *Biochemistry* **9**:1163.

Melchior, W. B., Jr., and Fahrney, D., 1970, *Biochemistry* **9**:251.

Menge, U., and Jaenicke, L., 1974, *Hoppe-Seyler's Z. Physiol. Chem.* **355**:603.

Metzger, H., Wofsy, L., and Singer, S. J., 1964, *Proc. Natl. Acad. Sci. U.S.A.* **51**:612.

Miles, E. W., 1975, *Biochem. Biophys. Res. Commun.* **64**:248.

Miles, L. E. M., and Hales, C. N., 1968, *Biochem. J.* **108**:611.

Miller, R. V., and Sypherd, P. S., 1973, *J. Mol. Biol.* **78**:527.

Misani, F., Fair, T. W., and Reiner, L., 1951, *J. Am. Chem. Soc.* **73**:459.

Modesto, R. R., and Pesce, A. J., 1971, *Biochim. Biophys. Acta* **229**:384.

Mole, J. E., and Horton, H. R., 1973a, *Biochemistry* **12**:5278.

Mole, J. E., and Horton, H. R., 1973b, *Biochemistry* **12**:5285.

Moore, G., 1975, *Can. J. Biochem.* **53**:328.

Moore, G., and Crichton, R. R., 1974, *Biochem. J.* **143**:607.

Moore, G. L., and Day, R. A., 1968, *Science* **159**:210.

Moore, J., Jr., and Fenselau, A., 1972a, *Biochemistry* **11**:3753.

Moore, J., Jr., and Fenselau, A., 1972b, *Biochemistry* **11**:3762.

Moore, J. E., and Ward, W. H., 1956, *J. Am. Chem. Soc.* **78**:2414.

Morgan, P. H., Robinson, N. C., Walsh, K. A., and Neurath, H., 1972, *Proc. Natl. Acad. Sci. U.S.A.* **69**:3312.

Morgan, W. T., and Müller-Eberhard, U., 1974, *Enzyme* **17**:108.

Morishita, M., Sakiyama, F., and Narita, K., 1967a, *Bull. Chem. Soc. Jpn.* **40**:433.

Morishita, M., Sowa, T., Sakiyama, F., and Narita, K., 1967b, *Bull. Chem. Soc. Jpn.* **40**:632.

Morrisett, J. D., and Drott, H. R., 1969, *J. Biol. Chem.* **244**:5083.

Morrison, M., and Bayse, G. S., 1970, *Biochemistry* **9**:2995.

Morrison, M., Steele, W., and Danner, D. J., 1969, *Arch. Biochem. Biophys.* **134**:515.

Moult, J., Eshdat, Y., and Sharon, N., 1973, *J. Mol. Biol.* **75**:1.

Mudd, J. B., Leavitt, R., and Kersey, W. H., 1966, *J. Biol. Chem.* **241**:4081.

Mueller, J. M., Pierce, J. G., and du Vigneaud, V., 1953, *J. Biol. Chem.* **204**:857.

Muhlard, A., Hegyi, G., and Toth, G., 1967, *Acta Biochim. Biophys.* **2**:19.

Murachi, T., and Yasui, M., 1965, *Biochemistry* **4**:2275.

Murachi, T., Inagami, T., and Yasui, M., 1965, *Biochemistry* **4**:2815.

Murachi, T., Miyake, T., and Yamasaki, N., 1970, *J. Biochem.* **68**:239.

Myer, Y., 1972, *Biochemistry* **11**:4195.

Nagradova, N. K., and Asryants, R. A., 1975, *Biochim. Biophys. Acta* **386**:365.

Naider, F., and Bohak, Z., 1972, *Biochemistry* **11**:3208.

Naider, F., Bohak, Z., and Yariv, J., 1972, *Biochemistry* **11**:3202.

Naik, V. R., and Horton, H. R., 1971, *Biochem. Biophys. Res. Commun.* **44**:44.

Nairns, R. C., ed., 1964, *Fluorescent Protein Tracing*, E. and S. Livingston, Edinburgh.

Nakae, Y., Ikeda, K., Azuma, T., and Hamaguchi, K., 1972, *J. Biochem.* **72**:1155.

Nakagawa, Y., and Bender, M. L., 1970, *Biochemistry* **9**:259.

Nakagawa, Y., Capetillo, S., and Jirgensons, B., 1972, *J. Biol. Chem.* **247**:5703.

Nakagawa, Y., Liaw, W.-Y. V., Hunt, A. H., and Jirgensons, B., 1974, *Immunochemistry* **11**:483.

Nakane, P. K., and Pierce, G. B., 1967, *J. Cell. Biol.* **33**:307.

Nakaya, K., Horinishi, H., and Shibata, K., 1967, *J. Biochem.* **61**:345.

Nakayama, H., Tanizawa, K., and Kanaoka, Y., 1970, *Biochem. Biophys. Res. Commun.* **40**:537.

Narita, K., 1970, *Protein Sequence Determination* (S. B. Needleman, ed.), Springer, New York.

Neet, K. E., and Koshland, D. E., Jr., 1966, *Proc. Natl. Acad. Sci. U.S.A.* **56**:1606.

Neims, A. H., Coffey, D. S., and Hellerman, L., 1966a, *J. Biol. Chem.* **241**:3036.

Neims, A. H., Coffey, D. S., and Hellerman, L., 1966b, *J. Biol. Chem.* **241**:5941.

Nelsestuen, G. L., Zytkovicz, T. H., and Howard, J. B., 1974, *Mayo Clin. Proc.* **49**:941.

Neri, P., Arezzini, C., Botti, R., Cocola, F., Tarli, P., 1973, *Biochim. Biophys. Acta* **322**:88.

Neumann, H., Steinberg, I. Z., Brown, J. R., Goldberger, R. F., and Sela, M., 1967a, *Eur. J. Biochem.* **3**:171.

Neumann, H., Shinitzky, M., and Smith, R. A., 1967b, *Biochemistry* **6**:1421.

Neumann, N. P., 1972, *Methods Enzymol.* **25B**:393.

Neumann, N. P., Moore, S., and Stein, W. H., 1962, *Biochemistry* **1**:68.

Nicolet, B. H., 1931, *J. Am. Chem. Soc.* **53**:3066.

Nigen, A. M., and Gurd, F. R. N., 1973, *J. Biol. Chem.* **248**:3708.

Niketic, V., Thomsen, J., and Kristiansen, K., 1974, *Eur. J. Biochem.* **46**:547.

Nishigaki, I., Chen, F. T., and Hokin, L. E., 1974, *J. Biol. Chem.* **249**:4911.

Nishimura, J. S., Mitchell, T., and Grinnell, F., 1973, *J. Biol. Chem.* **248**:743.

Nisonoff, A., 1967, *Methods in Immunology and Immunochemistry,* Vol. 1 (C. A. Williams and M. W. Chase, eds.), p. 120, Academic Press, New York.

Nixon, J., Spoor, T., Evans, J., and Kimball, A., 1972, *Biochemistry* **11**:4570.

Nureddin, A., and Inagami, T., 1975, *Biochem. J.* **147**:71.

Oakes, J., and Cafe, M. C., 1973, *Eur. J. Biochem.* **36**:559.

O'Brien, P. J., 1967, *Biochem. J.* **102**:28P.

Ogawa, S., and McConnell, H. M., 1967, *Proc. Natl. Acad. Sci. U.S.A.* **58**:19.

Oh, K.-J., and Churchich, J. E., 1974, *J. Biol. Chem.* **249**:4737.

O'Hern, D. J., Pal, P. K., and Myer, Y. P., 1975, *Biochemistry* **14**:382.

Ohta, M., and Hayashi, K., 1974a, *Biochem. Biophys. Res. Commun.* **56**:981.

Ohta, M., and Hayashi, K., 1974b, *Biochem. Biophys. Res. Commun.* **57**:973.

Ohtsuki, K., Liu, C. L., and Hatano, H., 1969, *J. Biochem.* **66**:863.

Okamoto, M., and Morino, Y., 1973, *J. Biol. Chem.* **248**:82.

Okumura, K., and Murachi, T., 1975, *J. Biochem. (Tokyo)* **77**:913.

Okuyama, T., and Satake, K., 1960, *J. Biochem. (Tokyo)* **47**:454.

O'Leary, M. H., and Samberg, G. A., 1971, *J. Am. Chem. Soc.* **93**:3530.

Omenn, G. S., Fontana, A., and Anfinsen, C. B., 1970, *J. Biol. Chem.* **245**:1895.

Ong, E. B., Shaw, E., and Schoellmann, G., 1965, *J. Biol. Chem.* **240**:694.

Oratz, M., Burks, A. L., and Rothschild, M. A., 1966, *Biochim. Biophys. Acta* **115**:88.

Osterman-Golkar, S., Ehrenberg, L., and Solymosy, F., 1974, *Acta Chem. Scand B* **28**:215.

Ozawa, H., 1967, *J. Biochem. (Tokyo)* **62**:531.

Ozawa, H., 1970, *Biochemistry* **9**:2158.

Palmer, J. L., Nisonoff, A., and Van Holde, K. E., 1963, *Proc. Natl. Acad. Sci. U.S.A.* **50**:314.

Panetta, C. A., and Casanova, T. G., 1970a, *J. Org. Chem.* **35**:2423.

Panetta, C. A., and Casanova, T. G., 1970b, *J. Org. Chem.* **35**:4275.

Parker, A. J., and Kharasch, N., 1959, *Chem. Rev.* **59**:583.

Parsons, S. M., and Raftery, M. A., 1969, *Biochemistry* **8**:4199.

Parsons, S. M., Jao, L., Dahlquist, F. W., Borders, C. L., Jr., Groff, T., Racs, J., and Raftery, M. A., 1969, *Biochemistry* **8**:700.

Patchornik, A., and Shaltiel, S., 1966, Peptides, in: *Proceedings of the Sixth European Symposium,* Athens, 1963 (L. Zervas, ed.), p. 177, Macmillan, New York.

Patchornik, A., and Sokolovsky, M., 1964a, *J. Am. Chem. Soc.* **86**:1206.

Patchornik, A., and Sokolovsky, M., 1964b, *J. Am. Chem. Soc.* **86**:1860.

Patchornik, A., Lawson, W. B., and Witkop, B., 1958, *J. Am. Chem. Soc.* **80**:4747.

Patchornik, A., Lawson, W. B., Gross, E., and Witkop, B., 1960, *J. Am. Chem. Soc.* **82**:5923.

Patchornik, A., Wilchek, M., and Sarid, S., 1964, *J. Am. Chem. Soc.* **86**:1457.

Patchornik, A., Wilchek, M., and Zioudrou, C., 1969, *Isr. J. Chem.* **7**:559.

Paterson, A. K., and Knowles, J. R., 1972, *Eur. J. Biochem.* **31**:510.

Patthy, L., and Smith, E. L., 1975a, *J. Biol. Chem.* **250**:557.

Patthy, L., and Smith, E. L., 1975b, *J. Biol. Chem.* **250**:565.

Pauly, H. Z., 1915, *Hoppe-Seyler's Z. Physiol. Chem.* **94**:284.

Paz, M. A., Henson, E., Rombauer, R., Abrash, L., Blumenfeld, O. O., and Gallop, P. M., 1970, *Biochemistry* **9**:2123.

Perham, R. N., 1973, *Biochem. J.* **131**:119.

Perham, R. N., and Richards, F. M., 1968, *J. Mol. Biol.* **33**:795.

Perham, R. N., and Thomas, J. O., 1971, *J. Mol. Biol.* **62**:415.

Perlstein, M. T., and Atassi, M. Z., 1974, *Immunochemistry* **11**:63.

Perlstein, M. T., Atassi, M. Z., and Cheng, S. H., 1971, *Biochim. Biophys. Acta* **236**:174.

Phillips, D. R., and Morrison, M., 1971, *Biochemistry* **10**:1766.

Philpot, J. S. L., and Small, P. A., 1938, *Biochem. J.* **32**:534.

Photaki, I., 1963, *J. Am. Chem. Soc.* **85**:1123.

Pihl, A., and Lange, R., 1962, *J. Biol. Chem.* **237**:1356.

Pinkus, L. M., and Meister, A., 1972, *J. Biol. Chem.* **247**:6119.

Plaut, A. G., and Tomasi, T. B., Jr., 1970, *Proc. Natl. Acad. Sci. U.S.A.* **65**:318.

Plummer, T. H., Jr., and Hirs, C. H. W., 1964, *J. Biol. Chem.* **239**:2530.

Pocker, A., 1973, *J. Org. Chem.* **38**:4295.

Podulso, J. F., Greenberg, C. S., and Glick, M. C., 1972, *Biochemistry* **11**:2616.

Poirier, L. A., Miller, J. A., Miller, E. C., and Sato, K., 1967, *Cancer Res.* **27**:1600.

Polyanovsky, O. L., Demidkina, T. V., and Egorov, C. A., 1972, *FEBS Lett.* **23**:262.

Poulos, T. L., and Price, P. A., 1974, *J. Biol. Chem.* **249**:1453.

Powell, W. S., and Heacock, R. A., 1972, *Can. J. Chem.* **50**:3360.

Powell, W. S., and Heacock, R. A., 1973, *Bio. Org. Chem.* **2**:191.

Powers, J. C., and Tuhy, P. M., 1972, *J. Am. Chem. Soc.* **94**:6544.

Press, E. M., Fleet, G. W. J., and Fisher, C. E., 1971, *Prog. Immunol.* **1971**:233.

Previero, A., Coletti-Previero, M. A., and Jòlles, P., 1966a, *Biochem. Biophys. Res. Commun.* **22**:17.

Previero, A., Coletti-Previero, M. A., and Jòlles, P., 1966b, *Biochim. Biophys. Acta* **124**:400.

Previero, A., Coletti-Previero, M. A., and Axelrud-Cavadore, C. L., 1967a, *Arch. Biochem. Biophys.* **122**:434.

Previero, A., Coletti-Previero, M. A., and Cavadore, J.-C., 1967b, *Biochim. Biophys. Acta* **147**:453.

Previero, A., Coletti-Previero, M. A., and Jòlles, P., 1967c, *J. Mol. Biol.* **24**:261.

Previero, A., Barry, L. G., and Previero, M. A., 1969a, *FEBS Lett.* **4**:255.

Previero, A., Coletti-Previero, M. A., and Barry, L. G., 1969b, *Biochim. Biophys. Acta* **181**:361.

Previero, A., Barry, L. G., and Coletti-Previero, M. A., 1972a, *Biochim. Biophys. Acta* **263**:7.

Previero, A., Prota, G., and Coletti-Previero, M. A., 1972b, *Biochim. Biophys. Acta* **285**:269.

Quiocho, F. A., and Olson, J. S., 1974, *J. Biol. Chem.* **249**:5885.

Quiocho, F. A., and Richards, F. M., 1964, *Proc. Natl. Acad. Sci. U.S.A.* **52**:833.

Quiocho, F. A., and Richards, F. M., 1966, *Biochemistry* **5**:4062.

Rachele, J. R., 1963, *J. Org. Chem.* **28**:2898.

Radomsky, N. A., Gibian, M. J., and Elliott, D. L., 1973, *J. Am. Chem. Soc.* **95**:8717.

Rafter, G. W., 1957, *Arch. Biochem. Biophys.* **67**:267.

Raftery, M. A., and Cole, R. D., 1963, *Biochem. Biophys. Res. Commun.* **10**:467.

Raftery, M. A., and Cole, R. D., 1966, *J. Biol. Chem.* **241**:3457.

Ram, J. S., 1963, *Biochim. Biophys. Acta* **78**:228.

Ramachandran, J., 1965, *Nature (London)* **206**:927.

Ramachandran, L. K., and Witkop, B., 1964, *Biochemistry* **3**:1603.

Rando, R. R., 1973, *J. Am. Chem. Soc.* **95**:4438.

Ray, A., and Cebra, J. J., 1972, *Biochemistry* **11**:3647.

Ray, W. J., Jr., and Koshland, D. E., Jr., 1962, *J. Biol. Chem.* **237**:2493.

Reimerdes, E. H., and Klostermeyer, H., 1973, *Milchwissenschaft* **28**:558.

Reisler, E., Burke, M., Himmelfarb, S., and Harrington, W. F., 1974, *Biochemistry* **13**:3837.

Reiss, A., and Lukton, A., 1975, *Bio. Org. Chem.* **4**:1.

Ressler, C., and Kashelikar, D. V., 1966, *J. Am. Chem. Soc.* **88**:2025.

Reynolds, J. H., 1968, *Biochemistry* **7**:3131.

Rice, R. H., and Means, G. E., 1971, *J. Biol. Chem.* **246**:831.

Riehm, J. P., and Scheraga, H. A., 1965, *Biochemistry* **4**:772.

Riehm, J. P., and Scheraga, H. A., 1966a, *Biochemistry* **5**:93.
Riehm, J. P., and Scheraga, H. A., 1966b, *Biochemistry* **5**:99.
Riley, M., and Perham, R. N., 1973, *Biochem. J.* **131**:625.
Rimon, S., and Perlmann, G. E., 1968, *J. Biol. Chem.* **243**:3566.
Riordan, J. F., 1973, *Biochemistry* **12**:3915.
Riordan, J. F., and Christen, P., 1968, *Biochemistry* **7**:1525.
Riordan, J. F., and Vallee, B. L., 1964, *Biochemistry* **3**:1768.
Riordan, J. F., and Vallee, B. L., 1972, *Methods Enzymol.* **25B**:500.
Riordan, J. F., Wacker, W. E. C., and Vallee, B. L., 1965, *Biochemistry* **4**:1758.
Riordan, J. F., Sokolovsky, M., and Vallee, B. L., 1966, *J. Am. Chem. Soc.* **88**:4104.
Riordan, J. F., Sokolovsky, M., and Vallee, B. L., 1967, *Biochemistry* **6**:358.
Robillard, G. T., Powers, J. C., and Wilcox, P. E., 1972, *Biochemistry* **11**:1773.
Robyt, J. F., Ackerman, R. J., and Chittenden, C. G., 1971, *Arch. Biochem. Biophys.* **147**:262.
Rochat, C., Rochat, H., and Edman, P., 1970a, *Anal. Biochem.* **37**:259.
Rochat, H., Rochat, C., Miranda, M., Lissitzky, S., and Edman, P., 1970b, *Eur. J. Biochem.* **17**:262.
Roger, R., and Neilson, D. G., 1961, *Chem. Rev.* **61**:179.
Roholt, O. A., and Pressman, D., 1967, *Biochim. Biophys. Acta* **147**:1.
Rohrbach, M. S., Humphries, B. A., Yost, F. J., Jr., Rhodes, W. G., Boatman, S., Hiskey, R. G., and Harrison, J. H., 1973, *Anal. Biochem.* **52**:127.
Rombauts, W. A., Shroeder, W. A., and Morrison, M., 1967, *Biochemistry* **6**:2965.
Rosén, C. G., and Fedorcsak, I., 1966, *Biochim. Biophys. Acta* **130**:401.
Rosen, N. L., Bishop, L., Burnett, J. B., Bishop, M., and Colman, R. F., 1973, *J. Biol. Chem.* **248**:7359.
Rosenthal, A. F., and Atassi, M. Z., 1967, *Biochim. Biophys. Acta* **147**:410.
Roskoski, R., Jr., 1974, *Biochemistry* **13**:5141.
Royer, G. P., Liberatore, F. A., and Green, G. M., 1975, *Biochem. Biophys. Res. Commun.* **64**:478.
Rudinger, J., and Ruegg, U., 1973, *Biochem. J.* **133**:538.
Ruegg, U. T., and Rudinger, J., 1974, *Int. J. Peptide Protein Res.* **6**:447.
Ruoho, A., Bartlett, P. A., Dutton, A., and Singer, S. J., 1975, *Biochem. Biophys. Res. Commun.* **63**:417.
Ruttenberg, M. A., King, T. P., and Craig, L. C., 1964, *Biochemistry* **3**:758.
Ruttenberg, M. A., King, T. P., and Craig, L. C., 1965, *Biochemistry* **4**:11.
Ryan, J., and Tollin, G., 1973, *Biochemistry* **12**:4550.
Sakiyama, F., and Sakai, S.-I., 1971, *Bull. Chem. Soc. Jpn.* **44**:1661.
Sakiyama, F., Morishita, M., Sowa, T., and Narita, K., 1966, *Bull. Chem. Soc. Jpn.* **39**:631.
Samy, T. S. A., Atreyi, M., Maeda, H., and Meienhofer, J., 1974, *Biochemistry* **13**:1007.
Sanger, F., 1945, *Biochem. J.* **39**:507.
Sarid, S., and Patchornik, A., 1963, *Isr. J. Chem.* **1**:63.
Schachter, H., and Dixon, G. H., 1964, *J. Biol. Chem.* **239**:813.
Schachter, H., Halliday, K. A., and Dixon, G. H., 1964, *J. Biol. Chem.* **238**:PC 3134.
Schaefer, F. C., Thurston, J. T., and Dudley, J. R., 1951, *J. Am. Chem. Soc.* **73**:2990.
Schaffer, N. K., May, S. C., and Summerson, W. H., 1954, *J. Biol. Chem.* **206**:201.
Schejter, A., and Aviram, I., 1970, *J. Biol. Chem.* **245**:1552.
Schick, A. F., and Singer, S. J., 1961, *J. Biol. Chem.* **236**:2477.
Schmall, B., Cheng, C. J., Fujmura, S., Gersten, N., Grunberger, D., and Weinstein, I. B., 1973, *Cancer Res.* **33**:1921.
Schmidt, E., and Fischer, H., 1920, *Chem. Ber.* **53**:1529.
Schmir, G. L., and Cohen, L. A., 1961, *J. Am. Chem. Soc.* **83**:723.
Schmir, G., Cohen, L., and Witkop, B., 1959, *J. Am. Chem. Soc.* **81**:2228.
Schöberl, A., Kawohl, M., and Hamm, R., 1951, *Chem. Ber.* **84**:571.

Schoellmann, G., and Shaw, E., 1962, *Biochem. Biophys. Res. Commun.* 7:36.

Schramm, V. H. J., 1967, *Hoppe-Seyler's Z. Physiol. Chem.* 348:232.

Schramm, V. H. J., and Lawson, W. B., 1963, *Hoppe-Seyler's Z. Physiol. Chem.* 97:332.

Schroder, E., and Lübke, K., 1965, *The Peptides*, Vol. 1, Academic Press, New York.

Schroeder, W. A., Shelton, J. R., and Robertson, B., 1967, *Biochim. Biophys. Acta* 147:590.

Schroeder, W. A., Shelton, J. B., and Shelton, J. R., 1969, *Arch. Biochem. Biophys.* 130:551.

Schultz, J., 1967, *Methods Enzymol.* 11:255.

Scoffone, E., Fontana, A., and Rocchi, R., 1966a, *Biochem. Biophys. Res. Commun.* 25:170.

Scoffone, E., Previero, A., Benassi, C. A., and Pajetta, P., 1966b, *Peptides* (L. Zervas, ed.), p. 183, Pergamon Press, New York.

Scoffone, E., Fontana, A., and Rocchi, R., 1968, *Biochemistry* 7:971.

Scouten, W. H., Lubcher, R., and Baughman, W., 1974, *Biochim. Biophys. Acta* 336:421.

Seela, F., and Cramer, F., 1975, *Hoppe-Seyler's Z. Physiol. Chem.* 356:1185.

Seiler, N., Schmidt-Glenewinkel, T., and Schneider, H. H., 1973, *J. Chromatog.* 84:95.

Sekine, T., Ando, K., Machida, M., and Kanaoka, Y., 1972, *Anal. Biochem.* 48:557.

Sela, M., and Arnon, R., 1972, *Methods Enzymol.* 25B:553.

Sela, M., White, F. H., Jr., and Anfinsen, C. B., 1957, *Science* 125:691.

Shafer, J., Baranowsky, P., Laursen, R., Finn, F., and Westheimer, F. H., 1966, *J. Biol. Chem.* 241:421.

Shafferman, A., 1972, *Isr. J. Chem.* 10:725.

Shaltiel, S., 1967, *Biochem. Biophys. Res. Commun.* 29:178.

Shaltiel, S., and Patchornick, A., 1963, *J. Am. Chem. Soc.* 85:2799.

Shaltiel, S., and Tauber-Finkelstein, M., 1970, *FEBS Lett.* 8:345.

Shamsuddin, M., Mason, R. G., Ritchey, J. M., Honig, G. R., and Klotz, I. M., 1974, *Proc. Natl. Acad. Sci. U.S.A.* 71:4693.

Shapiro, A. B., Suskina, V. I., Rozinov, B. Y., and Rozantzev, E. G., *Izv. Akad. Nauk S.S.S.R. Ser. Him.* 1969:2828.

Sharpless, N. E., and Flavin, M., 1966, *Biochemistry* 5:2963.

Shaw, E., 1970, *The Enzymes* 3rd ed., Vol. I (P. D. Boyer, ed.), p. 91, Academic Press.

Shaw, E., 1972, *Methods Enzymol.* 25B:655.

Shaw, E., and Ruscica, J., 1968, *J. Biol. Chem.* 243:6312.

Shaw, E., and Springhorn, S., 1967, *Biochem. Biophys. Res. Commun.* 27:391.

Shaw, E., Mares-Guia, M., and Cohen, W., 1965, *Biochemistry* 4:2219.

Shechter, Y., Burstein, Y., and Patchornick, A., 1972, *Biochemistry* 11:653.

Shechter, Y., Patchornik, A., and Burstein, Y., 1973, *Biochemistry* 12:3407.

Shechter, Y., Patchornik, A., and Burstein, Y., 1974, *J. Biol. Chem.* 249:413.

Sheehan, J. G., and Hlavka, J. J., 1956, *J. Org. Chem.* 21:43.

Sherman, M. P., and Kassell, B., 1968, *Biochemistry* 7:3634.

Shiao, D. D. F., Lumry, R., and Rajender, S., 1972, *Eur. J. Biochem.* 29:377.

Shiba, T., Koda, A., Kusumoto, S., and Kaneko, T., 1968, *Bull. Chem. Soc. Jpn.* 41:2748.

Shifrin, S., Solis, B. G., and Chaiken, I. M., 1973, *J. Biol. Chem.* 248:3464.

Shih, C. T., and Craven, G. R., 1973, *J. Mol. Biol.* 78:651.

Shimada, T., 1970, *J. Biochem. (Tokyo)* 67:185.

Shimizu, A., Watanabe, S., Yamamura, Y., and Putnam, F. W., 1974, *Immunochemistry* 11:719.

Signor, A., and Bordignon, E., 1968, *Tetrahedron* 24:6995.

Signor, A., Bonora, G. M., Biondi, L., Nisato, D., Marzotto, A., and Scoffone, E., 1971, *Biochemistry* 10:2748.

Simpson, R. T., Riordan, J. F., and Vallee, B. L., 1963, *Biochemistry* 2:616.

Singer, S. J., 1967, *Adv. Protein Chem.* 22:1.

Singer, S. J., and Schick, A. F., 1961, *J. Biophys. Biochem. Cytol.* 9:519.

Singh, A., Thornton, E. R., and Westheimer, F. H., 1962, *J. Biol. Chem.* 237:PC3006.

Singhal, R. P., and Atassi, M. Z., 1970, *Biochemistry* **9**:4252.
Singhal, R. P., and Atassi, M. Z., 1971, *Biochemistry* **10**:1756.
Sjoholm, I., Ekenas, A.-K., and Sjoquist, J., 1972, *Eur. J. Biochem.* **29**:455.
Slobin, L. I., 1972, *Proc. Natl. Acad. Sci. U.S.A.* **69**:3769.
Slobin, L. I., and Singer, S. J., 1968, *J. Biol. Chem.* **243**:1777.
Smith, G. D., and Schachman, H. K., 1971, *Biochemistry* **10**:4576.
Smithies, O., 1965, *Science* **150**:1595.
Smyth, D. G., 1967, *J. Biol. Chem.* **242**:1579.
Smyth, D. G., Nagamatsu, A., and Fruton, J. S., 1960, *J. Am. Chem. Soc.* **82**:4600.
Smyth, D. G., Blumenfeld, O. O., and Konigsberg, W., 1964, *Biochem. J.* **91**:589.
Sogin, D. C., and Plapp, B. V., 1975, *J. Biol. Chem.* **250**:205.
Sokolovsky, M., and Eisenbach, L., 1972, *Eur. J. Biochem.* **25**:483.
Sokolovsky, M., and Patchornik, A., 1963, *Isr. J. Chem.* **1**:215.
Sokolovsky, M., and Vallee, B. L., 1967, *Biochemistry* **6**:700.
Sokolovsky, M., Sadeh, T., and Patchornik, A., 1964, *J. Am. Chem. Soc.* **86**:1212.
Sokolovsky, M., Riordan, J. F., and Vallee, B. L., 1966, *Biochemistry* **5**:3582.
Sokolovsky, M., Riordan, J. F., and Vallee, B. L., 1967, *Biochem. Biophys. Res. Commun.* **27**:20.
Sokolovsky, M., Harell, D., and Riordan, J. F., 1969, *Biochemistry* **8**:4740.
Sokolovsky, M., Fuchs, M., and Riordan, J. F., 1970, *FEBS Lett.* **7**:167.
Spande, T. F., and Glenner, G. G., 1973, *J. Am. Chem. Soc.* **95**:3400.
Spande, T. F., Green, N. M., and Witkop, B., 1966, *Biochemistry* **5**:1926.
Spande, T. F., Wilchek, M., and Witkop, B., 1968, *J. Am. Chem. Soc.* **90**:3256.
Spande, T. F., Witkop, B., Degani, Y., and Patchornik, A., 1970, *Adv. Protein Chem.* **24**:97.
Sperling, R., and Steinberg, I. Z., 1971, *J. Biol. Chem.* **246**:715.
Sperling, R., Burstein, Y., and Steinberg, I. Z., 1969, *Biochemistry* **8**:3810.
Spikes, J. D., and MacKnight, M. L., 1970, *Ann. N.Y. Acad. Sci.* **171**:149.
Stallcup, W. B., and Koshland, D. E., Jr., 1973, *J. Mol. Biol.* **80**:63.
Stark, G. R., 1964, *J. Biol. Chem.* **239**:1411.
Stark, G. R., 1965a, *Biochemistry* **4**:588.
Stark, G. R., 1965b, *Biochemistry* **4**:1030.
Stark, G. R., 1970, *Adv. Protein Chem.* **24**:261.
Stark, G. R., 1972, *Methods Enzymol.* **25B**:579.
Stark, G. R., and Link, T. P., 1975, *Biochemistry* **14**:3476.
Stark, G. R., Stein, W. H., and Moore, S., 1960, *J. Biol. Chem.* **235**:3177.
Steers, E., Jr., Craven, G. R., Anfinsen, C. B., and Bethune, J. L., 1965, *J. Biol. Chem.* **240**:2478.
Stefanovsky, Y., and Westheimer, F. H., 1973, *Proc. Natl. Acad. Sci. U.S.A.* **70**:1132.
Stein, W. H., and Moore, S., 1946, *J. Org. Chem.* **11**:681.
Steiner, L. A., and Blumberg, P. M., 1971, *Biochemistry* **10**:4725.
Stender, W., Stutz, A. A., and Scheit, K. H., 1975, *Eur. J. Biochem.* **56**:129.
Stepanov, V. M., Lobareva, L. S., and Maltsev, N. I., 1968, *Biochim. Biophys. Acta* **151**:719.
Stevens, C. O., and Long, J. L., 1969, *Proc. Soc. Exp. Med.* **131**:1312.
Stevenson, K. J., 1973, *Anal. Biochem.* **56**:450.
Stewart, F. H. C., 1969, *Aust. J. Chem.* **22**:2451.
Stöhrer, G., Salemnick, G., and Brown, G. B., 1973, *Biochemistry* **12**:5084.
Strausbauch, P. H., Kent, A. B., Hedrick, J. L., and Fischer, E. H., 1967, *Methods Enzymol.* **11**:671.
Strausbauch, P. H., Weinstein, Y., Wilchek, M., Shaltiel, S., and Givol, D., 1971, *Biochemistry* **10**:4342.
Strumeyer, D. H., White, W. N., and Koshland, D. E., Jr., 1963, *Proc. Natl. Acad. Sci. U.S.A.* **50**:931.
Suzuki, S., Hachimori, Y., and Matoba, R., 1970, *Bull. Chem. Soc. Jpn.* **43**:3849.

Suzuki, T., Takenaka, O., and Shibata, K., 1969, *J. Biochem.* **66**:815.

Szabolcsi, G., Biszku, E., and Sajgo, M., 1960, *Acta Physiol.* **17**:183.

Takahashi, K., 1968, *J. Biol. Chem.* **243**:6171.

Takahashi, K., 1973, *J. Biochem.* **74**:1083.

Takahashi, K., Stein, W. H., and Moore, S., 1967, *J. Biol. Chem.* **242**:4682.

Takahashi, S., and Cohen, L. A., 1969, *Biochemistry* **8**:864.

Takenaka, A., Suzuki, T., Takenaka, O., Horinishi, H., and Shibata, K., 1969, *Biochim. Biophys. Acta* **194**:293.

Takenaka, A., Takenaka, O., Horinishi, H., and Shibata, K., 1970, *J. Biochem. (Tokyo)* **67**:397.

Tamaoki, H., Murase, Y., Minato, S., and Nakanishi, K., 1967, *J. Biochem. (Tokyo)* **62**:7.

Tang, J., 1971, *J. Biol. Chem.* **246**:4510.

Tarbell, D. S., and Harnish, D. P., 1951, *Chem. Rev.* **49**:1.

Tate, S. S., Relyea, N. M., and Meister, A., 1969, *Biochemistry* **8**:5016.

Taubman, M. T., and Atassi, M. Z., 1968, *Biochem. J.* **106**:829.

Taylor, R. P., Vatz, J. B., and Lumry, R., 1973, *Biochemistry* **12**:2933.

Teherani, J. A., and Nishimura, J. S., 1975, *J. Biol. Chem.* **250**:3883.

Telegdi, M., and Straub, F. B., 1973, *Biochim. Biophys. Acta* **321**:210.

Thomas, E. W., McKelvy, J. F., and Sharon, N., 1969, *Nature (London)* **222**:485.

Thompson, R. C., and Blout, E. R., 1973, *Biochemistry* **12**:44.

Thorpe, C., and Williams, C. H., Jr., 1975, *Biochemistry* **14**:2419.

Thorpe, N. O., and Singer, S. J., 1969, *Biochemistry* **8**:4523

Tietze, F., Gladner, J. A., and Folk, J. E., 1957, *Biochim. Biophys. Acta* **26**:659.

Todhunter, J. A., and Purich, D. L., 1974, *Biochem. Biophys. Res. Commun.* **60**:273.

Toennies, G., 1940, *J. Biol. Chem.* **132**:455.

Toennies, G., and Kolb, J. J., 1945, *J. Am. Chem. Soc.* **67**:849.

Toi, K., Bynum, E., Norris, E., and Itano, H. A., 1965, *J. Biol. Chem.* **240**:3455.

Toi, K., Bynum, E., Norris, E., and Itano, H. A., 1967, *J. Biol. Chem.* **242**:1036.

Tomasi, T. B., Jr., 1973, *Proc. Natl. Acad. Sci. U.S.A.* **70**:3410.

Traut, R. R., Bollen, A., Sun, T.-T., Hershey, J. W. B., Sundberg, J., and Pierce, L. R., 1973, *Biochemistry* **12**:3266.

Trundle, D., and Cunningham, L. W., 1969, *Biochemistry* **8**:1919.

Tsai, C. S., Tsai, Y. H., Lauzon, G., and Cheng, S. T., 1974, *Biochemistry* **13**:440.

Tsao, D., Azari, P., and Phillips, J. L., 1974, *Biochemistry* **13**:408.

Tsao, T.-C., and Bailey, K., 1953, *Biochim. Biophys. Acta* **11**:102.

Tschesche, H., and Jering, H., 1973, *Angew. Chem. Int. Ed. Engl.* **85**:765.

Tsukamoto, S., and Ohno, M., 1974, *J. Biochem.* **75**:1377.

Twu, J.-S., and Wold, F., 1973, *Biochemistry* **12**:381.

Udenfriend, S., and Velick, S. F., 1951, *J. Biol. Chem.* **190**:733.

Uehara, K., Mannen, S., and Kishida, K., 1970, *J. Biochem.* **68**:119.

van Rensburg, N. J. J., and Swanepoel, O. A., 1967, *Arch. Biochem. Biophys.* **118**:531.

Veeger, C., and Massey, V., 1962, *Biochim. Biophys. Acta* **64**:83.

Verma, K. K., and Bose, S., 1974, *Anal. Chim. Acta* **70**:227.

Veronese, F. M., Boccú, E., and Fontana, A., 1968, *Ann. Chim.* **58**:1309.

Veronese, F. M., Boccú, E., and Fontana, A., 1970, *Int. J. Protein Res.* **2**:67.

Veronese, F. M., Degani, Y., Nyc, J. F., and Smith, E. L., 1974, *J. Biol. Chem.* **249**:7936.

Vincent, J. P., Lazdunski, M., and Delaage, M., 1970, *Eur. J. Biochem.* **12**:250.

Virden, R., Bristow, A. F., and Pain, R. H., 1975, *Biochem. J.* **149**:397.

Volwerk, J. J., Pieterson, W. A., and de Haas, G. H., 1974, *Biochemistry* **13**:1446.

Wada, K., and Okunuki, K., 1968, *J. Biochem.* **64**:667.

Wagner, P. D., and Yount, R. G., 1975, *Biochemistry* **14**:1908.

Wagner, T. E., and Hsu, C.-J., 1970, *Anal. Biochem.* **36**:1.

Wallis, R. B., and Holbrook, J. J., 1973, *Biochem. J.* **133**:183.

Wang, K.-M., and Reichlin, M., 1974, *Immunol. Commun.* **3**:133.

Wang, K., and Richards, F. M., 1974*a, Isr. J. Chem.* **12**:375.

Wang, K., and Richards, F. M., 1974*b, J. Biol. Chem.* **249**:8005.

Waterman, M. R., 1974, *Biochem. Biophys. Acta* **371**:159.

Weber, G., 1952, *Biochem. J.* **51**:155.

Weeds, A. G., and Hartley, B. S., 1968, *Biochem. J.* **107**:531.

Weigele, M., DeBernardo, S. L., Tengi, J. P., and Leimgruber, W., 1972, *J. Am. Chem. Soc.* **94**:5927.

Weigele, M., DeBernardo, S., Leimgruber, W., Cleeland, R., and Grunberg, E., 1973, *Biochem. Biophys. Res. Commun.* **54**:899.

Weil, L., and Seibles, T. S., 1961, *Arch. Biochem. Biophys.* **95**:470.

Weil, L., Gordon, W. G., and Buchert, A. R., 1951, *Arch. Biochem. Biophys.* **33**:90.

Weiner, H., Batt, C. W., and Koshland, D. E., Jr., 1966*a, J. Biol. Chem.* **241**:2687.

Weiner, H., White, W. N., Hoare, D. G., and Koshland, D. E., Jr., 1966*b, J. Am. Chem. Soc.* **88**:3851.

Weinstein, Y., Shaltiel, S., Givol, D., and Strausbauch, P. H., 1973, *Immunochemistry* **10**:337.

Weitzman, P. D. J., 1975, *Biochem. J.* **149**:281.

Wells, M. A., 1973, *Biochemistry* **12**:1086.

Weltman, J., Frackelton, A., Jr., Szaro, R. P., and Dowben, R., 1972, *Biophys. Soc. Abst.* **12**:277a.

Weltman, J. K., Szaro, R. P., Frackelton, A. R., Jr., Dowben, R. M., Bunting, J. R., and Cathou, R. E., 1973, *J. Biol. Chem.* **248**:3173.

Werber, M. M., and Sokolovsky, M., 1972, *Biochem. Biophys. Res. Commun.* **48**:384.

Werber, M. M., Moldovan, M., and Sokolovsky, M., 1975, *Eur. J. Biochem.* **53**:207.

Westhead, E. W., 1972, *Methods Enzymol.* **25B**:401.

Wetz, K., Fasold, H., and Meyer, C., 1974, *Anal. Biochem.* **58**:347.

Weygand, F., Burger, K., and Engelhardt, K., 1966, *Chem. Ber.* **99**:1461.

White, E. H., and Branchini, B. R., 1975, *J. Am. Chem. Soc.* **97**:1243.

White, F. H., Jr., 1961, *J. Biol. Chem.* **236**:1353.

White, F. H., Jr., 1972*a, Methods Enzymol.* **25B**:387.

White, F. H., Jr., 1972*b, Methods Enzymol.* **25B**:541.

White, F. H., Jr., and Sandoval, A., 1962, *Biochemistry* **1**:938.

White, W. E., and Yielding, K. L., 1973, *Biochem. Biophys. Res. Commun.* **52**:1129.

Whitehead, J. K., and Bentley, H. R., *J. Chem. Soc.* **1952**:1572.

Wieghardt, T., and Goren, H. J., 1975, *Bioorg. Chem.* **4**:30.

Wilchek, M., and Witkop, B., 1967, *Biochem. Biophys. Res. Commun.* **26**:296.

Wilchek, M., Sarid, S., and Patchornik, A., 1965, *Biochim. Biophys. Acta* **104**:616.

Wilchek, M., Frensdorff, A., and Sela, M., 1967*a, Biochemistry* **6**:247.

Wilchek, M., Spande, T. F., Witkop, B., and Milne, G. W. A., 1967*b, J. Am. Chem. Soc.* **89**:3349.

Wilchek, M., Spande, T., Milne, G., and Witkop, B., 1968*a, Biochemistry* **7**:1777.

Wilchek, M., Spande, T., and Witkop, B., 1968*b, Biochemistry* **7**:1787.

Wilchek, M., Oka, T., and Topper, Y. J., 1975, *Proc. Natl. Acad. Sci. U.S.A.* **72**:1055.

Wilcox, P. E., 1972, *Methods Enzymol.* **25B**:596.

Williams, J. N., Jr., and Jacobs, R. M., 1968, *Biochim. Biophys. Acta* **154**:323.

Williams, J., and Lowe, J. M., 1971, *Biochem. J.* **121**:203.

Wilson, J. G., and Cohen, L. A., 1963*a, J. Am. Chem. Soc.* **85**:560.

Wilson, J. G., and Cohen, L. A., 1963*b, J. Am. Chem. Soc.* **85**:564.

Wilson, K. J., Birchmeier, W., and Christen, P., 1974, *Eur. J. Biochem.* **41**:471.

Witkop, B., 1961, *Adv. Protein Chem.* **16**:221.

Witkop, B., and Graser, G., 1944, *Ann. Chem. Liebigs* **556**:103.

Witter, A., and Tuppy, H., 1960, *Biochim. Biophys. Acta* **45**:429.

Witzemann, V., Koberstein, R., Sund, H., Rasched, I., Jörnvall, H., and Noack, K., 1974, *Eur. J. Biochem.* **43**:319.

Woenckhaus, C., Zoltobrocki, M., and Berghäuser, J., 1970, *Hoppe-Seyler's Z. Physiol. Chem.* **351**:1441.

Wofsy, L., and Singer, S. J., 1963, *Biochemistry* **2**:104.

Wofsy, L., Metzger, H., and Singer, S. J., 1962, *Biochemistry* **1**:1031.

Wolcott, M., Freeman, D. G., Schrohenloher, R. E., Hammack, W., and Bennett, J. C., 1975, *Immunochemistry* **12**:685.

Wold, F., 1961, *J. Biol. Chem.* **236**:106.

Wold, F., 1972, *Methods Enzymol.* **25B**:623.

Wolff, J., and Covelli, I., 1969, *Eur. J. Biochem.* **9**:371.

Wong, S.-C. C., Kandel, S. I., Kandel, M., and Gornall, A. G., 1972, *J. Biol. Chem.* **247**:3810.

Woodward, R. B., and Olofson, R. A., 1961, *J. Am. Chem. Soc.* **83**:1007.

Woodward, R. B., and Olofson, R. A., 1966, *Tetrahedron Lett. Suppl.* **7**:415.

Wu, C., and Stryer, L., 1972, *Proc. Natl. Acad. Sci. U.S.A.* **69**:1104.

Yang, S. F., 1970, *Biochemistry* **9**:5008.

Yankeelov, J. A., 1970, *Biochemistry* **9**:2433.

Yankeelov, J. A., 1972, *Methods Enzymol.* **25B**:566.

Yankeelov, J. A., and Acree, D., 1971, *Biochem. Biophys. Res. Commun.* **42**:886.

Yankeelov, J. A., and Jolley, C. J., 1972, *Biochemistry* **11**:159.

Yankeelov, J. A., Jr., Kochert, M., Page, J., and Westphal, A., 1966, *Fed. Proc.* **25**:590.

Yankeelov, J. A., Jr., Mitchell, C. D., and Crawford, T. H., 1968, *J. Am. Chem. Soc.* **90**:1664.

Yano, Y., Negi, T., and Irie, M., 1973, *J. Biochem.* **74**:67.

Yonemitsu, O., Hamada, T., and Kanaoka, Y., 1968, *Tetrahedron Lett.* **1968**:3575.

Yonemitsu, O., Hamada, T., and Kanaoka, Y., 1969a, *Tetrahedron Lett.* **1969**:1819.

Yonemitsu, O., Hamada, T., and Kanaoka, Y., 1969b, *Chem. Pharm. Bull.* **17**:2075.

Yoshida, N., Yamasaki, M., and Ishii, S.-I., 1973, *J. Biochem.* **73**:1175.

Young, J. D., and Leung, C. Y., 1970, *Biochemistry* **9**:2755.

Young, M., Blanchard, M. H., and Brown, D., 1968, *Proc. Natl. Acad. Sci. U.S.A.* **61**:1078.

Zahn, H., 1961, *Chimia (Aarav)* **15**:378.

Zahn, H., and Meienhofer, J., 1958, *Makromol. Chem.* **26**:153.

Zahn, H., and Zuber, H., 1953, *Chem. Ber.* **86**:172.

Zahn, H., Rouette, H.-K., and Schade, F., 1965, *Proc. Third Int. Wool Text. Res. Conf.* **2**:495.

Zappacosta, S., and Rossi, G., 1967, *Immunochemistry* **4**:122.

Zioudrou, C., Wilchek, M., and Patchornik, A., 1965, *Biochemistry* **4**:1811.

Zisapel, N., and Sokolovsky, M., 1974, *Biochem. Biophys. Res. Commun.* **58**:951.

Zytkovicz, T. H., and Nelsestuen, G. L., 1975, *J. Biol. Chem.* **250**:2968.

Influence of Conformation on Immunochemical Properties of Proteins

A. F. S. A. Habeeb

I. Introduction

The ability of foreign proteins to induce the production of antibody has formed the basis for both passive and active immunization of humans and animals against infectious diseases. Thus the observation of Behring and Kitasato (1890) that cell-free sera of rabbits and mice, which were injected with inactivated diphtheria or tetanus toxin, were capable of neutralizing the toxin led to the development of antitoxin therapy. In the early history of immunology, attention was focused on the development of methods to inactivate a toxin without affecting its antigenicity. The use of formalin to inactivate a toxin proved to be a valuable discovery (Salkowski, 1898) and had extensive application in the commercial production of antitoxins (Glenny and Südmersen, 1921).

Since then, extensive work has been carried out to determine the chemical basis of antigenicity (the ability of protein to induce antibody formation), and it has become evident that the conformation of the protein plays an important role (Landsteiner, 1945). Denaturation of proteins by heat (Rothen and Landsteiner, 1942) and by alkali (Dakin, 1912/1913) resulted in the production of antibody which reacted less efficiently with the native

A. F. S. A. Habeeb · Division of Clinical Immunology and Rheumatology. Department of Medicine and Departments of Microbiology and Biochemistry. The University of Alabama School of Medicine, Birmingham, Alabama 35294.

protein. Although the denatured proteins were poorly characterized, the conclusion emphasized the role played by the integrity of antigen in determining the immunochemical specificity of the antibody produced.

At the present time, immunochemical methods are used in many fields of biological sciences—e.g., characterizing proteins, testing for homogeneity of a protein, determining the phylogenetic relation among proteins from different species, and probing for macromolecules on the cell surface. In all cases it is essential that the protein used for immunization should be identical with that being characterized.

The fidelity with which an antibody to a protein is produced, in the animal or human, results in maximum immunochemical reaction with the homologous system. Therefore, any deviation in antigen conformation from that of the native molecule as a result of manipulation during isolation may result in changed immunochemical reactivity between antisera and the protein. This will undoubtedly reduce the meaningfulness and usefulness of immunochemical methods for characterization of macromolecules. Thus antibodies prepared against cell surface components may recognize them only when present on the cell or after isolation, if they were not changed during isolation.

The immunochemical behavior of globular proteins is highly influenced by changes in the native conformation of the antigen (Atassi, 1967; Atassi and Caruso, 1968; Habeeb, 1967b; Sela et al., 1967). Thus antibodies against native proteins react very little, if at all, with the respective reduced and alkylated proteins (Brown et al., 1959; Habeeb and Borella, 1966; Young and Leung, 1970).

Any modification of the native protein can be considered a potential source of producing conformational changes. This can be of great importance when immunochemical methods are used for characterization and identification of proteins.

The unique conformation of a protein is dictated by its amino acid sequence and stabilized by a complex network of both short-range and long-range noncovalent interactions (hydrogen bonds, electrostatic, and hydrophobic forces). As shown by X-ray diffraction pattern (Kendrew, 1962), most of the polar groups of native proteins are located at the surface, whereas hydrophobic side chains are buried inside the molecule. In some proteins, distant parts of the molecules are brought in close proximity and are further stabilized by disulfide bonds. The native stable structure is in a state of minimal conformational free energy and is critically dependent on the solvent environment and other extrinsic factors. Conditions for stability differ from one protein to another so that care has to be exercised in making generalizations about reactions and interactions that may take place as a result of given experimental conditions.

An understanding of protein structure and conformation is necessary in order to appreciate the potentials and pitfalls of immunochemical studies. This chapter will discuss the factors (thermodynamic and kinetic) that control protein folding and the dependence of the native conformation on almost the total amino acid sequence. This is shown by conformational studies on fragments from proteins of diverse structure (disulfide-free and disulfide-containing) and multisubunit enzymes. Such studies demonstrate the lack of structure or limited structural characteristics of such fragments. Native proteins may be subjected to scission of a peptide bond at a distinct site, and the resulting fragments will remain noncovalently bound, e.g., subtilisin digestion of ribonuclease between residues 20 and 21. An important point to be considered is the effect of a ligand on modifying the rate and path of enzymatic cleavage of a protein (trypsin on nuclease in the absence or presence of deoxythymidine $3',5'$-diphosphate and Ca^{2+}). Studies also have shown that peptides derived from a protein may associate to form stable complexes resembling, but not identical to, the original protein. In some cases no association of the peptides was possible.

The concept that conformational homology is exhibited by proteins which show chemical homology and that immunochemical cross-reaction among homologous proteins is correlated with their sequence similarity will be discussed. This concept is not sound and requires a restatement to the effect that proteins which show conformational homology may show sequence homology.

After discussing the above points, I will summarize the work dealing with the effect of protein conformation on immunochemical specificity.

II. Factors Responsible for Protein Folding

A. Factors Intrinsic to the Protein Molecule

The features by which a newly synthesized polypeptide chain folds into its native conformation have been under extensive study and two views are available.

1. The thermodynamic hypothesis: It argues that the polypeptide chain assumes the conformation that is associated with the lowest free energy.
2. The kinetic control of folding: The folding proceeds along limited paths through nucleation and the structure will be at a free energy minimum but not necessarily the global minimum.

1. The Thermodynamic Hypothesis

The information for acquiring the unique three-dimensional structure of a protein molecule resides in the linear amino acid sequence, and the folding of the polypeptide chain which gives the protein its native structure is thermodynamically controlled (Epstein et al., 1963). This hypothesis was based on documented work with ribonuclease (White, 1960, 1961; Anfinsen and Haber, 1961). Ribonuclease (mol. wt. 13,700 with 124 amino acid residues) was reduced with β-mercaptoethanol in 8 M urea, whereupon the molecule lost the native folding (White, 1960; Harrington and Sela, 1959). It was then oxidized by bubbling air in the solution (at a protein concentration of 2 mg/ml at ph 8) for 20–24 hr. Reduced-oxidized (reox) ribonuclease produced two main components (by chromatography on CM-cellulose corresponding to ribonuclease A and ribonuclease B) which were enzymatically active. The reox-ribonuclease showed 80–100% of the specific activity of native ribonuclease. Peptide maps of reox-ribonuclease produced a pattern nearly identical to that of native ribonuclease, thus indicating proper pairing of the disulfide bonds. The ultraviolet spectrum of reduced ribonuclease showed a shift caused by cleavage of the hydrogen bonds involving the hydroxyl groups of three tyrosine residues (Anfinsen et al., 1961). Upon oxidation, the spectrum returned to the native position (except for a deviation near 250 nm), indicating the participation of tyrosines in hydrogen bonding to the same degree as the native molecule. The optical rotatory dispersion constant dropped from 236 nm to 226 nm upon reduction (it reflects destruction of secondary structure), and upon air oxidation the constant returned to the native value because of re-formation of helical coiling, as in the native molecule. Intrinsic viscosity measurement showed a marked increase (from 0.033 to 0.186) upon reduction of ribonuclease due to increased asymmetry of the molecule, thus suggesting a random chain conformation. Upon air oxidation, the intrinsic viscosity returned to the value characteristic of the native molecule. Complement fixation and quantitative precipitin reactions indicated that reox-ribonuclease was immunochemically identical to native ribonuclease.

Lysozyme (Epstein and Goldberger, 1963; Goldberger and Epstein, 1963), insulin (Katsoyannis and Tometsko, 1966), Taka-amylase A (Isemura et al., 1963), poly-DL-alanyl trypsin (Epstein and Anfinsen, 1962), and alkaline phosphatase (Levinthal et al., 1962) were reduced and then refolded to their native conformation by reoxidation. Accuracy of refolding was dependent on the protein concentration, pH, temperature, and β-mercapto-ethanol concentration. Optimal conditions for the attainment of the native form varied for different proteins. A low concentration of reduced protein was necessary to allow maximal reactivation (0.01–0.1 mg/ml) in order to reduce the chance of intermolecular interaction and aggregation. In the initial work (Anfinsen *et al.*, 1961), the refolding of ribonuclease, as measured by the recovery of enzymatic activity, required 350 min for 50 % reactivation, far more than is necessary for synthesis of the polypeptide chain. Under optimal conditions of concentration, pH, and temperature, 50 % recovery of activity required 20 min of reoxidation. An enzyme system was found in the microsomal fraction of several tissue homogenates (Goldberger *et al.*, 1963, 1964) which was capable of accelerating the re-formation of ribonuclease (under physiological conditions, pH 7–7.4 and 37°C) from reduced ribonuclease or from ribonuclease with mismatched disulfide bonds. The enzyme functions as an exchange catalyst (Givol *et al.*, 1965), and it has been shown to catalyze the reactivation of reduced ribonuclease A, hen egg white lysozyme (Goldberger *et al.*, 1964), and soybean trypsin inhibitor (Steiner *et al.*, 1965). However, it was found to accelerate the rate of refolding of urea-denatured amylase, which had no disulfide bonds (Yutani *et al.*, 1967).

2. The Kinetic Control of Protein Folding

Levinthal (1968) argued that the time required to randomly sample all possible structures of a protein would be extremely long. Native protein is in a selected metastable state in which the conformational energy is at a local minimum but not necessarily at a global minimum. Folding requires a nucleation step by local condensations of segments of the unfolded polypeptide chains to form the unique three-dimensional structures in a biologically feasible time.

The presence of unique structural regions within the polypeptide chain suggests that in the early stages of re-formation of the three-dimensional structure nucleation occurs independently in separate parts of the molecule. Nucleation grows by adding segments of the polypeptide chains that are close to the nucleus to form the three-dimensional structure of the native protein. Wetlaufer (1973*b*) found that in several proteins compact regions exist, the size varying from about 40 to 150 amino acid residues, of which the nucleus can be as small as 8–18 residues.

Lewis *et al.* (1970) suggested that one of the initial steps for nucleation was the meeting of two distant sections to form a stabilized structure, around which the remainder of the chain folded. For cytochromes *c* of 27 species, the regions of high helical content were conserved among species (Lewis and Scheraga, 1971). These results were consistent with the proposal of invariance of conformation (Dickerson *et al.*, 1971), as well as the fact that these areas of high helical content directed the folding of the native structure (Lewis *et al.*, 1971). Lewis *et al.* (1971) proposed that certain segments of the polypeptide chain were responsible for bringing distant sections of the polypeptide chain into close proximity. The simplest example was the β-bend, which involved residues i to $(i + 3)$ and the formation of a hydrogen bond between the carbonyl group of i residue and the amide group of residue $(i + 3)$. They provided 180° reversal of chain direction and involved only four residues. Analysis of lysozyme, ribonuclease S, and the B- and C-chains of α-chymotrypsin showed that the β-bend occurred. Most of the observed β-bends appeared to be composed of polar amino acid residues and were located at the surface of the native protein. Kuntz (1972) developed a simple computer program for locating regions where the peptide backbone folds back on itself. From studies on carboxypeptidase and chymotrypsin, he concluded that turns occurred on the surface of the protein molecule, that turn segments were less hydrophobic than the protein as a whole, and that a sequence of three to eight hydrophilic residues was associated with folding of peptide chains. Carboxypeptidase studies (Kuntz, 1972) suggested that both backbone and side-chain hydrogen bonds were disrupted in turn regions, and that the solvent plays an important role in turn generation and stabilization.

Attempts to explore the possibility that the self-assembly of a polypeptide chain proceeds through a limited search of conformations by nucleation, rather than exhaustive random search, were conducted by Wetlaufer (1973a). Saxena and Wetlaufer (1970) developed a system for reoxidation of reduced lysozyme (at 1×10^{-6} M), consisting of oxidized glutathione/reduced glutathione (1:10 and GSH $= 5 \times 10^{-3}$ M), which corresponds with physiological levels. Reactivation of reduced lysozyme from 6 M guanidine, 8 M urea, and 0.1 N acetic acid by hundredfold dilution into reactivation medium produced identical regeneration kinetics. Reoxidized lysozyme gave three components on chromatography on Bio-Rex 70 columns. The major component (67%) was identical with native lysozyme by chromatography, circular dichroism (CD) spectrum, and specific activity of the recovered material. Recovery of the two other components was 20% and 13%, and their specific activity was 0% and 53%, respectively; these may represent proteins with mismatched disulfide bonds. The process of regeneration of lysozyme involved three steps: (1) a rapid chain folding where substantial native conformation was formed (from CD spectrum) before disulfide formation; (2) formation of intramolecular disulfide bonds either native or mismatched by sulfhydryl–disulfide exchange, unaffected by EDTA; and, finally, (3) shuffling of nonnative disulfide bonds to form the native conformation. Neither the initial folding nor the sulfhydryl–disulfide exchange seemed to be rate limiting. The rate-limiting reaction appeared to be the polypeptide backbone and side-chain folding that occurred during the disulfide interchange.

Protein biosynthesis either in intact cell (Long et al., 1961) or in cell-free extract (Matthaei and Nirenberg, 1961) occurred in reducing milieu. It was suggested that the cysteinyl residues in the growing polypeptide chain remained in the reduced form until it grew sufficiently, so that folding would provide the free energy for disulfide formation (Saxena and Wetlaufer, 1970). The regeneration of enzymatic activity from reduced human leukemia lysozyme was also achieved with a mixture of oxidized and reduced glutathione (Wetlaufer et al., 1974a). Moreover, ribonuclease (Ahmed, 1969; Schaffer, 1970) and Bowman-Birk trypsin inhibitor (Hogle and Liener, 1973) were regenerated using the same system.

Some evidence was obtained by Ristow and Wetlaufer (1973) that a limited number of conformations were formed in the early period of regeneration of lysozyme from the reduced form. They used the method of Yutani et al. (1968) for oxidation of reduced lysozyme (air in presence of Cu^{2+}). Samples were removed at intervals for sulfhydryl assay, and the regeneration was stopped by reaction with N-ethylmaleimide when the average number of disulfide bonds formed was 0.25–1.5. The protein was isolated and digested with pepsin, followed by chymotrypsin. Peptide maps of native lysozyme gave ten disulfide-containing spots when stained by the method of Maeda et al. (1970). Partially regenerated lysozyme showed three disulfide spots (when an average of 0.25 S—S formed), six disulfide spots (when 0.5 S—S formed), ten spots (when 1.0 S—S formed), and seven spots (when an average of 1.3 S—S formed), and the peptide pattern resembled somewhat that from native lysozyme. With complete regeneration (activity was 85 %), the peptide map was similar to that of native lysozyme but with an additional new spot. Based on the limited number of disulfide-containing peptides in peptide maps (a heterogeneous pairing would give 28 spots) during early regeneration of lysozyme, it was concluded that the results demonstrated a limited search of structures directed by nucleation during the formation of the native protein conformation (Ristow and Wetlaufer, 1973). The number of disulfide-containing spots did not support single folding pathway.

Further work by Wetlaufer et al. (1974b) showed that during regeneration of reduced lysozyme by oxidized glutathione/reduced glutathione system at high temperature, the native enzyme is formed as an intermediate. Regenerations at 37°C, 47°C, and 56°C were similar in rate and yield. A plateau of activity was demonstrated after 90 min at each temperature. However, regeneration at temperatures 60–90°C showed a maximum of activity followed by a decline in the activity. This was attributed to the conversion sequence: reduced lysozyme → enzymatically active protein → thermally inactivated lysozyme. Inactive lysozyme formed by regeneration at 75°C became enzymatically active when the temperature was lowered to 37°C. The fact that lysozyme was formed at high temperatures (when it was thermodynamically unstable) was in support of kinetic factors in the folding process.

A cyanogen bromide fragment from lysozyme, comprising residues 13–105 and containing disulfide bonds II–VI, was subjected to reduction and reoxidation (Johnson et al., 1975) by the glutathione system. The disulfide formation in the fragment was as rapid as in lysozyme, with the formation of two disulfide bonds after 5 min. The regenerated fragment was immunochemically reactive with anti-lysozyme serum, giving a reaction of 32% and 56% with two antisera compared to native lysozyme. The results were interpreted to demonstrate the formation of nativelike structure in the fragment and supported the hypothesis of independent folding of a segment of lysozyme.

Yutani et al. (1968) found that reoxidation of reduced lysozyme in 8 M urea by dilution resulted in complete recovery of enzymatic activity in the presence of Cu^{2+} at 10^{-7} to 10^{-6} M concentrations. The renaturation was studied by difference spectrum, optical rotatory dispersion, and circular dichroism. About 70% of the original helical content was reformed immediately after dilution (neither the enzymatic activity nor the disulfide bonds were re-formed), and one or two tryptophan residues were buried in the molecule. After 3 hr two disulfides were formed, 30% of the enzymatic activity was recovered, and the ORD spectrum for partially renatured lysozyme closely resembled that of the native enzyme. The original conformation was re-formed gradually from the partially folded form through disulfide interchange and through noncovalent bonds, and this interchange process was concomitantly followed by recovery of enzymatic activity.

Saxena (1971) studied the Cu^{2+}-catalyzed oxidation of reduced lysozyme. Fifty percent of enzymatic activity was recovered in 5 min (10^{-6} M reduced lysozyme, 2×10^{-6} M Cu^{2+}, 0.01 M tris-acetate, pH 8). Regeneration was monitored by CD spectra (245–210 nm) and sulfhydryl titration. As the first 4-SH groups were oxidized in a rapid regeneration, there was little change in CD spectra from that of reduced lysozyme and no enzymatic activity. Oxidation of the remaining 4-SH groups was accompanied by changes in CD to that characteristic of native lysozyme and by the development of enzymatic activity. The initial lag in the development of structure and enzymatic activity as the first 4-SH groups were oxidized was taken as evidence for a preferred regeneration pathway (Saxena, 1971). These results were at variance with those of Yutani et al. (1968), who found that 70% of the helical content was formed immediately and one or two tryptophan residues were buried as regeneration started.

Hantgan et al. (1974) examined the reoxidation of reduced ribonuclease under anaerobic conditions with equimolar concentrations of oxidized and reduced glutathione at 5×10^{-3} M. The time course of reoxidation was followed by measuring enzymatic activity, absorbance, fluorescence, sulfhydryl content, and disulfide bond formation from diagonal peptide maps for cystine peptides (Brown and Hartley, 1966). Disulfide bond formation took place in two steps, an initial fast step, where the sulfhydryl groups decreased from eight to one to form intrachain disulfide bonds within the ribonuclease molecule, followed by a slower decrease, until all sulfhydryl groups disappeared. Low enzymatic activity (2–3%) appeared after 5 min, 30% after 79 min, and 60% after 180 min of reoxidation. There were no detectable disulfide-containing peptides (after 5 min of incubation) because of formation of a large amount of incorrectly disulfide-paired RNase. After 17 min of reoxidation (8% of activity), disulfide-containing peptides were detected which corresponded to half-cystine III + IV–V, VI + VII, and II. On further oxidation (79 min and recovery of 30% enzymatic activity), all spots seen in native protein occurred, including off-diagonal spots corresponding to half-cystine VIII, VI + VII, and I. After 180 min of reoxidation, spectral properties of the enzyme and peptide maps were similar to those of the native molecule, and the recovered enzymatic activity was 60%. This reoxidation process involved formation of mixed disulfide between glutathione and reduced ribonuclease, followed by a rapid formation of a larger number of intermediates with incorrect intramolecular disulfide residues. These then underwent a disulfide exchange reaction catalyzed by reduced glutathione and led to the recovery of native conformation.

A simple model for protein folding was presented using β_2-microglobulin (Isenman et al., 1975). β_2-Microglobulin consists of a single polypeptide chain of 100 residues with one intrachain disulfide bond and molecular weight of 11,700. The molecule was reduced in 6 M guanidine (keeping it in the reduced form by excluding O_2) or reduced and alkylated using iodoacetic acid, iodoacetamide, or methyl iodide to introduce groups of different size and charge (to examine whether the blocking group was a factor in preventing the folding). None of the four derivatives showed characteristics of the native structure by CD; however, the CD spectra were not identical, thus suggesting differences in their conformation. Only upon reoxidation of the sulfhydryl groups was a native conformation formed, thus indicating the importance of disulfide bond formation for the recovery of native conformation. Disulfide bond formation occurred through a nucleation step which brought the two sulfhydryl groups in close proximity, thus facilitating oxidation. The formation of the disulfide bond stabilized the nucleus, and folding was brought to completion. In the absence of disulfide-bond formation, the nucleus was not stable enough for proper folding. This scheme was similar to that proposed by Saxena and Wetlaufer (1970).

The kinetics of thermal unfolding and refolding of ribonuclease (with intact disulfide bonds) was studied by the change in absorbance at 287 nm (Tsong et al., 1972), and a sequential model was proposed for nucleation-dependent protein folding, which was characterized by a rapid transient phase followed by a slow steady-state unfolding.

In the re-formation studies presented above, proteins with disulfide bonds were involved. The presence of disulfide bonds imposes certain restrictions on the refolding, whereas proteins devoid of disulfide bonds would present a simple model for studying the pathway of protein folding. Staphylococcal nuclease consists of one polypeptide chain of molecular weight 16,870, no disulfide bonds, and one tryptophan residue, which serves as a conformational probe. Reversible protein folding of acidified staphylococcal nuclease on neutralization was studied in a stopped-flow spectrofluorometer by measuring the increase in tryptophanyl fluorescence during renaturation (Epstein *et al.*, 1971*a*). Nuclease fluorescence as a function of pH showed a steepness of transition, thus suggesting a cooperative structural transition. The rate of folding was described by two rate-determining steps with a mean half-time of 56 ± 8 and 363 ± 15 msec, and it was independent of either the initial pH (from 3.2 to 3.8 corresponding to 0–50% of folding) or ionic strength (from 0.001 to 0.1). The acid-induced structural changes represented an extensive disruption of protein conformation, as demonstrated by CD spectra, intrinsic viscosity, and proton magnetic resonance spectra of histidine (Epstein *et al.*, 1971*a*). The half-time of the slow process decreased from 600 msec at 13°C to 150 msec at 38°C, while the half-time of the faster rate process did not change. The results suggested that two sequential processes were operating in refolding, a first step involving entropically driven nucleation of ordered structure (Schellman, 1958; Florey, 1969), followed by formation of hydrophobic bonds (Kauzmann, 1959; Richards, 1963). The structural changes occurring during the refolding of nuclease involved the nucleation of two helices that constituted the pocket where the indole ring was buried and would be represented by the fast rate process. This was followed by the slower process which resulted from the folding of one or more of the hydrophobic side chains or segments of side chains.

Several multisubunit enzymes, e.g., fumarase, enolase, aldolase, glyceraldehyde phosphate dehydrogenase, lactic dehydrogenase, and malic dehydrogenase, were subjected to reduction and renaturation in the presence and absence of substrates or cofactors. The renaturation was monitored by enzymatic activity, optical rotatory dispersion, and fluorescence spectra (Teipel and Koshland, 1971*a,b*). Reduction was done in 6 M guanidine, 0.01 M dithiothreitol, and 0.001 M EDTA at pH 7, for 2 hr at room temperature. Renaturation was performed by dialysis vs. 125 vol or dilution (101-fold) and monitored by recovery of enzymatic activity. Both the extent and rate of reactivation differed significantly among the enzymes. The presence of a substrate or cofactor in the reactivation medium at zero time resulted in increased activity. Delayed addition of the substrate increased the extent of reactivation of fumarase, enolase, and aldolase, but it had very little effect on glyceraldehyde phosphate dehydrogenase, lactic dehydrogenase, and malic dehydrogenase. An increase in recovery of activation with increase in concentration was observed with fumarase, enolase, and aldolase. In contrast, the behavior of glyceraldehyde phosphate dehydrogenase, lactic dehydrogenase, and malic dehydrogenase was the reverse. Optical rotation showed that the major regain of conformation upon renaturation was complete in 1 min, followed by a slow recovery of enzymatic activity and minor conformational change. Similarly, data from fluorescence spectra indicated that upon regeneration the initial increase in fluorescence intensity (associated with transfer of tryptophan residues from a hydrophilic to hydrophobic environment upon folding) was very rapid (half-time of 30 sec). However, emission spectra of renatured fumarase, enolase, and aldolase resembled more closely those of their native counterparts than did glyceraldehyde phosphate dehydrogenase, lactic dehydrogenase, and malic dehydrogenase. Small fluorescence changes were observed between 1 and 30 min after renaturation of the enzymes enolase, aldolase, and malic dehydrogenase, indicative of minor changes in the vicinity of aromatic residues. However, these changes did not affect the gross conformation, as revealed by optical rotation. Teipel and Koshland (1971b) presented a scheme for the refolding of denatured enzymes which involved the rapid folding (within 1 min) of a random polypeptide chain to an inactive intermediate, which was similar to the native molecule in its gross conformation. Similar results were found with lysozyme (Yutani et al., 1968; Wetlaufer, 1973a), ribonuclease (Tsong et al., 1972), and staphylococcal nuclease (Schechter et al., 1970; Epstein et al., 1971a). Minor conformational changes occurred very slowly (half-time up to 75 min) and were accompanied by recovery of enzymatic activity. Marked increase in the rate and extent of recovery occurred in the presence of substrates and other environmental conditions (e.g., ionic strength, protein concentration). According to Teipel and Koshland (1971b), refolding of fumarase, enolase, and aldolase was under thermodynamic control, whereas refolding of glyceraldehyde phosphate dehydrogenase, lactic dehydrogenase, and malic dehydrogenase was partly influenced by kinetic factors. They proposed that, for enzymes under thermodynamic control, the intermediate states were conformationally mobile, and the attainment of the thermodynamically most stable conformation occurred within hours. Thus the addition of substrate, initially or later, would displace equilibrium in favor of active species. For enzymes under kinetic control, the rate of formation of final conformational states was faster than the rate of equilibrium between the intermediate conformational states. The results of Teipel and Koshland (1971a) were obtained with multisubunit enzymes, and the mode of reassociation of subunits to form the native molecule may result in a complicated system for interpretation. They suggested that folding occurred as the polypeptide was synthesized (based on the fact that the synthesis of a polypeptide of molecular weight 35,000 took about 5 min compared to 1 min for the initial folding process), and that the nascent polypeptide chain, as it was being synthesized, would assume an initial folding distinct from that of the native protein. The role of the initial conformation, with respect to the final conformation of the protein, depended on whether thermodynamic or kinetic factors were more important in controlling the folding. If folding were under thermodynamic control, the initial folding would be incorrect, but the protein would quickly assume the active and most stable conformation. On the other hand, for enzymes under kinetic control, such as glyceraldehyde phosphate dehydrogenase and lactic dehydrogenase, the initial conformation assumed by the protein would be important in directing the final conformation. In this case, the native structure derived from folding of a partially complete chain *in vivo* might differ from that produced after refolding of a complete protein *in vitro*.

B. Dependence of Protein Conformation on Environment

Major conformational changes either reversible or irreversible are likely to take place under nonphysiological conditions, e.g., extremes of pH, presence of denaturing agents, inorganic salts, alcohols, organic acids, and thermal exposure. The magnitude of these changes will depend on the protein under investigation and the state of its disulfide bonds, whether they are intact or reduced.

Kauzmann (1959) defined denaturation as a process by which the conformation of the polypeptide chain within the molecule was changed from that typical of the native protein to a more disordered arrangement, and included changes that accompanied cleavage of disulfide bonds, but not peptide linkages. The distinction between denaturation and conformational reorganization, which accompanies the chemical modification of proteins by virtue of modifying the covalent and concomitantly the noncovalent interactions, was emphasized (Habeeb, 1966b).

Loss of the noncovalent structure of a protein can be complete, and the molecule assumes a random coil conformation which can be recognized by various physicochemical and chemical methods. However, the presence of intact disulfide bonds in the protein will exert constraints that restrict the unfolding during denaturation. Thus the viscosity, frictional ratio, reactivity of amino acid residues, and spectral properties will differ from those that occur if disulfide bonds were cleaved. Most of the irreversible denaturation conditions are due to chemical reactions where the sulfhydryl groups and/or disulfide bonds take part. Sulfhydryl–disulfide exchange, leading to intermolecular cross-linking and concomitant aggregation, has been observed during denaturation of various proteins in 8 M urea (Huggins *et al.*, 1951). Aggregation was also observed during alkali denaturation in 0.1 N NaOH of sulfhydryl-containing proteins, e.g., fetal hemoglobin (Robinson, 1965), due to oxidation of the sulfhydryl groups to disulfide bonds (Riggs and Wolbach, 1956). Heat denaturation (at 70°C and 90°C) of bovine serum albumin and β-globulin resulted in aggregation attributed to oxidation of sulfhydryl groups to form intermolecular disulfide bridges. Aggregation was prevented by blocking the sulfhydryl groups with iodoacetamide before heating (DiIeso and Verga, 1960; Kolthoff and Tan, 1965). When bovine serum albumin was heated at pH 7 to 70°C in the absence of air, a decrease in the sulfhydryl content was observed. This decrease was due to the masking of the sulfhydryl groups, since recovery of the sulfhydryl groups took place in 7–8 M urea (Kolthoff and Tan, 1965). On heating at pH greater than 8.5, an increase in the sulfhydryl content resulted from hydrolysis of the disulfide bonds. In the presence of air, heating at 70°C resulted in loss of the sulfhydryl groups caused by oxidation to disulfides. Conformational changes accompanying the intra- and intermolecular sulfhydryl–disulfide exchange caused an increase in reactive disulfides from 0 to 9, after heating of bovine serum albumin for 1 hr at 70°C. When it was heated in the presence of a sulfhydryl reagent, sulfhydryl–disulfide exchange was prevented and the resulting aggregation was attributed to intramolecular hydrogen bond formation (Kolthoff and Tan, 1965). Reactive disulfides reverted to those in the native protein when the protein solution was made 8 M in urea and diluted, indicating that heat denaturation of bovine serum albumin in the presence of sulfhydryl reagent was reversible (Kolthoff and Tan, 1965). In the absence of sulfhydryl reagents, heat denaturation was irreversible, and the molecules remained aggregated in 8 M urea or 4 M guanidine. However, depolymerization was possible in the presence of 0.03–0.05 M sodium sulfite, because of scission of inter- and intramolecular disulfide bonds.

Disulfide bonds in proteins undergo cleavage in alkaline solution (0.1 N NaOH or higher) to yield cysteine and a reactive intermediate, dehydroalanyl residue (Blackburn and Lee, 1956). The latter can undergo further reactions with amino and thiol groups in proteins, yielding lysinoalanine (Bohak, 1964) and lanthionine (Horn et al., 1941). Essentially all the disulfide bonds in ovomucoid were split by alkali at pH 13.5 and 22°C (Donovan, 1967). Exposure of various proteins (lysozyme, α-lactalbumin, human IgG, and bovine serum albumin) to 0.2 N sodium hydroxide for 3 hr at room temperature resulted in destruction of some of the disulfide bonds and some conformational changes, shown by changed susceptibility of the disulfide bonds to reduction as compared to the native protein (Habeeb and Bennett, 1971).

1. Effect of Guanidine

Optical rotatory dispersion studies on several proteins (lysozyme, insulin, pepsinogen, ribonuclease, chymotrypsinogen, Fab fragment from rabbit immunoglobulin, bovine serum albumin, aldolase, and β-lactoglobulin) in 6 M guanidine indicated that the polypeptide chains existed in a random coil. Noncovalent structures were absent regardless of whether the disulfide bonds were intact or ruptured (Tanford et al., 1967a, b; Nozaki and Tanford, 1967). However, disulfide-containing proteins showed intrinsic viscosity and sedimentation coefficients indicative of the restrictions imposed by the disulfide bonds on a random coil (Nozaki and Tanford, 1967).

2. Effect of Urea

Urea is a weaker denaturing agent than guanidine, and there are several proteins that scarcely show unfolding in urea at room temperature, e.g., lysozyme (Leonis, 1956) and the immunoglobulins (Buckley et al., 1963). Partial unfolding was shown for bovine serum albumin in 8–10 M urea (Kauzmann and Simpson, 1953). With β-lactoglobulin (Kauzmann and Simpson, 1953) and ribonuclease (Nelson and Hummel, 1962), complete denaturation was achieved with urea. The completeness of denaturation was influenced by changes in temperature, pH, or added salts. Thus an increase in temperature or the lowering of pH exerted a cooperative effect to bring the denaturation to completion. An increase in the pH during denaturation of sulfhydryl- or disulfide-containing proteins, e.g., β-lactoglobulin (Pace and Tanford, 1968), may lead to irreversible changes due to sulfhydryl–disulfide exchange.

3. Effect of Inorganic Salts

Several salts, e.g., $CaCl_2$, KSCN (at 2.5 M), LiBr, and NaI (at 4 M), were found to denature ribonuclease (Bigelow, 1964; Sarfare and Bigelow, 1967), serum albumin (Bigelow and Geschwind, 1961), and lysozyme (Hamaguchi et al., 1963). The conformational changes (intrinsic viscosity, optical rotation, and ultraviolet difference spectra) were lower than those achieved by 6 M guanidine, thus indicating residual ordered structures.

4. Thermal Denaturation

Exposure of proteins to heat at low pH (where no irreversible denaturation occurred) resulted in a highly disordered structure (shown by various physicochemical criteria), which was not a random coil. Thermally denatured proteins showed regions of ordered structure which were likely to be hydrophobic. Addition of guanidine to thermally denatured lysozyme, ribonuclease, and chymotrypsin (Aune *et al.*, 1967) resulted in a greater degree of denaturation. Similarly, urea can effect further unfolding of heat-denatured ribonuclease (Brandts and Hunt, 1967) and chymotrypsinogen (Biltonen *et al.*, 1965). Irreversible thermal denaturation due to formation of intermolecular disulfide bonds by disulfide interchange or by action of alkali on disulfide bonds was observed with bovine serum albumin (Frensdorff *et al.*, 1953; Warner and Levy, 1958). Bull and Breese (1973) developed a method to investigate thermal denaturation of proteins based on changes in pH of unbuffered protein solution due to net uptake or release of protons caused by changes in the environment of ionizable amino acid residues. This method was used for myosin which coagulated on thermal denaturation (Goodno and Swenson, 1975). By subjecting IgE, F(ab)$_2$, and Fc fragments to thermal denaturation at 56°C for 30 min, it was concluded (Dorrington and Bennich, 1973) that the irreversible thermal denaturation of IgE was restricted to the Fc region, since the thermal denaturation of the F(ab)$_2$ fragment was reversible. The pathway of the thermal unfolding of ribonuclease A was examined by an insoluble derivative of carboxypeptidase A (Burgess *et al.*, 1975). Initially, tyrosine-92 and -25 were exposed, followed by the unfolding of this *C*-terminal region, which was accompanied by exposure of tyrosine-97.

Some proteins show loss of activity and changed reactivity as a result of freezing and thawing. Aldehyde dehydrogenase (Bradbury and Jakoby, 1972) lost 91% of its activity after five cycles of freezing and thawing during the course of 1 hr. However, in the presence of either 30% glycerol or 50% sucrose, recovery of the enzymatic activity was 100%. Rabbit muscle aldolase contains eight sulfhydryl groups, two of which are accessible and react sluggishly on alkylation with concomitant loss of activity. Under the freeze–thaw cycle, in the presence of an alkylating agent (Friedrich *et al.*, 1974), the sulfhydryl groups acquired increased reactivity and the subsequent loss of activity (due to modification of sulfhydryl groups) was observed. Beef heart lactic dehydrogenase (Gold and Segal, 1964) and chicken heart lactic dehydrogenase (Chilson *et al.*, 1965) were inactivated when the enzymes were frozen with a sulfhydryl reagent. It was then suggested that loss of the activity of some enzymes during freezing was due to oxidation of exposed sulfhydryl groups (Zondag, 1963; Chilson *et al.*, 1965) and was prevented by the presence of β-mercaptoethanol.

5. Effect of Acid pH

Proteins vary in their susceptibility to unfolding (stable, unstable, and intermediate) as a result of lowering of the pH. Lysozyme, β-lactoglobulin, and ribonuclease were stable at a pH of 2 and retained their native conformations (Timasheff *et al.*, 1966; Bigelow, 1964; Brandts and Hunt, 1967). In contrast, glyceraldehyde 3-phosphate dehydrogenase (Shibata and Kronman, 1967) was dissociated below pH 4 into subunits which existed as a random coil with some residual structure. Similarly, native ferrimyoglobin underwent a transition, at room temperature, between pH 5 and 4, because of the exposure of six buried (uncharged) histidine residues (Breslow and Gurd, 1962). The acid denaturation of bovine serum albumin occurred in two stages (Foster, 1960). The first stage was observed between pH 4.5 and 3.5 and involved a limited expansion of the molecule, which left the major globular regions of the molecule intact (Foster, 1960; Herskovits and Laskowski, 1962). At low ionic strength, a further increase in intrinsic viscosity occurred. Relevant results were obtained when bovine serum albumin was succinylated, imparting a net negative charge (Habeeb, 1967a). A slight increase in the Stokes radius occurred with succinylation of up to 30 amino groups. At the same time, no change in the availability of the disulfide bonds to reaction with sodium sulfite was observed, indicative of limited conformational changes. As more amino groups were succinylated, there was a dramatic increase in the Stokes radius, with a concomitant increase in available disulfides (Habeeb, 1967a). Only about nine disulfide groups were available for reaction in the fully succinylated BSA, which indicated the presence of some residual native structure. In contrast to lysozyme, which was stable toward acid denaturation, α-lactalbumin exhibited conformational changes near pH 4 (Kronman *et al.*, 1966), suggesting conformational differences between these two proteins (Atassi *et al.*, 1970a; Habeeb and Atassi, 1971).

6. Alcohols, Chloroethanol, and Dioxane

Conformational changes, as a result of the addition of organic solvents (to 50%) to an aqueous protein solution (Weber and Tanford, 1959), occurred in two stages, an initial or partial unfolding followed by refolding. This was observed with ribonuclease in 2-chloroethanol (Weber and Tanford, 1959), with diisopropylphosphoryl chymotrypsin in 2-chlorethanol (Martin and Bhatnagar, 1967), and with β-lactoglobulin in dioxane (Tanford *et al.*, 1960). Proteins that exist as a random coil in the native state acquired an α-helix structure in organic solvents, e.g., α-casein in 2-chlorethanol or methanol plus 0.01 M HCl (Herskovits and Mescanti, 1965) and histone in 50% and 98% *n*-propanol (Jirgensons, 1967). At lower concentrations (10–20% of alcohol or dioxane), the conformation of a protein was not altered at room temperature, but the instability of the protein was demonstrated under different denaturing conditions, e.g., the low temperature necessary for thermal denaturation of ribonuclease (Schrier and Scheraga, 1962).

7. Ethylene Glycol and Other Polyhydric Alcohols

The stability of proteins in ethylene glycol was reported by Tanford *et al.* (1962), based on their findings that bovine γ-globulin and β-lacto-globulin did not show conformational changes (from optical rotation measurements). However, in anhydrous ethylene glycol, under alkaline conditions, ribonuclease showed conformational changes (Sage and Singer, 1962), while in a neutral solution it showed only partial exposure of the tyrosine residues (Herskovits and Laskowski, 1968). Studies on cardiac myosin, skeletal myosin, heavy meromyosin, and actomyosin (Brahms and Kay, 1962; Kay and Brahms, 1963) indicated that skeletal myosin A unfolded in 45% ethylene glycol, and the shape of the molecule changed (the length decreased from 1300 Å to 300 Å) in 67% glycol. In contrast, tropomyosin and heavy meromyosin did not show any conformation changes in ethylene glycol. Glycerol in high concentration was reported to protect proteins against heat denaturation (Beilinsson, 1929; Koide and Torres, 1964) and to protect aldolase (at 50% concentration) against proteolytic enzymes during fractionation by column chromatography (Wallevik, 1968). However, there is evidence that with some proteins, conformational changes take place (Bradbury and Jakoby, 1972; Klinman and Rose, 1971; Myers and Jakoby, 1973). Aldehyde dehydrogenase was stabilized by 30% glycerol (Bradbury and Jakoby, 1972). Stability was attributed to a change in the conformation induced by glycerol, in which sulfhydryl groups near the DPN-binding site became masked and protected by acquiring a reduced reactivity. The effects of glycerol on the kinetic parameters of 16 enzymes (Myers and Jakoby, 1973) showed essential changes in either the Michaelis constant (K_m) and/or the turnover rates, as shown in Table I. The results caution that glycerol can cause substantial changes in enzyme kinetic parameters in an unpredictable direction, despite its effect as a protein stabilizer. In 50% glycerol, yeast alcohol dehydrogenase (Myers and Jakoby, 1975) showed a decrease in K_m for several substrates, a decrease in its intrinsic fluorescence and ultraviolet absorption difference spectrum, and a decrease in the rate of reaction with 5,5'-dithiobis(2-nitrobenzoic acid); whereas circular dichroism failed to show any conformational changes. Taken as a whole, glycerol seems to be inert with some proteins and is capable of effecting subtle conformational changes with others.

8. Detergents

The binding of sodium dodecylsulfate (SDS) to proteins, and the concomitant conformational changes that accompany such binding, is dependent on the protein and whether its disulfide bonds are intact or reduced. With bovine serum albumin at pH > 10, binding of ten molecules

Table I. Effects of 30% Glycerol on Kinetic Constants of Enzymes[a]

Enzyme	Substrate[b]	Normal		With glycerol	
		K_m (mM)	Turnover[c]	K_m (mM)	Turnover[c]
Alcohol dehydrogenase	DPN	0.23	49,000	0.063	8,000
Alcohol dehydrogenase	Ethanol	11	37,000	2.8	13,000
Aldolase	FDP	0.62	750[d]	0.098	160[d]
Alkaline phosphatase	NPP	0.028	2,400	0.12	640
α-Chymotrypsin	ATEE	1.4	3,700	1.6	1,400
Diaphorase	DPNH	0.018	730	0.016	150
β-Galactosidase	ONPG	0.25	17,000	67	3,800
Glucose 6-phosphate dehydrogenase	G6P	0.013	1,900	0.014	980
Glutamate dehydrogenase	L-Glutamate	1.9	250	0.44	75
Glyceraldehyde 3-phosphate dehydrogenase	PGAL	0.17	3,500	0.20	1,100
Glyoxylate reductase	Glyoxylate	24	67[e]	26	13[e]
Hydroxypyruvate reductase	HP	19	1,500	36	320
Micrococcal nuclease	NPpdTp	0.023	4.2	0.019	1.8
Phosphodiesterase I	bisNPP	0.49	0.042[e]	3.3	0.14[e]
Sorbitol dehydrogenase	Fructose	300	1,000[e]	1,430	430[e]
Trypsin	BAA	1.8	3.5	8.0	16
Xanthine oxidase	Benzaldehyde	0.50	1,000	0.67	780

[a] From Myers and Jakoby (1973).
[b] The following abbreviations are used: FDP, fructose 1,6-diphosphate; NPP, p-nitrophenyl phosphate; ATEE, N-acetyltyrosine ethyl ester; ONPG, o-nitrophenyl β-galactoside; G6P, glucose 6-phosphate; PGAL, glyceraldehyde 3-phosphate; HP, hydroxypyruvate; NPpdTp, deoxythymidine 5'-p-nitrophenyl phosphate 3'-phosphate; bisNPP, bis (p-nitrophenyl) phosphate; BAA, benzoyl-L-arginine amide.
[c] Expressed as μmoles of product formed per minute per μmole of protein.
[d] Expressed as absorbance change per minute per μmole of protein.
[e] Expressed as μmoles of product formed per minute per milligram of protein.

of SDS per one molecule of protein resulted in a more compact structure (Lovrien, 1963).

The instability of interferons (from different species and even from the same species), caused by physical and chemical manipulation (Ng and Vilcek, 1972; Weil and Dorner, 1973), was prevented by SDS. A low concentration of SDS (0.0035 M) was found to stabilize a mouse L-cell interferon (Stewart et al., 1974a) and a human fibroblast interferon (Stewart et al., 1974b) against denaturation by heat (100°C for 2.5 min), freeze-thaw (30 cycle), and chemical manipulation. Human leukocyte interferon was stabilized by SDS against heat inactivation (Mogensen and Cantell, 1974). Similarly, low concentration of SDS (0.001–0.00015 M) had a protective effect on human serum albumin against 6 M urea (Markus and Karush, 1957). Markus et al. (1964) showed that human serum albumin had two distinct binding regions to detergents with a maximum molar binding ratio of 14 and 24. Neither a change in pH to 9.5 nor a urea concentration change to 6 M affected the binding at the first binding regions. Hydrodynamic measurements (sedimentation coefficients and intrinsic viscosity) and helical content measurements failed to show any conformational changes associated with the binding. Binding took place in the presence of urea and also when the amino groups were acetylated or modified by formalin. However, no protection against urea denaturation was afforded in the human serum albumins where the amino groups were modified. Thus the protection against urea denaturation required the presence of free amino groups in the protein and arose by stabilization of the native conformation by detergent cross-links between the positively charged amino groups and hydrophobic regions on the protein molecule. Direct evidence for the participation of the amino groups was shown by decreased reactivity of the free amino groups with trinitrobenzene sulfonic acid on the addition of SDS to bovine serum albumin, ovalbumin, and human IgG (Habeeb, 1966a), and to lysozyme and α-lactalbumin (Habeeb and Atassi, 1971). Subtle conformational changes accompanied the binding of SDS to bovine serum albumin (25 molar ratio) resulting in a relaxed conformation (shown by slight increase in availability of the disulfide bonds to reduction) and complete protection from the denaturing effect of urea up to 4 M concentration (Fig. 1). At greater concentrations of urea, partial protection was demonstrated (Habeeb, 1966b) by the differences in availability of the disulfide

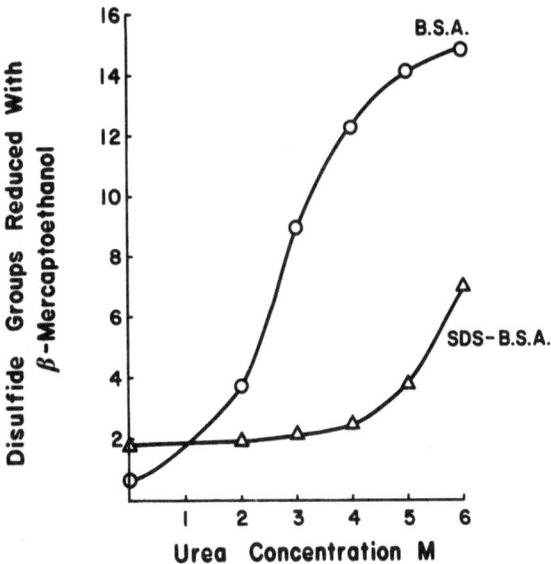

Figure 1. Availability of the disulfide bonds to reduction with 0.05 M β-mercaptoethanol in bovine serum albumin (BSA) and sodium dodecylsulfate bovine serum albumin (SDS-BSA) in the presence of different urea concentrations. From Habeeb (1966b).

bonds to reduction between BSA and SDS-BSA. With lysozyme a relaxed conformation resulted from SDS binding; in contrast, α-lactalbumin showed a constrained conformation (Habeeb and Atassi, 1971). In SDS, proteins tend to maintain their α-helical content and those that are randomly coiled, e.g., β-casein and histone, assume a helical structure (Jirgensons, 1967). SDS at $5-8 \times 10^{-4}$ M concentration produced a complex containing 0.4 g SDS per gram of protein (Reynolds and Tanford, 1970a) with a variety of reduced proteins, while at a concentration of SDS above 8×10^{-4} M, a second complex was formed containing 1.4 g SDS/g protein. The protein–SDS complex showed a helical structure demonstrated from optical rotation data (Reynolds and Tanford, 1970b). Hydrodynamic studies suggested that the complex is a rodlike particle, the length of which varies with the molecular weight of the protein. A plot of log Stokes radius, determined by gel chromatography, was linear with log molecular weight of the protein (Fish et al., 1970). The Stokes radii of unreduced protein–SDS complexes were smaller than those of their reduced counterparts, indicating decreased binding of SDS by proteins with intact disulfide bonds (Pitt-Rivers and Impiombato, 1968).

9. Binding of Ligands

Enzymes and other proteins undergo conformational changes as a result of the binding of inhibitors, substrates, or other ligands. The binding of N-acetylglucosamine and tri-N-acetylglucosamine to lysozyme resulted in the movement of the tryptophan-62 side chain by about 0.75 Å to narrow the cleft (Blake et al., 1967). The movement of this tryptophan side chain was accompanied by small shifts of other residues lining the cleft. When glycyl-L-tyrosine binds to carboxypeptidase A, the phenolic hydroxyl groups of tyrosine-248 moved 12 Å, the guanidinium group of arginine-145 moved 2 Å, and the carboxyl groups of glutamic-270 moved 2 Å (Reeke et al., 1967). Interaction of antibody with univalent hapten resulted in a more compact molecule, shown by an increase in the sedimentation coefficient (Warner et al., 1970), a decrease in the radius of gyration and the volume of antibody (Pilz et al., 1974), or reduced susceptibility to enzymatic digestion (Grossberg et al., 1965). Ligand binding to proteins may result in a more compact conformation, with a concomitant decrease in the rate of proteolysis. Markus (1965) showed that binding of one methyl orange molecule to human serum albumin caused a significant decrease in the rate of digestion. No further effect was observed beyond the binding of 5 moles of methyl orange per mole of human serum albumin. It is significant that the binding of 1 mole of methyl orange to human serum albumin produced a generalized conformational change, causing a decrease in accessibility of peptide bonds to digestion by various enzymes with different specificities (chymotrypsin, trypsin, papain, pronase, and subtilisin). Moreover, the attachment of six to eight lauroyl groups to human serum albumin resulted in 80% and 95% reduction in the rates of tryptic and chymotryptic digestion, respectively. Ligand binding to human serum albumin not only affected the rate of digestion but also changed the pathway of digestion, as demonstrated by chromatographic analysis of the breakdown products obtained in the presence and absence of ligands (Markus et al., 1967b). The fragmentation of human serum albumin by trypsin yielded two main fragments of 51,000 and 18,500 mol. wt. In addition, a second breakdown occurred, which liberated a 13,500 mol. wt. fragment and smaller peptides (Markus et al., 1967a). Interaction of human serum albumin with methyl orange reduced the yield of the 51,000 and 18,500 mol. wt. fragments. Although crystal violet, which produced a relaxed conformation, increased the digestibility of human serum albumin, the relative amount of 51,000 mol. wt. fragment was reduced, compared to the digestion of the native protein. The relative amounts of the fragments (51,000, 18,500, and 13,500 mol. wt., and the smaller peptides) produced during tryptic digestion of human serum albumin were different with various ligands. This indicated a profound influence of the ligand on the pathway of digestion, due to differences in the conformational changes induced by a given ligand.

Conformational changes, associated with the binding of the strong inhibitor 2'-cytidylate to the active center of ribonuclease, significantly reduced the rate of formation of ribonuclease S by subtilisin (Markus et al., 1968). Thus the bond between amino acids 20 and 21 (the site of subtilisin action), which is far removed from the site of binding of the inhibitor, became resistant to subtilisin attack. Moreover, the inhibitor conferred stability on ribonuclease against tryptic and chymotryptic digestion at 60°C. The conformational changes induced by the inhibitor affected nine defined peptide bonds which were not in the immediate vicinity of active site (Markus et al., 1968). Aspartate transcarbamylase acquired a relaxed conformation in the presence of the substrate aspartate as shown by increased digestibility with trypsin (McClintock and Markus, 1968). In contrast, in the presence of adenosine 5'-triphosphate (an allosteric activator) or cytidine 5'-triphosphate (an inhibitor), a constrained conformation resulted, which was demonstrated by reduced susceptibility to enzymatic digestion by trypsin, subtilisin, and pronase.

III. Dependence of Conformation on the Whole Amino Acid Sequence: Conformation of Unique Protein Fragments

There is disagreement as to the mode of the folding of a protein to form the native conformation during biosynthesis. Chantrenne (1961) and Phillips (1966, 1967) suggested that folding of the polypeptide chain to its native conformation starts from the *N*-terminal to form stable conformations, which act as centers around which the remainder of the chain folds. This hypothesis requires that fragments isolated from the NH_2-terminal end of the protein molecule possess a conformation similar to that in the intact molecule.

Crumpton (1968) isolated a peptide (sequence 1–55) from apomyoglobin by cleaving it with cyanogen bromide. Based on the ability of the peptide to precipitate half the antibody from antimetmyoglobin and the presence of 60% α-helix (from optical rotatory dispersion curves), Crumpton (1968) concluded that the peptide had a similar conformation to that of crystalline myoglobin. It is likely that the tendency of the peptide to aggregate permitted the re-formation of a conformation similar to native myoglobin.

The circular dichroism of the *S*-peptide from RNase was studied by Klee (1968) and was found to exhibit a stable negative peak near 225 nm, characteristic of α-helical structure (Holzwarth and Doty, 1965), and a much larger negative peak near 200 nm, characteristic of randomly coiled structure. The circular dichroism of *S*-peptide showed a mixed conformation of helical and random-type structures. The 225 nm peak of *S*-peptide was insensitive to temperatures 26–79°C and also to 1 M guanidine HCl. A higher concentration of guanidine caused a gradual conversion of *S*-peptide to a random coil. Free *S*-peptide therefore assumed a structure similar to that of the *S*-peptide segment in the intact protein. X-ray diffraction investigation by Kartha *et al.* (1967) and Wyckoff *et al.* (1967) showed that residues 2–12 of RNase were in an α-helical stretch. Later Brown and Klee (1969) examined, by circular dichroism, the conformation of small peptides (residues 1–8, 1–13, 1–15, 1–20) derived from the NH_2-terminal region of ribonuclease. This region contains a segment of α-helix in the intact molecule, which includes residues 2–12. The three longer peptides were partially helical, and helicity increased markedly in salt (by the suppression of charge interactions). Molar ellipticities of the three longer peptides at 224 nm in 0.033 M Na_2SO_4 were essentially the same at a low temperature. This suggested that the region between residues 1 and 12 is helical in the isolated peptide, as in the intact protein. The 14–20 region was not helical. Short-range interactions were sufficient to produce a structure similar to that of the NH_2-terminal region of the intact protein. The stability of the helices in the peptides was much lower than that in the protein, as shown by the low ellipticity. The peptide conformation was highly mobile, as demonstrated by the strong influence of ionic strength on ellipticity. Thus long-range interactions were important in stabilizing the conformation of segments within the protein molecule. Although peptide 1–8 contained the amino acid residues which formed part of the helix in intact ribonuclease, it was unable to form a helix because of its short length (Brown and Klee, 1969).

In contrast, the bulk of evidence from the extensive work on fragments and derivatives from ribonuclease, sperm whale myoglobin, and staphylococcal nuclease clearly demonstrates that the native conformation of the protein molecule and its stability are dependent on the integrity of the whole amino acid sequence and that folding to the native conformation does not occur until most of the polypeptide chain is biosynthesized.

1. Ribonuclease

Extensive work on ribonuclease fragments showed that conformational stability was greatly reduced and that derivatives lacking some amino acid residues, either from the N-terminal end or from the C-terminal end, had a changed conformation, resulting in loss of enzymatic activity. Richards and Vithayathil (1959) showed that exposure of ribonuclease A (RNase) to subtilisin for 3 hr resulted in the scission of the peptide bond between residues 20 and 21. Both the peptide part (S-peptide) and the protein part (S-protein) were strongly associated, noncovalently, and were dissociated only to the individual molecules in 3.33% trichloroacetic acid or by 8 M urea. Each fragment was enzymatically inactive, but activity was completely regained at a molar ratio of 1 when S-protein and S-peptide associated. It was significant that scission of one peptide bond in ribonuclease resulted in subtle changes in conformation of ribonuclease, as shown by susceptibility of ribonuclease S to trypsin digestion, with loss of activity in contrast to the stability of ribonuclease A. Chemical reactivity of histidine residues was changed, indicating that the reactivity depended on the conformational integrity of the protein molecule. Reaction of ribonuclease with iodoacetate at pH 5.5 (Gundlach et al., 1959) involved a unique histidine residue with concomitant loss of activity. Barnard and Stein (1959) identified the histidine residue as histidine-119 by reaction with bromoacetate. It was remarkable that the native conformation was essential for this reaction. When the molecule was denatured with urea, the reactivity of histidine dropped to zero, as the urea concentration increased to 8 M (Stark et al., 1961) and methionine residues became reactive. Both histidine and methionyl residues in ribonuclease S reacted with iodoacetate (Vithayathil and Richards, 1961), whereas, with S-protein, no reaction with histidine occurred, but one or more methionine residues reacted, resulting in inability of modified S-protein to bind S-peptide.

In contrast to native ribonuclease A, ribonuclease S and its separated fragments were susceptible to extensive digestion with carboxypeptidase A. The removal of the C-terminal valine-124 and serine-123 from S-protein resulted in the recovery of 45% enzymatic activity and 80–90% of binding affinity of S-protein (with respect to unmodified ribonuclease), when reconstituted with S-peptide (Potts et al., 1964). This partial loss of enzymatic activity was attributed to conformational changes (Potts and Young, 1963). S-protein lacking Val-124 to Phe-120 was inactive even in the presence of a hundredfold molar excess of S-peptide, despite binding with the S-peptide. These results demonstrated the essentiality of the C-terminal residues for the enzymatic activity of ribonuclease.

Residues between Ser-16 and Ala-20 in S-peptide were not essential for ribonuclease activity. A derivative of S-peptide, consisting of residues 1–13 (Hofmann, et al., 1963) and residues 1–12 plus homoserine at position 13 (Parks et al., 1963), restored considerable enzymatic activity, when mixed with S-protein at high molar ratios. Thus the dipeptide sequence aspartyl serine (residues 14–15) seemed to be important for optimal binding of S-peptide and S-protein for recovery of enzymatic activity.

Although the specific rotations in the absence of urea at $\lambda = 366$ Å for RNase, RNase S, and S-protein were similar ($-262°C$, $-267°C$ and $-263°C$, respectively), indicating similar conformation, subtle conformational changes were brought about by differences in the covalent structure of the three proteins. These changes were demonstrated by a decrease in the conformational stability observed when the derivatives were denatured by heat and urea. The midpoint of thermally induced conformational changes in the absence of urea was 62°C for RNase, 41.5°C for RNase S, and 35.5°C for S-protein. There was a decrease in the transition temperature as urea concentration increased (Sherwood and Potts, 1965a). Limited conformational changes may not be detected in aqueous buffers because of minor covalent alteration, but a marked deterioration in conformational stability became evident on denaturation by urea or heat.

Difference spectroscopy was used to investigate the molar absorbance changes of the buried tyrosine residues of RNase A, RNase S, and S-protein (Sherwood and Potts, 1965b). Both RNase and RNase S contain three buried tyrosines, two of which were exposed by heat alone; two abnormal tyrosines were observed with S-protein, one of which was heat labile. All three proteins had one abnormal tyrosine stable to heat, but it was exposed by performic acid oxidation, complete proteolytic digestion, or exposure to 8 M urea. These results indicated that the intramolecular environment in the vicinity of several tyrosine residues in RNase S and S-protein was similar to that of the native molecule, despite their reduced conformational stability.

Kato and Anfinsen (1969) demonstrated the conformational differences between RNase and RNase S-protein by the susceptibility of the disulfide bonds to disulfide interchange. Treatment of RNase S-protein with 0.001 M β-mercaptoethanol in the presence of the disulfide interchange enzyme resulted in rapid decrease in potential enzymatic activity when mixed with S-peptide, due to rapid scrambling and formation of mismatched disulfide bonds. The S-protein therefore did not have the information to direct the folding which is characteristic of the native protein. However, when the S-peptide was added to the scrambled S-protein and interchange enzyme, enzymatic activity was recovered. The results emphasized the importance of cooperative interactions between different parts of the molecule to create the native conformation.

Eaker *et al.* (1965*a,b*) isolated two structural homologues of bovine RNase A by countercurrent distribution. They were identified as des-lysylglutamyl RNase (lacking *N*-terminal lysine and having glutamic acid as *N*-terminal) and des-lysylpyroglutamyl RNase (where glutamyl residue cyclized to pyroglutamic acid). Although RNase A, as well as the two homologues, had similar overall conformation (similar ORD data and ultraviolet spectra), a subtle difference in the conformation was demonstrated by differences in enzymatic activity and susceptibility to tryptic digestion (Eaker *et al.*, 1965*c*). Glutamyl RNase was almost fully active, but it was slightly more susceptible to trypsin digestion than RNase A (11% digestion compared to 5% with RNase A), while pyroglutamyl RNase was considerably less active (40% of RNase activity with cytidine 2',3'-phosphate) and more susceptible to tryptic digestion (42% compared to 5% with RNase A). The results indicated that the *N*-terminal lysine played a minor role in maintaining an active and stable conformation, while glutamic acid-2 played a major role in the enzymatic activity and structural integrity of the RNase molecule. Eaker *et al.* (1965*c*) concluded that the des-lysyl RNases had greater conformational freedom, which may be the result of a decreased binding or an imperfect orientation of the *N*-terminal segment to the remainder of the molecule.

In the previous presentation, derivatives of RNase A lacking segments from *N*-terminal end were investigated for differences in their conformation. Similarly, derivatives of RNase deficient in some *C*-terminal residues showed conformational differences when compared to native RNase. A derivative of RNase A prepared by limited peptic digestion (RNase P) (Anfinsen, 1956) was found to lack residues 121–124, and was enzymatically inactive. Ribonuclease A and RNase P had similar hydrodynamic properties, but showed some differences in spectrophotometric and optical properties (Sela and Anfinsen, 1957). Taniuchi (1970) showed RNase P to form incorrect pairing of disulfide bonds on reduction and reoxidation. RNase P was reduced in 8 M urea with β-mercaptoethanol for 4 hr. The reduced RNase P was diluted and air reoxidized. The disappearance of the sulfhydryl groups was found to be complete in 21 hr as monitored by Ellman's reagent (1959). Circular dichroism data at 210–300 nm for RNase P and RNase A were similar, while that of reduced-reoxidized RNase P resembled that of a disordered structure (performic acid oxidized RNase). Moreover, in contrast to the stability of native RNase, RNase P showed conformational instability as detected by sulfhydryl–disulfide interchange reaction at 37°C (aggregation occurred with RNase P was incubated with 0.001 M β-mercaptoethanol, but not at 25°C). Evidence for incorrect pairing of disulfide bonds in reduced-reoxidized RNase P was also shown by cyanogen bromide cleavage at methionine (Taniuchi, 1970). Reduced-reoxidized RNase P gave a pattern on cyanogen bromide cleavage similar to that of RNase with incorrectly paired disulfide bonds. Therefore, the absence of the last four residues in RNase resulted in a protein which did not have the information for correct pairing of disulfide bonds. The ability to form disulfide bonds on reduction and reoxidation demonstrated that the polypeptide was flexible. These results show that the correct folding of polypeptide chain of RNase cannot be accomplished until all the molecule is biosynthesized.

Another approach was taken by Puett (1972b) to investigate the conformational differences between RNase A and RNase P (sequence 1–120). He examined the difference in the conformational stability of RNase P and RNase A by monitoring the reversible changes in CD spectrum and ultraviolet difference absorption spectrum of each protein at various guanidine concentrations. The near-ultraviolet CD spectra of the two proteins were almost identical, indicating that the local environment of the tyrosyl and disulfide residues did not alter significantly on removal of the four C-terminal residues. Changes in the ellipticity with guanidine or temperature suggested that small environmental differences occurred. The conformational free energy of RNase P was reduced by about 30% from that of RNase A (10.1 ± 0.7 kcal/mole compared to 14.4 ± 0.3 kcal/mole). RNase P with the disulfide bonds intact was able to refold to its native conformation. It was concluded that a stable conformation can occur only when most of the polypeptide chain is biosynthesized. Two more derivatives, RNase 1–119 and RNase 1–118, were prepared (Puett, 1972c) from RNase P by carboxypeptidase A. Under nondenaturing conditions, RNase 1–118 was found to have two buried tyrosine residues, indicating a stable conformation that may be similar to that of RNase A, which had more than two inaccessible tyrosines. However, the stability of the conformation was greatly reduced in RNase 1–119 and RNase 1–118, thus indicating the importance of the C-terminal region in stabilizing the native conformation.

Hayashi et al. (1973) found that RNase 1–114 and RNase 1–115, when mixed with 25–30 equivalents of synthetic RNase peptides, sequences 116–124, 113–124, and 111–124, restored about 50% of activity relative to an equimolar amount of RNase. The binding of the peptide was stronger when no overlapping segment was present. Partial recovery of enzymatic activity indicated that the re-formed active center was not identical to that in native RNase. Structural stabilities of various RNase derivatives and their complexes with peptides 116–124 were determined from heat-induced changes in ultraviolet absorption at 287 nm. RNase derivatives were unfolded at 25°C, but their transition temperature increased 37–38°C when they were mixed with 10 equivalents of the peptide.

2. Myoglobin

Atassi and Singhal (1970a) obtained fragments by specific cleavage of sperm whale myoglobin at arginine residues. Peptides 1–31, 46–118, and 119–139 were isolated. They were studied by ORD and CD, and their helical content was calculated (Table II). The peptides were less helical in the free state than in the intact protein. Peptide 119–139 gave less helical content in the free state, a fact attributed to decreased stability resulting from partial loss of short-range interactions (as it carried a portion of helix H) and minimal contribution of long-range interactions. Moreover, two separated fragments of a helix were not able to achieve a high degree of helicity. Overlapping fragments containing intact helices were obtained from sperm whale myoglobin by cleavage at a proline residue (prolines occur at four bends), with sodium in liquid ammonia (Atassi and Singhal, 1970b). Peptides comprising sequences 1–36, 37–87, 37–119, and 120–153 were isolated and studied by ORD and CD (Singhal and Atassi, 1970). Fragments 1–36, 1–87, and 37–87 showed lower helical content in the free state than in the intact protein and suggested that helicity was due to short-range interactions. In contrast, fragment 37–119 showed a very high helical content in the free peptide and suggested long-range interactions. Compari-

Table II. Helical Contents of Various Peptides of Myoglobin

Peptide segments or protein	Segment in molecule	Helical content of fragment	
		Free state (%)	Intact protein (%)
1–31[a]	Helix A and part of helix B	33	97
46–118[a]	Nonhelical segment CD, all helices D, E, and F and bends between them	38	62
119–139[a]	Nonhelical segment GH and a portion of helix H	15	71
1–36[b]	Helix A and helix B	28	97
1–87[b]	Overlap 1–36 and 37–87	30	79
37–87[b]	Helices C, D, E and bend EF	25	67
37–119[b]	Segment 37–87 and two complete helices F and G	42	74
120–153[b]	Helix H and nonhelical structure	19	71
Myoglobin			78
Apomyoglobin			58

[a] Obtained by cleavage at arginine residues (Atassi and Singhal, 1970a).
[b] Obtained by cleavage at proline residues (Singhal and Atassi, 1970).

son of fragment 120–153 with fragment 132–153, obtained by Epand and Scheraga (1968), indicated that the longer fragment 120–153 had a higher helical character than the shorter peptide 132–153. Cleavage of a helix into two fragments resulted in both fragments acquiring a lower helicity than the parent fragment. The helical contents of N-terminal peptides 1–36 and 1–87 in the free state were much lower than in the intact molecule. Data on the helix content of various fragments from sperm whale myoglobin (estimated from ORD measurements) were analyzed, using a model which treated proline residues as helix breakers (Puett, 1972a). The results indicated that the intrinsic helix potential of the N-terminal region (helices A and B) was slightly greater than that of the C-terminal region (helix H). Sequence 37–87 (helices C, D, and E) had the lowest helix fraction in the native protein. Helix G (sequence 100–119), had the highest helix-forming tendency in the protein and may represent the nucleus for chain folding (Hermans et al., 1969). The sequence corresponding to F and G helices was suggested to be present before stable folding occurred.

3. Staphylococcal Nuclease

Studies on staphylococcal nuclease fragments indicated that the free segments were structureless and that the entire amino acid sequence was essential for the correct folding of the protein. The results rule out sequential folding from the N-terminal as the protein is biosynthesized. Several fragments produced by limited digestion with trypsin were identified. Nuclease 6–149 was prepared by limited tryptic digestion in the presence of deoxythymidine $3',5'$-diphosphate and Ca^{2+} (Taniuchi and Anfinsen, 1968) and was fully active. On further digestion, nuclease T was formed and consisted of noncovalently bound fragments, nuclease 6–48, and nuclease 49, 50–149 (Taniuchi et al., 1967). The complex had 8–10% activity of native nuclease, while the individual fragments were inactive.

Two more fragments, nucleases 1–126 and 127–149, were produced by tryptic digestion of trifluoroacetyl nuclease for 8–10 min to effect cleavage of the bond between Arg-126 and Lys-127, followed by deblocking. The fragments were inactive, either alone or in combination (Taniuchi and Anfinsen, 1969).

Nuclease fragment sequence 6–149 was very similar to nuclease, as shown by its unchanged enzymatic activity, optical rotatory dispersion, and immunochemical reactivity by the Ouchterlony method (Taniuchi and Anfinsen, 1968). Therefore, sequence 1–5 from the N-terminal end was not required for enzymatic activity, and its removal was without effect on the conformation. However, cleavage of peptide bonds between residues 48 and 49 or 49 and 50 resulted in considerable decrease in the catalytic activity and heat stability. Individual fragments from nuclease, comprising sequences 1–126, 127–149, 6–48, and 49, 50–149, showed a loose and disorganized structure, as determined from CD and optical rotation (Taniuchi and Anfinsen, 1968, 1969). However, when fragments, 6–48 and 49, 50–149 were mixed, there was a recovery of enzymatic activity and helical content; the latter amounted to 9%, compared to 13% for unfractionated segments 6–48 and 49, 50–149 and 18% for nuclease. On the other hand, both fragments 1–126 and 127–149 were not reconstituted and showed no ability to associate. Stable structures can be formed from flexible and disordered segments when the minimal amino acid information is present. Fragment 49, 50–149 was capable of binding noncovalently to fragment 1–126 to form a conformation resembling nuclease T, and the overlapping sequence 49–126 from 1–126 protruded. Digestion with trypsin in the presence of thymidine $3',5'$-diphosphate and Ca^{2+} resulted in the production of small peptides sequence 1–5 and 49–126, derived from fragment 1–126, keeping the portion 6–48 bound to fragment 49, 50–149. Nuclease 1–126 was able to bind to a cyanogen bromide fragment 99–149 (which had a disordered structure by CD) to form a complex with ordered structure and with enzymatic activity similar to that of nuclease T (Taniuchi and Anfinsen, 1971). However, the helical content of the complex was almost half the helical content of nuclease and may indicate either a relative decrease in ordered structure or a decreased stability of the complex. Limited digestion with trypsin in the presence of deoxythymidine $3',5'$-diphosphate and Ca^{2+} removed residues 99–110 from the complex (sequence 1–126 and 111–149) without affecting the enzymatic activity. The interaction of the two fragments was reversible. Removal of residues 124–126 by carboxypeptidase from fragment 1–126 and residues 111–113 by aminopeptidase from fragment 111–149 did not affect the enzymatic activity of the complex. Two active complementing structures also were formed in equal amounts (within 1 min) when enzymatically inactive and disordered fragment, nuclease 49–149, was mixed with nuclease 1–126 (Taniuchi and Anfinsen, 1971). The structures contained sequence 1–48 from 1–126 + 49–149 and sequence 1–126 + 111–149 from 49–149. The redundant portions (residues 49–110 from segment 49–149 and residues 49–126 from segment 1–126) were susceptible to tryptic digestion in the presence of deoxythymidine $3',5'$-diphosphate and Ca^{2+}, because of their flexibility. Since nuclease 127–149 cannot form an active complex with 1–126, sequence 111–126 on fragment 127–149 was essential for noncovalent interactions with 1–126. The fragments nuclease 1–48 and 111–149 participated in the formation of the two active complexes by directing the necessary folding.

4. Proteins with Cleaved Disulfide Bonds

Disulfide bonds play an important role in stabilizing the native conformation. The intrachain disulfide bonds do, in many cases, form parts of stable ring structures (Cecil, 1963), stabilized by noncovalent interactions.

In most cases the disulfide bonds are buried inside the protein molecule and show very limited reactivity, if at all, in the absence of denaturing agents. It is very important to realize that differences exist with regard to the effect of the scission of one or more disulfide bonds on the conformation of the protein and its influence on its biological activity. Evidence was presented that not all of the disulfide bonds were essential for the biological activity of ribonuclease (Resnick *et al.*, 1959). Disulfide bonds were cleaved by reaction with sodium sulfite in the presence of different concentrations of urea, 0–8 M. Results showed that, despite the cleavage of 3.9 disulfide bonds in ribonuclease, about 30% of the enzymatic activity still remained. However, in this experiment, the absence of any unreduced ribonuclease was not established, which may account for the enzymatic activity. Staphylococcal enterotoxin, a toxin elaborated by *Staphylococcus aureus*, isolated in pure form (Schantz *et al.*, 1965) consists of one polypeptide chain (239 amino acid residues) of molecular weight 28,500 of known amino acid sequence, with one disulfide bond between residues 92 and 112 (Spero *et al.*, 1965; Huang and Bergdoll, 1970). Reduction of the single disulfide bond had no effect on the immunochemical reactivity, with antisera indicating no major conformational change as a result of this treatment (Spero *et al.*, 1973). It may be important to mention here that the liberated sulfhydryl groups were not blocked, and the solution was kept in 0.01 M β-mercaptoethanol. The directive, long-range interaction to achieve a folded structure similar to that of the native molecule was operative when sulfhydryl groups were free. A different result may have been obtained if the sulfhydryl groups were alkylated, in light of the work by Lee and Atassi (1973). Lysozyme was reduced in 8 M urea with β-mercaptoethanol for 4 hr at 37°C, and the sulfhydryl groups were blocked either with iodoacetic acid or with methyl *p*-nitrobenzene sulfonate to give *S*-carboxymethyl (SCM-) lysozyme or *S*-methyl (SM-) lysozyme (Lee and Atassi, 1973). Optical rotatory dispersion and circular dichroism measurements in water indicated that the two derivatives were greatly unfolded, relative to native lysozyme. However, SM-lysozyme was somewhat more folded than SCM-lysozyme (SM-lysozyme assumed some structural stability in 35% methanol while SCM-lysozyme showed no stabilized structure in 60% methanol). Further evidence for the formation of some native conformation in SM-lysozyme was obtained from immunochemical studies, where SCM-lysozyme showed no reaction with two antilysozyme sera, while SM-lysozyme gave 35% and 38% reaction with these antisera, compared to the native lysozyme. This work indicated that long-range interaction can direct the partial folding of the polypeptide chain which was cleaved at the disulfide bonds, so long as the blocking group is not sterically unfavored because of size or charge.

In the case of α-lactalbumin, one disulfide group (cystine I–VIII) was preferentially reduced with dithioerythritol in aqueous solution at pH 7 and carboxymethylated. There was no effect on the immunochemical reactivity with anti α-lactalbumin (Shechter *et al.*, 1973). Limited conformational changes were detected by susceptibility of the modified α-lactalbumin to tryptic digestion.

IV. Use of Immunochemical Methods as a Conformational Probe

A. Influence of Evolutionary Amino Acid Replacements on Conformation

The utilization of immunochemical methods to monitor sequence differences between homologous proteins from different species is fraught with pitfalls. It ignores a fundamental principle that the immune response is directed against an antigenic determinant in a certain conformation, and that the conformation of the protein is determined by its amino acid sequence. There has been a tendency to consider that homologous proteins having a distinct function or enzymatic activity will maintain this function by preserving the conformation. This is not the case, as great variation occurs in their amino acid sequence and conformation, but what is preserved is their catalytic site. Despite great variation by substitution, deletion, and addition of amino acid residues, the enzymatic function is maintained, e.g., human lysozyme where 53 amino acid residues are different from chicken egg white lysozyme.

Immunochemical reactivity was utilized to test the accuracy of the concept that sequence homology is associated with conformational homology. Such an idea was advanced (Neurath *et al.*, 1967, 1970; Bradshaw *et al.*, 1969) on the basis that several proteins with analogous functions had homologous amino acid sequences, and therefore would be expected to reveal similar three-dimensional features. Examples of these proteins were trypsin and chymotrypsin, which showed 40% sequence homology (Walsh and Neurath, 1964; Hartley, 1964; Hartley *et al.*, 1965), and elastase, trypsin, and chymotrypsin, where the disulfide bonds were homologous (Hartley *et al.*, 1965). The separation of two peptides (46 amino acid residues) from carboxypeptidases A and B, which showed 51% homology (Bradshaw *et al.*, 1969), was considered as an example that the two proteins have conformational homology.

As previously discussed, the native conformation of a protein is dependent on almost all of its amino acid sequence, and a deletion or substitution in only few amino acids will bring about detectable conformational changes. In addition, work on chemical modification of proteins indicates that modification of only few amino acid residues may result in pronounced conformational changes. In both of these cases, the sequence homology can be more than 90%, yet the proteins show no conformational identity and their immunochemical specificity is greatly modified. In this section, evidence will be presented to demonstrate that immunochemical specificity in a series of homologous proteins is not the direct result of sequence homology, but conformational factors play an important part. It is to be emphasized that amino acid replacement or deletion in a series of homologous protein has the potential to induce conformational changes that will affect the immunochemical reactivity.

1. Lysozyme and α-Lactalbumin

Lysozyme and α-lactalbumin appear to have very close primary structures (Brew and Campbell, 1967). The amino acid sequence of bovine α-lactalbumin (Brew et al., 1967) showed a high level of structural homology with lysozyme. Forty residues in α-lactalbumin were identical to corresponding residues in lysozyme, and an additional 27 residues, at corresponding positions, were chemically similar. To obtain maximum homology, six gaps, including two of two residues, were placed in α-lactalbumin sequence and two in lysozyme. It is remarkable that the four disulfide bonds in α-lactalbumin are homologous with the corresponding bonds in lysozyme. Based on this chemical homology, Brew et al. (1967) suggested that the conformation of the two proteins may be similar. Browne et al. (1969) constructed a model for α-lactalbumin based on the main chain conformation of lysozyme, and they concluded that the differences between the two molecules were not incompatible with their having closely similar conformation.

It is relevant to mention the statement by Browne et al. (1969) that "the proposed model for α-lactalbumin seems very likely to be substantially correct, though we must emphasize that the conformations of the two molecules may be different, even in those regions where the primary sequences are very similar (see Perutz et al., 1968)." Despite this cautionary remark, various workers have used the Browne et al. (1969) model as a fact and interpreted their results in its light (Castellino and Hill, 1970; Hill et al., 1974; Kronman et al., 1971). The near-ultraviolet circular dichroism (CD) spectrum for lysozyme and α-lactalbumin (Kronman, 1968) showed marked differences, which were assigned to differences in optical activity associated with side chains. Both ORD (Aune, 1968) and CD properties (Kronman, 1968) suggested similarities in their conformation. However, Kronman (1968) cautioned that the α-lactalbumin backbone conformation may not correspond in all detail to that of lysozyme. It is pertinent that the conformational similarities mentioned by Browne et al. (1968), Brew et al. (1967), Kronman (1968), and Aune (1968) had no direct evidence to support them unequivocally. It was therefore decided to compare the conformation of α-lactalbumin and lysozyme by immunochemical and chemical means (Atassi *et al.*, 1970*a*; Habeeb and Atassi, 1971). There was no cross-reaction between lysozyme and anti-α-lactalbumin or between α-lactalbumin and antilysozyme by quantitative precipitin reaction, using antisera from rabbits and goats. Immunochemical cross-reaction of proteins is a function both of similarity in sequence of the antigenic reactive sites and of their close conformations. The present immunochemical finding could therefore imply either that all the regions of sequence similarity are outside the antigenic sites or that the two proteins possess different conformations. Both factors may contribute simultaneously, and the correct interpretation cannot be based wholly on the immunochemical data alone. Chemical methods are highly sensitive to conformational changes and can detect the changes in the environment of certain side groups of amino acid residues. The chemical reactivities of functional groups are highly dependent upon their steric location within the molecule (Anfinsen, 1961). This was shown early by unmasking of sulfhydryl, disulfides, and other groups by denaturation. A very significant experiment is the reactivity of histidine-119 of ribonuclease with iodoacetic acid, which strictly depends on the native conformation (mentioned before in text). Differences in reaction of functional groups of α-lactalbumin and lysozyme were investigated. Of these, the reactivity of free amino groups with trinitrobenzene sulfonic acid and that of the tyrosine with tetranitromethane showed small differences in accessibility (these results were complicated by the differences in the number of amino groups and tyrosine residues in both proteins). However, the most compelling evidence of conformational differences between lysozyme and α-lactalbumin resulted from the reactivity of the disulfide bonds (which occupy homologous positions) with 0.05 M β-mercaptoethanol, in the absence and presence of various concentrations of guanidine hydrochloride at pH 7 (Atassi *et al.*, 1970*a*). Marked differences in disulfide reducibility were found (Fig. 2); 2.6 disulfide bonds were reduced in neutral solution in α-lactalbumin while almost no bonds were reduced in lysozyme. At a concentration of about 2.5 M guanidine, all four disulfide bonds of α-lactalbumin were reducible in 3 hr whereas only 1.4 bonds were reduced in lysozyme. Even at a guanidine concentration of 5.2 M, about 3.7 disulfide bonds were reduced in lysozyme. The results indicated that the conformations of the two proteins showed remarkable nonidentity. The lysozyme was more stable than α-lactalbumin and showed greater resistance to unfold and unmask the disulfide bonds in guanidine. The binding of sodium dodecylsulfate (SDS) to α-lactalbumin (13 moles SDS/mole protein) and lysozyme (7 or 13 moles SDS/mole protein) resulted in conformational changes which were different in both proteins and were reflected in the availability of the disulfide bonds to reduction (Habeeb and Atassi, 1971). The binding of SDS to α-lactalbumin resulted in a constrained conformation

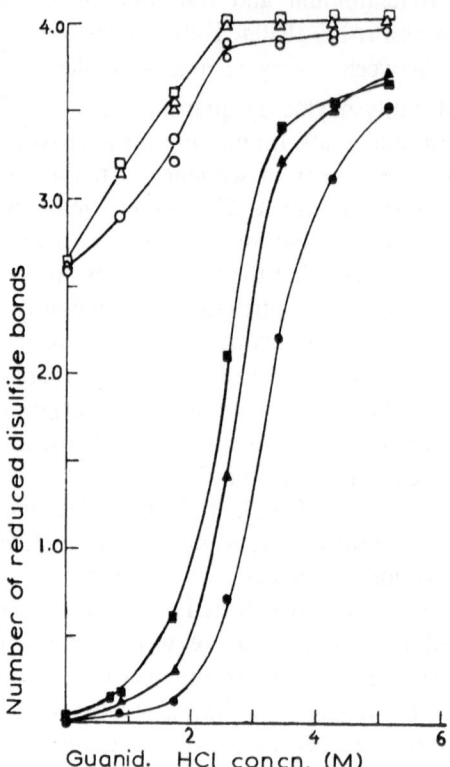

Figure 2. Effect of guanidine concentration on the number of disulfide bonds reduced with β-mercaptoethanol in lysozyme and α-lactalbumin. Open symbols: α-lactalbumin at 1 hr (○), 3 hr (△), and 6 hr (□). Closed symbols: lysozyme after 1 hr (●), 3 hr (▲), and 6 hr (■). From Atassi *et al.* (1970*a*).

accompanied by a decrease in disulfide availability, to β-mercaptoethanol reduction, whereas with lysozyme a relaxed conformation resulted, accompanied by an increase in disulfide reducibility (Fig. 3). The protection of SDS against the denaturing effect of guanidine was demonstrated in α-lactalbumin at concentrations as high as 4 M (Fig. 4). With lysozyme, after the initial expansion of the molecule due to SDS binding (at zero guanidine concentration), the presence of guanidine up to about 1.8 M resulted in the recovery of the constrained conformation. On further increase of guanidine concentration, the protective action of SDS against unfolding was less pronounced than with α-lactalbumin.

The chemical methods (Atassi *et al.*, 1970*a*; Habeeb and Atassi, 1971) demonstrated definite conformational differences between α-lactalbumin and lysozyme which indicated that the lack of immunochemical cross-reactivity was due to conformational dissimilarity between the two proteins.

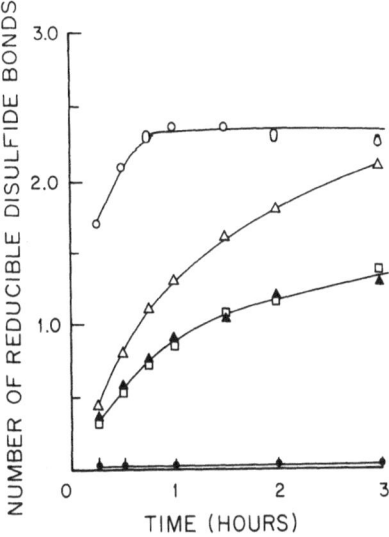

Figure 3. Effect of binding of sodium dodecylsulfate (SDS) to lysozyme and α-lactalbumin on the reducibility of the disulfide bonds. Symbols: ◯, α-lactalbumin in absence of SDS; △, in presence of SDS (13 moles SDS/mole α-lactalbumin); ●, lysozyme in absence of SDS; ▲,◻, in presence of SDS at 7 and at 13 mole SDS/mole lysozyme, respectively. From Habeeb and Atassi (1971).

Later work by other investigators corroborated our results. Krigbaum and Kügler (1970) concluded (from small-angle diffraction measurements) that lysozyme was a prolate ellipsoid, having dimensions 28 Å × 28 Å × 50 Å, while α-lactalbumin was oblate, with dimensions 22 Å × 44 Å × 57 Å. However, Achter and Swan (1971) attributed the differences in small-angle X-ray scattering from lysozyme and α-lactalbumin to the presence of a small percentage of α-lactalbumin dimer. A computed low-energy conformation of α-lactalbumin showed significant differences in shape. Lysozyme appeared a prolate ellipsoid, while α-lactalbumin was an oblate ellipsoid (Warme *et al.*, 1974).

Nearly all the carboxyl groups (20 residues) in α-lactalbumin were available for reaction with glycinimide in the presence of carbodiimide, compared to 8 out of 11 groups in lysozyme (Lin, 1970). Further treatment with 4 M guanidine resulted in additional modification of 0.6 and 2.1 residues in α-lactalbumin (residues 63–79) and lysozyme (Glu-35, Glu-7, and Asp-66), respectively (Lin, 1970). The regions not completely modified with the reagent (in nondenaturing conditions) were close to the disulfide bonds.

The single binding site of 2-*p*-toluidinyl naphthalene 6-sulfonate on α-lactalbumin had a more pronounced hydrophobic property than on lysozyme (Barel *et al.*, 1972). A nuclear magnetic resonance study of the denaturation (Bradbury and King, 1971) indicated that lysozyme was more

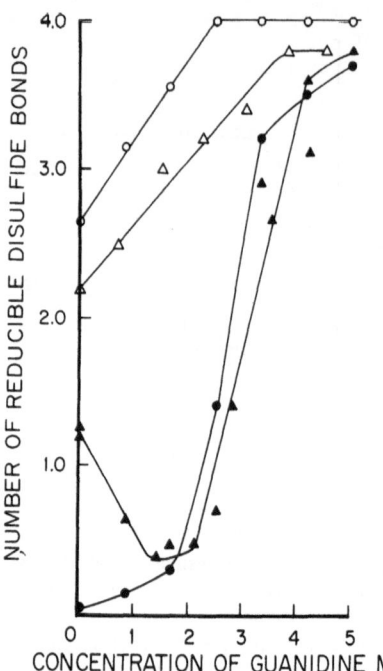

Figure 4. Effect of guanidine concentration on the number of disulfide bonds reduced with β-mercaptoethanol after 3 hr. Symbols: ○, α-lactalbumin in absence of SDS; △, in presence of SDS (13 moles SDS/mole α-lactalbumin); ● lysozyme in absence of SDS; ▲ in presence of SDS (7 moles SDS/mole lysozyme). From Habeeb and Atassi (1971).

stable toward unfolding by urea than was α-lactalbumin (midpoint of the transition of unfolding at pH 2.5–2.8 occurred at 3 M and 4.7 M urea, and at pH 6 it occurred at 3.5–6.5 M and above 8 M urea, respectively). The authors suggested that the abundance of aliphatic–aromatic interactions in lysozyme conferred stability on the molecule, whereas the scarcity of aliphatic aromatic interaction in α-lactalbumin accounted for its relaxed conformation. The rate of reoxidation of reduced α-lactalbumin (reduced in 6 M guanidine at 37°C for 12 hr) at pH 8, in the presence of 0.5 μM copper sulfate, was extremely slow (Tamburro et al., 1972). After 25 hr, complete recovery of native structure was not achieved, as shown from near- and far-ultraviolet CD spectra. In contrast, most of the structure of lysozyme was recovered in 90 min (Isemura et al., 1968). In the case of lysozyme, the second phase which was rate limiting in the reoxidation (Saxena and Wetlaufer, 1970) involved the folding of the polypeptide backbone and side chain that accompanied the disulfide interchange reaction. With α-lactalbumin, the rate for undergoing this localized conformational change was different from lysozyme.

Tryptophan-26, which is completely buried according to the model of Browne *et al.* (1969), was found to be accessible to modification by 2-hydroxyl-5-nitrobenzyl bromide, in addition to tryptophan-104 and -118 (Barman and Bagshaw, 1972) (in lysozyme tryptophan-62 or -63 was modified), and this was considered as evidence of differences in conformation between α-lactalbumin and lysozyme. Reaction with 2-nitrophenylsulfenyl chloride (Shechter *et al.*, 1974) resulted in modification of tryptophan-60 and -118 in α-lactalbumin and tryptophan-62 (which is homologous to 60 in α-lactalbumin) in lysozyme.

A *C*-terminal peptide (33 residues) from α-lactalbumin showed a high helix-forming potential which was not found in the proposed structure of Browne *et al.* (1969); this may suggest differences in folding of the *C*-terminal region of α-lactalbumin and lysozyme (Hermans and Puett, 1971).

2. α-Lactalbumins from Different Species

The amino acid sequence of α-lactalbumin taken from different species shows a high degree of sequence homology (72% of the amino acid residues are identical in comparing human to bovine and 64% are identical in guinea pig and bovine) (Hill *et al.*, 1974).

Some differences do exist in the reactivity of some amino acid residues, e.g., tyrosine and the amino groups in goat and bovine α-lactalbumin (Kronman *et al.*, 1972), and this fact may suggest conformational differences. However, no comparative study on the conformation of α-lactalbumins from different species has been undertaken. An immunochemical study (Tanahashi *et al.*, 1968) showed that α-lactalbumin from nonruminants (pig, guinea pig, and human) did not react with antiserum to bovine α-lactalbumin but that ruminant α-lactalbumins (bovine, buffalo, sheep, and goat) reacted with antibovine α-lactalbumin. These immunochemical differences were attributed to structural differences resulting from varied net charge of the proteins. A recent investigation (Prieels *et al.*, 1975) of the immunochemical cross-reactions of α-lactalbumin from different species (bovine, goat, sheep, and human) by immunoabsorbents (α-lactalbumin conjugated to Sepharose 4B) was reported. Antibodies that gave soluble antigen–antibody complexes were detected on immunoabsorbents. Table III shows the cross-reaction of α-lactalbumin and anti-α-lactalbumin by immunoabsorbents. Cross-reaction was detected between human, goat, bovine, and sheep α-lactalbumin and anti-human, anti-goat, and anti-sheep α-lactalbumin by precipitin formation in Ouchterlony plates. However, precipitin lines did not occur with human α-lactalbumin and anti-bovine α-lactalbumin, yet soluble antigen–antibody complexes formed between anti-bovine α-lactalbumin and human α-lactalbumin, as shown by immuno-absorption. Cross-reactivity did not reflect, in any simple fashion, the known sequence homology of the α-lactalbumins. The greater cross-reactivity

Table III. Immunological Cross-Reaction of α-Lactalbumins and Antisera to α-Lactalbumins, Determined by Use of Immunoabsorption[a]

Antigens	Cross-reaction with antibodies to α-lactalbumin from			
	Human(%)	Cow (%)	Goat (%)	Sheep (%)
Human α-lactalbumin	100	76	91	98
Bovine α-lactalbumin	68	100	68	87
Goat α-lactalbumin	79	82.5	100	96
Sheep α-lactalbumin	64	84	51	100

[a] From Prieels et al. (1975).

of human α-lactalbumin and goat α-lactalbumin than of human α-lactalbumin and bovine α-lactalbumin did not reflect sequence homology of these proteins. Such differences were attributed to conformational factors which may reduce or prevent the binding of antibody and antigen. It was surprising to find that human α-lactalbumin showed the highest immunochemical cross-reactivity with heterologous antisera, while sheep α-lactalbumin showed the lowest reaction.

3. Lysozyme from Different Species

The immunochemical cross-reactivity between lysozymes from egg white of several species of birds was examined by microcomplement fixation and quantitative precipitin (Arnheim and Wilson, 1967; Arnheim et al., 1969; Prager and Wilson, 1971a,b). Based on the amino acid analysis and peptide maps of chicken, quail, and pheasant lysozymes (chicken and quail lysozymes were similar, while the pheasant lysozyme showed seven interchanges), Arnheim et al. (1969) interpreted the differences in immunochemical cross-reaction on purely sequence homology. A correlation was observed by Prager and Wilson (1971a,b) between the immunochemical cross-reaction and sequence homology among the lysozymes from the eggs of seven different birds when sequence differences did not exceed 30–40%. Their antisera and the derivation of the immunological distance and index of dissimilarity were biased in favor of high cross-reactivity (Prager and Wilson, 1971a,b). The antisera were obtained after a long period of immunization, where the index of dissimilarity was low, and they averaged the results of reciprocal cross-reactivity. Late sera have been shown to demonstrate more immunochemical cross-reactivity than early sera, with both amidinated, guanidinated bovine serum albumin and native bovine serum albumin (Habeeb, 1968). Values of reciprocal cross-reactivity do not correspond, since the immunizing antigen in every case has its characteristic features (Habeeb, 1967b, 1968; Atassi and Saplin, 1971; Prieels et al., 1975). A demonstration of this point was shown by Atassi and Saplin (1971). The cross-reaction of finback whale myoglobin (FMb) with anti-sperm whale myoglobin (SMb) ranged from 34 to 41%, compared to the homologous system, while the reaction of SMb with anti-FMb was higher, 55–58%. Several peptides (Table IV) which showed cross-reaction with anti-SMb failed to react with anti-FMb, e.g., peptides S 1–55 and S 132–153. The central peptide S 56–113 reacted to a similar degree with both anti-SMb and anti-FMb, while the corresponding peptide F 55–129 from finback whale myoglobin reacted weakly with anti-SMb. It is significant that the cross-reaction of SMb with antisera to FMb was due to fragment S 56–131. Conversely, the cross-reaction of FMb with antisera to SMb resulted from peptide F 55–129, and another contribution was effected by a region within sequence 137–149 of FMb. Therefore, in considering reciprocal cross-reaction, it is important to consider that, whereas a given segment of a protein may elicit antibody formation, its corresponding structural counterpart may not even participate.

Prager and Wilson (1971a,b) reasoned that amino acid replacement occurred on the surface of the lysozyme molecule during evolution of the birds and that the conformation was strongly conserved during evolution. This line of reasoning is untenable, since homologous proteins do exist which show low conformational similarities and sequence homology (e.g., lysozymes), yet maintain their enzymatic activity. Amino acid replacements do occur in external, surface, and internal locations in the polypeptide chain, and one would expect that these may influence the conformation,

Table IV. Cross-Reactivity and Reciprocal Cross-Reactivity of
Fragments from Finback Whale Myoglobin and Sperm Whale
Myoglobin[a]

Peptide	Anti-sperm whale myoglobin			Anti-finback whale myoglobin	
	G1 (%)	G4 (%)	77 (%)	F6 (%)	F8 (%)
S 1–55[b]	27.6	8.2	25.6	0	0
S 56–131	62.6	80.5	49.0	60.4	55.8
S 132–153	21	13.3	21	0	0
F 1–54[c]	4.7	6.3	5.3	14.1	7.7
F 55–129	19.1	13.9	16.8	61.3	75
F 130–151	0	0	0	8.2	12.3

[a] From Atassi and Saplin (1971).
[b] S denotes peptides obtained from sperm whale myoglobin.
[c] F denotes peptides obtained from finback whale myoglobin.

and concomitantly the immunochemical specificity. Indeed, later work showed that conformational differences were responsible for the immuno- chemical differences in closely related lysozymes (Prager et al., 1974). Lysozyme from the egg whites of chicken and bobwhite quail differed at position 68 in the loop region (sequence 60–83) and also at positions 40, 55, and 91, the latter residues being fully buried in the lysozyme molecule. Chicken lysozyme has Thr-40, Ile-55, Arg-68, and Ser-91, and bobwhite quail lysozyme has Ser-40, Val-55, Lys-68, and Thr-91. When rabbit anti- chicken lysozyme was depleted of anti-loop antibodies (by absorption with insolubilized loop fragment), the absorbed antiserum was capable of distinguishing bobwhite lysozyme (and other bird lysozymes) as clearly as the unabsorbed serum. These results indicated that the ability of rabbit antiserum to distinguish differences between chicken and bobwhite lyso- zymes did not reside in the loop region, but was caused by the other amino acid replacements. It was remarkable that these replacements occurred in a region fully buried in the interior of the molecule and with amino acid residues that were conserved. Therefore, the differences in immunochemical reactivity were the result of conformational changes caused by the amino acid substitution, despite the fact that they were buried inside the molecule. It is most likely that the immunochemical cross-reactivity between lysozymes from different birds reported before will be greatly influenced by their conformation and will not be a result of sequence similarity.

Lysozymes from chicken, bobwhite quail, and turkey show a replace- ment of arginine by lysine (in the loop region 60–83) at position 68 in bob- white quail lysozyme and at position 73 in turkey lysozyme. Goat anti-loop antiserum (Fainaru et al., 1974) was able to reveal immunochemical dif- ferences between chicken and bobwhite quail lysozymes, indicating a low degree of immunochemical similarity in loop segment of hen and quail lysozyme. Whereas turkey lysozyme was immunochemically distinct from chicken lysozyme, its loop region was immunochemically similar to chicken lysozyme loop region. These results indicated that the replacement of arginine-68 by lysine-68 (in quail) was accompanied by considerable con- formational changes (while 33.5 ng of chicken lysozyme was required for inhibition of inactivation of loop–bacteriophage conjugate, more than 640 ng of quail lysozyme was needed). It is significant that in the loop region of turkey lysozyme, where arginine-73 is replaced by lysine, no change in the immunochemical reactivity was observed. The importance of the amino acid replacement on conformation and immunochemical reactivity is stressed in this work. Arginine-73 can be replaced by lysine (in turkey), without affecting the conformation and immunochemical specificity of the loop region. On the other hand, arginine-68 plays an important role in maintaining the native conformation and is indispensable. Its replacement by lysine results in conformational alteration. It may be relevant to indicate that goat antiserum (in contrast to rabbit antiserum) was capable of demonstrating the immunochemical differences between the loop region in quail and chicken lysozyme.

Sequence differences affect the immunochemical specificity, not in a simple, predictable way, but largely dependent on the number, nature, and location of the replaced residues. It is a complex effect and will depend on the interrelationship of various factors, e.g., the conformational reorganization as a result of the amino acid replacement with concomitant exposure and burying of groups.

4. Myoglobins

Myoglobins from sperm whale, horse, camel, beef, lamb, and goat showed nearly identical Stokes radii and sedimentation coefficients, indicating similar overall shape (Atassi, 1970). In contrast, human and monkey myoglobins had increased Stokes radii and decreased sedimentation coefficients, indicating increased asymmetry or less folded structure. Optical rotatory dispersion measurements indicated a helical structure lower in human and monkey myoglobins than in the other six myoglobins. These results showed that conformational differences existed as a result of amino acid replacement in a homologous group of proteins. The immunochemical cross-reactions of various myoglobins with anti-human myoglobin, anti-horse myoglobin, anti-goat myoglobin, and anti-beef myoglobin were extensively studied (Tables VA–VD) (Atassi et al., 1970b). An un-

Table VA. Structural and Immunochemical Similarity of Various Myoglobins to Human Mb[a]

Myoglobin	Total number of peptides	Peptides similar to human Mb peptides	% Cross-reaction relative to reaction with human Mb[b]	
			G7(%)	G8(%)
Human	29	29–30	100	100
Monkey	27	24	77.4	82.6
Camel	22	12[c]	75.2	76.4
Horse	22	12[c]	24.9	32.1
Beef	23	14	3.1	4.2
Lamb	23	13	3.4	3.2
Goat	23–24	13	2.9	0
Sperm whale	23	8–9	0	0

[a] From Atassi et al. (1970b).
[b] Results are expressed as percent precipitation by each component, at equivalence, relative to the homologous reaction. Values represent the average of three precipitin analyses each and ranged 1.4% or less.
[c] These two sets of peptides appear to be identical.

Table VB. Structural and Immunochemical Similarities to Horse Mb of Various Myoglobins[a]

Myoglobin	Total number of peptides	Peptides similar to horse Mb	% Cross-reaction relative to reaction with horse Mb[b]	
			G11 (%)	G12 (%)
Horse	22	22	100	100
Camel	22	20	36.8	39.7
Human	29	12[c]	32.8	29.9
Monkey	27	12[c]	32.6	29.2
Goat	23–24	11	6.8	5.1
Beef	23	9	6.1	7.0
Lamb	23	11	4.0	3.9
Sperm whale	23	9	0	0

[a] From Atassi et al. (1970b).
[b] Results are expressed as percent precipitation by each component, at equivalence, relative to the homologous reaction. Values represent the average of three precipitin analyses each and ranged 1.4% or less.
[c] These two sets of peptides appear to be identical.

Table VC. Structural and Immunochemical Similarities to Goat Mb of Various Myoglobins[a]

Myoglobin	Total number of peptides	Peptides similar to goat peptides	% Cross-reaction relative to reaction with goat Mb[b]	
			Serum AG$_1$ (%)	Serum AG$_2$ (%)
Goat	23–24	23	100	100
Lamb	23	21–22	89.6	91.0
Beef	23	18	89.6	90.3
Human	29	13	0	0
Monkey	27	13	0	0
Horse	22	11[c]	4.8	4.1
Camel	22	11[c]	3.9	3.2
Sperm whale	23	8	0	0

[a] From Atassi et al. (1970b).
[b] Results are expressed as percent precipitation by each component, at equivalence, relative to the homologous reaction. Values represent the average of three precipitin analyses each and ranged 1.4% or less.
[c] These two sets of peptides appear to be identical.

Table VD. Structural and Immunochemical Similarities
to Beef Mb of Various Myoglobins[a]

Myoglobin	Total number of peptides	Peptides similar to beef Mb peptides	% Cross-reaction relative to reaction of beef Mb[b]	
			Serum B_1 (%)	Serum B_2 (%)
Beef	23	23	100	100
Lamb	23	18[c]	87.1	89.9
Goat	23–24	18[c]	75.8	72.2
Human	29	14	<3	0
Monkey	27	14	3.6	0
Horse	22	9	0	0
Camel	22	9	0	0
Sperm whale	23	8	0	0

[a] From Atassi et al. (1970b).
[b] Results are expressed as percent precipitation by each component, at equivalence, relative to the homologous reaction. Values represent the average of three precipitin analyses each and ranged 1.4% or less.
[c] These two sets of peptides appear to be identical.

expected behavior was shown by camel and horse myoglobins. Both were structurally similar (12 out of 22 identical peptides), yet the camel myoglobin gave about 75% cross-reaction with anti-human myoglobin, while a 25–32% reaction was obtained with horse myoglobin. Myoglobin of beef, lamb, goat, and sperm whale reacted very poorly, if at all, with anti-human myoglobin. With anti-horse myoglobin, very poor reaction was obtained with goat, beef, lamb, or sperm whale myoglobin. On the other hand, camel myoglobin gave 37–40% cross-reaction with anti-horse myoglobin and the reactivities of human and monkey myoglobin were similar, 30–33%. Whereas 12 peptides were similar in human and monkey myoglobins, out of the 22 peptides in horse myoglobin, camel myoglobin showed 20 peptides identical to the 22. With anti-goat myoglobin, lamb and beef myoglobins showed identical cross-reactivities, although beef myoglobin had 18 similar peptides and lamb myoglobin 21–22 similar peptides out of 23 in goat myoglobins. Also with anti-beef myoglobin, lamb myoglobin showed a higher cross-reaction than goat myoglobin, despite a similar number of peptides (18 out of 23 in beef). The behavior of myoglobins from the camel, horse, beef, lamb, and goat indicated that immunochemical cross-reactivity was not directly the result of sequence homology, but that conformational changes secondary to evolutionary amino acid replacement played an important role. Further support of the conformational differences of myoglobins shown by Atassi (1970) was demonstrated by another investigation (Puett, 1973). The unfolding free energy of ferrimyoglobins from horse, bovine, seal, sperm whale, human, porpoise, and turtle demonstrated (Puett, 1973; Puett *et al.*, 1973) that the conformational stability differences among the various myoglobins were not correlated to the location, structural role, and chemical nature of substituted amino acids. Differences in total number of protein intramolecular and solvent interactions in the various myoglobins were likely to occur and resulted in minor conformational changes in restricted areas of the protein.

5. Cytochrome c

The immunochemical cross-reaction of three precipitating anti-cytochrome *c* sera (anti-human, anti-*Macaca mulatta*, and anti-horse cytochromes *c*) raised in rabbits with cytochrome *c* (mol. wt. 12,400) from 25 different eukaryotic species was investigated (Margoliash *et al.*, 1970) by quantitative complement fixation and by competition of unlabeled heterologous antigen with ^{125}I-labeled homologous antigen for its combination with antibody. A summary of the results is given in Table VI. The two rabbit anti-cytochrome *c* sera showed variation in their ability to distinguish the different cytochromes. Cytochromes *c* (from different species) with identical amino acid sequences had identical immunochemical cross-reactivities: e.g., (1) cow, sheep, and pig, (2) chicken and turkey, and (3) chimpanzee and human. Margoliash *et al.* (1970) reported a rough correlation between the immunochemical reactivity and amino acid sequence which was apparent when only few amino acid residues were involved. In a situation like this, the immunochemical cross-reactivity will be influenced by the conformation of the protein as well as the amino acid residues at the antigenic determinants. Unless a thorough evaluation of the conformational parameters of the cytochrome *c* is presented, it is difficult to attribute what variation in the immunochemical cross-reactivity was due to sequence dissimilarity and what was due to conformational changes. It should be emphasized that not every amino acid replacement is associated with a conformational change. The work on the effect of chemical modification of a particular amino acid side chain provides examples where the number of amino acids modified may or may not correlate with conformational changes and immunochemical cross-reactivity.

With anti-human cytochrome *c*, *M. mulatta* cytochrome *c* which differed in one residue (Thr-58, in human Ile-58) showed a decreased reaction (45–70%). Kangaroo cytochrome *c* showed 30–33% reaction, which was higher than the reaction with other nonprimates (elephant, dog, hippopotamus, and guanaco all gave 20% reaction). The high reactivity of kangaroo cytochrome was attributed to the presence of Ile-58, which was shared by the human cytochrome *c* (Nisonoff *et al.*, 1970). The extent of reaction of other cytochromes with anti-*M. mulatta* was similar to that of anti-human

Table VI. Immunochemical Cross-Reaction of Various Cytochromes c with Anti-Cytochromes c: Percentage of Homologous Reaction at Maximum[a]

	Anti-horse cytochrome c (%)	Anti-human cytochrome c (%)	Anti-$M.$ $mulatta$ cytochrome c (%)	Number of variant residues compared to horse cytochrome c (%)
Horse	100, 100[b]	10, 8	12	0
Donkey	100, 100	11, 12	N.R.[c]	1
Cow	60, 84	12, 17	16	3
Sheep	60, 87	12, 18	N.R.	3
Pig	60, 83	12, 18	16	3
Okapi	60, 84	N.R.	N.R.	N.R.
Impala	60, 88	N.R.	N.R.	N.R.
Finback whale	45, 44	N.R.	N.R.	5
Guanaco	39, 27	20, 11	16	N.R.
Rabbit	35, 22	13, 24	22	6
Kangaroo	38, 28	33, 30	20	7
Hippopotamus	26, 32	20, 18	25	N.R.
Dog	25, 12	20	N.R.	N.R.
Chicken	19, 10	4, 10	N.R.	11
Turkey	19, 10	4, 10	13	11
$M.$ $mulatta$	25, 0	70, 45	100	11
Chimpanzee	16, 0	100, 100	N.R.	12
Human	16, 0	100, 100	100	12
Tuna	27, 0	4, 5	8	17

[a] From Margoliash et al. (1970).
[b] The values were obtained from antisera from two different rabbits.
[c] Not reported.

cytochrome, except for the kangaroo cytochrome c. Nonprecipitating antibodies to cytochrome c (tuna, turkey, kangaroo, monkey, horse, and rabbit) were found to give precipitin reaction and to fix complement with the homologous glutaraldehyde-polymerized cytochrome c (Reichlin et al., 1970); the reaction was inhibited by the monomeric cytochrome. The effect of the heterogeneity of the immunizing antigen (a population of intermolecularly cross-linked polymerized cytochrome and intramolecularly cross-linked monomers) on the specificity of the antibodies produced was not examined by Reichlin et al. (1970). They reported that polymerized cytochromes (horse, human, tuna, $M.$ $mulatta$, and kangaroo) were good immunogens, and the antisera produced did not contain antibodies specific against the polymer. Moreover, homologous monomers inhibited more than 95% of the precipitin and complement fixation reaction of polymers, regardless of whether the antisera were raised against monomer or polymer. These results should be considered as characteristic of this system only and cannot be interpreted to mean that antibodies against glutaraldehyde-polymerized proteins will be devoid of antibodies to the polymer. Indeed, there was indication that antibodies against polymerized turkey cytochrome *c* showed two specificities, one against the monomer and the second against the polymer.

It is relevant to point out that glutaraldehyde is very reactive with lysine and cysteine residues in proteins and shows partial reactivity with histidine and tyrosine (Habeeb and Hiramoto, 1968). Whereas glutaraldehyde-modified ovalbumin and bovine serum albumin reacted completely with the respective antisera, with a shift of the equivalence point to a higher concentration these modified proteins exhibited distinct specificities when used as antigens in rabbits (Habeeb, 1969). Anti-glutaraldehyde-modified bovine serum albumin (GL-BSA) showed 47% specificity against BSA in early bleeding and increased to 67% in late bleeding, and the remainder was directed against new antigenic determinants created by polymerization. Moreover, it was possible to conjugate ovalbumin and BSA to form soluble polymers that were antigenic in rabbits (Habeeb, 1969). Antibodies to these polymers showed a specificity toward BSA, ovalbumin, polymerized BSA, and polymerized ovalbumin (Fig. 5).

Some workers observed some loss in the ability of tissues to react with their antibodies, after treatment with glutaraldehyde. Treatment of mouse

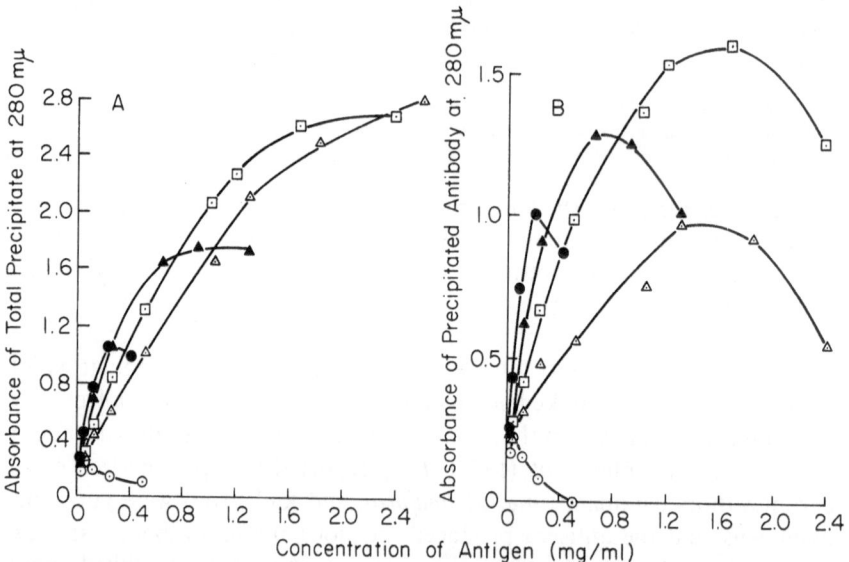

Figure 5. Quantitative precipitation of various antigens with anti-ovalbumin–bovine serum albumin conjugate (OA-BSA). Symbols: O, bovine serum albumin (BSA); △, glutaraldehyde-treated BSA; ●, ovalbumin (OA); ▲, glutaraldehyde-treated OA; □, OA-BSA conjugate. A shows absorbance of total precipitate, B shows absorbance of the precipitated antibody. From Habeeb (1969).

liver with 10% formaldehyde or 1% glutaraldehyde resulted in loss of its ability to react with anti-nuclear antibody. However, the inactivation was restored by incubation in 30% sucrose, and it was a result of the reversal of conformational changes induced by reaction with the aldehyde (Deng and Beutner, 1974). Treatment of feline lymphoid leukemia cells with formaldehyde (0.001%) or glutaraldehyde (0.0005%) resulted in a loss of 40% and 50% to bind with the antibody (Davis et al., 1974). This behavior resulted from certain distortion of the conformation due to introduction of intramolecular cross bonds (Davis et al., 1974).

6. Hemoglobins

The inability to obtain inhibitory peptides in the hemoglobin–anti-hemoglobin system has directed attention to the use of single amino acid mutants of hemoglobin to study the antigenic determinants (Reichlin et al., 1964, 1966). Several single and double amino acid mutants were investigated for their immunochemical cross-reactivity by quantitative complement fixation, using antisera against human hemoglobin A, as well as anti-α- and anti-β-chains (Reichlin, 1972). This approach was based on (1) the view that the amino acid substitution affects the antigenic determinant locally and has no effect on the conformation of the protein (which affects distal parts of the molecule, (2) the fact that mutants do not affect the interaction between the individual chains, and (3) the fact that β-mutant showed decreased reactivity with anti-A_1-serum and anti-β-serum but not with anti-α-serum, and the reverse was true for anti-α-chain mutant. In one case, with hemoglobin Riverdale (β mutant, Gly–Arg-24), a decreased reactivity was observed with both anti-α- and anti-β-chain sera, which may demonstrate a conformational change in the hemoglobin Riverdale. Seven of the 18 single amino acid mutants of human hemoglobin were immunochemically different from hemoglobin A_1 (Reichlin, 1972).

Local conformational differences need to be considered since they may influence the immunochemical cross-reactivity. Although the conformations of hemoglobin chains and myoglobin are similar over most of the length, some of the helical segments are more regular, and parts of the nonhelical segments have different conformations (Perutz et al., 1968).

7. Other Homologous Proteins

Immunochemical cross-reaction demonstrated the homology between papain and chymopapain in regions near their active sites. Antibodies to papain contained a population (32%) which was common to chymopapain (Arnon and Shapira, 1967), and antibodies to chymopapain contained a population (10%) which was common to papain (Arnon and Shapira,

1968). Both populations (despite their production by different antigens) showed complete identity in their immunochemical reaction and also in their inhibitory activity with papain and chymopapain. In addition to the common antibodies, additional antibodies were found which showed distinct specificity for one enzyme.

α-Amylases from various microorganisms exhibited differences in their cross-reaction with anti-α-amylase of *B. subtilis* (Sirisinha and Allen, 1965). *B. stearothermophilus* α-amylase precipitated only 18% of anti-*B. subtilis* α-amylase. Moreover, anti-*B. subtilis* α-amylase was able to inhibit 96% of the α-amylase activity of *B. stearothermophilus*. Despite the marked differences in both physical and chemical properties of α-amylase from both *B. subtilis* and *B. stearothermophilus* (Campbell and Cleveland, 1961; Campbell and Manning, 1961; Manning and Campbell, 1961), the immunochemical studies indicated that the regions at the active site were identical. A failure of reciprocal cross-reaction between *B. subtilis* α-amylase and anti-*B. stearothermophilus* α-amylase was observed. No immunochemical cross-reaction was observed among α-amylases from *Asperigillus oryzae, B, subtilis, B. polymyxa, B. macerans, Pseudomonas saccharophilia,* and *Euglena sangunis* (Sirisinha and Allen, 1965). With some bacterial enzymes, immunochemical cross-reaction did not follow strict taxonomic classification (Pollock, 1963); this may be due to conformational as well as sequence differences.

Carbonic anhydrase from human erythrocytes was compared immunochemically by quantitative complement fixation with the enzyme from other primates (Nonno *et al.*, 1970). The degree of serological activity agreed with the accepted primate taxa.

The immunochemical cross-reactivity of various thiol proteases was used as a tool to detect conformational as well as chemical homology among papain, ficin, stem bromelain, and fruit bromelain (Kato and Sasaki, 1974; Sasaki *et al.*, 1973). In some of the heterologous systems (where cross-reaction was below 10%), no precipitation occurred between the antigen and the antibody, but cross-reaction was demonstrated by use of enzyme immunoabsorbents. By preparing insoluble immunoabsorbents of papain, ficin, stem bromelain, and fruit bromelain. Kato and Sasaki (1974) were able to fractionate the antibody against one enzyme into different populations which had distinct reactivity and inhibited the enzymatic activity of the homologous or heterologous system. Anti-papain antibody was obtained by fractionating the IgG fraction of anti-papain antiserum on papain immunoabsorbent and eluting with 0.17 M glycine pH 2.3. Pure anti-papain antibody was applied on ficin immunoabsorbent and two populations of antibodies were obtained; 18% was absorbed and was cross-reacting with ficin [cFi(P)] and the nonabsorbed was non-cross-reacting with ficin (nFi(P)]. By subjecting anti-ficin to ficin immunoabsorbent followed by papain immunoabsorbent, two antibody populations were obtained; one (26%) was cross-reacting with papain [cP(Fi)] and the other non-cross-reacting with papain (nP(Fi)]. Non-cross-reacting antibodies [nFi(P)] and [nP(Fi)] did not inhibit the enzymatic activity of the heterologous enzymes, but they were capable of inhibiting the homologous enzymes to some extent. On the other hand, the cross-reacting antibodies [cFi(P)] and [cP(Fi)] were capable of inhibiting both the homologous and heterologous systems. Kato and Sasaki (1974) also were able to show, by immunochemical method, a common antigenic determinant to all four enzymes. When anti-stem bromelain antibody was passed over fruit bromelain immunoabsorbent, 18–23% cross-reacted and was designated [cF(S)]. When the cross-reacting antibody was applied to papain immunoabsorbent, 16% cross-reacted and was designated [cFcP(S)], and 84% did not cross-react (cFnP(S)]. The cross-reacting [cFcP(S)] was further applied to ficin immunoabsorbent. Twenty percent was absorbed and gave an antibody common to all four thiol proteases (cFcPcFi(S)], and 80% was unabsorbed, giving an antibody population with partial specificity (cFcPnFi(S)]. The ability to isolate an antibody population which was able to inhibit the enzymatic activity of all four proteases (papain, ficin, stem bromelain, and fruit bromelain) demonstrates the conservation of the conformational homology (among the four phylogenetically different proteases) at the active site and its vicinity, leading to preservation of the enzymatic function during the evolutionary process of these enzymes.

B. Conformational Equilibrium in Protein Fragments

An immunological approach to study of the conformational equilibrium of a protein molecule, or a fragment, has been suggested (Sachs et al., 1972; Furie et al., 1974, 1975; Anfinsen and Scheraga, 1975). It assumes that a polypeptide fragment exists in solution in a conformational equilibrium between disordered conformations and a native conformation. By using antibodies against either the native conformation (N) or random conformation (R), the conformational equilibrium of the system was calculated. Fragment 99–149 of nuclease which existed in disordered conformation was used as a model. Antibodies against the native conformation were prepared by passing antinuclease antiserum through an immunoabsorbent column of nuclease–Sepharose followed after elution by a passage on fragment 99–126 immunoabsorbent. The fraction of antibodies that was bound and then eluted from the latter immunoabsorbent was considered to be directed against the native conformation. The purified anti $(99–126)_N$, was used to determine the conformational equilibrium of fragment $(99–149)_R$.

The extent of binding of anti-$(99-126)_N$ with fragment $(99-149)_R$, due to native conformation in sequences 99–149, was determined from the ability of the remaining antibody to inactivate nuclease. A value of 0.02% was obtained for the fraction of fragment 99–149 that existed in the native conformation. By using anti-$(99-126)_R$ antibodies (Furie et al., 1975), the conformational constant for nuclease was found to be 2900 ± 1400.

While the principle is sound, the specificity of the antibodies and the results are in doubt. Anti-$(99-126)_N$ was obtained by subjecting pure anti-nuclease antibody to two immunoabsorbents bearing coupled fragment 99–149 and fragment 99–126. In solution, the fragments are disordered. If the conformation of a protein on an immunoabsorbent resembles the one it has in solution (as is commonly believed), then these fragments will also be disordered on the immunoabsorbent. Therefore, anti-$(99-126)_N$ will represent only a population of antibodies capable of cross-reacting with both native nuclease and fragment 99–126 which is in a disordered conformation. It cannot represent an antibody population against a native conformation in the true sense. The immunochemical behavior of nuclease is somewhat unusual since a highly disorganized derivative (performic acid treated nuclease) precipitated as much antibody as nuclease (Omenn et al., 1970). Similarly, anti-$(99-126)_R$ was prepared by immunization using nuclease fragment 99–149 and fractionation on Sepharose–nuclease followed by Sepharose–fragment 99–126. They cannot truly be considered as antibodies against a random conformation, but as antibodies that cross-react with both native and disordered conformation.

In order to obtain antibodies directed against conformational determinants to study the conformational equilibrium with peptides, we are using the myoglobin system (Habeeb and Atassi, unpublished results). Myoglobin contains five antigenic reactive regions comprised of sequences 16–21, 56–62, 94–99, 113–119, and 146–151 (Atassi, 1975). In selected myoglobin derivatives in which the chemical modification caused no conformational change, each of the reactive regions had been made immunochemically inert in one or more derivatives. Therefore, by using immunoabsorbents of specifically modified myoglobin derivatives, each with a single region being made unreactive, antibodies directed against the unreactive region will be unbound and will elute from the immunoabsorbent unchanged. These antibodies are being used in combination with peptides of various lengths obtained by specific chemical cleavage at certain peptide bonds to study the conformational equilibrium of these fragments. This approach is best suited for proteins whose antigenic sites have been accurately delineated.

V. Influence of Conformational Changes on Immunochemical Behavior

The immunochemical specificity of globular proteins is strongly influenced by changes in the native conformation. Therefore, when immunochemical methods are used as a tool of investigation it becomes essential to determine the magnitude of the conformational changes and their effect on the interpretation of the results. Studies with reduced and alkylated proteins or performic acid oxidized proteins do not offer a precise and discriminating approach for studying the relationship between conformation and immunochemical specificity. If the disulfide bond is either a part of or is essential for constituting the antigenic determinant, then the decrease or loss of the immunochemical reactivity of the protein on breaking the disulfide bond is due to direct effect on the antigenic site, rather than due to conformational factors. Performic acid oxidation, in addition to splitting the disulfide bonds, affects methionine, tryptophan, tyrosine, serine, and threonine residues (Hirs, 1967), and therefore the changes of immunochemical reactivity may be due to modification of these amino acids.

In order to systematically investigate the contribution of conformation to the immunochemical reactivity of proteins, two approaches were taken: (1) the study of conformational changes induced by modification of the nonimmunogenic prosthetic group of hemoproteins and (2) the induction of conformational changes in a protein by modification of amino acid residues that are not part of the antigenic determinant.

A. Conformational Changes Induced by Modification of Nonimmunogenic Prosthetic Groups

In hemoglobin and myoglobin, the heme group contributes greatly to the native conformation. Removal of heme group from sperm whale myoglobin resulted in slight swelling and increased asymmetry of the molecule as shown by a decrease in sedimentation and diffusion coefficients and an increase in the intrinsic viscosity (Crumpton and Polson, 1965). There was also about 15–20% loss of helical folding (Breslow, et al., 1965; Harrison and Blout, 1965).

Antibodies to porcine hemoglobin and to horse muscle myoglobin react less with the corresponding globin (Reichlin et al., 1963). However, on addition of hematin to the globin solution, there was a gradual increase in the reactivity, reaching a maximum which corresponded to the reformation and restoration of the native conformation of the heme proteins. The immunochemical method was capable of detecting the transfer of the heme moiety from rabbit hemoglobin to the globin moieties of porcine hemoglobin and horse muscle myoglobin. The heme group was not part of an antigenic reactive site, since 30,000 and 100,000 M excess was not capable of inhibiting the immunochemical reaction of hemoglobin–anti-hemoglobin and myoglobin–antimyoglobin systems, respectively, but it provides the necessary conformation for the immunochemical reactivity of myoglobin (Reichlin et al., 1963) and hemoglobin (Atassi et al., 1965).

Crumpton (1966) reported that two types of antibodies were produced against sperm whale metmyoglobin and horse metmyoglobin; the first type precipitated more antibodies with metmyoglobin than with apomyo-globin, while the second type showed no such difference. Re-formation of metmyoglobin (by addition of hematin to apomyoglobin–antimetmyo-globin precipitate) was incomplete with antibodies of the first type and complete with those of the second type. The immunochemical reaction between antiapomyoglobin or its Fab fragments and metmyoglobin resulted in liberation of free hemin, and was attributed to conformational changes in metmyoglobin caused by reaction with the antibody (Crumpton, 1966).

Atassi (1967) prepared several artificial myoglobins by complexing whole apomyoglobin with different metalloporphyrins (manganese, iron, cobalt, nickel, copper, zinc, ferriheme dipyrid-4-yl propylester, and proto-porphyrin IX). Very little complex formation was obtained with nickel, cobalt, manganese metalloporphyrin, and apomyoglobin. With the excep-tion of copper myoglobin, which was immunochemically indistinguishable from native ferrimyoglobin, all other artificial myoglobins were less immuno-chemically reactive to varying extents. The immunochemical differences in reactivity were attributed to conformational reorganization induced by the different coordination tendencies of the various metals, or by modifi-cation of the side chains of the heme. The conformation of these derivatives [in addition to a derivative prepared by combination of apomyoglobin with ferriheme previously nitrated at the vinyl group (N-heme-Mb)] was studied by optical rotatory dispersion and circular dichroism. In addition, their relative stabilities were evaluated from changes in optical rotatory behavior with increasing pH (Andres and Atassi, 1970). Results showed that the conformations of copper–myoglobin and the reconstituted myoglobin were identical with that of native myoglobin, whereas N-heme-Mb showed a small conformational change and zinc myoglobin showed an appreciable degree of unfolding. The structural stabilities showed the zinc derivative to be the least stable. Since the heme group was not part of an antigenic site, the change in immunochemical reactivity was due to the conformational alteration introduced by the modified prosthetic groups. Some artificial hemoglobins were similarly prepared by complexing globin with zinc metalloporphyrin, protoporphyrin IX, and ferriheme dipyrid-4-yl propyles-ter (Atassi and Skalski, 1969) to yield Zn-Hb, proto-Hb, and PP-Hb, respectively. While a decrease in the Stokes radius (22.45 Å) occurred with PP-Hb, indicating a more compact molecule, an increase was observed for Zn-Hb (34.4 Å) and proto-Hb (51 Å) which was large compared to native hemoglobin (25.5 Å). These conformational changes were accompanied by a decrease in the immunochemical reactivity in the case of Zn-Hb and a surprisingly increased reactivity with proto-Hb and PP-Hb; the latter was attributed to the presence of nonprecipitating antibodies which did not precipitate with hemoglobin but precipitated with proto-Hb and PP-Hb (Atassi and Skalski, 1969).

B. Conformational Changes Induced by Controlled Modification of Amino Acid Residues

Several derivatives of bovine serum albumin were prepared by succinylation (Habeeb, 1967a), guanidination, amidination, and nitroguanidination (Habeeb, 1967b) and by paired modification by succinylation, followed by guanidination or nitroguanidination (Habeeb, 1967b), or by succinylation, followed by amidination (Habeeb, 1968). The conformational changes were assessed (1) by determination of the Stokes radius (Habeeb, 1966c), which provides a workable dimension for comparison of the overall shape of the molecule, and also (2) by the availability of the disulfide bonds for reaction with β-mercaptoethanol or sodium sulfite as a parameter for the changes in conformation which affect the vicinity of the disulfide bonds (Habeeb, 1966b). Upon succinylation of bovine serum albumin, a progressive increase in Stokes radius of the protein, with increased modification, was observed. The initial increase in Stokes radius was slow, up to 34 amino groups succinylated (0.322 nm per ten amino groups succinylated); then it was followed by a steeper increase (1.44 nm per ten amino groups modified) on further modification (Fig. 6). The availability of the disulfide bonds to sulfitolysis remained unchanged, up to succinylation of about 30 amino groups; then it was followed by a pronounced increase in reacting disulfides with further succinylation (Fig. 7). Cherry (1964) observed a sharp increase in the electrophoretic mobility with increasing degrees of succinylation (up to about 30 groups) followed by a plateau. The electrophoretic mobility in the initial stage increased from -5 to -9.3 cm^2/V/sec $\times 10^{-5}$ (up to 50% succinylation), and it then reached -9.8 cm^2/V/sec $\times 10^{-5}$ with complete succinylation. When the results were taken as a whole, it was concluded that the first 30–34 amino groups occupied surface positions, and their succinylation was accompanied by minor shape changes, despite the considerable increase in the net negative charge. Moreover, the availability of the disulfide bonds to reaction was unchanged, indicating retention of major native conformation. On further succinylation of more than 34 groups

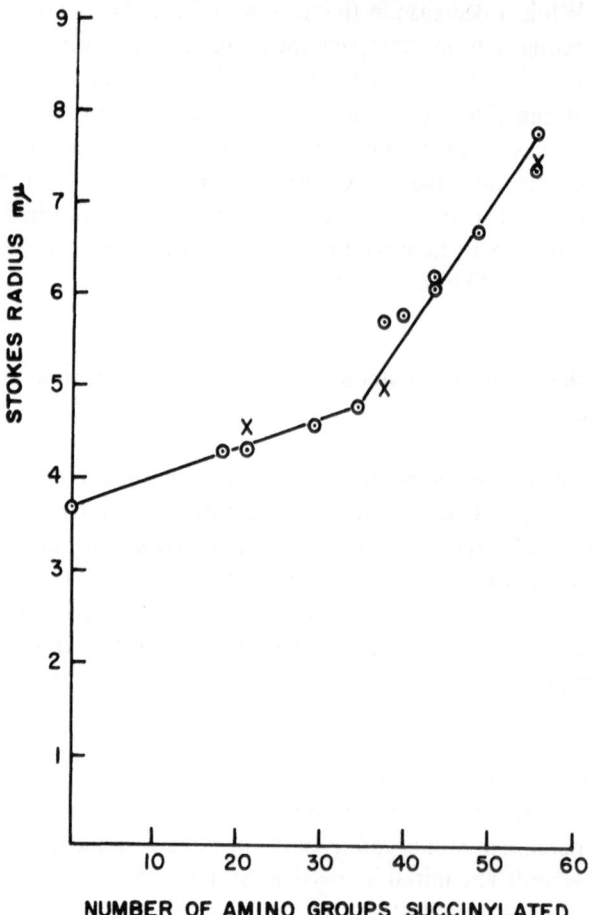

Figure 6. Relationship between Stokes radius and the number of amino groups succinylated in bovine serum albumin. Symbols: O, values obtained from a calibrated Sephadex G200 column; ×, values calculated from diffusion coefficient determined with the ultracentrifuge. From Habeeb (1967a).

(which occupy internal position), the native conformation was disrupted, as shown by the steep increase in both the Stokes radius and the susceptibility of the disulfide bonds to reaction. The ability of various succinylated bovine serum albumins to react with anti-bovine serum albumin was investigated, as a function of the amino groups modified and the Stokes radius as a conformational parameter. Figure 8 shows that the amount of precipitated antibody decreased slowly, followed by a sharper decrease with increase in the number of amino groups modified. The initial region corresponded to minimal conformational changes in the antigen, while the latter part was associated with significant conformational changes due to modification.

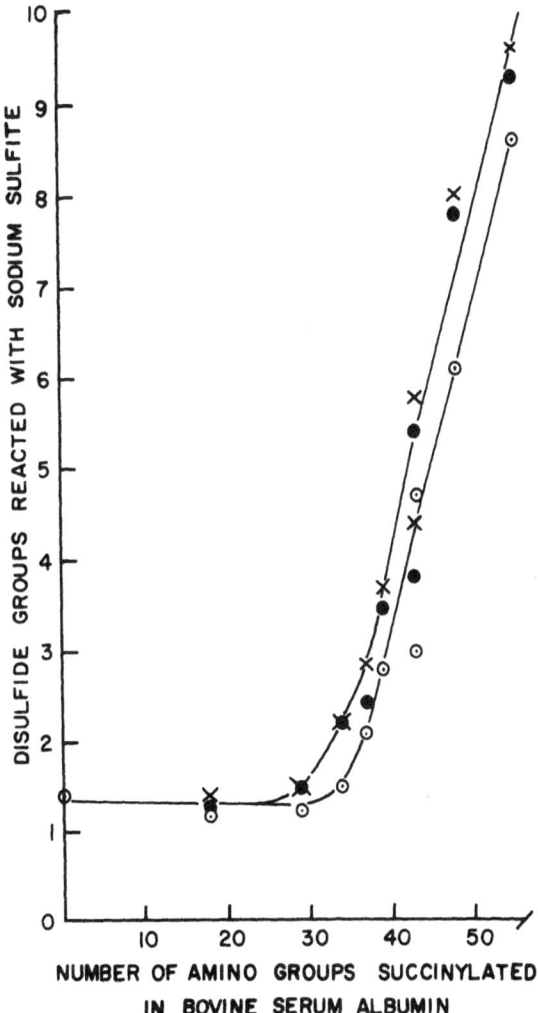

Figure 7. Number of disulfide bonds susceptible to sulfitolysis in bovine serum albumin as a function of amino groups succinylated. Symbols: ○, sulfitolysis for 1 hr; ●, sulfitolysis for 3 hr; ×, sulfitolysis for 6 hr. From Habeeb (1967a).

Immunochemical reactivity was influenced by the conformational changes rather than charge effect, since the initial region where the change in the net charge was maximal and the conformational change was minimal exhibited minimal decrease in immunochemical reactivity. On the other hand, in the second region, where the change in net charge was minimal but showed major conformational change, considerable drop in the immunochemical reactivity was demonstrated. A recovery of about 50% of the native precipitating capacity for fully succinylated BSA was achieved

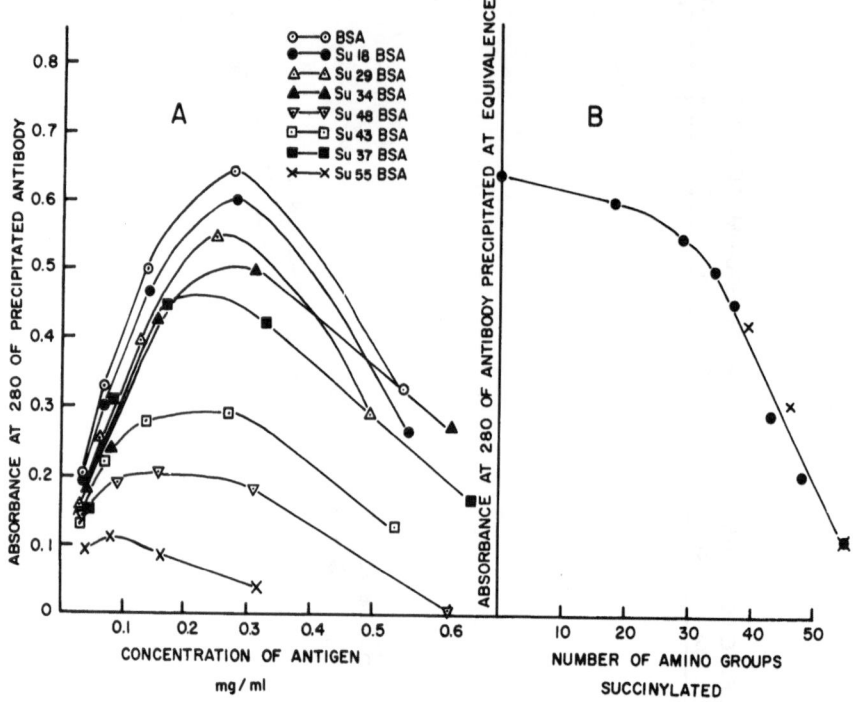

Figure 8. (A) Quantitative precipitin curves obtained with various succinylated bovine serum albumin (Su-BSA) and anti-bovine serum albumin. The subscript indicates the number of amino groups modified. (B) Amount of anti-BSA antibodies precipitated with various Su-BSA at equivalence as a function of amino groups succinylated. Symbols: ●, monomer; ×, aggregate. From Habeeb (1967a).

by performing the precipitation reaction at pH 5.3 (Cherry, 1964), a pH at which renaturation was 72% (from optical rotation). Similar results were obtained with succinyl derivatives of human IgG and anti-human IgG antibodies (Habeeb, 1967a). However, the increase in Stokes radius with succinylation was less dramatic and was accompanied by moderate drop in the precipitated antibody. The amino groups of bovine serum albumin were shown not to be part of the antigenic determinants, since 90% modification by amidination, guanidination, and nitroguanidination resulted in retention of 85–91% of the ability of modified BSA to precipitate with anti-BSA antibodies (Table VII) (Habeeb, 1967b). Amidination and guanidi-nation of BSA did not affect its electrophoretic mobility (Habeeb, 1960; Wofsy and Singer, 1963) or its overall shape, as determined from Stokes radius (Habeeb, 1966c) and intrinsic viscosity (Habeeb, 1966b). In contrast, nitroguanidinated BSA (NG$_{54}$-BSA) was more electronegative than succinyl BSA (Su$_{57}$-BSA) (Habeeb, 1964; Habeeb et al., 1958), yet it showed limited

Table VII. Properties of Modified Bovine Serum Albumin and
Their Immunochemical Reactivity with Anti-Bovine Serum
Albumin[a]

Antigen[b]	Stokes radius (nm)	Number of disulfide groups reacted	Percent reactivity with anti-BSA
Bovine serum albumin (BSA)	3.7	1.2	100
Su_{21}-BSA	4.3	1.0	93
Su_{32}-BSA	4.7	1.23	93
Su_{37}-BSA	5.2	2.1	87
Su_{39}-BSA	5.5	2.6	80
Su_{43}-BSA	6.1	3.1	81
Su_{57}-BSA	6.8	9.6	38
$Su_{21}Gu_{33}$-BSA	4.3	1.02	88
$Su_{21}NG_{34}$-BSA	5.7	6.5	80
Am_{58}-BSA	3.9	1.9	84
Gu_{54}-BSA	3.8	2.7	91
NG_{54}-BSA	4.5	1.9	84

[a] From Habeeb (1967b).
[b] Su, succinyl; Gu, guanyl; NG, nitroguanyl; Am, amidinated; the numerical
subscript denotes the number of amino groups modified.

unfolding compared to Su_{57}-BSA, as seen from the Stokes radius and
availability of disulfide groups to reaction (Habeeb, 1966b,c). Various
succinylated bovine serum albumins Su-BSA were tested against anti-BSA
serum, anti-Su_{32}-BSA serum, and anti-Su_{57}-BSA serum. Su_{21}-BSA and
Su_{32}-BSA retained about 93% of their ability to precipitate with anti-BSA
serum, despite the increase in the net negative charge due to the limited
conformational change. The relationship between the amount of antibody
precipitated as a function of Stokes radius is shown in Fig. 9. Maximum
precipitation occurred with the homologous system. Initially, the decrease
in the precipitated antibody was small, as the Stokes radius either increased
or decreased (compared to the homologous antigen) and was then followed
by a sharp reduction in the precipitated antibody. This was attributed
to the extensive unfolding of the antigen, which would drastically impede
the complementarity of the antigen–antibody reactive sites, and not to
the high net negative charge on the antigen. With anti-Su_{57}-BSA, the marked
loss of reaction with BSA was due to the fact that a major part of the antibody was directed against the haptenic succinyl groups, and against the
succinyl groups comprised in antigenic patches of BSA, which reacted only
with succinyl BSA.

A series of chemically modified human serum albumins (Jacobsen
et al., 1972) were prepared by modification of the amino groups (with acetic
anhydride, N-acetylimidazole, methyl acetimidate, and succinic anhydride),

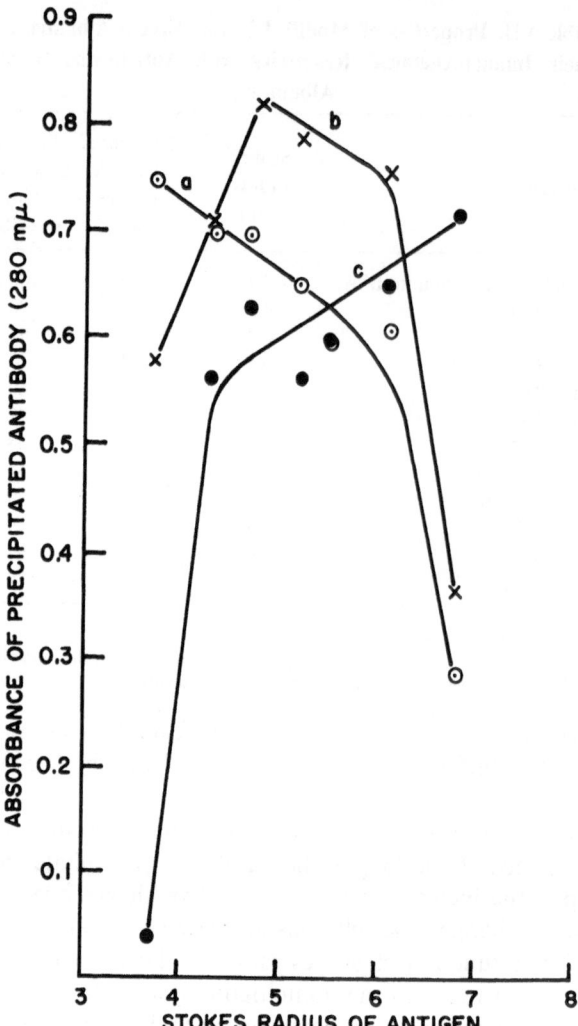

Figure 9. Relationship between the antibody precipitated at equivalence and the Stokes radius of different preparations of succinylated BSA by using (a) anti-BSA, (b) anti-Su_{32}-BSA, and (c) anti-Su_{57}-BSA. From Habeeb, (1967b).

histidine residues (by diethyl pyrocarbonate), tyrosine (by N-acetylimidazole and tetranitromethane), and tryptophan (2-nitrophenyl sulfenyl chloride). There was a distinct relationship between the immunochemical reactivities of the various derivatives and the Stokes radius (Jacobsen *et al.*, 1972). The results showed a considerable decrease in the immunochemical reactivity on modification of the amino groups, which was in contrast to the behavior with BSA reported by Habeeb (1967a).

RNase, RNase S, and S-protein when tested with anti-RNase serum

(Singer and Richards, 1959) showed reduced reactivity of RNase S. Both RNase and RNase S had similar gross conformation, but subtle differences were present. A marked decrease (33–60%) in immunochemical reactivity occurred with the S-protein. It was remarkable that minor conformational changes, as a result of scission of one peptide bond, were detected by immunochemical means. The removal of S-peptide from RNase S resulted in a major conformational change, which was detectable by a considerable decrease in the immunochemical reactivity. Although the S-peptide had no intact antigenic site, it was necessary for the folding of S-protein to recover the immunochemical reactivity characteristics of RNase S. Using double diffusion in agar, Merigan and Potts (1966) showed partial reaction of RNase S and S-protein with anti-RNase antiserum and the formation of a spur with RNase. Reversible conformational changes of RNase, RNase S, and S-protein with heat and urea were accompanied by a decrease in antibody precipitation. The thermal and urea stability showed that S-protein was the most unstable, losing most of the reactivity with antibody at about 60°C or in 1 M urea, conditions at which minor loss of precipitated antibody occurred with RNase S. The loss of the immunochemical reactivity was due to conformational changes of the antigen since the reaction was reversible, and RNase–anti-RNase served as a control and excluded effects on the antibody in explaining the influence of denaturants on the precipitation reaction.

Reduction and reoxidation of bovine serum albumins yielded several components (Peters and Goetzl, 1969) which varied in their elution volumes on Sephadex G100 and in their electrophoretic patterns. A stable monomer was obtained in 40–50% yield, which differed significantly in conformation from native BSA (shown by optical rotatory dispersion). Despite this conformational difference, it precipitated about 15% more antibody than did BSA with anti-bovine serum albumin. Possibly, the increase in precipitated antibody was due to either an internal determinant exposed or a new determinant re-formed in the reoxidized albumin. This behavior is rather unusual and may result from certain features characteristic of BSA. Recovery of the native antigenic determinants in reoxidized albumin (despite differences in conformation) may be due to conformational changes which occurred only after binding with the antibody, resulting in regeneration of all the antigenic determinants of the native albumin.

VI. Conclusion

The advances in immunochemical research within the last two decades resulted from the development of new techniques and methodologies.

The basic question that faces immunochemistry is, What constitutes an antigenic determinant? What are the characteristic features that cause a given arrangement of amino acids in a given sequence and conformation (different from a multitude of other sequences within the protein molecule) to be recognized as foreign and to stimulate synthesis of antibodies? Thus in sperm whale myoglobin (the only protein whose antigenic structure is completely mapped), out of the 153 amino acid residues which comprise the protein, the antigenic reactivity is due to five regions, each containing six or seven amino acid residues. The reasons for their immunogenicity are not presently apparent. In globular proteins, the conformation of the proteins plays an important part. Seemingly innocuous manipulation or treatment may have a significant effect on the conformation, and concomitantly on the immunochemical reactivity. In this chapter, I presented the current views on protein folding, with evidence to show that the complete amino acid sequence is necessary for the native folding of the polypeptide chain. In some cases, the deletion of a few amino acids from a polypeptide chain will result in a protein with low conformational stability. Some physicochemical methods (ORD and CD) may not always be able to detect conformational changes that accompany certain modifications of the protein molecule. The most valuable and sensitive methods that we have used to detect the conformational changes that accompany modification include the Stokes radius method, which evaluates changes in the overall shape of the molecule, the availability of the disulfide bonds to reduction, and the susceptibility to proteolytic digestion. Evidence has been presented that, in a series of homologous proteins, sequence homology does not imply conformational homology. The effect of changes in the conformation of a protein on the immunochemical reactivity has been assessed by controlled modification of the protein, to effect only conformational changes without affecting amino acid residues at the antigenic sites.

The complete determination of the antigenic structure of myoglobin is encouraging that such endeavors can come to fruition. With the methods available at hand and with new innovations, it is anticipated that the antigenic determinants of several proteins will be accurately mapped out in the next decade. It will be a rewarding undertaking, as it will undoubtedly reveal some of the mysteries that lie in the protein molecule; it may also be full of surprises.

ACKNOWLEDGMENTS

I greatly appreciate the assistance of Mrs. Sharon O'Brien in typing the manuscript and Mrs. Hilda G. Harris in checking the references.

VII. References

Achter, E. K., and Swan, I. D. A., 1971, *Biochemistry* **10**:2976.

Ahmed, A. K., 1969, Ph.D. thesis, University of Minnesota, Minneapolis.

Andres, S. F., and Atassi, M. Z., 1970, *Biochemistry* **9**:2268.

Anfinsen, C. B., 1956, *J. Biol. Chem.* **221**:405.

Anfinsen, C. B., 1961, *J. Polym. Sci.* **49**:31.

Anfinsen, C. B., and Haber, E., 1961, *J. Biol. Chem.* **236**:1361.

Anfinsen, C. B., and Scheraga, H. A., 1975, *Adv. Protein Chem.* **29**:205.

Anfinsen, C. B., and White, F. H., Jr., 1961, in: *The Enzymes*, Vol. V, 2nd ed., Part B (P. D. Boyer, H. Lardy, and K. Myrbäck, eds.), p. 95, Academic Press, New York.

Anfinsen, C. B., Haber, E., Sela, M., and White, F. H., Jr., 1961, *Proc. Natl. Acad. Sci. U.S.A.* **47**:1309.

Arnheim, N., Jr., and Wilson, A. C., 1967, *J. Biol. Chem.* **242**:3951.

Arnheim, N., Prager, E. M., and Wilson, A. C., 1969, *J. Biol. Chem.* **244**:2085.

Arnon, R., and Shapira, E., 1967, *Biochemistry* **6**:3942.

Arnon, R., and Shapira, E., 1968, *Biochemistry* **7**:4196.

Atassi, M. Z., 1967, *Biochem. J.* **103**:29.

Atassi, M. Z., 1970, *Biochim. Biophys. Acta* **221**:612.

Atassi, M. Z., 1975, *Immunochemistry* **12**:423.

Atassi, M. Z., and Caruso, D. R., 1968, *Biochemistry* **7**:699.

Atassi, M. Z., and Saplin, B. J., 1971, *Biochemistry* **10**:4740.

Atassi, M. Z., and Singhal, R. P., 1970a, *J. Biol. Chem.* **245**:5122.

Atassi, M. Z., and Singhal, R. P., 1970b, *Biochemistry* **9**:3854.

Atassi, M. Z., and Skalski, D. J., 1969, *Immunochemistry* **6**:25.

Atassi, M. Z., Brown, R. K., and McEwan, M., 1965, *Immunochemistry* **2**:379.

Atassi, M. Z., Habeeb, A. F. S. A., and Rydstedt, L., 1970a, *Biochim. Biophys. Acta* **200**:184.

Atassi, M. Z., Tarlowski, D. P., and Paull, J. H., 1970b, *Biochim. Biophys. Acta* **221**:623.

Aune, K., 1968, Ph.D. dissertation, Duke University, Durham, N.C.

Aune, K. C., Salahuddin, A., Zarlengo, M. H., and Tanford, C., 1967, *J. Biol. Chem.* **242**:4486.

Barel, A. O., Turner, M., and Dolmans, M., 1972, *Eur. J. Biochem.* **30**:26.

Barman, T. E., and Bagshaw, W., 1972, *Biochim. Biophys. Acta* **278**:491.

Barnard, E. A., and Stein, W. D., 1959, *J. Mol. Biol.* **1**:339.

Behring, E., and Kitasato, S., 1890, *Dtsch. Med. Wochenschr.* **16**:1113.

Beilinsson, A., 1929, *Biochem. Z.* **213**:399.

Bigelow, C. C., 1964, *J. Mol. Biol.* **8**:696.

Bigelow, C. C., and Geschwind, I. I., 1961, *C. R. Trav. Lab. Carlsberg* **32**:89.

Biltonen, R., Lumry, R., Madison, V., and Parker, H., 1965, *Proc. Natl. Acad. Sci. U.S.A.* **54**:1412.

Blackburn, S., and Lee, G. R., 1956, *Biochim. Biophys. Acta* **19**:505.

Blake, C. C. F., Johnson, L. N., Mair, G. A., North, A. C. T., Phillips, D. C., and Sarma, V. R., 1967, *Proc. Roy. Soc.* (*London*) *Ser. B* **167**:378.

Bohak, Z., 1964, *J. Biol. Chem.* **239**:2878.

Bradbury, J. H., and King, N. L. R., 1971, *Aust. J. Chem.* **24**:1703.

Bradbury, S. L., and Jakoby, W. B., 1972, *Proc. Natl. Acad. Sci. U.S.A.* **69**:2373.

Bradshaw, R. A., Neurath, H., and Walsh, K. A., 1969, *Proc. Natl. Acad. Sci. U.S.A.* **63**:406.

Brahms, J., and Kay, C. M., 1962, *J. Biol. Chem.* **237**:3449.

Brandts, J. F., and Hunt, L., 1967, *J. Am. Chem. Soc.* **89**:4826.

Breslow, E., and Gurd, F. R. N., 1962, *J. Biol. Chem.* **237**:371.

Breslow, E., Beychok, S., Hardman, K. D., and Gurd, F. R. N., 1965, *J. Biol. Chem.* **240**:304.

Brew, K., and Campbell, P. N., 1967, *Biochem. J.* **102**:258.

Brew, K., Vanaman, T. C., and Hill, R. L., 1967, *J. Biol. Chem.* **242**:3747.

Brown, J. E., and Klee, W. A., 1969, *Biochemistry* **8**:2876.

Brown, J. R., and Hartley, B. S., 1966, *Biochem. J.* **101**:214.

Brown, R. K., Durieux, J., Delaney, R., Leikhim, E., and Clark, B. J., 1959, *Ann. N.Y. Acad. Sci.* **81**:524.

Browne, W. J., North, A. C. T., Phillips, D. C., Brew, K., Vanaman, T. C., and Hill, R. L., 1969, *J. Mol. Biol.* **42**:65.

Buckley, C. E., III, Whitney, P. L., and Tanford, C., 1963, *Proc. Natl. Acad. Sci. U.S.A.* **50**:827.

Bull, H. B., and Breese, K., 1973, *Arch. Biochem. Biophys.* **156**:604.

Burgess, A. W., Weinstein, L. I., Gabel, D., and Scheraga, H. A., 1975, *Biochemistry* **14**:197.

Campbell, L. L., and Cleveland, P. D., 1961, *J. Biol. Chem.* **236**:2966.

Campbell, L. L., and Manning, G. B., 1961, *J. Biol. Chem.* **236**:2962.

Castellino, F. J., and Hill, R. L., 1970, *J. Biol. Chem.* **245**:417.

Cecil, R., 1963, in: *The Proteins,* Vol. 1, 2nd ed. (H. Neurath, ed.), p. 379, Academic Press, New York.

Chantrenne, H., 1961, in: *The Biosynthesis of Proteins,* Pergamon Press, New York, p. 122.

Cherry, M., 1964, Ph.D. thesis, Yale University, New Haven.

Chilson, O. P., Costello, L. A., and Kaplan, N. O., 1965, *Biochemistry* **4**:271.

Crumpton, M. J., 1966, *Biochem. J.* **100**:223.

Crumpton, M. J., 1968, *Biochem. J.* **108**:18P (abst.).

Crumpton, M. J., and Polson, A., 1965, *J. Mol. Biol.* **11**:722.

Dakin, H. D., 1912/1913, *J. Biol. Chem.* **13**:357.

Davis, S., Boone, C. W., Radin, R., Wade, M. J., and Kleiner, G., 1974, *Immunol. Commun.* **3**:189.

DeLorenzo, F., Goldberger, R. F., Steers, E., Jr., Givol, D., and Anfinsen, C. B., 1966, *J. Biol. Chem.* **241**:1562.

Deng, J. S., and Beutner, E. H., 1974, *Int. Arch. Allergy Appl. Immunol.* **47**:562.

Dickerson, R. E., Takano, T., Eisenberg, D., Kallai, O. B., Samson, L., Cooper, A., and Margoliash, E., 1971, *J. Biol. Chem.* **246**:1511.

DiIeso, F., and Verga, E., 1960, *Ital. J. Biochem.* **9**:117.

Donovan, J. W., 1967, *Biochem. Biophys. Res. Commun.* **29**:734.

Dorrington, K. J., and Bennich, H., 1973, *J. Biol. Chem.* **248**:8378.

Eaker, D. L., King, T. P., and Craig, L. C., 1965a, *Biochemistry* **4**:1473.

Eaker, D. L., King, T. P., and Craig, L. C., 1965b, *Biochemistry* **4**:1479.

Eaker, D. L., King, T. P., and Craig, L. C., 1965c, *Biochemistry* **4**:1486.

Edelhoch, H., 1967, *Biochemistry* **6**:1948.

Ellman, G. L., 1959, *Arch. Biochem. Biophys.* **82**:70.

Epand, R. M., and Scheraga, H. A., 1968, *Biochemistry* **7**:2864.

Epstein, C. J., and Anfinsen, C. B., 1962, *J. Biol. Chem.* **237**:3464.

Epstein, C. J., and Goldberger, R. F., 1963, *J. Biol. Chem.* **238**:1380.

Epstein, C. J., Goldberger, R. F., and Anfinsen, C. B., 1963, *Cold Spring Harbor Symp. Quant. Biol.* **28**:439.

Epstein, H. F., Schechter, A. N., Chen, R. F., and Anfinsen, C. B., 1971a, *J. Mol. Biol.* **60**:499.

Epstein, H. F., Schechter, A. N., and Cohen, J. S., 1971b, *Proc. Natl. Acad. Sci. U.S.A.* **68**:2042.

Fainaru, M., Wilson, A. C., and Arnon, R., 1974, *J. Mol. Biol.* **84**:635.

Fish, W. W., Reynolds, J. A., and Tanford, C., 1970, *J. Biol. Chem.* **245**:5166.

Flory, P. J., 1969, in: *Statistical Mechanics of Chain Molecules,* p. 291, Interscience, New York.

Foster, J. F., 1960, in: *The Plasma Proteins* (F. W. Putman, ed.), p. 179, Academic Press, New York.

Frensdorff, H. K., Watson, M. T., and Kauzmann, W., 1953, *J. Am. Chem. Soc.* **75**:5157.

Friedrick, P., Földi, J., and Varadi, K., 1974, *Acta Biochim. Biophys. Acad. Sci. Hung.* **9**:1.

Furie, B., Schechter, A. N., Sachs, D. H., and Anfinsen, C. B., 1974, *Biochemistry* **13**:1561.

Furie, B., Schechter, A. N., Sachs, D. H., and Anfinsen, C. B., 1975, *J. Mol. Biol.* **92**:497.

Givol, D., De Lorenzo, F., Goldberger, R. F., and Anfinsen, C. B., 1965, *Proc. Natl. Acad. Sci. U.S.A.* **53**:676.

Glenny, A. T., and Südmersen, H. J., 1921, *J. Hyg.* **20**:176.

Gold, A. H., and Segal, H. L., 1964, *Fed. Proc.* **23**:424 (abst.).

Goldberger, R. F., and Epstein, C. J., 1963, *J. Biol. Chem.* **238**:2988.

Goldberger, R. F., Epstein, C. J., and Anfinsen, C. B., 1963, *J. Biol. Chem.* **238**:628.

Goldberger, R. F., Epstein, C. J., and Anfinsen, C. B., 1964, *J. Biol. Chem.* **239**:1406.

Goodno, C. C., and Swenson, C. A., 1975, *Biochemistry* **14**:867.

Grossberg, A. L., Markus, G., and Pressman, D., 1965, *Proc. Natl. Acad. Sci. U.S.A.* **54**:942.

Gundlach, H. G., Stein, W. H., and Moore, S., 1959, *J. Biol. Chem.* **234**:1754.

Habeeb, A. F. S. A., 1960, *Can. J. Biochem. Physiol.* **38**:493.

Habeeb, A. F. S. A., 1964, *Biochim. Biophys. Acta* **93**:533.

Habeeb, A. F. S. A., 1966a, *Anal. Biochem.* **14**:328.

Habeeb, A. F. S. A., 1966b, *Biochim. Biophys. Acta* **115**:440.

Habeeb, A. F. S. A., 1966c, *Biochim. Biophys. Acta* **121**:21.

Habeeb, A. F. S. A., 1967a, *Arch. Biochem. Biophys.* **121**:652.

Habeeb, A. F. S. A., 1967b, *J. Immunol.* **99**:1264.

Habeeb, A. F. S. A., 1968, *J. Immunol.* **101**:505.

Habeeb, A. F. S. A., 1969, *J. Immunol.* **102**:457.

Habeeb, A. F. S. A., and Atassi, M. Z., 1971, *Biochim. Biophys. Acta* **236**:131.

Habeeb, A. F. S. A., and Bennett, J. C., 1971, *Biochim. Biophys. Acta* **251**:181.

Habeeb, A. F. S. A., and Borella, L., 1966, *J. Immunol.* **97**:951.

Habeeb, A. F. S. A., and Hiramoto, R., 1968, *Arch. Biochem. Biophys.* **126**:16.

Habeeb, A. F. S. A., Cassidy, H. G., and Singer, S. J., 1958, *Biochim. Biophys. Acta* **29**:587.

Hamaguchi, K., Kurono, A., and Goto, S., 1963, *J. Biochem. (Tokyo)* **54**:259.

Hantgan, R. R., Hammes, G. G., and Scheraga, H. A., 1974, *Biochemistry* **13**:3421.

Harrington, W. F., and Sela, M., 1959, *Biochim. Biophys. Acta* **31**:427.

Harrison, S. C., and Blout, E. R., 1965, *J. Biol. Chem.* **240**:299.

Hartley, B. S., 1964, *Nature (London)* **201**:1284.

Hartley, B. S., Brown, J. R., Kauffman, D. L., and Smillie, L. B., 1965, *Nature (London)* **207**:1157.

Hayashi, R., Moore, S., and Merrifield, R. B., 1973, *J. Biol. Chem.* **248**:3889.

Heins, J. N., Suriano, J. R., Taniuchi, H., and Anfinsen, C. B., 1967, *J. Biol. Chem.* **242**:1016.

Hermans, J., Jr., and Puett, D., 1971, *Biopolymers* **10**:895.

Hermans, J., Jr., Puett, D., and Acampora, G., 1969, *Biochemistry* **8**:22.

Herskovits, T. T., and Laskowski, M., Jr., 1962, *J. Biol. Chem.* **237**:2481.

Herskovits, T. T., and Laskowski, M., Jr., 1968, *J. Biol. Chem.* **243**:2123.

Herskovits, T. T., and Mescanti, L., 1965, *J. Biol. Chem.* **240**:639.

Hill, R. L., Steinmann, H. M., and Brew, K., 1974, in: *Lysozyme* (E. F. Osserman, R. E. Canfield, and S. Beychok, eds.), p. 55, Academic Press, New York.

Hirs, C. H. W., 1967, *Methods Enzymol.* **11**:197.

Hofmann, K., Finn, F., Haas, W., Smithers, M. J., Wolman, Y., and Yanaihara, N., 1963, *J. Am. Chem. Soc.* **85**:833.

Hogle, J. M., and Liener, I. E., 1973, *Can. J. Biochem.* **51**:1014.

Holzwarth, G., and Doty, P., 1965, *J. Am. Chem. Soc.* **87**:218.

Horn, M. J., Jones, D. B., and Ringel, S. J., 1941, *J. Biol. Chem.* **138**:141.

Huang, I.-Y., and Bergdoll, M. S., 1970, *J. Biol. Chem.* **245**:3518.

Huggins, C., Tapley, D. F., and Jensen, E. V., 1951, *Nature (London)* **167**:592.

Isemura, T., Takagi, T., Maeda, Y., and Yutani, K., 1963, *J. Biochem. (Tokyo)* **53**:155.

Isemura, T., Yutani, K., Yutani, A., and Imanishi, A. I., 1968, *J. Biochem. (Tokyo)* **64**:411.

Isenman, D. E., Painter, R. H., and Dorrington, K. J., 1975, *Proc. Natl. Acad. Sci. U.S.A.* **72**:548.

Jacobsen, C., Funding, L., Møller, N. R. H., and Steensgaard, J., 1972, *Eur. J. Biochem.* **30**:392.

Jirgensons, B., 1967, *J. Biol. Chem.* **242**:912.

Johnson, E. R., Anderson, W. L., Atassi, M. Z., Lee, C.-L., and Wetlaufer, D. B., 1975, *Fed. Proc.* **34**:597 (abst.).

Kartha, G., Bello, J., and Harker, D., 1967, *Nature (London)* **213**:862.

Kato, I., and Anfinsen, C. B., 1969, *J. Biol. Chem.* **244**:1004.

Kato, T., and Sasaki, M., 1974, *J. Biochem. (Tokyo)* **76**:1021.

Katsoyannis, P. G., and Tometsko, A., 1966, *Proc. Natl. Acad. Sci. U.S.A.* **55**:1554.

Kauzmann, W., 1959, *Adv. Protein Chem.* **14**:1.

Kauzmann, W., and Simpson, R. B., 1953, *J. Am. Chem. Soc.* **75**:5154.

Kay, C. M., and Brahms, J., 1963, *J. Biol. Chem.* **238**:2945.

Kendrew, J. C., 1962, *Brookhaven Symp. Biol.* **15**:215.

Klee, W. A., 1968, *Biochemistry* **7**:2731.

Klinman, J. P., and Rose, I. A., 1971, *Biochemistry* **10**:2253.

Koide, S. S., and Torres, M. T., 1964, *Biochim. Biophys. Acta* **89**:150.

Kolthoff, I. M., and Tan, B. H., 1965, *J. Am. Chem. Soc.* **87**:2717.

Krigbaum, W. R., and Kügler, F. R., 1970, *Biochemistry* **9**:1216.

Kronman, M. J., 1968, *Biochem. Biophys. Res. Commun.* **33**:535.

Kronman, M. J., Blum, R., and Holmes, L. G., 1966, *Biochemistry* **5**:1970.

Kronman, M. J., Holmes, L. G., and Robbins, F. M., 1971, *J. Biol. Chem.* **246**:1909.

Kronman, M. J., Hoffman, W. B., Jeroszko, J., and Sage, G. W., 1972, *Biochim. Biophys. Acta* **285**:124.

Kuntz, I. D., 1972, *J. Am. Chem. Soc.* **94**:4009.

Landsteiner, K., 1945, in: *The Specificity of Serological Reactions,* Dover Publications, New York.

Lee, C.-L., and Atassi, M. Z., 1973, *Biochemistry* **12**:2690.

Leonis, J., 1956, *Arch. Biochem. Biophys.* **65**:182.

Levinthal, C., 1968, *J. Chim. Phys.* **65**:44.

Levinthal, C., Signer, E. R., and Fetherolf, K., 1962, *Proc. Natl. Acad. Sci. U.S.A.* **48**:1230.

Lewis, P. N., and Scheraga, H. A., 1971, *Arch. Biochem. Biophys.* **144**:576.

Lewis, P. N., Gō, N., Gō, M., Kotelchuck, D., and Scheraga, H. A., 1970, *Proc. Natl. Acad. Sci. U.S.A.* **65**:810.

Lewis, P. N., Momany, F. A., and Scheraga, H. A., 1971, *Proc. Natl. Acad. Sci. U.S.A.* **68**:2293.

Lin, T.-Y., 1970, *Biochemistry* **9**:984.

Long, C., King, E. J., and Sperry, W. M., eds., 1961, in: *The Biochemists' Handbook,* p. 682, Van Nostrand, New York.

Lovrien, R., 1963, *J. Am. Chem. Soc.* **85**:3677.

Lumry, R., Biltonen, R., and Brandts, J. F., 1966, *Biopolymers* **4**:917.

Maeda, H., Glaser, C. B., and Meienhofer, J., 1970, *Biochem. Biophys. Res. Commun.* **39**:1211.

Manning, G. B., and Campbell, L. L., 1961, *J. Biol. Chem.* **236**:2952.

Margoliash, E., Nisonoff, A., and Reichlin, M., 1970, *J. Biol. Chem.* **245**:931.

Markus, G., 1965, *Proc. Natl. Acad. Sci. U.S.A.* **54**:253.

Markus, G., and Karush, F., 1957, *J. Am. Chem. Soc.* **79**:3264.

Markus, G., Love, R. L., and Wissler, F. C., 1964, *J. Biol. Chem.* **239**:3687.

Markus, G., McClintock, D. K., and Castellani, B. A., 1967a, *J. Biol. Chem.* **242**:4395.

Markus, G., McClintock, D. K., and Castellani, B. A., 1967b, *J. Biol. Chem.* **242**:4402.

Markus, G., Barnard, E. A., Castellani, B. A., and Saunders, D., 1968, *J. Biol. Chem.* **243**:4070.

Martin, C. J., and Bhatnagar, G. M., 1967, *Biochemistry* **6**:1638.

Matthaei, J. H., and Nirenberg, M. W., 1961, *Proc. Natl. Acad. Sci. U.S.A.* **47**:1580.

McClintock, D. K., and Markus, G., 1968, *J. Biol. Chem.* **243**:2855.

Merigan, T. C., Jr., and Potts, J. T., Jr., 1966, *Biochemistry* **5**:910.

Mogensen, K. E., and Cantell, K., 1974, *J. Gen. Virol.* **22**:95.

Myers, J. S., and Jakoby, W. B., 1973, *Biochem. Biophys. Res. Commun.* **51**:631.

Myers, J. S., and Jakoby, W. B., 1975, *J. Biol. Chem.* **250**:3785.

Nelson, C. A., and Hummel, J. P., 1962, *J. Biol. Chem.* **237**:1567.

Neurath, H., Walsh, K. A., and Winter, W. P., 1967, *Science* **158**:1638.

Neurath, H., Bradshaw, R. A., and Arnon, R., 1970, in: *Structure–Function Relationships of Proteolytic Enzymes* (P. Desnuelle, H. Neurath, and M. Ottesen, eds.), p. 113, Munksgaard, Copenhagen.

Ng, M. H., and Vilcek, J., 1972, *Adv. Protein Chem.* **26**:173.

Nisonoff, A., Reichlin, M., and Margoliash, E., 1970, *J. Biol. Chem.* **245**:940.

Nonno, L., Herschman, H., and Levine, L., 1970, *Arch. Biochem. Biophys.* **136**:361.

Nozaki, Y., and Tanford, C., 1967, *J. Am. Chem. Soc.* **89**:742.

Omenn, G. S., Ontjes, D. A., and Anfinsen, C. B., 1970, *Biochemistry* **9**:304.

Pace, N. C., and Tanford, C., 1968, *Biochemistry* **7**:198.

Parks, J. M., Barancik, M. B., and Wold, F., 1963, *J. Am. Chem. Soc.* **85**:3519.

Perutz, M. F., Muirhead, H., Cox, J. M., and Goaman, L. C. G., 1968, *Nature (London)* **219**:131.

Peters, J. H., and Goetzl, E., 1969, *J. Biol. Chem.* **244**:2068.

Phillips, D. C., 1966, *Sci. Am.* **215**:78.

Phillips, D. C., 1967, *Proc. Natl. Acad. Sci. U.S.A.* **57**:484.

Pilz, I., Kratky, O., and Karush, F., 1974, *Eur. J. Biochem.* **41**:91.

Pitt-Rivers, R., and Impiombato, F. S. A., 1968, *Biochem. J.* **109**:825.

Pollock, M. R., 1963, *Ann. N.Y. Acad. Sci.* **103**:989.

Potts, J. T., Jr., and Young, D. M., 1963, *Fed. Proc.* **22**:418 (abst.).

Potts, J. T., Jr., Young, D. M., Anfinsen, C. B., and Sandoval, A., 1964, *J. Biol. Chem.* **239**:3781.

Prager, E. M., and Wilson, A. C., 1971*a*, *J. Biol. Chem.* **246**:5978.

Prager, E. M., and Wilson, A. C., 1971*b*, *J. Biol. Chem.* **246**:7010.

Prager, E. M., Fainaru, M., Wilson, A. C., and Arnon, R., 1974, *Immunochemistry* **11**:153.

Prieels, J.-P., Poortmans, J., Dolmans, M., and Leonis, J., 1975, *Eur. J. Biochem.* **50**:523.

Puett, D., 1972*a*, *Biochim. Biophys. Acta* **257**:537.

Puett, D., 1972*b*, *Biochemistry* **11**:1980.

Puett, D., 1972*c*, *Biochemistry* **11**:4304.

Puett, D., 1973, *J. Biol. Chem.* **248**:4623.

Puett, D., Friebele, E., and Hammonds, R. G., Jr., 1973, *Biochim. Biophys. Acta* **328**:261.

Reeke, G. N., Hartsuck, J. A., Ludwig, M. L., Quiocho, F. A., Steitz, T. A., and Lipscomb, W. N., 1967, *Proc. Natl. Acad. Sci. U.S.A.* **58**:2220.

Reichlin, M., 1972, *J. Mol. Biol.* **64**:485.

Reichlin, M., Hay, M., and Levine, L., 1963, *Biochemistry* **2**:971.

Reichlin, M., Hay, M., and Levine, L., 1964, *Immunochemistry* **1**:21.

Reichlin, M., Bucci, E., Fronticelli, C., Wyman, J., Antonini, E., Ioppolo, C., and Rossi-Fanelli, A., 1966, *J. Mol. Biol.* **17**:18.

Reichlin, M., Nisonoff, A., and Margoliash, E., 1970, *J. Biol. Chem.* **245**:947.

Resnick, H., Carter, J. R., and Kalnitsky, G., 1959, *J. Biol. Chem.* **234**:1711.

Reynolds, J. A., and Tanford, C., 1970*a*, *Proc. Natl. Acad. Sci. U.S.A.* **66**:1002.

Reynolds, J. A., and Tanford, C., 1970*b*, *J. Biol. Chem.* **245**:5161.

Richards, F. M., 1963, *Annu. Rev. Biochem.* **32**:269.

Richards, F. M., and Vithayathil, P. J., 1959, *J. Biol. Chem.* **234**:1459.

Richards, F. M., and Vithayathil, P. J., 1960, *Brookhaven Symp. Biol.* **13**:115.

Riggs, A. F., and Wolbach, R. A., 1956, *J. Gen. Physiol.* **39**:585.

Ristow, S. S., and Wetlaufer, D. B., 1973, *Biochem. Biophys. Res. Commun.* **50**:544.

Robinson, E. A., 1965, *Biochem. Biophys. Res. Commun.* **20**:573.

Rothen, A., and Landsteiner, K., 1942, *J. Exp. Med.* **76**:437.

Rupley, J. A., 1967, *Methods Enzymol.* **11**:905.

Sachs, D. H., Schechter, A. N., Eastlake, A., and Anfinsen, C. B., 1972, *Proc. Natl. Acad. Sci. U.S.A.* **69**:3790.

Sage, H. J., and Singer, S. J., 1962, *Biochemistry* **1**:305.

Salkowski, E., 1898, *Berl. Klin. Wochenschr.* **35**:545.

Sarfare, P. S., and Bigelow, C. C., 1967, *Can. J. Biochem.* **45**:651.

Sasaki, M., Kato, T., and Iida, S., 1973, *J. Biochem.* (*Tokyo*) **74**:635.

Saxena, V. P., 1971, *Fed. Proc.* **30**:1287 (abst.).

Saxena, V. P., and Wetlaufer, D. B., 1970, *Biochemistry* **9**:5015.

Schaffer, S. W., 1970, Ph.D. thesis, University of Minnesota, Minneapolis.

Schantz, E. J., Roessler, W. G., Wagman, J., Spero, L., Dunnery, D. A., and Bergdoll, M. S., 1965, *Biochemistry* **4**:1011.

Schechter, A. N., Chen, R. F., and Anfinsen, C. B., 1970, *Science* **167**:886.

Schellman, J. A., 1958., *J. Phys. Chem.* **62**:1485.

Schrier, E. E., and Scheraga, H. A., 1962, *Biochim. Biophys. Acta* **64**:406.

Sela, M., and Anfinsen, C. B., 1957, *Biochim. Biophys. Acta* **24**:229.

Sela, M., Schechter, B., Schechter, I., and Borek, F., 1967, *Cold Spring Harbor Symp. Quant. Biol.* **32**:537.

Shechter, E., and Blout, E. R., 1964, *Proc. Natl. Acad. Sci. U.S.A.* **51**:695.

Shechter, Y., Patchornik, A., and Burstein, Y., 1973, *Biochemistry* **12**:3407.

Shechter, Y., Patchornik, A., and Burstein, Y., 1974, *J. Biol. Chem.* **249**:413.

Sherwood, L. M., and Potts, J. T., Jr., 1965a, *J. Biol. Chem.* **240**:3799.

Sherwood, L. M., and Potts, J. T., Jr., 1965b, *J. Biol. Chem.* **240**:3806.

Shibata, Y., and Kronman, M. J., 1967, *Arch. Biochem. Biophys.* **118**:410.

Singer, S. J., and Richards, F. M., 1959, *J. Biol. Chem.* **234**:2911.

Singhal, R. P., and Atassi, M. Z., 1970, *Biochemistry* **9**:4252.

Sirisinha, S., and Allen, P. Z., 1965, *J. Bacteriol.* **90**:1120.

Spero, L., Stefanye, D., Brecher, P. I., Jacoby, H. M., Dalidowicz, J. E., and Schantz, E. J., 1965, *Biochemistry* **4**:1024.

Spero, L., Warren, J. R., and Metzger, J. F., 1973, *J. Biol. Chem.* **248**:7289.

Stark, G. R., Stein, W. H., and Moore, S., 1961, *J. Biol. Chem.* **236**:436.

Steiner, R. F., De Lorenzo, F., and Anfinsen, C. B., 1965, *J. Biol. Chem.* **240**:4648.

Stewart, W. E. II, De Somer, P., and De Clercq, E., 1974a, *Biochim. Biophys. Acta* **359**:364.

Stewart, W. E. II, De Clercq, E., and De Somer, P., 1974b, *Nature* (*London*) **249**:460.

Tamburro, A. M., Jori, G., Vidali, G., Scatturin, A., and Saccomani, G., 1972, *Biochim. Biophys. Acta* **263**:704.

Tanahashi, N., Brodbeck, U., and Ebner, K. E., 1968, *Biochim. Biophys. Acta* **154**:247.

Tanford, C., 1970, *Adv. Protein Chem.* **24**:1.

Tanford, C., De, P. K., and Taggart, V. G., 1960, *J. Am. Chem. Soc.* **82**:6028.

Tanford, C., Buckley, C. E., III, De, P. K., and Lively, E. P., 1962, *J. Biol. Chem.* **237**:1168.

Tanford, C., Kawahara, K., and Lapanje, S., 1967a, *J. Am. Chem. Soc.* **89**:729.

Tanford, C., Kawahara, K., Lapanje, S., Hooker, T. M., Jr., Zarlengo, M. H., Salahuddin, A., Aune, K. C., and Takagi, T., 1967b, *J. Am. Chem. Soc.* **89**:5023.

Taniuchi, H., 1970, *J. Biol. Chem.* **245**:5459.

Taniuchi, H., and Anfinsen, C. B., 1968, *J. Biol. Chem.* **243**:4778.

Taniuchi, H., and Anfinsen, C. B., 1969, *J. Biol. Chem.* **244**:3864.

Taniuchi, H., and Anfinsen, C. B., 1971, *J. Biol. Chem.* **246**:2291.

Taniuchi, H., Anfinsen, C. B., and Sodja, A., 1967, *Proc. Natl. Acad. Sci. U.S.A.* **58**:1235.

Teipel, J. W., and Koshland, D. E., Jr., 1971a, *Biochemistry* **10**:792.

Teipel, J. W., and Koshland, D. E., Jr., 1971b, *Biochemistry* **10**:798.

Timasheff, S. N., Townend, R., and Mescanti, L., 1966, *J. Biol. Chem.* **241**:1863.

Tsong, T. Y., Baldwin, R. L., and McPhie, P., 1972, *J. Mol. Biol.* **63**:453.

Urnes, P., and Doty, P., 1961, *Adv. Protein Chem.* **16**:401.

Vithayathil, P. J., and Richards, F. M., 1961, *J. Biol. Chem.* **236**:1386.

Wallevik, K., 1968, *Protides Biol. Fluids Proc. Colloq.* **15**:561.

Walsh, K. A., and Neurath, H., 1964, *Proc. Natl. Acad. Sci. U.S.A.* **52**:884.

Warme, P. K., Momany, F. A., Rumball, S. V., Tuttle, R. W., and Scheraga, H. A., 1974, *Biochemistry* **13**:768.

Warner, C., Schumaker, V., and Karush, F., 1970, *Biochem. Biophys. Res. Commun.* **38**:125.

Warner, R. C., and Levy, M., 1958, *J. Am. Chem. Soc.* **80**:5735.

Weber, R. E., and Tanford, C., 1959, *J. Am. Chem. Soc.* **81**:3255.

Weil, R., and Dorner, F., 1973, in: *Selective Inhibitors of Viral Functions* (W. A. Carter, ed.), p. 107, CRC Press, Cleveland.

Wetlaufer, D. B., 1973a, *J. Food Sci.* **38**:740.

Wetlaufer, D. B., 1973b, *Proc. Natl. Acad. Sci. U.S.A.* **70**:697.

Wetlaufer, D. B., Johnson, E. R., and Clauss, L. M., 1974a, in: *Lysozyme* (E. F. Osserman, R. E. Canfield, and S. Beychok, eds.), p. 269, Academic Press, New York.

Wetlaufer, D. B., Kwok, E., Anderson, W. L., and Johnson, E. R., 1974b, *Biochem. Biophys. Res. Commun.* **56**:380.

White, F. H., Jr., 1960, *J. Biol. Chem.* **235**:383.

White, F. H., Jr., 1961, *J. Biol. Chem.* **236**:1353.

Wofsy, L., and Singer, S. J., 1963, *Biochemistry* **2**:104.

Wyckoff, H. W., Hardman, K. D., Allewell, N. M., Inagami, T., Tsernoglou, D., Johnson, L. N., and Richards, F. M., 1967, *J. Biol. Chem.* **242**:3749.

Young, J. D., and Leung, C. Y., 1970, *Biochemistry* **9**:2755.

Yutani, K., Yutani, A., and Isemura, T., 1967, *J. Biochem. (Tokyo)* **62**:576.

Yutani, K., Yutani, A., Imanishi, A., and Isemura, T., 1968, *J. Biochem. (Tokyo)* **64**:449.

Zimmerman, S. B., and Schellman, J. A., 1962, *J. Am. Chem. Soc.* **84**:2259.

Zondag, H. A., 1963, *Science* **142**:965.

Investigation of Immunochemical Reactions by Fluorescence Polarization

Walter B. Dandliker

I. Introduction

Fluorescence polarization provides the biologist and the chemist with a highly sensitive and versatile probe for investigating both the structural features and molecular motions of macromolecules. It provides information on the individual isolated molecule, as well as on the interactions occurring with other molecules, and is hence adaptable to a diversity of equilibrium and kinetic measurements over extremely wide ranges of concentration and time. The magnitude of the steady-state polarization (or the anisotropy) observed in the fluorescent light emitted from solutions is a function of several variables. It depends upon the relaxation time of the rotary Brownian motion, the decay time of the electronically excited state, and the relative orientations of the transition moments for absorption and emission. If the transient-state polarization is observed after the excitation has been cut off, then the polarization is a function of time as well. Measurements of both the steady-state and transient-state polarization are well known (Dandliker and deSaussure, 1970; Yguerabide, 1972) and are usually analyzed in terms of rotational motions of the fluorescent unit and of relaxation phenomena involving the macromolecule or solvent. The latter effects may be, in part, induced by the difference in free energy between the ground

Walter B. Dandliker · Department of Biochemistry, Scripps Clinic and Research Foundation, La Jolla, California 92037.

and the electronically excited states. In the last few years, there have been substantial advances in the theory of fluorescence polarization (Tao, 1969; Weber, 1971; Belford et al., 1972; Chuang and Eisenthal, 1972) together with improvements in instrumentation both for transient-state (Yguerabide, 1972) and for steady-state measurements (Kelly, Dandliker, and Williamson, 1976).

In addition to the applications of fluorescence polarization directed toward elucidation of the detailed motions of molecules, there is an important area in which the polarization is used in an empirical fashion to monitor the rates and equilibria of chemical reactions involving a fluorescent species. Other optical parameters such as light absorption, optical rotation, circular dichroism, wavelength dependence of fluorescence, fluorescence intensity, and light and low-angle X-ray scattering may be applied similarly, in special cases for monitoring chemical reactions. Some of these have been used in immunochemical investigations (Holowka et al., 1972; Pollet et al., 1974; Pilz et al., 1973). This chapter is concerned mainly with the utilization of fluorescence polarization and intensity as sensitive measures of the progress and equilibria of immunochemical reactions, especially in conjunction with fluorescent labels covalently attached to one reactant.

The simplest prototype reaction representative of antigen–antibody or hapten–antibody interaction may be written as

$$\mathscr{F} + \mathscr{R} \rightleftharpoons \mathscr{F}\mathscr{R} \tag{1}$$

in which $\mathscr{F}$ is a fluorescent ligand reacting with $\mathscr{R}$, a nonfluorescent receptor, to form a complex, $\mathscr{F}\mathscr{R}$. In such a reaction, the polarization of fluorescence will normally be expected to rise, as the reaction proceeds from left to right, because of the larger molecular volume of the complex, as compared to that of the fluorescent ligand. The expected increase in polarization may be altered by changes in decay time or by changes in molecular geometry of the emitting unit as the reaction proceeds, but these influences are usually small and are allowed for in the treatment below.

A more general type of reaction than that given in equation (1) may be called an inhibition reaction in which the ligand is present also in a non-fluorescent (unlabeled) form, $\mathscr{N}$, so that a competing reaction occurs:

$$\mathscr{N} + \mathscr{R} \rightleftharpoons \mathscr{N}\mathscr{R} \tag{2}$$

For describing the equilibrium state, alternative classical or modified mass law treatments can be formulated embodying equations (1) and (2), as in the discussion below.

If instead of equilibrium measurements alone, rate measurements are made, then the kinetic parameters of reactions represented by equations (1) and (2) may be deduced. Data processing is usually adequately done by simple graphical methods (Dandliker and Levison, 1968; Levison and

Dandliker, 1969; Levison *et al.*, 1970, 1975; Dandliker *et al.*, 1973; Portmann *et al.*, 1975), except for systems with nonuniform binding sites for which numerical methods have been devised (Dandliker *et al.*, 1964; Kierszenbaum *et al.*, 1969; Dandliker, 1971; Mavis *et al.*, 1974).

II. Symbols

In this chapter, the following symbols will be used to summarize the most useful relationships. These have been based upon some simple initial assumptions, *viz.*, that a particular molecule of the fluorescent ligand is in one of two distinct chemical states, either free or bound to receptor, and that the free and bound states can be fully characterized optically by four constants, Q_f, Q_b, p_f, and p_b.

a heterogeneity index, equations (14) and (15).

b subscript indicating "bound."

e subscript indicating value at equilibrium.

F molar concentration of $\mathscr{F}$.

$\mathscr{F}$ chemical symbol for the fluorescent-labeled antigen or hapten.

f subscript indicating "free."

$F_{b,\max}$ the maximum value of F_b, taken to be a measure of the total concentration of antibody binding sites.

$\mathscr{F}\mathscr{R}$ chemical symbol for the fluorescent antigen–antibody or hapten–antibody complex.

k empirical rate constant, equations (16) and (17).

k' empirical rate constant, equation (16).

k_1 second-order rate constant for the forward reaction.

k_{-1} first order rate constant for the back-reaction.

K_F the association constant for the reaction between $\mathscr{F}$ and $\mathscr{R}$.

K_N the association constant for the reaction between $\mathscr{N}$ and $\mathscr{R}$.

M the total molar concentration of $\mathscr{F}$ in both bound and free forms.

N molar concentration of $\mathscr{N}$.

$\mathscr{N}$ chemical symbol for the unlabeled antigen or hapten.

N_1 order of reaction with respect to receptor.

N_2 order of reaction with respect to ligand.

N_3 order of reaction with respect to complex.

$\mathscr{N}\mathscr{R}$ chemical symbol for the nonfluorescent antigen–antibody or hapten–antibody complex.

$_0$ subscript indicating value at zero time.

p the polarization of the excess fluorescence, that is, $p = (\Delta V - \Delta H)/(\Delta V + \Delta H)$, where ΔV and ΔH are the intensities, in arbitrary units, of the components in the excess fluorescence

(above that of the blank) polarized in the vertical and hori-
zontal directions, respectively.

Q molar fluorescence of the equilibrium mixture of the free and
bound forms of $\mathscr{F}$, i.e., $Q = (\Delta V + \Delta H)/M$.

$\mathscr{R}$ chemical symbol for the receptor (antibody).

s subscript to K indicating a Sips distribution.

t time.

W the total molar concentration of $\mathscr{N}$ in both bound and free
forms.

x the ratio of F_b/F_f.

III. Equations Relating Fluorescence Polarization and Intensity to Concentration

(Dandliker *et al.*, 1964; Dandliker and Levison, 1968; Levison and
Dandliker, 1969)

$$\frac{F_b}{F_f} = \frac{Q_f}{Q_b}\left(\frac{p - p_f}{p_b - p}\right) \tag{3}$$

Substituting $M = F_b + F_f$ gives

$$F_b = \frac{MQ_f(p - p_f)}{Q_b(p_b - p) + Q_f(p - p_f)} \tag{4}$$

and

$$F_f = \frac{MQ_b(p_b - p)}{Q_f(p - p_f) + Q_b(p_b - p)} \tag{5}$$

Differentiation of the expression for F_f yields

$$\frac{dF_f}{dt} = \frac{-MQ_fQ_b(p_b - p_f)}{[Q_f(p - p_f) + Q_b(p_b - p)]^2}\left(\frac{dp}{dt}\right) \tag{6}$$

For initial rates, if $p \approx p_f$, then

$$\left(\frac{dF_f}{dt}\right)_0 \approx \frac{-MQ_f}{Q_b(p_b - p_f)}\left(\frac{dp}{dt}\right)_0 \tag{7}$$

If the reaction between receptor and ligand produces changes in fluorescence
intensity, then useful information may be obtained from the relationships

$$\frac{F_b}{F_f} = \frac{Q_f - Q}{Q - Q_b} \tag{8}$$

$$\frac{dF_f}{dt} = \frac{F_f^2}{M}\left(\frac{Q_f - Q_b}{[Q - Q_b]^2}\right)\frac{dQ}{dt} \tag{9}$$

and at $t = 0$

$$\left(\frac{dF_f}{dt}\right)_0 \approx \frac{M}{Q_f - Q_b}\left(\frac{dQ}{dt}\right)_0 \tag{10}$$

IV. Equilibrium Equations

A. Classical Mass Law, Uniformly Binding Sites, No Site–Site Interactions
(Dandliker *et al.*, 1973)

$$\frac{F_b}{F_f} = K_F(F_{b,\max} - F_b - N_b) \tag{11}$$

$$\frac{N_b}{N_f} = K_N(F_{b,\max} - F_b - N_b) \tag{12}$$

These two equations assume that both $\mathscr{F}$ and $\mathscr{N}$ compete for the same sites, but bind to $\mathscr{R}$ with different association constants. Equations (11) and (12) form the basis of equilibrium immunoassay procedures.

The constants K_F and $F_{b,\max}$ can be most readily evaluated from Scatchard plots with $W = 0$. Knowing these two constants then permits the determination of K_N by means of the equation

$$K_N = K_F\left[F_{b,\max} - \frac{Mx}{x+1} - \frac{x}{K_F}\right]\bigg/ x\left[W - \left(F_{b,\max} - \frac{Mx}{x+1} - \frac{x}{K_F}\right)\right] \tag{13}$$

B. Nonuniformly Binding Sites Characterized by a Sips Distribution of Binding Affinities (Kierszenbaum *et al.*, 1969)

$$\log F_f = \frac{1}{a_F}\log\left(\frac{F_b}{F_{b,\max} - F_b - N_b}\right) - \log K_{0,F} \tag{14}$$

$$\log N_f = \frac{1}{a_N}\log\left(\frac{N_b}{F_{b,\max} - F_b - N_b}\right) - \log K_{0,N} \tag{15}$$

V. Kinetic Equations

(Dandliker and Levison, 1968; Levison and Dandliker, 1969; Levison et al., 1975; W. Dandliker and J. Dandliker, unpublished results.) The analysis of the kinetics of immunochemical reactions has been based upon a general form of the rate equation applicable to equation (1):

$$\frac{-dF_f}{dt} = \frac{dF_b}{dt} = k \, (F_{b,max} - F_b)^{N_1} (F_f)^{N_2} - k' \, (F_b)^{N_3} \qquad (16)$$

Relationships for the general case in which arbitrary initial concentrations of $\mathscr{F}$ and $\mathscr{R}$ react and progress toward equilibrium, as well as for various specialized circumstances, are discussed below. In calculating rate constants, there is a possibility of confusion depending upon whether site concentration (of antibody which may be either univalent or divalent) or molar concentration is used in the expressions. In the present treatment, all concentrations have been expressed in terms of site concentration. If the receptor sites act independently, and if the ligand is univalent, this convention is the most convenient and perfectly adequate.

A. Reaction Order

The reaction order can be determined from initial rate measurements using the equation

$$\left(\frac{dp}{dt}\right)_0 = \frac{Q_b}{Q_f}(p_b - p_f) \, k(F_{b,max})^{N_1} (F_{f,0})^{N_2 - 1} \qquad (17)$$

where k is the empirical forward rate constant. If the receptor (e.g., antibody) is in such great excess that its concentration can be regarded as constant, then equation (17) can be written

$$\log\left(\frac{dp}{dt}\right)_0 = (N_2 - 1)\log F_{f,0} + a \text{ constant} \qquad (18)$$

allowing easy evaluation of N_2 from a linear plot of data at varying $F_{f,0}$. Conversely, if the ligand is in large excess, then equation (17) becomes

$$\log\left(\frac{dp}{dt}\right)_0 = N_1 \log F_{b,max} + a \text{ constant} \qquad (19)$$

from which N_1 can be obtained. If the reaction between a ligand and a receptor produces changes in fluorescence intensity, then an equation analogous to equation (17) may be written by combining equations (16) and (9). Application of equations (18) and (19) does not require knowledge of absolute concentrations, but only of relative concentrations.

B. Evaluation of Rate Constants

From the initial rate equation: Use equation (17) to obtain k, or if $N_1 = N_2 = 1$ then k_1 can be found from

$$\left(\frac{dp}{dt}\right)_0 \approx \frac{Q_b}{Q_f}(p_b - p_f)k_1(F_{b,max}) \tag{20}$$

From the integrated rate equation, assuming that $N_2 = N_3 = 1$ and that the receptor concentration is sufficiently high to be considered constant throughout the reaction:

$$\log\left(\frac{F_{b,e}}{F_{b,e} - F_b}\right) \approx \left[\frac{k_1(F_{b,max})^{N_1} + k_{-1}}{2.3}\right]t \tag{21}$$

If $Q_f \approx Q_b$, then the combination of equations (21) and (3) results in the following relationship:

$$\log(p_e - p) \approx \log(p_e - p_f) - \left[\frac{k_1(F_{b,max})^{N_1} + k_{-1}}{2.3}\right]t \tag{22}$$

Hence, a plot of $\log(p_e - p)$ versus time should be linear with a slope equal to $-1/2.3[k_1(F_{b,max})^{N_1} + k_{-1}]$. Furthermore, a plot of this latter quantity versus $F_{b,max}$ will be linear if the order with respect to receptor concentration is 1. The rate constants k_1 and k_{-1} are obtained as the slope and intercept, respectively, of the latter plot.

The rate constants can be determined from the half-time as follows. If in equation (22), $F_{b,max}^{N_1} \gg k_{-1}/k_1$, and if the half-time is defined as the time when $(p_e - p)/(p_e - p_f) = 1/2$, then equation (22) becomes $0.692 = k_1(F_{b,max})^{N_1}t_{1/2}$ and

$$\log t_{1/2} = -N_1\log F_{b,max} + \log\left[\frac{0.692}{k_1}\right] \tag{23}$$

Equation (16) is a general form of the rate equation applicable to equation (1). As shown above, N_1 and N_2 are readily determined from initial rate measurements. Under conditions where $N_1 = N_2 = N_3 = 1$, and where the reaction is started with $F_{b,0} = 0$, equation (16) may be integrated analytically. From the expression for equilibrium, one can write

$$k_{-1} = \frac{k_1(F_{b,max} - F_{b,e})(F_{f,0} - F_{b,e})}{F_{b,e}} \tag{24}$$

Substituting equation (24) into equation (16) gives, after rearrangement, the rate equation as

$$\frac{-dF_f}{dt} = k_1 [F_f - F_{f,e}] \left[(F_f - F_{f,e}) + \frac{F_{f,0} F_{b,\max} - (F_{f,0} - F_{f,e})^2}{F_{f,0} - F_{f,e}} \right] \quad (25)$$

or as the equivalent expression

$$\frac{-dF_f}{dt} = k_1 [F_{b,e} - F_b] \left[(F_{b,e} - F_b) + \frac{F_{b,\max} F_{f,0} - (F_{b,e})^2}{F_{b,e}} \right] \quad (26)$$

After the partial fractions have been formed, integration is readily accomplished to give

$$\ln \left\{ \frac{F_{f,0} F_{b,\max} [F_f - F_{f,e}]}{[F_{f,0} - F_{f,e}][(F_f - F_{f,e})(F_{f,0} - F_{f,e}) + F_{f,0} F_{b,\max} - (F_{f,0} - F_{f,e})^2]} \right\}$$
$$= -k_1 t \left[\frac{F_{f,0} F_{b,\max} - (F_{f,0} - F_{f,e})^2}{F_{f,0} - F_{f,e}} \right] \quad (27)$$

or the equivalent expression

$$\ln \left\{ \frac{F_{b,\max} F_{f,0} [F_{b,e} - F_b]}{F_{b,e}[(F_{b,e} - F_b)(F_{b,e}) + F_{b,\max} F_{f,0} - F_{b,e}^2]} \right\}$$
$$= -k_1 t \left[\frac{F_{b,\max} F_{f,0} - F_{b,e}^2}{F_{b,e}} \right] \quad (28)$$

In the limit when the receptor is present in very large excess, equations (27) and (28) reduce to

$$\ln \left[\frac{F_f - F_{f,e}}{F_{f,0} - F_{f,e}} \right] = \ln \left[\frac{F_{b,e} - F_b}{F_{b,e}} \right] = -k_1 t F_{b,\max} \quad (29)$$

In the limit of very high ligand concentration, equations (27) and (28) become

$$\ln \left[\frac{F_f - F_{f,e}}{F_{f,0} - F_{f,e}} \right] = \ln \left[\frac{F_{b,e} - F_b}{F_{b,e}} \right] = -k_1 t F_{f,0} \quad (30)$$

It may be noted that a similar set of equations containing k_{-1} could be obtained by solving for k_1, instead of k_{-1}, in equation (24).

C. Dissociation of Complexes

Information on the backward rate constant, k_{-1}, may be obtained by direct observation on the dissociation of complexes following rapid dilution (dilution jump). A dilution jump at present requires at least a few milliseconds, but if the complexes to be investigated are reasonably stable, the rates will be small enough to permit ready observation, often even with manual dilution. Hence, the reaction may be still represented by equation (1), where the reaction starts with $\mathscr{F}\mathscr{R}$ only. Denoting the rate constant for dissociation by k_{-1}, and assuming, as before, that $N_3 = 1$, the integrated rate equation (Frost and Pearson, 1961, p. 187) becomes

$$\ln\left\{\frac{F_{b,\max}^2 - F_{b,e}F_b}{(F_b - F_{b,e})(F_{b,\max})}\right\} = k_{-1}\left\{\frac{F_{b,\max} + F_{b,e}}{F_{b,\max} - F_{b,e}}\right\}t \qquad (31)$$

An alternative form is

$$\ln\left\{\frac{F_{b,\max}^2 - (F_{b,\max} - F_{f,e})(F_{b,\max} - F_f)}{[(F_{b,\max} - F_f) - (F_{b,\max} - F_{f,e})]F_{b,\max}}\right\}$$

$$= k_{-1}\left\{\frac{2F_{b,\max} - F_{f,e}}{F_{b,\max} - (F_{b,\max} - F_{f,e})}\right\}t \qquad (32)$$

This equation reduces to the form

$$\ln\left\{\frac{F_{b,\max}(F_{f,e} + F_f) - F_{f,e}F_f}{F_{b,\max}(F_{f,e} - F_f)}\right\} = -k_1 t\left(\frac{2F_{b,\max} - F_{f,e}}{F_{f,e}}\right) \qquad (33)$$

If the dilution is so large that dissociation goes practically to completion, then equation (31) or (33) takes on its limiting first-order forms:

$$\ln\left(\frac{F_{b,\max}}{F_b}\right) = \ln\left(\frac{F_{b,0}}{F_b}\right) = \ln\left(\frac{M}{F_b}\right) = k_{-1}t \qquad (34)$$

In terms of the polarization, equation (34) becomes

$$\ln\left\{\frac{Q_b[p_b - p] + Q_f(p - p_f)}{Q_f(p - p_f)}\right\} = k_{-1}t \qquad (35)$$

If $Q_f \approx Q_b$, then

$$\ln\left(\frac{p_b - p_f}{p - p_f}\right) \approx k_{-1}t \qquad (36)$$

which permits the evaluation of k_{-1} from a linear plot.

VI. Relaxation Methods

The term "relaxation methods" is usually applied to measurements on systems near equilibrium, which have been perturbed in any one of a variety of ways. After the perturbation, the rate of return to a new equilibrium state is observed. In principle, both k_1 and k_{-1} can be found in this way. Relaxation methods lend themselves to the study of fast reactions, but suffer from the disadvantage that only a small concentration region is usually accessible for experimentation. Hence, results from relaxation methods should be supplemented by data from other types of kinetic experiments whenever possible. The most usual means of perturbing the equilibrium is by a temperature jump, produced by a capacitor discharge. In systems where the ΔH of reaction is small, it is sometimes possible to couple the reaction to another with a large ΔH, e.g., by a pH change. Other means of perturbation include rapid changes in pressure or electric field.

The general concept of relaxation time arose originally in considering the rate of response of a physical system after it has been strained or deformed by some external agency. The relaxation time is the time required for the system to traverse all but $1/e$ of its path to the new equilibrium state. To apply these ideas to the reaction represented by equation (1), let the concentrations of $\mathscr{F}$, $\mathscr{R}$, and $\mathscr{FR}$ be denoted by α, β, and γ, respectively. Then, the rate equation can be written

$$\frac{-d\alpha}{dt} = \frac{-d\beta}{dt} = \frac{d\gamma}{dt} = k_1\alpha\beta - k_{-1}\gamma \tag{37}$$

Now, after the perturbation, the conditions for equilibrium have changed so that the existing concentrations differ from the equilibrium values by the amounts $\Delta\alpha$, $\Delta\beta$, and $\Delta\gamma$. Hence, the rate of approach to the new equilibrium state is

$$\frac{-d\alpha}{dt} = k_1(\alpha_e + \Delta\alpha)(\beta_e + \Delta\beta) - k_{-1}(\gamma_e + \Delta\gamma)$$

$$= k_1(\alpha_e\beta_e + \alpha_e\Delta\beta + \beta_e\Delta\alpha + \Delta\alpha\Delta\beta) - k_{-1}(\gamma_e + \Delta\gamma) \tag{38}$$

Neglecting the higher-order term $(\Delta\alpha\Delta\beta)$ and utilizing the equilibrium expression

$$k_1\alpha_e\beta_e - k_{-1}\gamma_e = 0 \tag{39}$$

gives the rate as

$$\frac{-d\alpha}{dt} = k_1(\alpha_e\Delta\beta + \beta_e\Delta\alpha) - k_{-1}\Delta\gamma \tag{40}$$

Since $\Delta\alpha = \Delta\beta = -\Delta\gamma$, and since $d\alpha/dt \equiv d\Delta\alpha/dt$, equation (40) becomes

$$\frac{-d(\Delta\alpha)}{dt} = \Delta\alpha[k_1(\alpha_e + \beta_e) + k_{-1}] \tag{41}$$

This equation is of the same form as that of a first-order rate law, with a rate constant of $[k_1(\alpha_e + \beta_e) + k_{-1}]$. The relaxation time for a first-order reaction is equal to the reciprocal of the rate constant so that

$$\frac{1}{\tau} = k_1(\alpha_e + \beta_e) + k_{-1} \tag{42}$$

Hence, k_1 and k_{-1} are evaluated as the slope and intercept, respectively, of a plot of $1/\tau$ versus a series of values of $(\alpha_e + \beta_e) = (F_{f,e} + F_{b,\max} - F_{b,e})$. The relaxation time, τ, is equal to the reciprocal of the slope of a plot of $(-\ln \Delta F_f)$ versus time. In terms of the polarization

$$\Delta F_f = \frac{MQ_b(p_b - p)}{Q_f(p - p_f) + Q_b(p_b - p)} - \frac{MQ_b(p_b - p_e)}{Q_f(p_e - p_f) + Q_b(p_b - p_e)} \tag{43}$$

If Δp is small, then $p \approx p_e$ and

$$\Delta F_f \approx \frac{-MQ_bQ_f(p_b - p_f)\,\Delta p}{[Q_f(p_e - p_f) + Q_b(p_b - p_e)]^2} \tag{44}$$

and

$$\ln \Delta F_f = \text{const.} + \ln \Delta p \tag{45}$$

Hence, the relaxation time, τ, is equal to the reciprocal of the slope of a plot of $\ln \Delta p$ versus t.

VII. Results Obtained on Immunochemical Reactions by Means of Fluorescence Polarization and Intensity Measurements

A. Determination of Binding Affinities and Site Concentration from Equilibrium Titrations

The reaction between fluorescein, acting as a hapten, and its antibody has been thoroughly studied by means of fluorescence methods. Antifluorescein obtained by relatively short-term immunization via the intravenous route is heterogeneous and of relatively low binding affinity (Fig. 1). A similar antibody was also obtained by Lopatin and Voss (1971). Under conditions of long immunization using adjuvants and intracutaneous administration, antifluorescein is obtained which is uniformly binding and which has an extremely high binding affinity ($K \sim 10^{11}$ M^{-1}). During the "maturation" process leading to this very tight binding antibody, the value of both K and a increases with time (Fig. 2). Scatchard plots of early antibody show marked curvature (Fig. 3), while those from late bleedings are linear (Fig. 4). The first antigen–antibody reaction to be studied by fluorescence polarization was that between fluorescein-labeled ovalbumin and

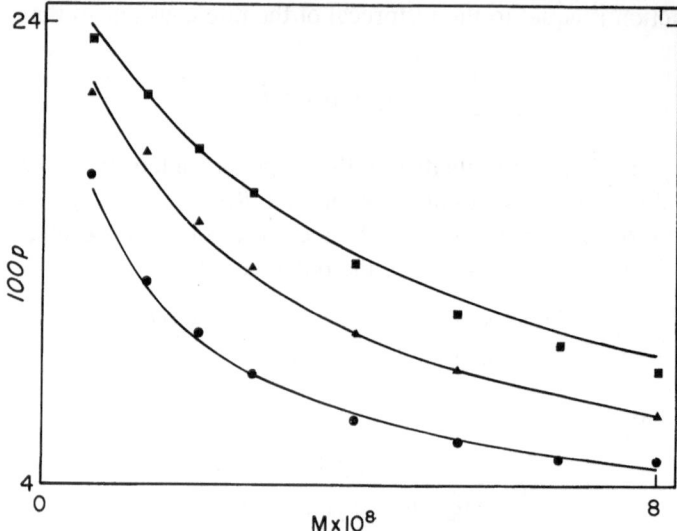

Figure 1. Titration of antifluorescein–ovalbumin with fluorescein. Unpolarized incident light, 436 nm. Antibody protein concentration (μg/ml) calculated from precipitation with fluorescein ovalbumin. Symbols: ●, 11.3; ▲, 17.0; ■, 22.6. Solid curves calculated from $Q_f = 28.0$; $Q_b = 3.6$; $p_f = 0.016$; $p_b = 0.290$; $K_0 = 5.5 \times 10^6 \, M^{-1}$; $a = 0.51$; $F_{b,\max} = 13.5 \times 10^{-8} \, M$ for lowest antibody concentration. From Dandliker et al. (1964).

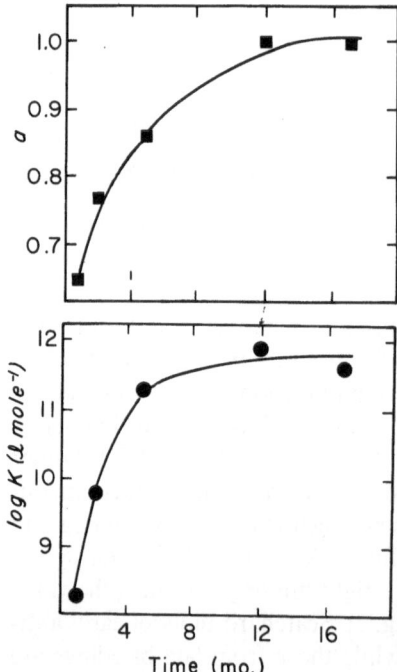

Figure 2. Behavior of the association constant and the heterogeneity index of antifluorescein antibody at different times during the immune response of a single rabbit. Both parameters increased with the duration of immunization and it was found that the binding data could always be fitted to a Sips plot. From Portmann et al. (1975).

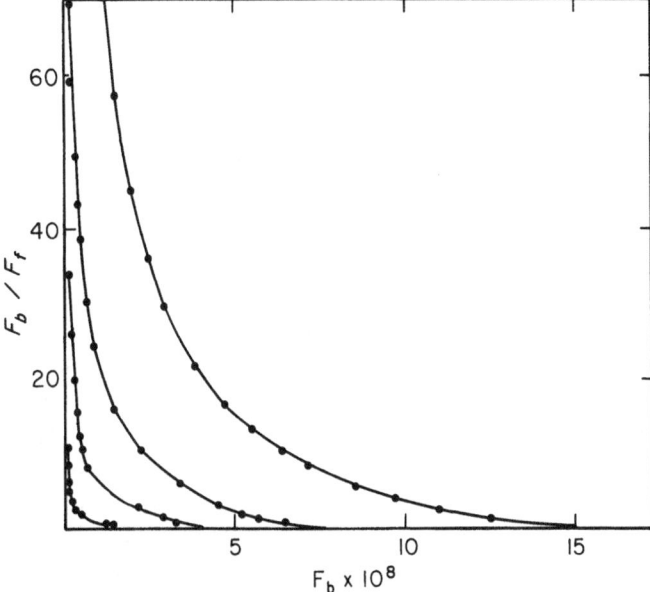

Figure 3. Scatchard plots obtained from fluorescence polarization data performed at various dilutions on an IgG preparation from an early (1 month) antifluorescein antiserum from an individual rabbit. Reaction was with free fluorescein. The strong curvature indicates a high degree of heterogeneity in this antifluorescein antibody. Dilution factors correspond to serum volumes and reading from top to bottom are $31 \times$, $61 \times$, $121 \times$, and $301 \times$. For example, in the lowermost curve, 1 ml of the Ig dilution was derived from 1/301 ml of original serum. The quenching factor, Q_f/Q_b, was 17. From Portmann et al. (1975).

Figure 4. Scatchard plots from fluorescence polarization data on different dilutions of an IgG fraction from a late bleeding (18 months) of the same rabbit as in Fig. 3. The linearity of these plots indicates the absence of binding heterogeneity over wide ranges of concentration of both hapten and antibody. Dilution factors for the curves reading from right to left are 9,000, 18,000, 36,000, and 72,000. These numbers have the same significance as those in Fig. 3. The quenching factor, Q_f/Q_b, was 17. From Portmann et al. (1975).

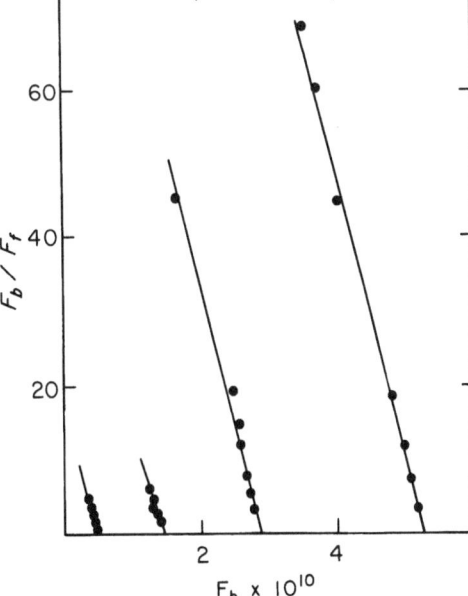

antiovalbumin. These data showed many qualitative similarities to the hapten–antibody reaction discussed above and were fitted by numerical methods to theoretical curves (Fig. 5). In the fluorescein–antifluorescein reaction, the hapten is itself also the fluorescent indicator. A different type of hapten reaction is that in which the fluorescent molecule is immuno-chemically uninvolved, but serves only to tag the hapten. Such a reaction was investigated using a penicilloyl group coupled to a fluorescein molecule via an interconnecting four-carbon chain. Equilibrium data obtained on this system indicated a relatively low binding affinity and heterogeneity in the antibody (Fig. 6).

In employing an added fluorescent label to follow a reaction, there is always a question as to what degree the native immunochemical reactivity may have been altered, either by the labeling procedure or by the mere presence of the fluorescent label. This question was studied experimentally utilizing dansyl-labeled BSA reacting with anti-BSA. To assess the effect of labeling, inhibition experiments with added native BSA were performed. In this case, the effect of labeling was found to be small: 2.7 dansyl residues per BSA molecule lowered the association constant from 3.7×10^8 M^{-1}

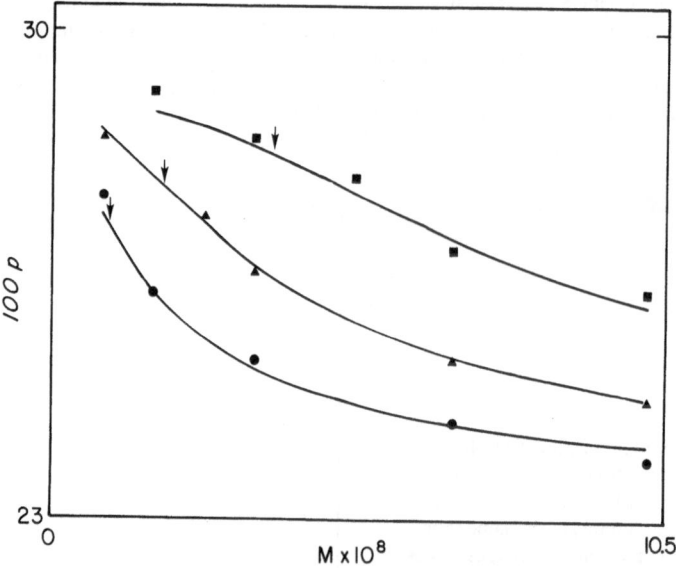

Figure 5. Titration of anti-native ovalbumin with fluorescein ovalbumin. Polarized incident light, 487 nm. Antibody protein concentration (μg/ml) calculated from precipitation with native ovalbumin. Symbols: ●, 3.3; ▲, 6.6; ■, 13.2. Vertical arrows indicate points at which the antigen–antibody ratio corresponds to that found in precipitates at maximum precipitation. Solid curves calculated from $Q_f = 4.36$; $Q_b = 3.90$; $p_f = 0.234$; $p_b = 0.293$; $K_0 = 1.83 \times 10^8$ M^{-1}; $a = 0.65$; $F_{b,\max} = 1.5 \times 10^{-8}$ M for lowest antibody concentration. From Dandliker et al. (1964).

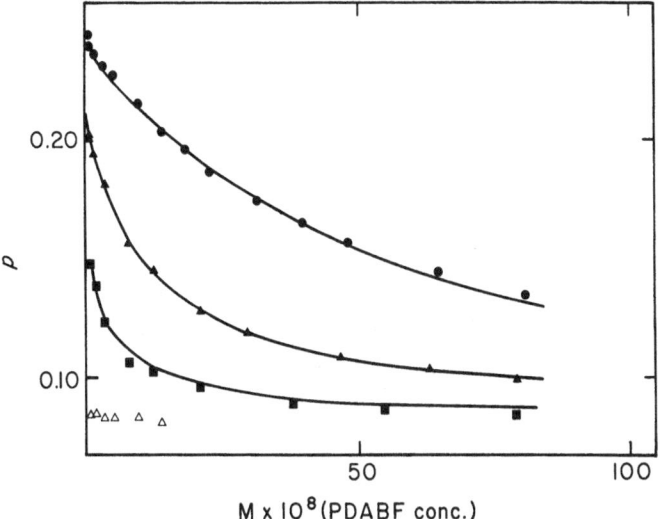

Figure 6. Fluorescence polarization titration data for rabbit anti-penicilloyl γ-globulin from a single rabbit. Symbols: ●, immune globulin, 1.2 mg/ml; ▲, immune globulin, 0.40 mg/ml; ▪, immune globulin, 0.13 mg/ml; △, normal globulin control, 0.4 mg/ml. Avidity $(K_0) = 9 \times 10^6$ M^{-1}; heterogeneity $(a) = 0.71$; antibody site concentration $(F_{b,\text{max}}$ lowest curve$) = 4.3 \times 10^{-8}$ M. From Dandliker *et al.* (1965).

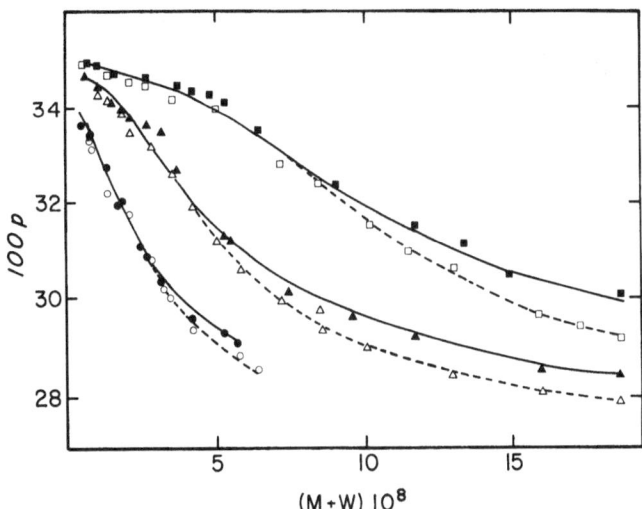

Figure 7. Fluorescence polarization data as a function of antigen concentration showing competition between dansyl-BSA and BSA for rabbit anti-BSA. Both antigens were purified by acrylamide gel electrophoresis. Closed symbols, dansyl-BSA, only; open symbols, dansyl-BSA/BSA. 1.12. Precipitable antibody concentrations were as follows: ○/●, 6.0 (AB = 1); △/▲, 12.0 (AB = 2); □/▪, 24.0 μg/ml (AB = 4). From Kierszenbaum *et al.* (1969).

for the native molecule to 2.1×10^8 M^{-1} for the labeled one. The form of the experimental curves corresponded closely with those predicted theoretically (Fig. 7).

B. Immunoassay

The application of inhibition experiments to fluorescence polarization immunoassay was investigated theoretically and experimentally (Dandliker et al., 1973). Depending upon antibody binding affinity, the sensitivity of immunoassays can readily attain the ng/ml range. The practical limit of sensitivity which may be much less than this depends upon the magnitude of the background fluorescence, e.g., in serum or serum fractions. In one example, the assay of human chorionic gonadotropin, the sensitivity was of the order of 10 ng/ml (Fig. 8).

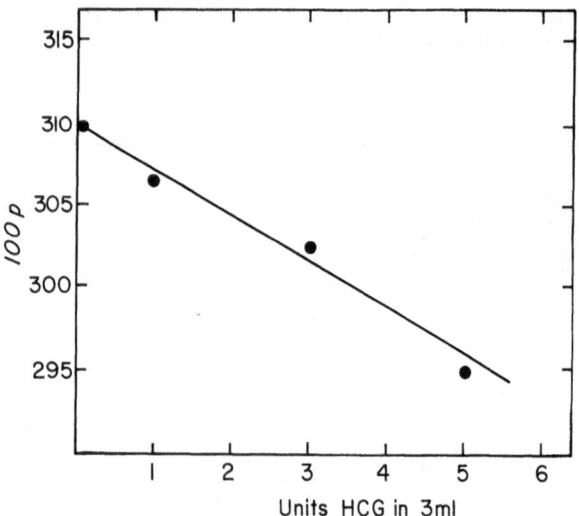

Figure 8. Standard curve for the fluorescence polarization immunoassay of human chorionic gonadotropin (HCG). The polarization, p, is shown as a function of the concentration of unlabeled (HCG) present in the final mixture. The concentration of antibody, as total γ-globulin, was held constant at 0.1 mg/ml. Van Hell et al. (1966) found that the activity of the hormone is 19,000 IU/mg. One unit of HCG is therefore 50 ng. On this basis, the concentration of fluorescein-labeled HCG (which was held constant) was 80 ng/ml. The line shown is empirical only; from its slope the sensitivity of the assay (dp/dw) is estimated to be -0.0002 ml ng^{-1}, meaning that a change of 1 ng/ml gives a polarization change of -0.0002. From Dandliker et al. (1973).

C. Determination of Reaction Order

Typical data showing the determination of reaction order with respect to ligand concentration (equation 18) and with respect to receptor concentration (equation 19) are shown for the dansyl-BSA–anti-BSA system (Figs. 9 and 10). Different ions exert vastly different effects on both the rates and order of reaction. Relatively nonchaotropic ions promote fractional order dependence upon the antibody if the antibody is divalent, while chaotropic ions lead to an order of 1 (Fig. 11). If the antibody is univalent, the antibody order is always 1, regardless of the ions present (Fig. 12). However, with both univalent and divalent antibody, chaotropic ions slow down the rate of combination. The order with respect to antigen has always been found to be 1.

D. Determination of the Forward- and Back-Reaction Rate Constants

Results on the ovalbumin–antiovalbumin reaction, utilizing equation (22), are shown in Fig. 13. Initial rate behavior for the dansyl-BSA–anti-BSA reaction is represented in Fig. 14. Tables of similar data for various systems are given in Levison *et al.* (1970).

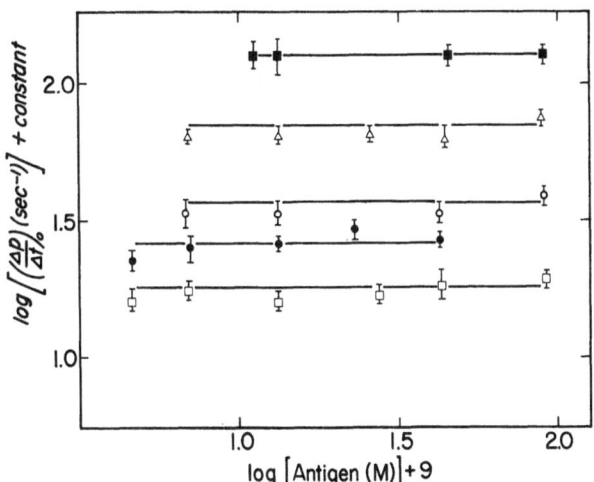

Figure 9. Determination of the order of reaction with respect to antigen for the dansyl-labeled bovine serum albumin–divalent anti-bovine serum albumin system in various ionic media at 1.5 ± 0.5 C (see equation 18). All solutions were buffered at pH 7.0. Symbols: ●, 1.0 M phosphate; ■, 0.15 M NaCl–0.01 M tris; △, 0.5 M NaF–0.01 M tris; ○, 0.5 M NaCl–0.01 M tris; □, 0.5 M NaSCN–0.01 M tris. From Levison *et al.* (1970).

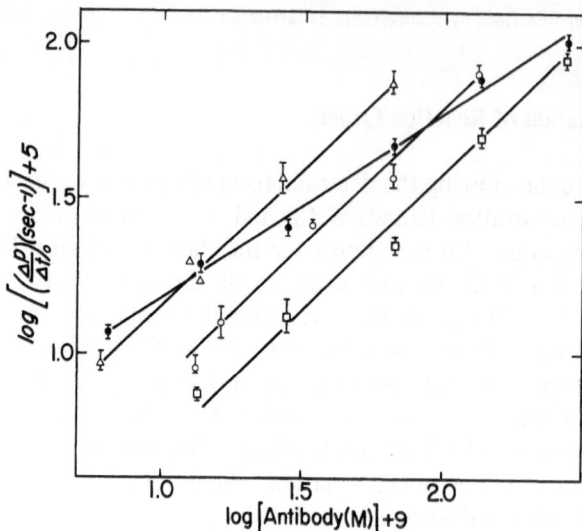

Figure 10. Determination of the order of reaction with respect to antibody concentration for the dansyl-labeled bovine serum albumin–divalent anti-bovine serum albumin system in various ionic media (see equation 19). All of the studies were performed in pH 7.0, 0.01 M tris solutions at $1.5 \pm 0.5°C$. Symbols: ●, 0.5 M NaF; ○, 0.5 M NaCl; □, 0.5 M NaSCN; △, 0.15 M NaCl. From Levison et al. (1970).

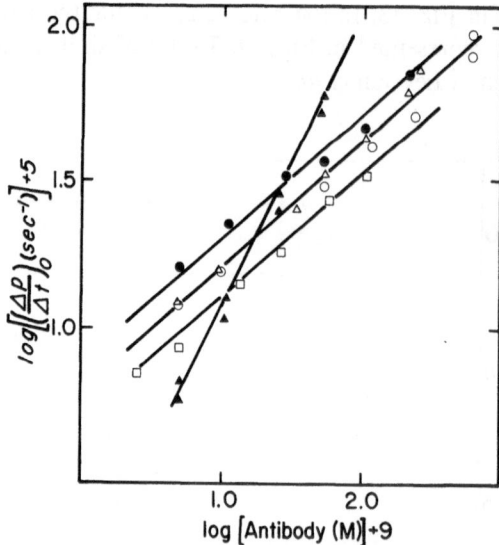

Figure 11. Effect of nonchaotropic ions on the order of reaction with respect to antibody concentration for the fluorescein-labeled ovalbumin–divalent antiovalbumin system (see equation 19). The antigen was a narrow fraction of fluorescein-labeled ovalbumin, purified on Sephadex G-100. The antibody was an IgG preparation isolated by DEAE-cellulose chromatography. Similar results were obtained with immunospecifically purified antibody (Levison and Dandliker, 1969). All of the studies were performed in pH 7.0 solutions at $1.5 \pm 0.5°C$. Symbols: ▲, 1.5 M KCl–0.01 M tris; □, 1.5 M KCl–0.1 M K_2SO_4–0.01 M tris; △, 1.5 M KF–0.01 M tris; ●, 1.5 M KCl–0.01 M K_2HPO_4–0.005 M KH_2PO_4; ○, 1.5 M KCl–0.01 M K_2HPO_4–0.05 M KH_2PO_4. From Levison et al. (1970).

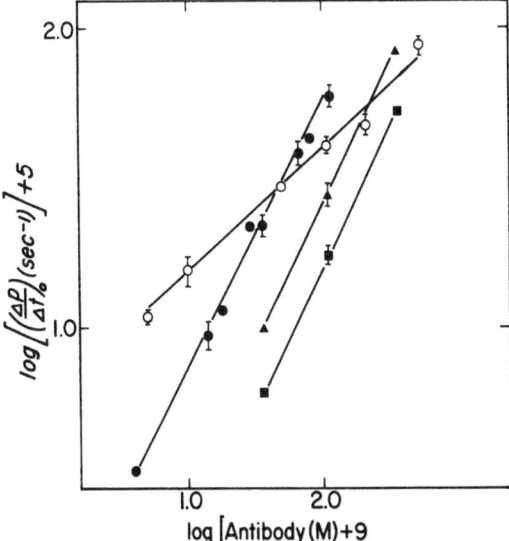

Figure 12. Initial rate behavior for the fluorescein-labeled ovalbumin–univalent antiovalbumin system in various ionic media at $1.5 \pm 0.5°C$. All solutions were buffered at pH 7.0. The order of reaction with respect to antibody concentration was determined by means of equation 19. Symbols: ●, 0.15 M NaCl–0.015 M phosphate–univalent antibody; ▲, 1.5 M KCl–0.15 M phosphate–univalent antibody; ■, 1.5 M KF–0.01 M tris–univalent antibody; ○, 1.5 M KCl–0.15 M phosphate–divalent antibody. From Levison *et al.* (1970).

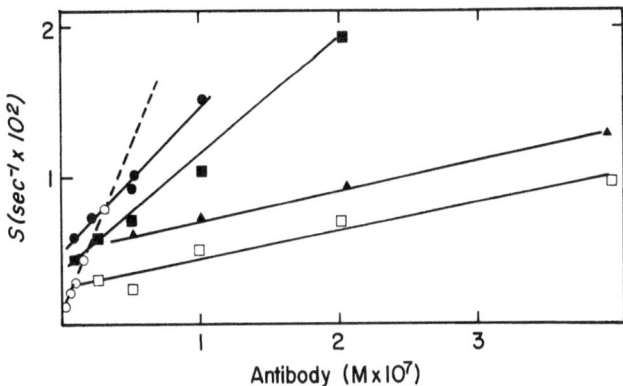

Figure 13. Plots of pseudo-first-order rate constants versus divalent antiovalbumin concentration in various ionic media. The symbol S denotes pseudo-first-order parameter, $k_1(AB) + k_{-1}/2.3$ (see equation 22). The slope and intercept of these plots yield the second-order association constant, k_1, and the first-order dissociation constant, k_{-1}, respectively, for the ovalbumin–antiovalbumin reaction. All experiments were performed in pH 7.0, 0.01 M tris at $1.5 \pm 0.5°C$. Antigen–antibody preparations were the same as those in Fig. 11. Symbols: ○, 0.15 M NaCl; ●, 1.5 M KCl; ■, 1.5 M NaCl; ▲, 1.5 M NaSCN; □, 1.5 M NaClO$_4$. From Levison *et al.* (1970).

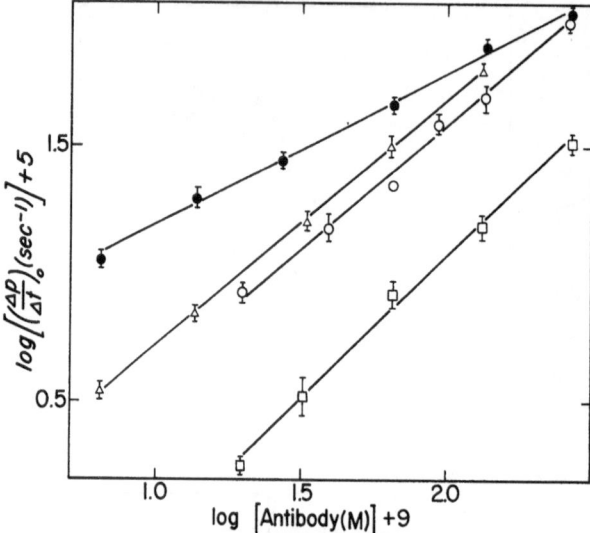

Figure 14. Initial rate behavior for the dansyl-labeled bovine serum albumin–univalent anti-bovine serum albumin system in various ionic media at $1.5 \pm 0.5°C$; $\Gamma/2 = 0.50$. All solutions were buffered at pH 7.0. The order of reaction with respect to antibody concentration was determined by means of equation (19). Symbols: ●, NaF–divalent anti-bovine serum albumin; Δ, univalent antibovine serum albumin; ○, NaCl–univalent antibovine serum albumin; □, NaSCN univalent anti-bovine serum albumin. From Levison *et al.* (1970).

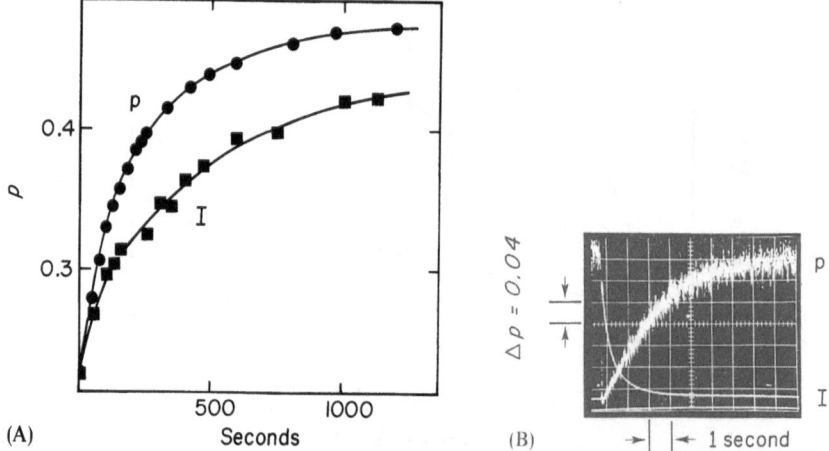

Figure 15. Kinetic polarization and intensity curves involving the primary binding of fluorescein to antifluorescein. (A) Fluorescein, 1.9×10^{-9} M, and antifluorescein, 4.2×10^{-8} M (late, uniformly binding), were hand-mixed within a few seconds in 1 M sodium salicylate–0.015 M sodium phosphate (pH 7.0) buffer at 14.5°C, and the fluorescence polarization and enhancement were monitored. The polarization, p, is in the units shown, while the intensity, I, is in arbitrary units. (B) Stopped flow trace, fluorescein, 2.5×10^{-8} M, and antifluorescein (same as in A), 2.6×10^{-8} M, were mixed in 0.15 M NaCl–0.015 M phosphate at pH 7.0 in a stopped flow device, and the fluorescence polarization, as well as the fluorescence intensity, was observed as a function of time. From Levison *et al.* (1970).

The fluorescein–antifluorescein reaction, which is much faster than the antigen–antibody reactions studied, has been investigated at very low concentrations by manual methods and at higher concentrations by stopped flow measurements (Fig. 15). Rate constants were evaluated from both intensity and polarization measurements (Fig. 16).

E. Activation Parameters

The reaction of fluorescein with antifluorescein has been studied in different ionic media as a function of temperature. In this way, effects not only on the rate constants but also on the activation parameters (activation energy and entropy) have been determined. The results are shown as bar graphs in Fig. 17.

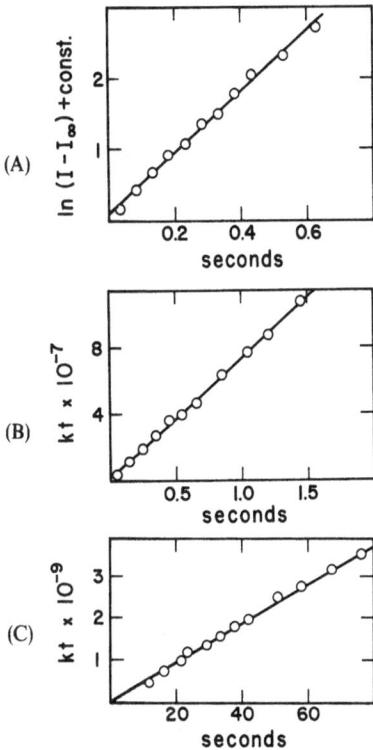

Figure 16. Representative integrated rate plots for the fluorescein–antifluorescein reaction in 0.15 M NaCl–0.015 M phosphate (pH 7.0) at 18.5°C. k = second-order rate constant (M^{-1} sec^{-1}). (A) Fluorescence quenching of fluorescein under pseudo-first-order conditions; antifluorescein (late, uniformly binding), 5.0×10^{-8} M, fluorescein, 2.9×10^{-9} M; I and I_∞ denote fluorescence intensity at times t and infinity. The pseudo-first-order rate constant k' (sec^{-1}) is obtained from the slope of the plot in (A) and equals k times the initial antibody concentration. (B) Fluorescence quenching, second-order kinetics, antifluorescein, 2.6×10^{-8} M (same as in A), fluorescein, 1.5×10^{-8} M. (C) Fluorescence polarization, second-order kinetics. Antifluorescein, 2.6×10^{-9} M (same as in A and B), fluorescein, 1.5×10^{-9} M. From Levison et al. (1975).

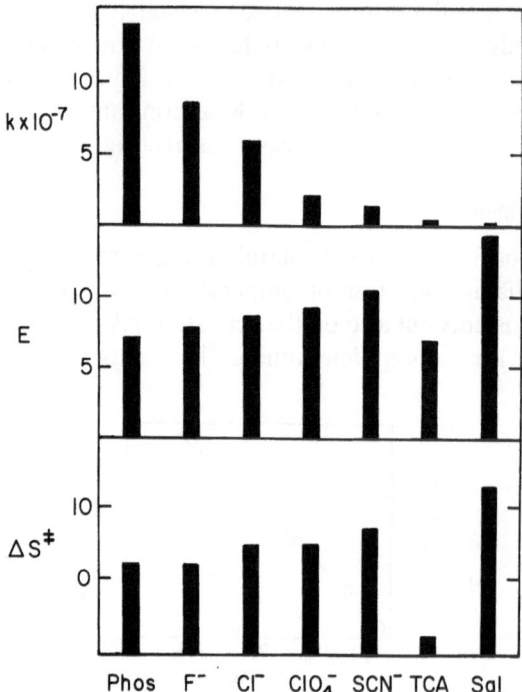

Figure 17. Salt effects on the second-order rate constant. k_1 (M^{-1} sec^{-1}), at 18.5°C, the activation energy, E_a (kcal/mole), and the activation entropy, $\Delta S^{\ddagger}$ (cal/mole deg), for the fluorescein–antifluorescein reaction. The antibody here is late and uniformly binding. Each solution contained the appropriate anion at 1.0 M concentration and was buffered with 0.015 M phosphate (pH 7.0). Phos, TCA, and Sal denote phosphate, trichloroacetate, and salicylate ions, respectively. E_a was determined from $\ln k_1$ versus $1/T$ plots, whereas $\Delta S^{\ddagger}$ was estimated from k_1 at 18.5°C and E_a, using the Eyring equations. $\ln k_1 = \ln(k^*/T/h) - (\Delta S^{\ddagger}/R) - (E_a/RT)$. From Levison *et al.* (1975).

VIII. What Has Been Learned from Fluorescence Polarization Measurements on Antigen–Antibody and Hapten–Antibody Reactions?

A. Antibody Binding Affinity and Specificity

Results of equilibrium binding measurements show that the binding affinity as measured by the association constant of antibody for antigen or hapten can vary over wide limits, perhaps from 10^6 M^{-1} at least to 10^{11} M^{-1}. The most striking example of very tightly binding antibody is that of antifluorescein, which has the highest association constant ever reported for what appears to be a univalent hapten. Since even the large binding constant of 10^{11} M^{-1} represents the free energy of interaction of only a relatively few groups, the theoretical question arises as to what is the maximum possible binding strength of an antibody for a univalent ligand. The univalency is important to keep in mind. If, for example, a divalent ligand were combining with divalent antibody, the association constant for reaction of the second ligand group with an antibody site would generally be changed considerably by the steric constraints imposed by the connection between the two groups of the ligand. This connection may lead to increased probability of reaction, if the distance between the two ends of the ligand is favorable (positive cooperativity), or to a decreased probability of reaction (negative cooperativity), if the distance between the two groups on the ligand is too small, or if the ligand is not sufficiently flexible.

In the case of the univalent ligand, it is evident that the strength of the interaction has an upper limit imposed by the nature and limited number of the various amino acid residues in the combining site regions of the H and L chains, and by the complementary groups in the ligand. As was pointed out some time ago (Karush, 1962; Dandliker et al., 1967), the predominant kinds of interactions which contribute to the stability of antigen–antibody or hapten–antibody complexes are electrostatic forces, hydrogen bonds, hydrophobic bonding, and weak dispersion forces. The free energy of interaction between the antibody site and the antigen or hapten is a net effect determined by the number and type of these interactions, which can be brought into play as the interacting molecules collide, stick, and then slowly rearrange to give the complex of minimum free energy. From a very basic viewpoint, all such possible interactions are completely determined by the time-averaged, three-dimensional distribution of electron density in the antibody site and in the complementary determinant group. These distributions have some particular form in the isolated reactants where the determinant group and the antibody combining site are in contact with solvent molecules and ions. It is almost axiomatic that when combination between antigen or hapten and antibody takes place both distributions will accommodate to the new environment in which solvent and ions are gradually pressed out as the complementary groups come into close contact, allowing the entire structure to relax to the equilibrium configuration of minimum free energy. As an example of how these principles may apply, we have found that high-affinity antifluorescein ($K \sim 10^{10}$ to 10^{11}) shows no measurable tendency to combine with rhodamine B, even at 5×10^{-5} M antibody (Levison et al., 1975). The structure of fluorescein differs from that of rhodamine mostly in the presence of the negatively charged phenoxide ion and the quinoidlike oxygen, which produce peaks in the local and hence specific electron density distribution. At the geometrically corresponding locations in rhodamine, the negative peaks have disappeared and have, perhaps, even become valleys (at the positively charged diethylammonium group). At first it might seem unreasonable to attribute such importance to the charge of one or two electrons in the face of the background electron density, but it must be kept in mind that monopolar forces are very much more important than dipolar or multipolar forces, and can so exert overwhelming effects. In antifluorescein, for example, such groups as ε-amino or guanidino would be expected in positions complementary to the negative regions on the fluorescein molecule, while in antirhodamine there are probably negatively charged regions corresponding to the positive regions on rhodamine. This is not to say that other types of interactions, especially hydrophobic bonding, are unimportant. Hydrophobic interactions contributing to the free energy via entropy terms are present in all regions of contact between organic molecules and in the absence of large energy terms (e.g., those due to monopolar fields) may then necessarily emerge as the predominant type of interaction. Still it is the topography of electron density that determines not only electric field effects but also all the other types of interaction. In other words, the strength of interaction of an antigenic or hapten determinant with antibody is determined by the electronic topography of the interacting partners, and it is in the complexity of the pattern of this topography, together with the magnitudes of the interactions achieved, that antibody specificity resides.

B. Antibody "Maturation" during the Immune Response

The immunochemical parameters of antifluorescein antibody have been followed by both equilibrium and kinetic measurements over more than a year of immunization (Portmann et al., 1971, 1975, Levison et al., 1971, 1975). At the early stages of immunization (2–3 months), the antibody is of low affinity and is very heterogeneous. This type of antibody was first investigated by Dandliker et al. (1964) and then by Lopatin and Voss (1971). After a year of immunization, the binding affinity has risen to a plateau, and the antibody is uniformly binding, as evidenced by linear Scatchard plots over wide ranges of concentration. This maturation process is explained rationally on the basis that only one or a very few clones of B cells are being stimulated by virtue of the small immunizing and booster doses of antigen. Only those clones of high affinity finally can respond, since, as the concentration of high-affinity antibody rises, the concentration of antigen available for stimulation becomes less and less. However, tight-binding antibodies from different rabbits are not necessarily of the same structure. This was realized when it was found that the extent of quenching of the fluorescein fluorescence by antibody could be markedly different from rabbit to rabbit, even though all the binding affinities were about the same (10^{11} M^{-1}). These differences show that high binding affinities can be achieved by more than one unique amino acid sequence in the H and L chains, and probably reflect genetic differences in the immune response in the outbred rabbits used. It would be most interesting to repeat similar experiments with highly inbred animals. To what extent the observations on antifluorescein are general for antibody to other determinants is not known. However, it is reasonably certain that determinants lacking ionic or highly polar atomic groupings are incapable of exciting antibody of very high binding affinity, since in those cases only hydrophobic interactions and dispersion forces could be operative.

C. Effects of Fluorescent Labeling upon Immunochemical Reactivity

In principle, the addition of a fluorescent label to a molecule must necessarily alter its chemical and physical properties, and in particular its ability to react with antibody. The important question is not whether the effect exists, but how large it is. In one case, the effect of label has been carefully studied, and the results showed that the presence of about three dansyl groups per BSA molecule lowered the association constant for reaction with anti-BSA to about one-half the value of that for the native molecule. This difference is not much greater than the uncertainty in K imposed by experimental error. The method used to measure the effect of dansyl labeling involved quantitative inhibition measurements interpreted by means of equations (14) and (15). Other approaches to assessing the effect of label could also be used. For example, the immunochemical reactivity as measured by the association constant could be measured as a function of the degree of labeling and then an empirical extrapolation to zero label could be made. In all systems thus far studied, there has been no case in which fluorescent labeling was found to have a large effect on the reaction being studied, except of course in the case of antifluorescein reacting with fluorescein, where the label and the hapten are the same. In this case, the combination with antibody gives rise not only to an increase in polarization but also to a drastic decrease in fluorescence yield.

D. Why Does Antifluorescein Quench the Fluorescence of Fluorescein?

As pointed out in Sections VIIIB and VIIIC, antifluorescein antibodies all show large quenching effects on the fluorescence of fluorescein. In other cases when the fluorescent label is not a part of the immune reaction, minimal quenching or enhancement effects are present. An explanation of the large quenching effect observed in the fluorescein–antifluorescein reaction was offered by Lopatin and Voss (1971). They suggested that the decrease was due to the low dielectric constant of the antibody site or to the close positioning of the ligand with amino acid residues leading to nonfluorescent loss of the electronic excitation energy. The latter explanation amounts essentially to paraphrasing the observation.

It would seem more likely that the quenching effect has to do with interaction of the ionized form of the fluorescein molecule with ionic and polar groups in the antibody site. This type of interaction would be expected to produce partial neutralization of the electric fields on the fluorescein molecule, e.g., at the phenoxide ion and the quinoid oxygen by the antibody (see Section VIIIA). It follows that groups which strongly interact will tend to produce a partial neutralization of any electric fields present. In the fluorescein molecule, this could produce quenching in much the same way as does the addition of protons to the ionized form of the molecule.

The role of low dielectric constant can be perhaps better interpreted as follows: that in media of low dielectric constant, electrostatic interactions are stronger and hence protons would tend to bind to the ionizing groups of fluorescein, thus producing the un-ionized, relatively nonfluorescent form. Fluorescein probably owes its strong fluorescence to the symmetry of the two extreme resonance forms of the molecule; that is, the electron normally denoted by the negative charge on the phenoxide oxygen is strongly delocalized. When this molecule is put into a medium of low dielectric constant, the consequent increase in the strength of electrostatic interactions will tend to protonate one of the oxygens, but not both, since to do so would then produce a cation. Thus the symmetry of the molecule is lost, the electron becomes localized, and the fluorescence disappears. As is well known, if fluorescein is put into strongly acidic media a symmetrical cationic structure is formed by protonation of both oxygens. This structure shows a bluish fluorescence, reflecting restoration of the symmetry. All of these arguments, while rational, touch upon the basic mechanisms involved in the nonfluorescent loss of the electronic excitation energy only at a superficial level.

E. The Mechanism of Antigen–Antibody and Hapten–Antibody Reactions

A variety of lines of evidence indicates that antigen–antibody and hapten–antibody reactions consist of a primary collision, probably diffusion controlled, an incipient adhesion of the two molecules at one or a few points, and then a rearrangement to give the stable primary complex. The simplest type of evidence, and probably the least convincing, that immunochemical reactions are not diffusion controlled is that the magnitudes of the forward rate constants are considerable and significantly smaller than the theoretical values. For the ovalbumin–antiovalbumin reaction, the forward rate constant was found to be 2×10^5 M sec^{-1}. The value, estimated from Smoluchowski's equation, is 1.7×10^7 M sec^{-1}, even after insertion of a reaction probability factor of 3×10^{-3} to take care of nonfruitful collisions due to unfavorable molecular orientations. It seems very unlikely that the difference of a factor of nearly 100 can be due to inadequacies in the theory. The experimental error in k is probably not more than 30% at most, and the conclusion is that the reaction is not diffusion controlled (Dandliker and Levison, 1968). Originally, it was believed that hapten–antihapten reactions were diffusion controlled, or nearly so, on the basis of the small activation energies observed in the DNP system (Day et al., 1963).

The idea that hapten–antibody and antigen–antibody reactions are, in fact, not diffusion controlled is supported by several other types of evidence. One of the most dramatic of these deals with specific ionic effects on both hapten–antibody and antigen–antibody reactions. These ionic effects are correlated with the position of the ion in the Hofmeister or chaotropic series (Hamaguchi and Geiduschek, 1962; Dandliker and de Saussure, 1971). The effects include both a change in the rate of the forward reaction and, in some cases, a change in the rate law. Strongly chaotropic ions such as thiocyanate and perchlorate decrease the forward rate constant, as compared, say, to chloride, while ions at the other end of the series, such as fluoride and phosphate, tend to increase the forward rates. However, reactions involving univalent and divalent antibody can be affected quite differently by specific ions (Levison et al., 1970). In the case of divalent antiovalbumin reacting with fluorescein-labeled ovalbumin, the presence of nonchaotropic ions produces a rate law depending upon a fractional (~ 0.5–1) power of the antibody concentration. In chaotropic media, the dependence is upon the first power of divalent antibody concentration, as it is for univalent Fab fragments in all media examined. In the case of the antifluorescein reaction, however, no fractional orders of reaction have ever been observed. Also, in none of the systems have fractional power dependencies ever been observed for antigen or hapten concentration (Levison et al., 1975). The fractional order behavior was explained theoretically on the basis of an encounter pair mechanism, in which antigen and antibody are in rapid equilibrium with a loose encounter pair, which in turn slowly rearranges to the final stable complex (Levison and Dandliker, 1969). A necessary condition for this type of mechanism to produce a fractional order rate law is that the sites involved in the formation of the encounter pair are nonuniform and have, for example, a Sips distribution of binding free energies (Levison and Dandliker, 1969). Why then, is it that fractional orders are found only with divalent antibody, and then only in very nonchaotropic media? This question has not yet been fully answered, but it may be that the observed effects have to do with folded conformations of the divalent antibody molecule, and that in chaotropic media, the molecule is more unfolded; no fractional orders have ever been observed with Fab. Also, weakly binding sites are inhibited from reaction in chaotropic media, so that the distribution of binding affinities should be consequently sharpened. The absence of fractional order dependencies in the fluorescein–antifluorescein system may also be due to the fact that the antibody most studied is uniformly binding and hence lacks one of the essential characteristics to give fractional order.

F. Specific Ionic Effects on Reaction Rates and Activation Parameters

As mentioned in Section VIIIE, highly chaotropic ions decrease the forward rate of reaction by as much as 3 orders of magnitude. An explanation of this effect can be given in terms of two apparently different but somewhat equivalent concepts (Levison et al., 1975). One is that the formation of the transition state involves solvent reorganization and loss; the importance of these factors in antigen–antibody reactions was pointed out long ago by Haurowitz (1952). If the activated complex is less solvated than the isolated reactants, then ions which compete more effectively for water molecules will tend to promote the reaction. This is what is observed experimentally. Anions with high charge densities, such as fluoride and phosphate, tend to enhance the reaction rate, while anions with low charge densities (thiocyanate and perchlorate) lower the forward rate of reaction. The same effects can be discussed using the second concept, that of hydrophobic bonding. Highly chaotropic ions render hydrophobic interactions weaker (Dandliker and de Saussure, 1971). If such interactions are involved in the formation of the transition state, then the rate of the forward reaction will be lowered in chaotropic media, which is what is observed. Effects such as binding of chaotropic ions to the reactants themselves, with a consequent change in the free energy of activation, would give similar results and cannot presently be ruled out.

The above considerations tie in with the well-known "dissociating" effect of chaotropic media on antigen–antibody complexes (Dandliker et al., 1967). The presence of chaotropic ions impedes the process of combination, but has relatively little effect on the rate of dissociation of antigen–antibody complexes (Levison et al., 1970). Probably the same is true of hapten–antihapten complexes in view of the common difficulty encountered in attempting to dissociate high avidity hapten–antihapten complexes. The molecular picture suggested by these phenomena is that chaotropic ions can act primarily only when reactants are separated. However, once they are firmly bound, and solvent and ions have been squeezed out, there is no obvious means by which the chaotropic ions can exert a direct effect. Obviously, an effect on the forward rate alone is sufficient to produce an observed lowering of the equilibrium constant. The effects of chaotropic ions on hydrophobic bonding are superimposed on the weakening of hydrogen bonds and electrostatic interactions which would be produced nonspecifically by high concentrations of any ion. Specific ion effects on the activation energy and entropy give a type of insight into immuno-chemical reactions which has not been hitherto available for any macro-molecular reaction. The essential findings are shown in Fig. 17. First, the forward rates decrease monotonically in the order: phosphate $> F^- > Cl^- > ClO_4^- > SCN^- >$ salicylate. In the same order of ions, the activation energies increase, which indicates that it is energetically more difficult to form the transition state complex in strongly chaotropic media than in less chaotropic media. This fact, perhaps, argues for the picture involving solvent loss from ionic and polar groups, which could invoke energetic terms rather than hydrophobic bonding alone, which should be mainly entropic. The effects on the activation entropies fit more logically into the hydrophobic bond concept. All the entropies are positive, although some are near zero. They increase with the same order of the ions previously mentioned. Since the entropy change in introducing nonpolar groups into water is negative, the positive entropies would seem to correspond to transfer of nonpolar groups of the hapten or antibody out of water before the activated complex can form. The signs of the contributions of the energy and entropy to the free energy of activation are in opposite directions, if interpreted in the context of the Eyring equation; the increasing entropies tend to make it faster. The behavior of trichloroacetate seems atypical, in that the activation energy is lower than anticipated on the basis of the observed rate, but the activation entropy is lower than in any other ion tested, and is in fact negative instead of positive. Various *ad hoc* explanations could be offered, but there is no clear criterion for choosing, at present, the correct one. Perhaps the most constructive attitude is to emphasize the need for more work on the effects of solvent and ion environments on the activation parameters of macromolecular reactions.

G. Manipulation of the Binding Affinity of Antibody by Changing Either the Forward- or Backward-Rate Constants of the Binding Reaction

As the antibody maturation process discussed in Section VIIIB proceeds, measurements of the forward rate constants show but little change, with time of immunization, while the equilibrium constant changes by several orders of magnitude (Portmann *et al.*, 1975; Levison *et al.*, 1975).

The conclusion is clear that it is the rate constant for dissociation that is decreasing and it is this decrease that is intimately related to the increase in strength of the hapten–antibody interaction.

In contrast, the effect of chaotropic ions discussed in Section VIIIF is mainly to influence the forward rate constant (Levison *et al.*, 1970). A logical explanation of this effect already given is that the influence of the medium is most effective as combination occurs and as the medium is squeezed out. Once formed, the complex is relatively unresponsive to changes in medium, since it is then essentially absent from the locale of the bonds binding the antigen or hapten to the antibody molecule.

ACKNOWLEDGMENTS

This work was supported by Research Grant No. GB-31611 from the National Science Foundation. The author wishes to express his gratitude to colleagues whose efforts have helped to make this review possible. especially Dr. Stuart Levison, Dr. Anton Portmann, and Dr. Felipe Kierszenbaum.

IX. References

Belford, G. G., Belford, R. L., and Weber, G., 1972, *Proc. Natl. Acad. Sci. U.S.A.* **69**:1392.

Chuang, T. J., and Eisenthal, K. B., 1972, *J. Chem. Phys.* **57**:5094.

Dandliker, W. B., 1971, in: *Methods in Immunology and Immunochemistry,* Vol. III (C. A. Williams and M. W. Chase, eds.), p. 435, Academic Press, New York.

Dandliker, W. B., and de Saussure, V. A., 1970, *Immunochemistry* **7**:799.

Dandliker, W. B., and de Saussure, V. A., 1971, in: *The Chemistry of Biosurfaces,* Vol. I (M. L. Hair, ed.), p. 1, Dekker, New York.

Dandliker, W. B., and Levison, S. A., 1968, *Immunochemistry* **5**:171.

Dandliker, W. B., Schapiro, H. C., Meduski, J. W., Alonso, R., Feigen, G. A., and Hamrick, J. R., Jr., 1964, *Immunochemistry* **1**:165.

Dandliker, W. B., Halbert, S. P., Florin, M. C., Alonso, R., and Schapiro, H. C., 1965, *J. Exp. Med.* **122**:1029.

Dandliker, W. B., Alonso, R., de Saussure, V. A., Kierszenbaum, F., Levison, S. A., and Schapiro, H. C., 1967, *Biochemistry* **6**:1460.

Dandliker, W. B., Kelly, R. J., Dandliker, J., Farquhar, J., and Levin, J., 1973, *Immunochemistry* **10**:219.

Day, L. A., Sturtevant, J. M., and Singer, S. J., 1963, *Ann. N.Y. Acad. Sci.* **103**:611.

Gafni, A., and Steinberg, I. Z., 1972, *Photochem. Photobiol.* **15**:93.

Hamaguchi, K., and Geiduschek, E. P., 1962, *J. Am. Chem. Soc.* **84**:1329.

Haurowitz, F., 1952, *Biol. Rev. Cambridge Philos. Soc.* **27**:247.

Holowka, D. A., Strosberg, A. D., Kimball, J. W., Haber, E., and Cathou, R. E., 1972, *Proc. Nat. Acad. Sci. U.S.A.* **69**:3399.

Karush, F., 1962, *Adv. Immunol.* **2**:1.

Kelly, R. J., Dandliker, W. B., and Williamson, D. E., 1976, *Anal. Chem.* **48**:846.

Kierszenbaum, F., Dandliker, J., and Dandliker, W. B., 1969, *Immunochemistry* **6**:125.

Levison, S. A., and Dandliker, W. B., 1969, *Immunochemistry* **6**:253.

Levison, S. A., Kierszenbaum, F., and Dandliker, W. B., 1970, *Biochemistry* **9**:322.

Levison, S. A., Portmann, A. J., Kierszenbaum, F., and Dandliker, W. B., 1971, *Biochem. Biophys. Res. Comm.* **43**:258.

Levison, S. A., Hicks, A. N., Portmann, A. J., and Dandliker, W. B., 1975, *Biochemistry* **14**:3778.

Lopatin, D. E., and Voss, E. D., 1971, *Biochemistry* **10**:208.

Mavis, D., Schapiro, H. C., and Dandliker, W. B., 1974, *Anal. Biochem.* **61**:528.

Pilz, I., Kratky, O., Licht, A., and Sela, M., 1973, *Biochemistry* **12**:4998.

Pollet, R., and Edelhoch, H., 1974, *J. Biol. Chem.* **249**:5188.

Portmann, A. J., Levison, S. A., and Dandliker, W. B., 1975, *Immunochemistry* **12**:461.

Schlessinger, J., and Steinberg, I. Z., 1972, *Proc. Natl. Acad. Sci. U.S.A.* **69**:769.

Tao, T., 1969, *Biopolymers* **8**:609.

Van Hell, H., Goverde, B. C., Schuurs, A. H. W. M., De Jager, E., Matthijsen, R., and Homan, J. D. H., 1966, *Nature (London)* **212**:261.

Weber, G., 1971, *J. Chem. Phys.* **55**:2399.

Yguerabide, J., 1972, in: *Methods in Enzymology* Vol. XXVI (C. H. W. Hirs and S. N. Timasheff, eds.), p. 498, Academic Press, New York.

4

In Vitro Immune Responses of Lymphoid Cell Populations to Proteins and Peptides

Abram B. Stavitsky

I. Introduction

A. Scope

A great deal of valuable information about the immune response has been obtained through studies employing hapten–protein and synthetic peptide systems. Relatively less is known about the immune response to the determinants on proteins. Therefore, in the context of this volume, this chapter considers selected aspects of recent *in vitro* studies of immune responses to proteins *per se*—or as carriers for haptens—and to the peptides derived from these proteins. Some genetic, cellular, and molecular aspects of the cooperation of T and B lymphocytes, macrophages, and dendritic-type cells in the induction and maintenance of the antibody response to proteins are stressed. Also summarized are the antibody, proliferative, and differentiative responses and the generation of macrophage inhibitory factor—an *in vitro* correlate of cellular immunity—upon addition of peptides to lymphoid cells from animals immunized previously with the native proteins from which these peptides were derived. The section on regulation focuses upon the newly emergent findings on the nonspecific modulation of the antibody response by heterologous antigens and by cyclic nucleotides. Finally, the discussion section attempts to put these observations into perspective, and, with broad

Abram B. Stavitsky · Department of Microbiology, School of Medicine, Case Western Reserve University, Cleveland, Ohio 44106.

brush strokes, to paint the rather impressionistic picture of the antibody response that is possible with the available limited infromation about detailed mechanisms.

In vitro observations are emphasized because of the many advantages of this approach over studies in intact animals, including more ready analysis of cellular and/or molecular mechanisms, better contact of antigen with the cellular and molecular elements of the immune response, absence of cell traffic into and out of the lymphoid organ, and less catabolism of antigen–antibody complexes. However, because of the many artifactual potentialities of *in vitro* systems, the *in vitro* observations are compared with data obtained from studies in intact animals. Also, for completion of the picture and for comparison the immune responses to particulate antigens such as foreign erythrocytes and to synthetic peptides are sometimes described.

B. Historical

The recent explosion of new information and ideas has revolutionized immunology and turned it into one of the most exciting fields of modern molecular and biological investigation. This explosion was sparked by the development of much new knowledge about the structure and function of antigens and antibodies; the genetic control of immunoglobulin structure; the phylogeny and ontogeny, morphology, and ultrastructure of lymphoid cells; protein and nucleic acid syntheses and inhibitors of these processes. Until 8 years ago, studies of the antibody response *in vitro* were limited to observations on the continued antibody synthesis that was initiated *in vivo*. Then Dutton and Mishell (1967) developed a dissociated mouse lymphoid cell system for inducing a primary antibody response to foreign erythrocytes, utilizing the newly developed plaque methods (Ingraham, 1963; Jerne and Nordin, 1963) for enumerating antibody-forming cells. With this system, they were able to obtain additional evidence for the importance of cell proliferation in the antibody response. At about the same time, Marbrook (1967) developed another culture technique and Diener (1968) developed another method for enumerating antibody-forming cells which were employed by Feldmann (1972a) to analyze the primary antibody response to dinitrophenyl-flagellin. Many investigations (e.g., Claman *et al.*, 1966; Davies *et al.*, 1967; Miller and Mitchell, 1967; Mitchison, 1971) then established the requirement for the cooperation of T and B lymphocytes in the induction of the antibody response. Later significant developments include reagents and techniques for identifying and separating T- and B-cell populations, the development of systems and methods for demonstrating the genetic control of the immune response to certain determinants, and, finally, the studies of specific and nonspecific regulation of the antibody response.

Perhaps, the most promising development to date of the new molecular immunology is the isolation of many soluble factors—too many and in too crude a form at this time—that can induce many of the inductive and regulatory events of the antibody response.

II. *In Vitro* Consequences of the Reaction of Proteins or Peptides with Lymphoid Cell Populations

Parts A, B, and C of this section deal with some cellular events that occur following the reaction of proteins and/or peptides with the various cells involved in the antibody response. Some of these events are of interest because they may provide clues to the sequence of mechanisms whereby the superficial binding of antigen to cell receptors leads to the expression of the genetic information for antibody synthesis. Part D deals with events and mechanisms that appear to be related to the regulation, i.e., the enhancement and/or suppression of the antibody reponse, including both specific and nonspecific mechanisms. The relationship of the inductive events to the regulatory ones is obscure, but, because there is some evidence that inductive and regulatory phenomena are at least partially separable, they are discussed separately.

A. Cellular Events, Requirements, and Kinetics of Responses to Proteins

The separation of Part A, into subparts 1, 2, etc., is artificial, because these events merge into one another temporally and sometimes almost imperceptibly. However, their separation permits consideration of many separate questions, such as the nature and specificity of cell receptors and the possible relation of each event to the induction of antibody synthesis.

1. Antigen Binding

The study of antigen is of interest since it relates to the nature and function of the receptors on the various cells involved in the antibody response. There is considerable evidence that the antigen-binding receptor on the B lymphocyte is immunoglobulin in nature and may belong to one of several classes of immunoglobulins, including at least IgM, IgG, and IgD (Vitetta and Uhr, 1975a,b). There is much indirect evidence for the presence of specific receptors on T lymphocytes (Roelants and Askonas, 1971), but the nature of this receptor is still the subject of controversy, one group providing evidence that it is also an immunoglobulin, a monomeric IgM of molecular weight about 180,000 (Cone and Marchalonis, 1974), and the other group supporting the theory that T cells either lack surface immunoglobulin or display so little that it is undetectable (Vitetta *et al.*, 1972; Grey *et al.*, 1972). The resolution of this argument is complicated by the finding that, at least occasionally, much of surface immunoglobulin on T cells may be of exogenous origin (Hudson *et al.*, 1974).

The question of whether the receptor on lymphocytes is uni- or multispecific is still unsettled. DeLuca *et al.* (1974) determined the median frequency of antigen-binding cells for β-galactosidase (GZ) in mouse organs as thymus 0.1%, lymph nodes 3.5%, spleen 2.0%, and bone marrow 4.8%. They presented evidence that this binding is specific and that it involves specific receptors for this antigen. They attributed the relatively high frequencies to the incubation of the cells with saturating concentrations of antigen, the multimeric nature of this enzyme, and the retention of receptors by fixation. They concluded that the high frequency of antigen-binding cells is not consistent with a model of unispecificity in precursor cells of either the T- or B-cell lines.

Decker *et al.* (1974a) found that 0.3–1.4% of the cells from the lymphoid organs of germ-free, colostrum-deprived piglets bound GZ specifically. They speculated that these cells acquired their specificity spontaneously, before contact with GZ. They also considered these data consistent with the view that some cells may bind antigens of more than one specificity; i.e., some cells may have receptors of more than one specificity. Indeed, in another study (Decker *et al.*, 1974b), the presence of antigen-binding cells for GZ, keyhole limpet hemocyanin, horse spleen ferritin, horseradish peroxidase, and ovalbumin was noted at the onset of lymphoid development, i.e., by half term in mouse, rabbit, and chick embryos. Binding was by immunoglobulinlike receptors, as it was inhibited by anti-immunoglobulin sera. Moreover, a proportion of the cells bound two different antigens noncompetitively. These findings were interpreted as evidence for the presence of the relevant genes in the germ line.

Antigen-binding experiments utilizing polymerized flagellin (POL) and the phenomenon of capping support the conclusion that all of the immunoglobulin on B lymphocytes is specific for POL (see Section IIA3).

2. Handling of Antigen by Macrophages

There is much evidence that macrophages are required for the induction of the antibody response to many, if not most, antigens (Unanue, 1972). However, the nature of the role played by this cell type is still obscure. The possible role played by soluble factors produced by these cells is discussed in Section III. Here attention is focused on the nature of the reactions that occur between antigens and macrophages. Elsewhere, the interactions of macrophages with T and/or B lymphocytes is considered (Section IIA4).

The uptake and trapping of antigen in lymphoid organs is strictly correlated with its immunogenicity (Unanue, 1972). Thus highly polymerized proteins are highly immunogenic and monomeric proteins less so; the former are trapped more efficiently than the latter. Most trapping in these sites is accomplished by macrophages. A variety of antigens when bound to macrophages are more highly immunogenic *in vivo* or *in vitro* than the same antigen in soluble form (Katz and Unanue, 1973).

There is much interest in identifying the process whereby macrophage-bound antigen is produced and in determining its fate, especially in relation to its immunogenicity (Unanue, 1972; Unanue and Calderon, 1975). The initial event is the binding of the antigen to the cell surface membrane. Most of the antigen is then rapidly interiorized and degraded by lysosomes; there is an early phase of rapid degradation having a half-life of 0.5–2 hr and a later, slow phase with a half-life of 8–22 hr. From 1 to 10% of large protein molecules such as hemocyanin persisted on the plasma membrane for a period with a half-life of more than 24hr, while smaller molecules like albumins tended to disappear more rapidly. At least the surface-bound hemocyanin could be utilized to induce antibody synthesis in a lymphocyte culture. Removal of the surface antigen by trypsinization abolished most immunogenicity of some macrophage-bound protein immunogens (Unanue and Cerottini, 1970). Calderon and Unanue (1974) found that hemocyanin and rabbit IgG can be released from the interior of murine macrophages following interiorization. Their evidence suggests that the released antigen is derived from intracellular vesicles. The molecular size of the released proteins was smaller than that of the native molecules; most immunogen did not react with antibody to native protein, indicating that most of it had lost its native conformation. Nevertheless, some of the released hemocyanin was still immunogenic. However, they concluded that further study is required to assess the significance of the released molecules in the induction of the antibody response. Certainly, in view of the important role of steric conformation in the antigenic and immunogenic specificity of proteins and of synthetic polypeptides (Sela, 1969), no significant degradation by proteolytic enzymes may occur between the time an immunogen is introduced and when it is recognized by the cells involved in the antibody response.

Fishman (1961) and Fishman and Adler (1963) reported that RNA isolated from peritoneal exudate cells exposed to T2 phage induced lymphocytes to produce neutralizing antibody for this phage; neither the phage *per se* nor RNA extracts of macrophages alone induced antibody. On the basis of this type of evidence, it was concluded that for a particulate structure such as a phage to be immunogenic it had somehow to be "processed" by macrophages. Subsequently, antigen or fragments of antigen were found in association with RNA isolated from macrophages that had taken up tobacco mosaic virus, has induced patching and capping *in vitro* and patch-hemocyanin (Askonas and Rhodes, 1965) or T2 phage (Friedman *et al.*, 1965). The authors of these studies ascribed the immunogenicity of these RNA preparations to their antigenic content, but more recent observations on the immunogenicity of RNA extracted from macrophages exposed to antigens are not explicable merely on the basis of an RNA–antigen complex (Adler *et al.*, 1966; Bell and Dray, 1970). The significance of the latter observations is still the subject of much controversy. A monograph by Friedman (1973) reviews many old and new aspects of this controversy without resolving it.

3. Lymphocyte Surface Events

Cell membranes were long considered rigid structures. However, recent findings suggest that the cell membrane is a dynamic envelope or fluid mosaic (Singer and Nicolson, 1972). These findings include the lymphocyte surface membrane. Thus anti-immunoglobulin antibody reacts with this membrane on B cells to induce the movement of immunoglobulin molecules to form a polar "cap" (Taylor *et al.*, 1971; Unanue *et al.*, 1972). This movement is preceded by the formation of aggregates or patches of variable sizes on the cell surface, a temperature- but not energy-dependent step (Loor, *et al.*, 1972; Raff and de Petris, 1973). At about the time of capping, the translational motility of the cell is increased (Unanue *et al.*, 1974). The redistribution of immunoglobulin is followed by pinocytosis of the aggregates near the Golgi apparatus, with subsequent partial degradation of the membrane immunoglobulin molecules (Taylor *et al.*, 1971; Engers and Unanue, 1973). Capping, stimulation of translation, and internalization are both temperature and energy dependent. It has been proposed that the movement of these complexes on the cell surface may be the result of some form of cell surface "activity," perhaps in the form of "waves" or "membrane" flow" (Unanue *et al.*, 1974). Immunoglobulin receptor movement was dependent on crosslinkage by a bivalent ligand, since bivalent F(ab)2, but not monovalent Fab', fragments of anti-immunoglobulin induced capping (Taylor *et al.*, 1971).

More relevant than the induction of capping in response to antibody against immunoglobulin would be the induction of similar events by the binding of antigen to these immunoglobulin molecules. It has been found that multivalent conjugates of dinitrophenylated bovine serum albumin (DNP_8-BSA), but not monovalent conjugates (DNP_1-BSA), cause capping on living lymphocytes (Taylor *et al.*, 1971). Another highly polymeric antigen, tobacco mosaic virus, has induced patching and capping *in vitro* and patching *in vivo* (Loor *et al.*, 1972). In view of the requirement for bivalent anti-immunoglobulin reagents to cause receptor capping, Diener and Langman (1975) have raised the question of whether or not the direct triggering of B cells by polymeric antigens such as polymerized flagellin is correlated with capping. Diener and Paetkau (1972) have shown that polymerized flagellin (POL) did cause capping, but there were two important differences between POL- and anti-immunoglobulin-induced capping: (1) anti-immunoglobulin-caused caps were pinocytosed, whereas antigen–receptor complexes were shed from the surface after capping (Diener, Lee, and Paetkau, cited in Diener and Langman, 1975); (2) prolonged incubation of lymphocytes with antigen induced the production of new receptors within 1 hr after capping and an increase in receptor density during a 4–6 hr period (Diener and Paetkau, 1972). When anti-immunoglobulin was present for long periods, the receptors did not reappear (Taylor et al., 1971; Perkins et al., 1972). Observations by Diener et al. (1974) may help to resolve these discrepancies. They found that rabbit lymphocytes treated with antiallotype sera specific for the Fc portion of the receptor immunoglobulin did not cause reappearance of receptors, whereas sera specific for the Fab moiety did. Presumably, antisera directed against the Fab region induce events that simulate those that occur following the interaction of antigen with the Fab region of the receptor. Thus ligand–receptor interaction at or near the antibody-combining site may activate cells differently from interaction that occurs elsewhere on the receptor molecule.

It is reasonable to speculate that the redistribution of receptors on the lymphocyte membrane triggers this cell in much the same way that immunoglobulin activation is required to mediate biological reactions, such as complement fixation and activation (Hyslop et al., 1970; Muller-Eberhard, 1968). However, it seems unlikely that pinocytosis provides the signal, because mitogens (Greaves and Bauminger, 1972) and antigens (Feldmann et al. 1974) on insoluble particles can activate lymphocytes. There does not seem to be a correlation between capping and activation; under certain in vitro conditions antilymphocyte sera and mitogens cap but do not trigger or trigger but do not cap (Greaves and Janossy, 1972). Moreover, Lee et al. (1973) showed that concanavalin A inhibited capping by B cells in vitro without affecting their immune response to POL. However, as Con A-induced capping involves a receptor, distinct from the immunoglobulin receptor, this finding is not conclusive. Further, by analogy with the finding that monovalent anti-immunoglobulin does not cause capping and blast transformation (Taylor et al., 1971) it might be expected that monomeric antigens would not activate B cells. Yet, it has been found that monomeric proteins are immunogenic in the apparent absence of T cells (Hunter and Munro, 1972; Armstrong et al., 1974). Diener and Langman (1975) conclude on the basis of this and additional evidence that it is unlikely that capping is an obligatory event in the induction of the immune response. They speculate that capping exists as a mechanism to keep the cell surface cleared of antigen that might otherwise accumulate and attain tolerigenic levels.

Regardless of its relevance to the activation of lymphocytes for the antibody response, the surface events described in this section, especially capping, have already proven very valuable as experimental tools for the analysis of many structure–function relationships in the lymphocyte membrane.

Diener and Paetkau (1972) observed striking differences in the frequency of cap formation following exposure of antigen-binding lymphocytes to immunogenic and tolerigenic concentrations of POL.

Roelants et al. (1973) took advantage of the phenomenon of capping to determine whether murine T cells contain surface immunoglobulin. Antigen-binding T and B lymphocytes were incubated with $[^{125}I]$hemocyanin, and then with rhodamine-labeled anti-immunoglobulin (Ig) reagents or with a rhodamine-labeled fraction of anti-θ serum. B cells were identified as Ig + or $\theta-$, T cells as Ig− or θ +. It was found that 20–30% of the antigen-binding cells were T cells, depending on the interval that had elapsed between priming and the antigen-binding tests. When Ig at the surface of T or B cells was induced to cap, by noninhibiting concentrations of anti-Ig reagents, and the cells were then expossed to $[^{125}I]$antigen under noncapping conditions, the $[^{125}I]$antigen silver grains were localized in caps superimposed on the Ig fluorescent cap. Since anti-μ- and anti-light-chain-capped T cells showed such silver grains, it was concluded that T cells have antigen-specific receptors, probably of IgM nature. However, the authors did adduce evidence that antigen binding by T cells was much lower than that of B cells, a finding which may explain reports of a lack of surface Ig on T cells (e.g., Lamelin et al., 1972).

4. Cellular, Genetic, and Antigenic Requirements and Kinetics and Nature of in Vitro Antibody Responses

The cell cooperation hypothesis states that the induction of an antibody response to most antigens requires that two distinct antigenic determinants on the same molecule be recognized by two different cell populations. In vivo and in vitro studies employing hapten–protein conjugates as model antigens indicate that T lymphocytes recognize the protein component and thereby provide helper activity for the B lymphocytes, which recognize the haptenic determinant and also serve as the precursors of the cells which actually synthesize the antibodies (Feldmann and Nossal, 1972; Greaves et al., 1973). Other experiments indicate that macrophages may be required in the response to certain antigens (Unanue, 1972). Moreover, the requirement for T-helper cells depends on the nature of the antigen. Rapidly accumulating evidence suggests that certain interactions of T and B cells and of T cells with macrophages may be under genetic control. By now the role of cell cooperation, i.e., T-B cell interactions, in the IgM, IgG, and IgE antibody responses, have been extensively studied in in vitro systems, and studies of the IgA response have begun. It is especially encouraging that thus far there do not appear to be any major discrepancies in the pictures of cell collaboration derived from *in vivo* and *in vitro* experiments. This section describes recent experimental studies of the topics just summarized. To facilitate the presentation and to aid investigators in selecting systems that suit their purposes, this reasearch is categorized according to the cellular requirements for the demonstration of antibody responses to different types of antigens.

a. *Primary and/or Secondary T-Cell- and Macrophage-Independent Responses.* Shortman and Palmer (1971) found that an antiserum to mouse macrophages blocked the antibody response of mouse spleen cells to sheep erythrocytes, but did not affect the response to a polymerized flagellin from *Salmonella* (POL). Feldmann and Basten (1972a) induced a primary IgM antibody response to POL or the dinitrophenyl (DNP) determinant coupled to POL in mouse spleen cells deprived of T cells. In contrast, the response to monomeric flagellin required T cells. Feldmann (1972a,c) then showed that the primary anti-DNP response elicited in mouse spleen cell suspensions by DNP-POL or DNP-flagella was both T-cell- and macrophage-independent. Feldmann *et al.* (1974) were directly able to induce unprimed or antigen-primed mouse splenic B cells to produce antibodies to the trinitrophenyl (TNP) determinant by exposing these cells to TNP-KLH conjugated to Sepharose beads. Exposure of these cells to soluble TNP-keyhole limpet hemocyanin (KLH) did not induce a primary response. Thus unless some soluble antigen was dissociated from the beads, interiorization of antigen did not appear to be required for induction of antibody synthesis. Both the primary and secondary responses of spleen cells to DNP-POL occur rapidly, with peak responses by day 3 (Feldmann, 1972b). DNP-POL with few DNP groups was immunogenic, but even at very high concentrations did not induce tolerance, whereas highly conjugated DNP-POL tolerized but did not immunize (Feldmann, 1972b). DNP-POL conjugated with intermediate concentrations of hapten, and, like POL itself, hapten was tolerigenic at high concentrations and immunogenic at lesser levels (Feldmann, 1972b).

b. *Primary and/or Secondary T-Cell- and Macrophage-Dependent Responses.* Feldmann and his colleagues have shown that both T cells and macrophages are required for the induction of antihapten antibody to DNP and TNP conjugated to proteins other than POL. Cultures of mouse lymphoid cells primed to DNP-fowl γ-globulin (FGG) did not produce antibody upon addition of homologous conjugate if macrophages had been removed from the cell suspension or were not present, e.g., thoracic duct cells (TDC). Moreover, the antibody response was restored if the macrophage-depleted populations or TDC were fortified with 5×10^5 macrophages (Feldmann, 1972c). Antibody production was initiated promptly and attained a peak on the fourth day of culture.

Feldmann and Basten (1972a) obtained specific cell collaboration across a cell-impermeable membrane using a double-chamber setup. The top chamber contained mouse thymocytes primed to DNP-FGG or DNP-KLH plus the homologous DNP conjugate. The bottom chamber contained macrophages and DNP-KLH or DNP-flagella-primed spleen cells plus DNP-FGG or DNP-KLH. Antibody to DNP was produced if the B cells in the lower chamber were presented with DNP on the same protein as recognized by the T cells in the upper chamber. Specific activation of thymocytes by antigen in the upper chamber was required for efficient cooperation across the membrane. The response of both unprimed and hapten-primed B cells was enhanced by the T-cell "factor," but, as expected, the hapten-primed cells gave greater responses. Subsequently, it was shown (Feldmann and Basten, 1972c) that antigen-activated T cells produced a factor which acted indirectly on B cells through the intervention of macrophages. Thus macrophages cultured with antigen-activated T cells acquired the ability to specifically induce B cells to produce antibody. The macrophages appeared to acquire complexes of antigen and a T-cell component that contained antigenic determinants of both κ- and μ-chains. Evidence was then adduced (Feldmann and Basten 1972d) that T cells participated actively, not merely to present antigen to B cells. Two drugs were utilized at concentrations which did not affect B cells. These included actinomycin D, which inhibits DNA-dependent synthesis of at least some species of RNA, and antimycin, which blocks electron transfer reactions required to generate energy for protein synthesis. These drugs inhibited the helper activity of T cells and thus prevented the antibody response.

Unanue and Katz (1973) showed that cultures of DNP-KLH-primed mouse spleen cell suspensions and macrophages bearing the homologous conjugate on their surface yielded strong antihapten antibody responses. Cultures containing this hapten bound to an unrelated carrier did not respond. Lymphocyte cultures from DNP-KLH-primed mice responded only feebly to macrophages that contained both DNP-bovine γ-globulin and KLH; collaboration was optimal when both determinants were on the same molecule. Utilizing the same system, Katz and Unanue (1973) obtained additional evidence for the role of macrophages in the *in vitro* secondary response. The antibody response utilizing antigen bound to macrophages was much greater than that to soluble antigen. Antigen bound to fibroblasts was as effective as antigen bound to macrophages in inducing antibody synthesis. An even greater antibody response was generated if the macrophages bound complexes of DNP-KLH and antibody to DNP. The response to DNP-KLH of 1×10^7 primed spleen cells was augmented considerably by the addition of 5×10^5 macrophages bearing only 0.003 μg of DNP KLH.

Katz *et al.* (1973) presented evidence of genetic restrictions for optimal collaboration of murine T and B cells, both *in vivo* and *in vitro*. In a typical *in vitro* experiment BALB/c DNP-KLH-primed spleen cells developed very good IgG anti-DNP PFC responses to soluble DNP-KLH, whereas treatment of such cells with anti-θ serum plus complement virtually abolished antibody production. The response of anti-θ-inactivated cells was restored by syngeneic, KLH-primed helper cells, but not by allogeneic, A/J, KLH-primed cells. Katz *et al.* (1974*a*) utilized DNP-Asc-primed cells for challenge with DNP-Asc in a similar experiment. They observed cooperative interactions between T and B cells sharing gene identities in the K and I regions, but differing in the S and D regions, of the H-2 locus. They postulated that the B-lymphocyte surface possesses "acceptor" molecules either for the T cell *per se* or for a product of the T cell. Presumably, it is these "acceptor" structures that are under genetic control. Katz *et al.* (1974*b*) then raised the possibility that the failure of histoincompatible T and B cells to cooperate was due to nonspecific suppressive influences. They established the absence of such suppressive effects by the finding that histoincompatible T cells did not interfere with physiological cooperation between syngeneic T and B lymphocytes upon adoptive transfer into X-irradiated hosts. However, Heber-Katz and Wilson (1975) have obtained evidence for such suppressive effects with respect to the *in vitro* primary IgM antibody response of rat lymphoid cells to SRBC. This response was inhibited when large numbers of allogeneic T cells were mixed with constant numbers of B cells. The response was not inhibited when they employed either smaller numbers of allogeneic T cells or allogeneic T cells from which B-reactive cells had been removed. Additional evidence for cooperation between allogeneic T cells—at least T-cell factor—and B cells comes from a recent study by Taussig *et al.* (1975). They further mapped the mouse T-cell factor for the antibody response to poly(Tyr, Glu)–poly DL(Ala)–poly(Lys) (see Section III2). They found that this factor cooperates across allogeneic barriers, i.e., when the factor produced by one strain is added to bone marrow cells of other H-2 incompatible strains. Obviously, further study is required to reconcile these divergent results obtained in such admittedly different experimental systems.

c. Secondary T-Cell-Dependent, Apparently Macrophage-Independent Responses. These responses clearly require T cells, but *apparently* do not require macrophages. The word *apparently* is used because it appears that the participation of small numbers of macrophages was not rigorously excluded.

Kishimoto and Ishizaka studied the antihapten antibody response of primed rabbit lymph node cell suspensions to hapten–protein conjugates. Although they have not directly demonstrated that the cells providing helper activity are T cells, the indirect evidence for this conclusion is very strong. Ishizaka and Kishimoto (1972) injected rabbits intraperitoneally with DNP-*Ascaris* extract (Asc) and removed the mesenteric lymph nodes for culture some monthes later. Addition of homologous DNP-Asc for 24 hr induced the formation of IgG and IgM antibodies. Lymph nodes obtained from rabbits that formed IgE antibodies after primary immunization also produced this antibody upon *in vitro* challenge with homologous antigen. The removal of more than 95% of the adherent cells from the lymph node cell suspension—which would include most of the macrophages—did not have a significant effect on the level of synthesis of IgG, IgM, and IgE antibodies. Kishimoto and Ishizaka (1972) then observed that primed cells challenged with DNP-homologous carrier (DNP-Asc) produced much greater amounts of IgM and IgG antihapten antibody than when challenged with DNP-heterologous carrier (DNP-bovine γ-globulin, BGG). If the rabbit was primed with DNP-Asc and BGG, incubation of these primed lymph node cells with DNP-BGG yielded enhanced IgG and IgM, but not IgE anti-DNP antibody. The DNP-Asc-primed cells gave maximal antibody responses when stimulated with certain concentrations of antigen, the optimal concentration being dependent upon the interval between priming and *in vitro* challenge. However, with aliquots of the same cell suspension, the same optimal antigen concentration induced maximal synthesis of IgG, IgM, and IgE antibodies. Since IgE antibody was not formed when DNP-Asc + BGG-primed cells were incubated with DNP-BGG, it was interpreted that BGG-specific helper cells for IgG and IgM antibody responses did not serve in this capacity for the IgE response. Other evidence was adduced to support the conclusion that the optimal concentration of antigen and the ratio of IgG to IgM antibodies were a function of the hapten-specific memory cells rather than the carrier-specific helper cells.

Subsequently, Kishimoto and Ishizaka (1973*a,b*) observed that the type of adjuvant employed in priming may determine whether the synthesis of a particular class of immunoglobulin antibody occurs or, if it occurs, the level of synthesis. They primed rabbit lymph node cells *in vivo* with (1) alum-DNP-Asc followed by DNP-Asc, (2) alum-Asc, then alum-DNP-Asc, (3) Asc in complete Freund's adjuvant (CFA) followed by alum-DNP-Asc, and (4) alum-DNP-Asc. These variously primed cell populations were then challenged with DNP-Asc in culture. The cells primed by regimens (1), (2), and (3) produced much more IgG than IgM antibody, whereas those primed as in (4) produced much more IgM than IgG antibody. Moreover, the cells primed with alum-Asc, but not with CFA-Asc, produced IgE antibody. Kishimoto and Ishizaka concluded that carrier-specific T cells may regulate the class distribution of antihapten antibodies through effects on the production of hapten-specific B cells. In the second study, Kishimoto and Ishizaka (1973*b*) provided evidence that the helper function of the carrier-specific cell population for IgE antibody production was not related either to the helper function of this cell population for the IgG antibody production or to the size of the carrier-specific cell population, as estimated by the uptake of [^{3}H]thymidine. Thus additional evidence was obtained to indicate that carrier-specific helper cells for the IgE antibody response were distinct from those for the IgM/IgG antibody response. This interpretation is also supported by the results of experiments (Section III) that indicate that there are different enhancing soluble factors for the IgG and IgE antibody responses (Kishimoto and Ishizaka, 1973c).

Systems and reagents have been developed which demonstrate directly the role of T cells in the secondary antibody response of rabbit lymph node cells to KLH. Herscowitz and Stavitsky (1970) primed these cells by the injection of alum-KLH. When removed some months later and challenged with optimal concentrations of KLH (200 μg/2×10^7 cells), these cells were induced to produce IgG antibody. Stavitsky and Cook (1974) immunized rabbits with alum-KLH and removed the draining lymph nodes 6 days or 2 months later. The addition of 1 μg KLH/10^7 cells (for 0–24 hr of culture) induced antibody synthesis several days later. This antibody response was totally abolished by the inclusion in the culture of highly specific IgG goat antibody to rabbit thymocytes (ATG). This T-cell-dependent phase of the antibody response lasted 24–36 hr. The response of the 6-day-primed cells to KLH was about 60% IgG and 40% IgM; the response of the 2-month-primed cells was virtually all IgG. Both responses were highly antigen concentration dependent with maximal antibody synthesis induced by 1 μg KLH and higher concentrations generating much less antibody. Cook *et al.* (1975) removed most of the macrophages from these primed lymph node cell suspensions on glass bead columns so that only about 100,000 macrophages/culture remained. These macrophage-depleted cell populations yielded antibody responses virtually identical to the control cell suspensions in regard to peak antibody levels, IgM/IgG ratio, and the response to optimal (1 μg) and supraoptimal (100 μg) concentrations of KLH. However, Kim *et al.* (1975) have utilized the lymph node primed cell system described by Herscowitz and Stavitsky (1970)—KLH added to 2×10^7 cells—to determine whether macrophages are required for this anamnestic antibody response. They prepared a goat anti-rabbit macrophage serum (AMS) and made it specific by absorptions with rabbit tissues and serum proteins. When suitable concentrations of this AMS were added to KLH-primed cells at the same time as KLH, the antibody response was largely inhibited, suggesting that macrophages were required. The discrepancy between the results of this study utilizing antibody to destroy macrophages and that employing only a slightly different system—1×10^7 cells/culture—and a glass bead column to remove macrophages (Cook *et al.*, 1975) is unexplained at present. However, the question of the macrophage requirement in this type of system is obviously worthy of further study and resolution.

d. Primary and Secondary T-Cell-Dependent Responses; No Study of Macrophage Dependence. Most of these systems presumably require macrophages because they employ antigens and murine spleen cells, which have been found to require this cell type. Moreover, most of these organ culture or cell systems contain macrophages. The T-cell requirements have not been directly determined in some systems, but since they employ hapten–protein conjugates and require carrier protein priming it is most likely that T helper activity is involved.

Bullock and Rittenberg (1970) developed the first *in vitro* model of the anamnestic antibody response to a hapten. They primed mice several times with TNP-KLH-bentonite and removed their spleens 3–7 wk later. When challenged with suitable concentrations of either soluble TNP-KLH or TNP-KLH-bentonite, cultures of these primed cells produced both IgM and IgG antibodies to TNP. Subsequently, Rittenberg and Bullock (1972), by inactivating T cells with anti-θ serum plus complement, showed that the carrier-primed and reactive cell was a T cell. Cheers *et al.* (1971) presented the first evidence for *in vitro* collaboration between carrier-reactive and hapten-sensitive cells to generate an antihapten antibody. Mice were immunized with fowl IgG (FGG), ovalbumin (OV), or these proteins conjugated with the hapten 3, 4-dinitro-4-hydroxyphenylacetic acid (NNP). Spleen cells were then removed for culture. When cultured with the NNP-homologous protein, but not NNP-heterologous protein, the cells were induced to produce antibody to NNP. Carrier-primed spleen cells could be replaced with thymus cells activated with the same antigen, indicating that carrier-specific T cells were required for the induction of antibody to the hapten.

Segal *et al.* (1970) exposed spleen organ explants to DNP-hemocyanin and assayed the resulting antibody to DNP by the neutralization of DNP-conjugated T4 bacteriophage. IgM antibodies appeared in the medium between days 4 to 6 and IgG between days 8 to 10. Segal *et al.* (1971*a*) induced an *in vitro* primary response to DNP upon addition of DNP-rabbit serum albumin (RSA) to spleen fragments from mice immunized with RSA or a secondary response by adding this antigen to tissue from mice primed with DNP-RSA. Much greater responses were obtained with the DNP-RSA-primed fragments. Spleens from mice rendered tolerant to RSA did not produce antibody to DNP when challenged with DNP-RSA, strongly suggesting that carrier-specific helper cells were required (Segal *et al.*, 1971*b*). Kunin *et al.* (1971) reconstituted lethally irradiated mice with bone marrow and thymus cells, with thymus cells alone, or with bone marrow cells alone, and then injected them with RSA. Their spleens were removed 6–8 days later and then challenged with DNP-RSA. Those reconstituted with both marrow and thymus cells produced antibody to DNP, and those reconstituted with either of these populations did not, indicating that T-sensitive carrier cells were required.

A similar system has been utilized by Klinman and co-workers to approach some of the same questions as well as others. Mice were primed with DNP-hemocyanin (HC) and their spleens were removed in 4–8 months for spleen fragment cultures (Klinman, 1971). When challenged with DNP-HC these cultures first produced antibody to DNP and to HC on days 6–8, reached peak production on days 12–14, and continued to synthesize antibody for at least a month. The induction of antibody production by DNP-HC was partially inhibited in the presence of high concentrations of DNP-lysine or HC. Antibody production to DNP was antigen-dose dependent: 0.1 μg DNP-HC inducing maximal production, some induction occurring when from 0.000001 to 100 μg was added, but much less antibody produced with 10 or 100 μg. Significant, but much less stimulation occurred when DNP-BGG was added to DNP-HC-primed cells. By equilibrium dialysis, it was shown that the binding of $\alpha,N[^{3}H]$-acetyl-ε-DNP-L-lysine at 7°C by antibody present in the serum of secondarily stimulated mice and the binding in culture media of fragments stimulated with DNP-HC were essentially the same. The K_a of serum antibody was 2.4×10^7 M^{-1}, whereas that of antibody from pooled media of fragments stimulated with 1 μg of DNP-HC was 2.1×10^7 M^{-1} and antibody produced by fragments stimulated with 10^{-3} μg/ml of this conjugate was 2.6×10^7 M^{-1}. The finding that the secondary response to DNP was induced at equally low concentrations of the hapten on homologous and nonhomologous carriers indicated that the affinity of the hapten–cell interaction was independent of the carrier protein molecule. Since the hapten was presented in multivalent form, it was considered possible that the affinity of the cell receptor for hapten was greatly enhanced by multivalent binding (Klinman et al., 1969). Klinman (1972) then utilized the same system for in vitro stimulation of clonal precursors of anti-DNP antibody-producing cells derived from both immune and nonimmune mice. The principal conclusions of this study were that (1) foci derived from single precursors from nonimmune (primary) foci or immune (secondary) foci produced homogeneous antibody, (2) carrier-specific enhancement is required for the stimulation of primary precursor cells and increases both the size and number of detectable foci derived from secondary precursors, (3) the K_a of primary, monofocal antibodies is less than tenfold lower than that of secondary clonal antibody, and (4) the antigen receptors of primary cells interact with antigen as if they are monovalent, while receptors of secondary cells evidence multivalence.

Rabbit spleen cell cultures were employed by Sela and his collaborators to reach some of the same conclusions as those of other studies (Bustin et al., 1972; Strausbauch et al., 1972). Cells primed by immunization with DNP-proteins produced antibody to DNP upon stimulation either with DNP-homologous protein or by the homologous protein alone, but not response to DNP-heterologous protein or unrelated protein.

Two recent studies utilized limiting dilution analysis of helper T-cell function. Waldmann et al. (1973) determined the anti-TNP antibody response when KLH-primed mouse spleen cells were mixed with TNP-FGG or TNP-OV-primed spleen cells and then challenged with TNP-KLH. They found the frequency of KLH-primed cells capable of specific helper function to be $9-11 \times 10^{-6}$. They concluded that only one helper cell was needed to engage a single B cell in the production of antibodies to TNP-KLH. Hunter *et al.* (1974) utilized a similar approach and system. They concluded that upon immunization the frequency of cells primed with KLH was 12.5×10^{-6}.

Schmiege and Miller (1974) developed a system for the culture of mouse bone marrow cells and thymocytes in which maturation of the various lymphoid cell types occurs. The T cells collaborated with B cells to develop a biphasic antibody response (IgM and IgG) to TNP-BGG that resembled the primary and secondary responses that occur *in vivo*. It appeared that during the first 9 days T cells divided rapidly and many times before developing into functional T lymphocytes. These cells could then collaborate in the induction of terminal differentiation of B cells into antibody producing cells. In addition, these T cells supported the proliferation of Newcastle disease virus which serves as a correlate of delayed hypersensitivity (Bloom *et al.*, 1970).

Hurme *et al.* (1975) found that hapten–protein conjugates (4-hydroxy-3-iodo-5-nitophenylacetyl–ovalbumin, NIP-OV) induced very poor anti-hapten antibody responses in mouse spleen fragment cultures from unimmunized mice, but strong antihapten responses when the donors of the fragments were primed with OV. This carrier-primed response consisted mainly of IgA antibodies of 9–13 S, but also IgM at the beginning and IgG at the end of these responses.

e. Carrier-Independent T-Cell Helper Effects in Antigenic Stimulation (Klinman and Doughty, 1973). Cells from the spleens of donor mice immunized either with DNP-hemocyanin or DNP-BSA were transferred to nonimmune recipients before or after treatment with antiserum and complement in order to destroy T cells. Fragment cultures of the recipient spleens were incubated with homologous or heterologous antigen. At low antigen concentrations, the antiserum treatment of the transferred cells diminished the anti-DNP antibody response to both DNP-heterologous and DNP-homologous antigens, suggesting that these responses were dependent upon T cells. These findings were interpreted to indicate a role for hapten-specific T cells with B cells specific for the same determinant. Klinman and Doughty considered this system a possible model of the antibody response to viruses and to other agents that display multiple repeating determinants.

f. Primary and/or Secondary Antibody Responses; No or Incomplete Study of Cellular Requirements. Panijel *et al.* (1971) induced a primary response to phage ϕX174 in cultures of rabbit and germ-free mouse spleen cells. They obtained peak responses in 3–5 days and average peak k values (phage neutralization) of 19.5×10^{-4}. Jonard and Panijel (1973) developed a microculture system in which fewer than 50,000 mouse spleen cells yielded a primary IgM antibody response to $\phi17$ phage. By limiting dilution analysis, 1 "response" unit for this antigen was present in a frequency of 3×10^{-5}, a frequency much higher than previously reported *in vivo* or *in vitro* (Shearer *et al.*, 1968; Cunningham, 1969). Tao (1972) initiated primary and secondary responses in rabbit lymph node fragments to phage ϕX174. The primary IgM antibody response occurred in 5–9 days. If the node was removed from a rabbit that had received phage 4 days earlier, restimulation with phage resulted in mainly IgM antibody, whereas if immunized 14 days previously, restimulation yielded mainly IgG antibody. Thus IgM memory appeared transient. Adler *et al.* (1973) prepared a soluble extract by treatment of phage T2 with detergent. This soluble preparation induced a vigorous primary-type IgM antibody response after only a lag of 1 day and reached a peak in 5 days. Secondary challenge of primed cells yielded mainly IgG antibody. Another study of this system showed that adherent cells were not required when the soluble antigen was employed, but were needed for a response to intact T2 phage. As found with a number of other systems, antibody formation was induced by only a rather narrow range of antigen concentrations and supraoptimal doses induced less or no antibody production.

    g. Macrophage-Dependent in Vitro Induction of T Helper Activity. Erb and Feldmann (1975a) have described an *in vitro* system in which soluble protein antigens activated unprimed-mouse T cells to develop into T helper cells. Purified T cells were obtained from cortisone-resistant thymus cell populations (CRT) by the nylon wool technique (Greaves and Brown, 1974), which removes macrophages and B cells. To generate helper cells, the CRT were incubated with KLH for 4 days with or without syngeneic, allogeneic, or semiallogeneic macrophages. In a second step, these cells were cultured for days with normal spleen cells and with TNP-KLH. The anti-TNP response then provided a measure of the helper activity generated during the first step. Helper cells were not developed in the absence of macrophages, but appeared in the presence of adequate numbers of syngeneic macrophages. Semiallogeneic macrophages did generate helper activity, but more of them were required than of syngeneic macrophage, and the response was less than with the syngeneic macrophages. Subsequently (Erb and Feldmann, 1975b), it was shown that the macrophages and T cells must share the I-A region of the H-2 complex for the induction of T helper activity. These findings recall those of Rosenthal and Shevach (1973), who primed guinea pig T lymphocytes with antigen (PPD or DNP-guinea pig albumin), and challenged them with specific antigen. They found that antigen recognition by specific macrophages was required for stimulation of DNA synthesis. Moreover, for stimulation of DNA synthesis by the lymphocytes, the macrophages and T lymphocytes must share some portion of the major histocompatiblility locus. Thus strain 13 macrophages cooperated with strain 13 lymphocytes, but not with strain 2 lymphocytes.

5. Cellular Differentiation and Proliferation during the Antibody Response

The reaction of immunogen with immunocompetent lymphocytes initiates a series of biochemical events in T and/or B lymphocytes that culminates in the antibody response. Mitogens, which activate a greater percentage of lymphocytes than immunogens, have been employed as model inducers to gain further information about these biochemical events. Cellular activation generally has been assayed by the capacity of the mitogen to induce DNA or RNA synthesis, both late expressions of activation. Earlier expressions of mitogenic activation of lymphocytes, especially at the membrane level, include a very rapid increase in the turnover of the phosphate group of phosphatidylinositol (Fisher and Mueller, 1969) and increases in the uptake of amino acids (Mendelsohn et al., 1971), sugars (Peters and Hausen, 1971), and small ions (Quastel and Kaplan, 1970). To date, studies of antigenic activation of lymphocytes mainly have dealt with the stimulation of DNA or RNA synthesis. Vaughan et al. (1960) and then O'Brien and Coons (1963) observed a connection between antibody synthesis and DNA synthesis in vitro. Subsequently, Dutton (1961) incorporated very high specific activity tritiated thymidine into lymphoid cells from an immunized animal and thereby reduced the subsequent antibody synthesis. This finding provided evidence that some of the antibody-forming cells were derived from the proliferation of precursor cells. Thereafter, different types of evidence were adduced to indicate that cell proliferation was both a prominent and a necessary feature of the inductive phase of the antibody response. Nossal and Makela (1962) observed that the cell population responding to secondary in vivo challenge with Salmonella already had synthesized DNA before the reinjection of antigen. Dutton and Mishell (1967) developed a dissociated cell system for the induction of a primary IgM antibody response to foreign erythrocytes. These spleen cells from unimmunized mice were subjected—at various times after antigen—to a pulse of 10 μCi of tritiated thymidine to selectively irradiate those cells which synthesize DNA. Presumably, if these irradiated cells had been destined to develop into antibody-producing cells or if their division was somehow required for the antibody response, this lethal internal irradiation would inhibit the antibody response. These experiments indicated that (1) DNA synthesis is initiated 24–32 hr after antigenic stimulation and (2) essentially all of the antibody-producing cells arise by cell division. The addition of highly radioactive antigen to selectively irradiate only those cells which bind that antigen has also abrogated the antibody response (Roelants and Askonas, 1971). The *in vivo* tissue culture studies from the Makinodan laboratory (Urso and Makinodan, 1963) contributed greatly to the fund of information that supports the importance of proliferation in the immunological response.

In vitro proliferative responses to antigen were first reported by Dutton and Pearce (1962), who added specific antigens to lymphoid cell suspensions obtained from previously immunized rabbits. Proliferation was assayed by the rate of incorporation of radioactive thymidine and was easily measurable 24 hr after the addition of antigen.

Mach and Vassalli (1965a) first correlated nucleic acid syntheses with the antibody response. They showed that the rate of DNA and RNA synthesis was increased in the spleens and lymph nodes of rats after the primary and secondary injections of antigen. After primary immunization, there was a peak at 2–3 days, presumable associated with proliferation, and a second at 9–10 days, assumed to be associated more closely with antibody synthesis. Following secondary stimulation, there was also a peak at 3 days. A large fraction of the newly synthesized RNA had the properties of ribosomal RNA, but a smaller fraction had characteristics of mRNA (Mach and Vassalli, 1965b). Lazda *et al.* (1968) presented further evidence for the synthesis of mRNA during the early inductive phase of the antibody response. Experiments with metabolic inhibitors of RNA synthesis such as actinomycin D indicated that the synthesis of at least some species of RNA was essential for the antibody response (Wust *et al.*, 1964; Herscowitz *et al.*, 1971).

Thus the bulk of the experimental evidence indicates that generally the same series of events is involved in the induction and synthesis of antibody globulin as for other proteins in mammalian systems. One difference, however, may be the requirement for the collaboration of more than one cell type in the antibody response. Moreover, it is not always clear when a given biochemical event in the antibody response is T cell dependent, i.e., requires particular function(s) of T cells, or is actually performed by T cells *per se*.

Although it is certain that both proliferation and differentiation are essential events in the antibody response, it is not clear what precise roles are played by the synthesis of DNA and different species of RNA. This section summarizes recent information about these syntheses under two headings (a) studies in which the correlation with antibody synthesis has not been attempted, but many aspects of these syntheses have been investigated, and (b) studies in which the correlation with antibody synthesis has been analyzed. The role of RNA–antigen complexes in the antibody response (Friedman, 1973) has not been discussed. The stimulation of DNA and RNA synthesis by peptides is taken up in Section IIB.

a. Various Parameters of Proliferative and Differentiative Responses to Antigen. Siskind and Thorbecke (1971) studied the proliferative response of DNP-BGG-primed rabbit lymph node cells to DNP-BGG. Cultures set up early (1–4 wk) after immunization gave a peak response on days 1–2 of culture, whereas those set up late (2–8 months) after immunization showed a peak response on days 3–4. Through use of the metabolic inhibitor 5-bromodeoxyuridine, it appeared that these results were at least partially caused by a greater recruitment of cells into this response during the third day, when lymph node cells removed late after immunization were used. Rubin and Wigzell (1974) found that DNP-guinea pig albumin (GPA) primed guinea pig lymph node cells responded to DNP-GPA by an increase in DNA synthesis. The addition of increasing concentrations of antigen induced increased stimulation of DNA synthesis, with the threshold often being as low as 0.02 μg/culture. In contrast, lymph node cells from guinea pigs given complete Freund's adjuvant alone responded only to very high concentrations (20 mg/culture) of antigen.

Several laboratories have studied the question of whether T and/or B cells proliferate in response to antigen. Rubin and Wigzell (1974) found that column-purified T lymphocytes from guinea pig lymph nodes immunized with DNP-GPA proliferated in response to the addition of DNP-GPA. Piguet and Vassalli (1973) studied the proliferative response of unprimed or primed mouse spleen cells to T4 phage. Both primary and secondary proliferative responses involved primarily B cells, although there was more mitosis of T cells in the primed populations. Osborne and Katz (1973a) observed that KLH induced mitosis in cultures of normal as well as KLH-primed cells, the activity being much greater in primed cells. Cells removed 1–3 months after primary immunization showed a peak DNA synthetic response 48 hr after the addition of KLH. However, spleen cultures from normal mice did not respond to DNP-KLH, whereas cells from DNP-KLH-sensitized mice showed an active, dose-dependent response to this conjugate. The latter response required DNP coupled to the homologous carrier. This response was also hapten specific, since KLH *per se* induced only low levels of DNA synthesis. Osborne and Katz (1973b) then utilized these systems to determine which cells were involved in DNA synthesis. They depleted the cell suspensions either of T or B cells and then challenged them with antigen. They observed that the KLH-induced DNA synthetic response of DNP-KLH-primed cells was primarily B, whereas the DNP-KLH-induced response was a mixed response, but again largely involved the B-lymphocyte population. The depletion of adherent cells did not affect DNP-KLH-induced replication. Moorhead *et al.* (1973) similarly found that the proliferative response of NIP-mouse globulin (MGG) primed mouse spleen cells involved B lymphocytes to a great extent.

Greenberg *et al.* (1975) incubated purified and HL-A serotyped human peripheral human lymphocytes with varying concentrations of streptokinase/streptodornase. They found a significant association between the ability to incorporate tritiated thymidine in response to antigen and the HL-A5 serotype.

b. Correlation between DNA and/or RNA Synthesis and the Antibody Response. Tao and Leary (1969) determined the effects of irradiation on the primary and secondary antibody responses of rabbit lymph node fragments to phage ϕX174. The primary antibody response was inhibited when the fragments were irradiated 1 day before to 2 days after introduction of the antigen. For instance, when irradiated on day 1—antigen having been cultured from day 0 to day 1—50, 250, 500, and 1,000 rads depressed the antibody response to 61, 55, 19, and 16% respectively, of the nonirradiated control. These cultures never showed the phenomenon of radiation-induced enhancement of the primary response seen in the whole animal (Dixon and McConahey, 1963). The secondary response was initiated by incubation with phage for 24 hr when some cultures received 500 rads; other cultures received 500 rads 3 hr before antigen. Irradiation before antigen depressed the response to 15% and after antigen to 4% of the control.

Kettman and Dutton (1971) investigated the *in vitro* primary response of mouse spleen cell suspensions to trinitrophenyl (TNP) erythrocytes. They found that the number of anti-TNP plaque-forming cells that develop after *in vitro* immunization was greatly augmented by utilizing cells that had been immunized *in vitro*, with the carrier erythrocyte. The carrier-primed cells that mediate this enhancement are thymus derived. The enhancing effect of the carrier-primed cells was radioresistant, suggesting that additional DNA synthesis was not required for the helper function of these cells. Katz *et al.* (1970) had previously presented evidence for the radioresistance of T-cell helper function in an *in vivo* system. However, Miller *et al.* (1971) treated T cells from unprimed mice with mitomycin C, which inhibited DNA synthesis and impaired the capacity of these cells to collaborate with B cells upon transfer into irradiated hosts.

The secondary antibody and proliferative responses of rabbit spleen cells to DNP-BSA were investigated by Tarrab *et al.* (1971). Thymidine uptake preceded the appearance of both PFC for DNP and neutralizing antibody for DNP-phage. Thymidine and the number of PFC were dependent on the amount of added antigen, but the level of neutralizing antibody was not. Segal *et al.* (1971a) induced the primary anti-DNP antibody response by exposing RSA-primed mouse spleen organ cultures to DNP-RSA. Exposure of these cells to antigen together with vinblastine, which inhibits DNA synthesis, suppressed the antibody response. Exposure to antigen for 24 hr, followed by vinblastine, did not affect the ensuing antibody response. Nakamura *et al.* (1972) utilized cytosine arabinoside (CA) to inhibit DNA synthesis in the same system. The addition of CA for 0–26 hr and after 48 hr of culture with antigen did not inhibit antibody synthesis, whereas the presence of this agent during 36–48 hr inhibited this response. It was concluded that the helper function required one critical replication 36–48 hr after antigenic stimulation. However, Feldmann and Basten (1972*d*) approached the same question with quite a different experimental design. They studied cell cooperation between murine T and B cells in the induction of the primary antibody response to SRBC. Mitomycin 4 wk earlier markedly reduced helper activity, as reflected in the antibody response. In contrast, activated T cells which had recently divided upon exposure to SRBC were resistant to mitomycin; thus effective cooperation with B cells could occur in the absence of further division of T cells. All of these T cell populations (normal, primed, or activated) were susceptible to inhibition by actinomycin D, however, indicating that active RNA synthesis by T cells was required for cell cooperation.

Kishimoto and Ishizaka (1973*b*) analyzed the secondary IgG and IgE antibody and the proliferative responses of DNP-protein-primed rabbit lymph node cells to the DNP-proteins (Section IIA4c). The level of carrier function of the carrier-specific cells for the IgE response did not bear any relationship with the size of this population, as estimated by the uptake of tritiated thymidine. Moreover, the optimal concentration of protein for the uptake of thymidine by DNP-protein-primed cells was different from the concentration of carrier for the formation of IgG antibody to this protein. Ambrose (1973) induced a secondary antibody response to diphtheria toxoid in rabbit lymph node fragments. Exposure of these organ cultures to hydroxyurea (which inhibits DNA synthesis) during the productive phase, the second week, markedly inhibited antibody synthesis. Waldmann *et al.* (1973) utilized microcultures of KLH-primed helper cells to study the generation of antibody to TNP-KLH. In this system, helper activity was resistant to irradiation with 1200 rads. Adler *et al.* (1973) inhibited the primary antibody response of rabbit spleen cells to soluble T2 phage antigen with vinblastine and rifampicin, the latter an inhibitor of RNA synthesis.

Herscowitz and Stavitsky (1970) exposed KLH-primed rabbit lymph node cells to 100 μg KLH. This antigen stimulated RNA synthesis beginning on about day 2 and peaking on day 5, enhanced DNA synthesis by day 3 and peaking on day 4, and induced antibody synthesis by day 3 and peaking by day 5. Herscowitz *et al.* (1971) then determined the effect of various drugs on these syntheses. In agreement with a previous study (Stavitsky and Gusdon, 1966), the presence of 1 μg actinomycin (AD) with an immunogenic concentration of antigen for 0–24 hr of culture inhibited DNA synthesis about 85%, RNA synthesis 95%, and antibody synthesis completely. However, paradoxically, the incorporation of 0.00001 μg AD with antigen enhanced the antibody response. Mitomycin C (0–24 hr) inhibited the antibody response completely, and nucleic acid syntheses were inhibited over 90%.

Stavitsky and Cook (1974) modified the KLH *in vitro* anamnestic system to sharpen its antigen-concentration dependence and to induce the synthesis of both IgM and IgG antibody by (1) reducing the number of cells/culture from 2×10^7 to 1×10^7 and (2) removing the lymph node cells for antigenic challenge only 6 days after priming *in vivo*. The addition of KLH to these cells induced the synthesis, within 2 days, of both DNA and RNA, followed by the synthesis of IgG and IgM antibody to KLH. When a highly specific goat antibody to rabbit thymus cells was present together with KLH for the first 24 hr of culture, the subsequent induction of all of these syntheses was almost completely inhibited. Thus it appears that in this system the antigen-induced DNA and RNA syntheses are mediated by T lymphocytes. It is not known, however, whether these syntheses are carried out by the T memory cells *per se*, by T blasts derived from these memory cells, by B lymphocytes or B blasts dependent upon information derived from KLH-stimulated T cells, or by a combination of these cell types.

Schmiege and Miller (1974) cultured mouse bone marrow and thymus cells together under conditions that allowed the maturation of the various types of lymphoid cells. When challenged with antigens like TNP-BGG, these cultures yielded a biphasic anti-TNP antibody response. They interpreted their observations to indicate that a carrier-specific proliferation of thymocytes occurred during the first 9 days of culture prior to the development of carrier-specific helper activity required for the antibody response to the hapten.

Delespesse *et al.* (1975) studied the increase in DNA synthesis when DNP-Asc- or DNP-Rag-primed rabbit lymph node cells were stimulated with the priming antigen, with free homologous carrier protein, or with DNP-rabbit serum albumin (RSA). Both free carrier and DNP-RSA stimulated DNA synthesis. The proliferative response to DNP-homologous carrier was slightly higher than to the free carrier, but the optimal concentration of both antigens was 10–100 µg/ml. This concentration was about 100 times higher than the optimal concentration of the same antigens for the maximal antibody response. The lymph node cells were fractionated with antigen-coated or anti-Ig-coated columns and the fractions were subjected to antigenic challenge. The results indicated that the hapten-specific, immunoglobulin-bearing (presumably) B cells are responsible for the DNA synthetic response to DNP-RSA, whereas these cells play only a minimal role in this response to free carrier.

6. Maturation of the Antibody Response

Studies of antibodies isolated from serum at various intervals after immunization with DNP-proteins have shown that the affinity of these antibodies for simple DNP-haptens is greater the longer the interval between immunization and bleeding and the lower the concentration of immunogen (Eisen and Siskind, 1964). Steiner and Eisen (1967) showed that these changes in affinity represent sequential alterations in the nature of the antibodies synthesized by lymphoid cells. Bullock and Rittenberg (1970) injected mice with TNP-KLH every 2 wk for a total of three injections; the mice were then rested for 1–4 months, when spleen cells were challenged with different concentrations of TNP-KLH and their IgM and IgG PFC responses assayed. Cell populations with increasing avidity for antigen emerged with time. This avidity increased a thousandfold in a 4-month period, 18-wk cells being maximally stimulated by that much less antigen than 6-wk cells. Macario and de Macario (1974) have studied the maturation of the antibody response in an *in vitro* rabbit lymph node fragment system. Fragments from immunized mice were challenged and cultured for periods of up to 6 wk, and the association constant of the secreted antibody was determined at various times. The immunogen was β-galactosidase (GZ) of *Escherichia coli*. The procedure for measuring the affinity of the antibody to GZ was based on the property of these antibodies to activate the enzymatic activity of a point-mutant defective enzyme. Early secondary antibodies comprised a wide range of affinities. Later on, a gradual increase in affinity with progressive restriction occured, especially in multifragment cultures, and in cultures challenged with 50 μg/ml rather than 5 μg/ml of GZ. Pelley and Stavitsky (1975) determined that the type of adjuvant employed for priming may influence the maturation of the antibody response. They immunized rabbits with KLH in complete Freund's adjuvant (CFA), removed the draining lymph nodes at different times for *in vitro* challenge with different concentrations of KLH, and then assayed the level of antibody synthesis. These KLH-CFA-primed cells yielded a maximal antibody response to the following concentrations of KLH: after 7 days of priming, 10 μg; after 9–11 days, 1 μg; after 60 days, 100 ng. Thus there was a hundredfold rise in sensitivity in 2 months. By way of contrast, lymph node cells removed 6 days or 2 months after immunization of rabbits with alum-KLH give a maximal antibody response to 1 μg KLH at both times (Stavitsky and Cook, 1974). The data from these various studies support the hypothesis that memory cells of high avidity result from the selection pressure of diminishing antigen concentration.

B. *In Vitro* Immunological Responses to Peptides

Four different antigenic systems have been employed to determine whether peptides will trigger specific immunological responses in *in vitro* systems. In each instance, the peptides have been added to cultures of lymphoid cells from animals previously immunized with the native protein from which the peptides had been prepared or to which they were structurally related or identical, e.g., synthetic peptides. In each system, substantial studies had shown that these peptides were antigenic; i.e., each reacted serologically with one or more antisera to the native protein. The single exception is the N-terminal peptide (1–6) of sperm whale myoglobin (MB), which thus far has not been shown to be antigenic (Pai and Atassi, 1975). Table I summarizes the results of these studies. In all four systems the addition of peptides to these cultures induced the production of macrophage inhibitory factor (MIF). The production of MIF was induced in the oxidized ferredoxin (O-Fd) systems by a tetrapeptide, in the tobacco mosaic virus protein (TMVP) system by a pentapeptide, and in the myoglobin (MB) system by heptapeptides. In two systems, TMVP and O-Fd, the addition of these same small peptides did not induce the incorporation of radioactive thymidine into the cells. In the glucagon system, the C-terminal peptide (11–12 amino acids) stimulated thymidine incorporation, but the N-terminal NM peptides (17 amino acids) did not. The MB system has been studied with respect to several other syntheses. Unlike the data with the other three systems, the findings with this system have not been published; therefore, representative data are shown in Table II. The data indicate that the putative nonantigenic peptide 1–6 (for structures of the MB peptides and evidence for their antigenic independence, see Atassi, 1975) induced the synthesis of antibody, IgG, and other nonantibody proteins, but not MIF production. Peptides from region 15–21 induced thymidine incorporation, MIF production, and the synthesis of antibody, IgG, and nonantibody proteins. Peptides from regions 56–62 and 146–151 evoked all six events, including uridine incorporation. Peptide 94–100 stimulated MIF production and the formation of antibody, IgG, and other nonantibody proteins. Peptide 113–120 elicited the formation of MIF, antibody, and IgG.

Table III summarizes the data that indicate that great molar excesses of peptide over native protein are required to induce thymidine incorporation, protein synthesis (MB system), and MIF production (TMVP and O-Fd systems).

C. Roles of Persisting Immunogen and Accessory and Thymus-Derived Cells in the Maintenance of the Antibody Response

Antibody synthesis may continue for months or even years after immunization, even with nonreplicating antigens (Sterzl, 1959; Weigle, 1966). It is assumed that this continued synthesis depends upon persistent immunogen, which has been demonstrated in association with macrophages and/or dendritic-type cells in lymphoid organs (Nossal and Ada, 1971). There is much indirect evidence that this retained immunogen functions

Table I. *In Vitro* Induction of Thymidine and Uridine Incorporation, MIF Production, and Antibody, IgG, and Protein Synthesis upon Addition of Proteins and Tryptic or Synthetic Peptides to Protein-Primed Lymphoid Cells

Sources of cells			Additions to cell cultures[c]	Results[a]						Reference
Species	Organ[a]	Priming[b]		Tdr	Ur	MIF	Antibody	IgG	Protein	
GP	Spleen PEC	TMVP	TMVP	+		+				Spitler et al. (1970)
			93–112	−		+				
			C deca	−		+				
			C penta	−		+				
			N octanoyl–C tri	−		+				
GP	LN	G	G	+		+				Senyk et al. (1971)
			C	+		+				
			N			+				
			M			−				
			NM	−		+				
			Undeca synthetic	+		+				
GP	LN	O-Fd	O-Fd	+		+				Levy et al. (1972)
			C octa + N hepta	−		+				Waterfield et al. (1972)
			C octa	−		+				Kelly et al. (1973)
			C tetra	−		+				
			N hepta	−		+				
			N + C-SBSA	+		+				

	Immunogen	Peptide							Reference
	N-10-C	N-10-C	+						
		N-8-N	+						
		C-Mal-10-C	−						
		N	−						
	N-8-N	N-8-N	+						
		N-10-C	+						
		C-Mal-10-C	−						
		N	−						
RBT	C-mal-10-C	C-mal-10-C	+						
		N-10-C	−						
LN	MB	MB	+	+	+	+	+	+	+
		1–6	+	−	+	+	+		+
		15–21	+	+	+	+	+		+
		56–62	+	+	+	+	+		+
		94–100		+	+	+	+		
		113–120		+	+	+	+		
		146–151	+	+	+	+	+		+

Stavitsky *et al.* (1975); unpublished observations (Gooch *et al.*, 1976)

[a] PEC, peritoneal exudate cells; LN, lymph node.
[b] TMVP, tobacco mosaic virus protein; G, glucagon; O-Fd, oxidized ferredoxin of *Clostridium pasteurianum*; MB, sperm whale myoglobin.
[c] C, C-terminal peptide; N, N-terminal peptide; M, interior peptide; SBSA, succinylated BSA; mal, malonic acid; 10, 10 glycine residues.
[d] Tdr and Ur, thymidine and uridine incorporation; antibody, IgG, and protein synthesis.

Table II. *In Vitro* Induction of Thymidine and Uridine Incorporation, MIF Production, and Antibody, IgG, and Protein Synthesis upon Addition of Synthetic Peptides Containing Antigenic Regions of Myoglobin to Myoglobin-Primed Rabbit Lymph Node Cells[a]

| Expt. number | Days | Additions | Results (cpm × 10^{-3}) | | | | | MIF (%) |
			Tdr	Ur	Protein	Antibody	IgC	
7399	60	—				0.15		
		15–23				0.5		
		54–62				1.0		
		146–151				0.6		76 ± 2
7423	50	—	1.3	1.4	30.6			
		56–62	12.2	3.5	71.8			
		46–153	11.4		73.4			
7425	103	—	2.8	25.0	34.0			
		56–62	13.2	44.0	67.0	5.1		
7463	30	—				0.9		
		15–22						26 ± 5
		57–63				2.0		80 ± 4
		146–151						46 ± 5
7491	175	—				0.5	1.8	
		1–6				1.5	12.4	
		16–23				2.2	15.3	
		56–62				1.8	13.7	
		94–100				1.6	18.4	
		146–151				2.0	14.0	
7500	86	—	2.6				3.2	
		1–6						14 ± 5
		15–22						47 ± 21
		16–23						
		94–100						31 ± 11
		146–151	5.6				9.2	34 ± 9
7604	35	—				0.2		
		1–6				0.7		
		16–23				0.9		
		94–100				0.9		
		113–119				0.7		26 ± 5

[a] From Stavitsky *et al.* (1975) and unpublished observations (Gooch *et al.* 1976).

Table III. Relative Concentrations of Native Protein and Synthetic Peptides Required for *in Vitro* Induction of Thymidine Incorporation, MIF Production, and Protein Synthesis

Source of cells			Additions	Molar ratio: peptide/protein for equivalent			Reference
Species	Organ	Priming		Tdr	MIF	Protein	
GP	Spleen PEC	TMVP	C deca		1600		Spitler *et al.* (1970)
GP	LN	O-Fd	C octa N-10-C		3000 1		Waterfield *et al.* (1972)
Rbt	LN	MB	56–62	4000		400	Gooch *et al.* (1976)
			146–153	4000		400	

at least for a few weeks or months. Thus the passive transfer of cells or subcellular preparations from immunized to nonimmunized animals may induce antibody synthesis in the latter (Stavitsky, 1954). Passive antibody given 3–4 wk after immunogen inhibits the induction of optimal immunological memory (Cerottini and Trnka, 1970). Cyclic fluctuations occur in the number of antibody-forming cells after a single injection of some immunogens (Britton and Moller, 1968; Romball and Weigle, 1973). The blood antibody level of an immunized animal that was reinfused with its plasma, from which specific antibody was removed *in vitro*, rises promptly (Graf and Uhr, 1969). There is also evidence for long-term persistence of immunogen. Occasionally, when spleen or thoracic duct cells from mice injected 7 months earlier with a hapten–protein conjugate were transferred into irradiated, nonimmunized mice, antibody synthesis to hapten occurred (Mitchison, 1969). Several laboratories (Michaelides and Coons, 1963; Stecher and Thorbecke, 1967; Kishimoto and Ishizaka, 1971) found that cultures of cells or fragments from lymphoid organs of protein-immunized animals—after a lag—began to synthesize antibodies to these specific proteins, presumably because of residual immunogen.

Based on these observations and the presumption that residual immunogen was functional for a long time after immunization, an *in vitro* system has been developed to investigate the roles of persistent immunogen and various cell types in the maintenance of the antibody response (Tew *et al.*, 1973). Rabbits were injected in the hind foot pads with glutaraldehyde-polymerized HSA (POL-HSA). Months later, the draining popliteal lymph nodes were removed for the preparation of cell suspensions, which were washed and then cultured in the absence of additional antigen. The incorporation of $[^{14}C]$leucine into antibody provided the measure of antibody synthesis. IgG antibody synthesis of appreciable proportions occurred in these cultures ofter a lag of only several days, suggesting that a spontaneous anamnestic antibody response had occurred. The addition of antibody—either hyperimmune or taken from the same animal as provided the nodes—inhibited this induction of antibody synthesis. This so-called spontaneous antibody response has been observed with cells removed as late as $12\frac{1}{2}$ months after the injection of POL-HSA, and the magnitude of this response suggests that this type of response can be obtained even later than 1 yr after immunization. Similar spontaneous responses to KLH (Stavitsky et al., 1974) and myoglobin (Stavitsky et al., 1975) have been observed. Utilizing a highly specific goat IgG antibody to rabbit thymus cells, it was established that the spontaneous antibody responses to at least HSA and KLH require T cells (Stavitsky et al., 1974). Induction of this response also requires accessory, presumably dendritic-type cells. Thus the spontaneous synthesis was abrogated when these accessory cells were removed by exposing the cell suspensions to carbonyl iron particles and then to a magnet (Tew and Stavitsky, 1974); this synthesis was then restored by the addition of nanogram amounts of HSA. Moreover, treatment of the cells from POL-HSA-primed animals with ethylenediamine tetracetate, which removes antigen bound to cell surfaces, also inhibited spontaneous induction, and this inhibition was reversed by the addition of HSA.

In a subsequent study, it was found that a spontaneous proliferative response also occurred following the removal and culture of cells from POL-HSA-immunized rabbits (Greene et al., 1975). The spontaneous antibody and proliferative responses were markedly higher in cells from lymph nodes draining the site of injection (DLN) than from nondraining lymph nodes (NDLN). The NDLN generally required at least a hundredfold more HSA to achieve maximal antibody and proliferative responses than DLN. The local factor implicated in the antibody response and exogenously added HSA acted additively to induce antibody synthesis, thereby providing further evidence for the existence of persistent immunogen. These data may be explained by the retention of greater amounts of HSA immunogen in the DLN than NDLN and/or the presence of greater numbers of T and B memory cells in the DLN than NDLN.

On the basis of these observations, the induction of the spontaneous antibody response was attributed to persistent immunogen—associated with accessory cells—whose immunogenicity is subject to an antibody feedback mechanism. Possible mechanisms whereby this residual immunogen maintains the levels of circulating antibody for long periods will be discussed in Section IV.

D. Regulation of the Antibody Response

The antibody response can be regulated by antigen, by antibody, by T cells, and by macrophages. These forms of regulation, while potentially of great importance, will not be reviewed here. Attention is rather focused on two other aspects, one of them known and discussed for many decades, but only recently beginning to be understood, *regulation by heterologous antigen*; the other, a more recent product, also apparently reflecting non-specific regulation, *regulation by cyclic nucleotides*. The regulation by heterologous antigen appears to require soluble factor(s) generated by antigen-stimulated T lymphocytes. These factors are discussed in Section III.

1. Heterologous Antigen

In parallel with many observations of the striking specificity of the antibody response are many different kinds of evidence for nonspecific enhancement (Wilson and Miles, 1964) or suppression (Adler, 1964) of this response. However, only recently have newer systems, reagents, and techniques permitted a more detailed analysis of these phenomena. Nonspecific enhancement or suppression of the antibody response has been achieved by the injection into animals or the addition to lymphoid cell cultures of non-cross-reactive antigens or immunocompetent cells (reviewed in Katz and Benacerraf, 1972). The observed effects can be divided into two categories, enhancement and suppression.

a. Enhancement of Synthesis of Protein and Nonantibody and Antibody Globulin. Recent studies show that during the *in vitro* anamnestic antibody response there is much synthesis of nonantibody immunoglobulin and nonimmunoglobulin. Kishimoto and Ishizaka (1975a) added DNP-Rag to DNP-Rag-primed rabbit lymph node cells and promoted total IgG synthesis from 4.2 to 80 μg/ml, whereas IgG anti-DNP antibody synthesis was enhanced from only 0.7 to 48 μg/ml. Stavitsky and Cook (1974), performing a similar experiment with KLH, raised total protein synthesis from 38,000 to 92,000 cpm (incorporated radioactivity from [^{14}C]leucine), whereas anti-KLH antibody synthesis was raised from only 1000 to 12,000 cpm. An earlier similar study (Herscowitz and Stavitsky, 1970) showed that the *in vitro* anamnestic antibody response to KLH comprised the production of α, β, and γ nonantibody globulins. Pelley and Stavitsky (1975) have shown that this KLH response also includes the production of much nonantibody IgG and IgM. The specificity of these nonantibody globulins has not been determined.

Table IV summarizes the results of a number of recent studies in which nonspecific enhancement of *in vitro* primary and secondary antibody

Table IV. Nonspecific Enhancement of *in Vitro* Primary and Secondary Antibody Responses

Species	Organ	Antigen[a]	Challenge antigen[b]	Results	References
Mouse	Spleen	TT	TT + SRBC	Enhanced IgM anti-SRBC antibody	Rubin and Coons (1972a,b)
	Thymus	OV	OV + SRBC		
Rabbit	Spleen	DNP-OV	OV	Enhanced IgG anti-DNP antibody	Strausbauch et al. (1972)
		DNP-BSA	BSA		
Rabbit	LN	KLH + HSA	KLH	Enhanced IgG anti-HSA antibody	Stavitsky and Self (1972)
			HSA	Enhanced IgG anti-KLH antibody	
Mouse	Spleen	KLH	KLH + SRBC	Enhanced IgM anti-SRBC antibody	Waldmann et al. (1973)
	Thymus	FGG	FGG + SRBC		
Rabbit	LN	DNP-Rag	Rag + DNP-KLH	Enhanced IgG and IgE anti-DNP antibody	Kishimoto and Ishizaka (1973c)
		DNP-Asc	Asc + DNP-KLH		
Mouse	Spleen	KLH	TNP-KLH + SRBC[c]	Enhanced IgM anti-SRBC antibody	Hunter and Kappler (1975)
				Enhanced IgM anti-TNP antibody	
Mouse	Spleen	TNP-KLH	TNP-KLH + SRBC	Enhanced IgM anti-SRBC antibody	Waldmann (1975)
		TNP-FGG	TNP-FGG + SRBC		
		TNP-OV	TNP-OV + SRBC		
		TNP-FGG	FGG[d]	Enhanced IgG and IgM anti-TNP antibody	
Rabbit	LN	KLH + MB	KLH	Enhanced IgG anti-MB antibody	Gooch et al. (1976)
		KLH + MB	MB	Enhanced IgG anti-KLH antibody	
		KLH + T2	KLH	Enhanced IgG anti-T2 antibody	
		KLH + DNP-BGG	KLH	Enhanced IgG anti-DNP antibody	

[a] TT, tetanus toxoid; OV, ovalbumin; BSA, bovine serum albumin; KLH, keyhole limpet hemocyanin; MB, sperm whale myoglobin; T2, T2 bacteriophage; BGG, bovine globulin; TNP, trinitrophenyl group; DNP, dinitrophenyl group.

[b] Antigens added to cultures of primed cells; SRBC, sheep red blood cells.

[c] These antigens were added to DNP-BSA-primed B-cell preparations.

[d] Enhancement was observed only when FGG was added to TNP-FGG primed cells from mice primed 5 wk previously. Inhibition was observed when this antigen

responses was achieved. Not included (although undoubtedly very important in suggesting these experiments) are observations *in vitro* (Munro and Hynter, 1970; Hirst and Dutton, 1970; Ekpaha-Mensa and Kennedy, 1971; Feldmann and Basten, 1972*b*) and *in vivo* (McCullagh, 1970; Katz *et al.*, 1971) that interactions between allogeneic lymphoid cell populations nonspecifically augmented the antibody response. This so-called *allogeneic effect* is considered in Section III, in terms of the soluble enhancing factors generated by these allogeneic cell populations.

These studies with a number of different systems reveal certain features of the phenomena of nonspecific enhancement by antigen: (1) Both primary and secondary responses can be enhanced, including the synthesis of at least IgM, IgG, and IgE antibodies. (2) The responses to diverse antigenic determinants, including erythrocytes, T2 phage, haptens and large (KLH) and small (MB) proteins can be augmented. (3) Primed T cells appear to be responsible for the nonspecific activation of B cells. Thus nonspecific enhancement is abolished by treating the primed rabbit lymph node cells with specific antibody to rabbit T cells (Stavitsky and Self, 1972; Stavitsky, *et al.*, 1975). Moreover, primed thymocytes can be utilized (Rubin and Coons, 1972*b*; Waldmann *et al.*, 1973). Indirect evidence is provided by the utilization of carrier protein to promote an antihapten antibody response (Kishimoto and Ishizaka, 1973*a*; Waldmann, 1975). The most convincing evidence that T cells directly influence the response of B cells comes from the experiments of Hunter and Kappler (1975), who utilized DNP-BSA-primed B cells as targets and, most certainly, as the source of the cells that produced IgM antibody to SRBC. (4) Nonspecific enhancement is antigen-concentration dependent; frequently, antigen concentrations which result in a lower specific antibody response markedly enhance the nonspecific response (Stavitsky and Self, 1972; Waldmann, 1975). (5) The extent of nonspecific enhancement is very impressive, especially in those systems in which the IgG or IgE antibody syntheses are promoted. The primary IgM responses are enhanced up to twofold (Rubin and Coons, 1972*c*), the secondary IgG responses to HSA (Stavitsky and Self, 1972) and MB (Stavitsky *et al.*, 1975) up to fifteenfold and tenfold, respectively. Indeed, greater synthesis of antibody to MB has been achieved by the addition of KLH to KLH- and MB-primed lymph node cells than by the addition of MB *per se* (Stavitsky *et al.*, 1975). The secondary IgG antibody response to DNP was enhanced up to twentyfold by free carrier (Kishimoto and Ishizaka, 1973*c*). (6) Both homologous and heterologous antigenic determinants must be presented for the cells to elicit nonspecific enhancement. However, in one system (Stavitsky and Self, 1972; Stavitsky, *et al.*, 1975) only the heterologous antigen was added and the homologous antigen was provided by antigen persisting from the original immunization. (7) In one study (Waldmann, 1975), the interval between priming and *in vitro* challenge was critical: enhancement was observed when FGG was added to TNP-FGG cells primed 5 wk earlier, but inhibition was observed when cells primed 14 wk earlier were used. (8) Hunter and Kappler (1975) presented evidence for the conclusion that the T helper cells that collaborate specifically with B cells are distinct from those T cells that nonspecifically enhance antibody production.

b. *Inhibition of the Synthesis of Antibody*. There is much less information on the nonspecific inhibition than on enhancement of the antibody response. There is also much confusion about the relations between the cells and mechanisms involved in these two types of regulation, including the role of macrophages and of suppressor T cells in these phenomena. Soluble factors can mediate suppression and will be discussed in Section III. Here some of the experimental systems and results are briefly described and discussed.

Schrader and Feldmann (1973) developed a model to study antigenic competition *in vitro*. Mice were primed with FGG 3 wk before use as a source of spleen cells. Two days before sacrifice, they were injected with donkey erythrocytes (DRC). The response of their spleen cells to DNP-FGG *in vitro* was used as an assay of antigenic competition. The cells primed with DRC did not produce antibody to DNP, but did respond to a thymus-independent antigen, DNP-flagella of *Salmonella adelaide*. The function of B cells in this system was normal, as judged by the normal anti-DNP antibody response elicited by DNP-flagella. It appeared that the site of suppression was the macrophage since small numbers (3000) of peritoneal cells depleted of T cells restored the response to DNP-FGG. It was proposed that antigenic competition was due to the release by T cells of complexes of antigen and a T-derived immunoglobulin, IgT. These complexes then bind to macrophages and thereby initiate the response to that antigen by antigen-reactive B cells. However, the binding of IgT complexes formed with a subsequently administered antigen is competitively inhibited so that the macrophage–IgT–second antigen complex required to trigger B cells reactive with the second antigen is not formed and the response to the second antigen does not occur.

Kishimoto and Ishizaka (1973b, 1974) and Klinman (1971) observed inhibition of the anti-DNP antibody response when DNP-protein-primed cells were challenged with high concentrations of DNP-heterologous carrier.

Essentially the same generalizations can be applied to the nonspecific suppressive phenomena as to nonspecific enhancement, including the diversity of responses that can be suppressed (IgM, IgG, IgE), the putative role of T cells, the magnitude of suppression, the requirement for both heterologous and homologous antigens, the importance of interval between priming and challenge, and the significance of antigen concentration.

2. Cyclic Nucleotides

The regulation by cyclic AMP of the *in vitro* anamnestic antibody response to KLH has been studied in this laboratory (Cook and Stavitsky, 1975, 1976). Rabbits were immunized with alum-KLH. Cells from the draining lymph node were removed 6 days later for culture. When optimal amounts of KLH were added to these cells for 24 hr, within the next 5 days they were induced to synthesize IgM and IgG antibody. When cholera enterotoxin (CT) and prostaglandins E_1 and E_2 (PGE_1, PGE_2)—which raise levels of intracellular cyclic AMP—and dibutyryl cyclic AMP (DBcAMP) were added to these cultures with 1–100 μg KLH for the first 24 hr, the ensuing antibody synthesis was enhanced at least 200%. When these agents were added to cultures during 72–120 hr of culture, the antibody response was inhibited. The addition of cyclic GMP or prostaglandin $F_{1\alpha}$ to these cultures for 0–24 hr did not affect the antibody response. T cells, but not macrophages, were required for enhancement of antibody synthesis by CT and DB. T cells were not required for inhibition of the response by these agents.

Two types of experiment served to indicate that at least a partial separation of inductive and regulatory events could be achieved. First, fractionation of the lymph node cell populations on nylon fiber columns yielded cell populations, which were not subject to enhancement of antibody synthesis by CT or DBcAMP, but were induced by KLH to synthesize antibody. Second, induction of the antibody response by KLH, but not enhancement of this response by CT, DBcAMP, and PGE_1, occured in calcium-free culture media.

Enhancement of the antibody response by these agents seemed specific; i.e., only antibody synthesis was enhanced. Also, KLH had to be added before DBcAMP to achieve enhancement, strongly suggesting that antigen-induced event(s) were required for regulation by this agent. One such event might be the KLH-induced uptake of DBcAMP. Indeed, it was observed that the addition of KLH to KLH-primed lymph node cells for 0–24 hr enhanced manyfold the uptake of [^{3}H]DBcAMP during the next 24 hr. This uptake was inhibited by a specific goat IgG antibody to rabbit T cells and thus appears to require T cells. Uptake was also inhibited by KCN and iodoacetate and must involve active transport.

III. Induction and Regulation of *in Vitro* Immune Responses by Soluble Factors

A. Production of Soluble Factors from T Cells

Davies *et al.* (1967) first suggested that mediators released from antigen-stimulated T cells might increase the antibody response of B-line cells. Since then, a good deal of evidence has been obtained for such factors produced by T cells (Katz and Benacerraf, 1972) or macrophages (Unanue, 1972). These factors are categorized according to their cellular sources and their nature.

B. Soluble Factors with Helper and/or Regulatory Activity Generated by or Prepared from T Lymphocytes

1. Immunoglobulin Molecules

Feldmann and Basten (1972*b*) have described antigen-specific murine T-cell products that mediate cell collaboration by binding to macrophages as antigen–IgT complexes that trigger antigen-specific B cells to develop into antibody-forming cells. This T-cell factor was shown to have the mobility of an immunoglobulin in polyacrylamide gel, a molecular weight of 180,000 daltons, two polymeric chains with the electrophoretic mobility of light and μ-chains, and specificity for the T-cell activating antigen (Feldmann *et al.*, 1973). Like the complex that mediates cell collaboration, the factor was cytophilic for macrophages, but not for T or B cells. The existence of this monomeric IgM immunoglobulin as a product of, or in association with, T lymphocytes is disputed (Vitetta *et al.*, 1972). Cone and Marchalonis (1974) have suggested some possible reasons for the discrepancy between their findings and those of others.

Feldmann (1974*a*) reported that supernatants of cultures of antigen-stimulated T cells were just as inhibitory of specific and nonspecific antibody responses as on direct contact of T and B cells. These supernatants induced partial tolerance in both T- and B-cell populations. Both specific and nonspecific suppression occurred only in the absence of macrophages and were abrogated by the addition of these cells. Thus far Feldmann (1974*b*) has not separated the specific (helper) and nonspecific (suppressor) factors. Both factors were absorbed by Sepharose conjugated with anti-mouse, anti-μ, and anti-k antibody and were cytophilic for macrophages. Both activities were generated only when hapten was linked to the same carrier with which the T cells were primed and were specific for that carrier protein.

Further biochemical study is required to determine whether both activities are connected with the same molecule.

2. Nonimmunoglobulin Molecules

Kishimoto and Ishizaka (1973c) incubated DNP-Asc-primed rabbit lymph node cells with DNP-KLH and with a soluble factor (SF) generated by incubating DNP-Rag-primed cells with Rag. They enhanced the anti-DNP IgG and IgE antibody responses in some experiments and only the IgG response in others. They suggested that different T helper cells for IgG and IgE released different SF, with triggered DNP-primed B cells for IgG or IgE antibody synthesis. Kishimoto and Ishizaka (1974) were able to generate both enhancing and suppressive SF. Suppression apparently was not due to an excess of enhancing SF. Kishimoto and Ishizaka (1975a) adduced evidence that the SF was nonspecific in its action: carrier specificity was not involved and SF enhanced the IgG and/or IgE antihapten antibody responses of DNP-carrier-primed cells to DNP-heterologous carrier. The production of SF was inhibited by pantamycin, which inhibits protein synthesis, but not by cytosine arabinoside, which suppresses DNA synthesis (Kishimoto and Ishizaka, 1975b). The SF was produced by incubation of carrier-primed cells with carrier-conjugated Sepharose. The enhancing SF activity for IgG and IgE was not absorbed by carrier-coated immunosorbent, by antibody to carrier, or by anti-Fab, anti-γ-chain, or anti-u-chain immunosorbents. Enhancing activity for IgG response had a molecular weight of 20,000-40,000 and that for IgE 150,000 daltons, although both were β-globulins electrophoretically.

Munro et al. (1974) described a SF which replaces mouse T cells in inducing the antibody response of B cells to poly (tyrosyl, glutamyl)-poly DL (alanyl-polylysyl) (TGAL) in irradiated recipients. This SF was induced by the reaction of primed thymocytes and TGAL, had a molecular weight of 50,000, was antigenspecific, but was not absorbed by anti-Fab or anti-u columns. However, it was removed by alloantisera to the H-2 antigen of the strain of mouse producing the factor—only antisera to the K side of the H-2 locus. Taussig et al. (1975) further mapped this SF and showed that it was a product of the I-A subregion of the H-2 complex. The factor crossed allogeneic barriers: SF produced by one strain cooperated with B cells of H-2 incompatible strains.

Of the variety of factors extracted from thymus (Friedman, 1975), only one is described here because of its demonstrated effect on the antibody response (Armerding and Katz, 1975). This SF appears identical to thymosin (fraction V) of Goldstein et al. (1972). In the presence of this SF spleen cells from athymic mice were induced to synthesize IgM anti-DNP antibody upon challenge with DNP-KLH, DNP-FGG, or DNP-OV. This SF

appeared to promote induction and differentiation of precursor T lymphocytes in nude spleen cell populations, but not to influence B cell functions.

3. Soluble Enhancing and Inhibitory Factors of Unknown Nature

It has not been determined whether the remainder of SF generated
by antigen-stimulated T cells are immunoglobulin or not. Rubin and Coons
(1972a,c) produced a SF by incubating tetanus toxoid-primed mouse thymocytes or spleen cells with that toxoid. This SF—which nonspecifically
enhanced the IgM antibody response of normal spleen cells to SRBC—had
a molecular weight of about 75,000 daltons, was degraded by a protease,
and was heat stable (56°C/30 min). A factor with similar properties was
found in the supernatant fluid of cultures of equal numbers of histoincompatible mouse spleen cells. Gisler et al. (1973) induced specific and nonspecific
SF by adding KLH to KLH-primed mouse spleen cells. The nonspecific
factor potentiated the antibody response to fully or partially T-independent
antigens (DNP-dextran or foreign erythrocytes) and required macrophages,
which were replaceable by 2-mercaptoethanol. The specific helper factor
required the physical presence of macrophages.

Waldmann and Munro (1974) also released SF by culturing KLH-
primed mouse thymus or spleen cells with KLH. Their SF augmented the
in vitro IgM antibody response to SRBC of splenic B cells. This factor was
heat stable (56°C/30 min), did not require KLH for its action, and was not
absorbed by the SRBC, and its activity was not inhibited by a protease
inhibitor. Optimal activation of the B cells occurred when the SF was added
to B cell cultures on day 0 or day 1. Adherent cells were required for production but not for action of this factor. Lefkovits et al. (1975) generated
SF by adding KLH to KLH-primed mouse spleen cells. In a microculture
system, this SF promoted the IgM antibody response of B cells. It was felt
that the SF activated B cells directly and recruited many SRBC-specific B
cells into the antibody response, the number of PFC being dependent on
the concentration of SF.

Thomas et al. (1975) added OV-primed mouse spleen cells to SRBC-
primed mouse spleen cells and observed a dramatic decrease in the number
of direct PFC to SRBC. This inhibition was shown to be due to a SF induced
by the reaction of OV and OV-primed T cells. This SF was inactivated by
trypsin and by heating to 80°C, but not 70°C, and had a molecular weight
of 55,000–60,000. A nonspecific helper SF for SRBC antibody also was
demonstrated and by differential heat inactivation was shown to be different
from the suppressor SF.

4. Nonspecific Factors Generated in Mixtures of Allogeneic Murine Lymphoid Cells

In vitro (Dutton *et al.*, 1971) and *in vivo* (Katz *et al.*, 1971; Kreth and Williamson, 1971) experiments indicated that T cells reacted to allogeneic cells by producing SF that stimulated the antibody response of B cells to foreign erythrocytes and to hapten–protein conjugates. These nonspecific helper SF could replace T-cell function in both IgM (Schimpl and Wecker, 1972*a*) and IgG (Schimpl and Wecker, 1972*b*) antibody responses. The SF reconstituted the IgM response more efficiently when added on day 2 of a 4-day culture than on day 0 (Schimpl and Wecker, 1972*a*), but had to be present from the onset to enhance the IgG response of SRBC-primed B cells (Schimpl and Wecker, 1972*b*). Thus a SF for IgM acted only upon antigen-triggered cells, but the SF for IgG response could activate the already primed cells. Feldmann and Basten (1972*b*) described a mouse allogeneic factor which is dialyzable, does not show antigenic specificity, and acts directly on B cells at a later stage in their development to antibody-forming cells than does the specific helper SF. Rubin *et al.* (1973, 1974) produced a murine allogeneic factor which had similar properties to a nonspecific SF that appeared when tetanus toxoid-primed lymphoid cells were incubated with toxoid. Gorczynski *et al.* (1973) described a mouse allogeneic factor produced by long incubation (48–60 hr) of allogeneic cells with lymphocytes already primed with those cells. This SF had a molecular weight of 150,000, and unlike all SF described to date required SRBC-specific T cells to promote the IgM antibody response to this antigen. Hunter and Kettman (1974) produced a murine allogeneic SF that contained three active fractions, a dialyzable component, one of high molecular weight (150,000), and one of 27,000. The nondialyzable fractions increased both the frequency of B cells responding to SRBC and the size of the responding unit. The dialysate was only able to increase the number of PFC from B cells already triggered by T cells. Armerding and Katz (1974) produced an allogeneic SF with a molecular weight of 30,000–40,000, acting directly upon B cells, with added SRBC, to promote the IgM antibody response. This SF showed no specificity for SRBC, and was inactivated by trypsin and heating (56°C/1 hr). Armerding *et al.* (1974) showed that this SF was removed by an immunosorbent prepared with an anti-Ia antiserum, indicating that the components implicated in T-B cell cooperation were probably products of genes in the I region of the H-2 complex.

IV. Discussion

In this section, information presented earlier is woven together with some new information to illuminate some aspects of the antibody response, to speculate, to reconcile apparent differences, to suggest new experimental approaches, and to indicate some biological and clinical implications.

A. Antigen-Binding Receptors on Lymphocytes

Knowledge of the nature and specificity of the antigen-binding and activatable receptors on T and B lymphocytes is vital for a more complete understanding of the immune response. There is much agreement about the globulin nature and the number of receptors on B lymphocytes, but there is much disagreement about the receptors on T lymphocytes. Studies with with proteins, peptides, and small synthetic antigenic determinants are adding to this knowledge. Utilizing very high concentrations of different antigens, some lymphocytes bound more than one antigen (Decker et al., 1974a), but the physiological significance of this binding is in doubt. In another approach, polymerized flagellin capped more than 95% of surface Ig on lymphocytes from unimmunized and immunized mice, suggesting that all of the Ig receptors on these cells were specific for this multi-determinant antigen (Raff et al., 1973). Weinbaum et al. (1974) have shown through a combination of in vitro and in vivo experiments that murine T and B cells have similar specificity toward albumins from a number of species. However, the most illuminating experiments have been done with peptides synthesized corresponding to the NH_2-terminal heptapeptide (N) and the COOH-terminal pentapeptide (C) of O-Fd; joined by spacers of eight or ten glycine residues to form a bivalent monospecific peptide (N-8-N) or a bispecific peptide (N-10-C). The injection of both peptides into guinea pigs induced both humoral and cellular immunity, indicating that such small determinants can be recognized by receptors on lymphocytes and that when two determinants—of the same or different specificities—are recognized, the antibody response can be induced (Kelly et al., 1973). Autoradiographic and reconstitution experiments with T and/or B cells indicated that both populations could bind the N and C determinants and that both populations were required for the antibody response to both determinants (Kelly et al., 1974). However, the addition of small MB peptides to MB-primed cells induced IgG antibody formation to MB. Very high concentrations of these peptides were required, presumably to increase the probability of finding a conformation approaching the conformation of the peptide in the native protein (Atassi and Saplin, 1968). Thus the receptors on lymphocytes can combine productively, e.g., to induce cellular and humoral immunity, with peptides as small as a pentapeptide (Table I), which is close in size to the tetrapeptide which is the minimal size of determinant for binding to antibody (Schechter *et al.*, 1966).

B. Cellular and Molecular Aspects of Induction

1. Interactions of T and B Cells and Macrophages

The introduction of molecules with repeating units like POL—or determinants like DNP conjugated to these molecules—elicits a T-independent antibody response to both the DNP and the carrier. This response may also be macrophage-independent (Feldmann, 1972*a,c*). The T-dependent responses require T cells, and often MP, and appear to be mediated by soluble factors (SF) (Section III). There general agreement stops. Feldmann and his colleagues (Section IIA4) propose that the MP bearing an AG–IgT complex induces the antibody response by B cells. They also found that in the absence of MP this complex tolerizes B cells. Finally, they produced evidence that inhibition of the antibody response to AG1 by the non-cross-reacting AG2 also involves MP; the binding of AG1–IgT1 to the MP surface saturates the sites that would have bound AG2–IgT2 for the antibody response to AG2. However, it has been questioned whether T cells possess or produce an immunoglobulin receptor. (Vitetta *et al.*, 1972). It has also been questioned whether an immune complex on MP is a better inducer of antibody formation than AG alone on MP (Unanue and Katz, 1973). Feldmann (1972*d*) found that *in vitro* unprimed or primed T cells can be triggered by free AG to produce IgT, but Katz and Unanue (1973) recall that T cells were rapidly tolerized in unprimed animals by the injection of deaggregated proteins which were poorly taken up by MP (Dresser and Mitchison, 1968). Katz and Unanue (1973) showed that MP bearing DNP-protein conjugates can trigger both T and B cells for the antibody response to DNP in an *in vitro* system. Indeed, Katz and Unanue (1973) envision at least two roles for MP in the antibody response, the destruction of excess and possible tolerizing concentrations of AG, and the more efficient presentation of AG to T and B cells than in the form of soluble AG. These divergent views may be reconciled by postulating that AG, free or on MP, induces SF production by T cells and also initiates certain B-cell events that are required for the action of IgT or another SF. Indeed, it would be expected that *in vivo* even deaggregated proteins would be partially taken up and displayed on the surface of MP and could then initiate the T and B cell reactions needed for antibody synthesis.

2. Genetic Control

The immune response to various AG is under genetic control (McDevitt and Benacerraf, 1969; Schreffler and David, 1975). The studies summarized in Section III indicate that some helper and/or regulatory SF may reflect this genetic control (Munro et al., 1974; Taussig, 1975). There is evidence that histocompatibility between T and B cells is required for the induction of the antibody response (Katz et al., 1973, 1974a), histocompatibility between macrophages and T cells for *in vitro* induction of helper activity (Erb and Feldmann, 1975b) and for antigenic recognition for T-cell proliferation (Rosenthal and Shevach, 1973). However, it is difficult to reconcile the findings of Katz et al. (1973, 1974a) with the report that T-cell helper SF can operate across allogeneic barriers (Taussig et al., 1975). Indeed, the findings of Katz and his colleagues suggest still another requirement for T-B cooperation, i.e., the possession by B cells of specific surface acceptor molecules for T-cell products. The alternative explanation and evidence (Heber-Katz and Wilson, 1975) that these genetic restrictions are simply due to antogonism of histoincompatible T cells toward B cells will need further study, especially since Katz et al. (1974b) previously considered and experimentally rejected this explanation.

3. Cellular Mechanisms of Induction of Antibody Synthesis

There is much evidence that T cells are involved in both the induction and regulation of the antibody response (Gershon, 1974; Katz and Benacerraf, 1972), but the mechanisms of these effects are only superficially understood. Clearly, much cell proliferation and differentiation occur (Mach and Vassalli, 1965a); there is also evidence that some proliferation (Dutton and Mishell, 1967), perhaps one critical replication of T cells (Nakamura et al., 1972), is required for induction. However, much evidence is presented in Section IIA5b for a disjunction between DNA synthesis and induction of antibody formation. For instance, there are several reports that helper activity can be exhibited by highly irradiated T cells and that helper or regulatory SF can be produced by T cells that were exposed to cytosine arabinoside, an inhibitor of DNA synthesis. Perhaps the most insightful results were obtained by Feldmann and Basten (1972d). They found that mitomycin C treatment (which inhibits DNA synthesis of normal T cells or T cells from mice primed to SRBC at least 4 wk earlier) markedly reduced their helper function, as reflected in the antibody response to SRBC. In contrast, treatment with this drug of T cells recently induced to divide by exposure to SRBC did not affect their helper function, suggesting that perhaps a critical transcription of DNA had occurred and sufficient information was now available for completion of the antibody response. However, the helper activity of all of these T-cell populations (normal, primed, and recently activated) was inhibited by actinomycin D, indicating that active synthesis of at least some species of RNA was required. These questions probably can only be resolved by detailed analysis of the composition and functions of the various DNA and RNA species in different subcellular fractions utilizing a much more active and refined cell-free system for antibody synthesis than has been developed to date.

4. Induction and Regulation

The relationship between inductive and regulatory events of the antibody response is very obscure. This response can be regulated by appropriate concentrations of specific antigen and antibody, by T cells (Gershon, 1974), and by MP (Unanue, 1972). However, many questions are unanswered: Are there separate populations of inductive (helper) and regulatory T cells or separate helper and regulatory SF? In one study (Feldmann, 1974b) the helper and suppressor SF could not be distinguished. Are there different helper and suppressor SF? Kishimoto and Ishizaka (1974) found evidence for separate factors with these activities. How many different species of SF are there? At present—as indicated in Section III—there is a bewildering array of different SF acting on T cells, on the early phase of the B-cell response, and on the already triggered B cell. The purification and further study of the SF promises to clear up some of this confusion. Of particular interest is the nature of the factor described by Munro et al. (1974) and Taussig (1975) which—although not reactive with antisera to Fab or u determinants—has specificity for the synthetic peptide TGAL. It is encouraging that at least one study (Fauci and Johnson, 1971) presents evidence for the activity of a circulating inhibitor of the antibody response in a whole animal system.

Recent evidence (Cheers et al., 1971; Kishimoto and Ishizaka, 1974) indicates that there are specific T-cell populations that regulate the production of Ig of different classes, in contrast to the earlier view that this regulation was exclusively the function of B cells. The studies of Waldmann (1975) suggest that, depending upon the interval between priming with TNP-FGG and antigenic challenge, helper (5 wk) or suppressor (14 wk) populations develop, providing further indirect evidence for a distinction between these populations. Finally, the studies of Feldmann (1974a) and others suggest a quantitative factor may determine whether enhancement or inhibition occurs, namely, the number of T cells—perhaps expressed in the amounts of SF of one type or another produced by these cells.

The evidence reviewed in Section IIA2 suggests that antigen-induced capping and patching of receptors and interiorization of antigen are not required for induction of the antibody response. That capping may, however, serve a regulatory function was suggested by the observation that the induction of tolerance in B cells is associated with a failure of capping to occur (Diener and Paetkau, 1972). Exposure of B cells to some concentrations of polymerized flagellin resulted in the shedding of the antigen–receptor complex from the cell surface (Diener, Lee, and Paetkau, cited in Diener and Langman, 1975). Diener and Langman (1975) speculate that capping may be a mechanism to clear the surface of potentially tolerigenic amounts of antigen. New approaches are needed to understand how the reaction of antigen with receptors on T and B cells is transduced to the expression of the relevant information for the antibody response contained in these cells. It may be fruitful to investigate antigen-induced alterations in structure and function of the T- and B-lymphocyte cell membranes, along the lines of the studies on the effects of mitogens, e.g., phospholipid metabolism (Fisher and Mueller, 1969). The experiments on polyvalent inducers of the antibody response by B cells and on lymphocyte activation by bivalent antibody to surface Ig (Fanger et al., 1970) on B cells strongly suggest that crosslinking of receptors by ligands plays an important role. These observations should be taken advantage of in conjunction with the analysis of lymphocyte structure–function relations.

C. Maintenance of the Antibody Response

Section IIC described experiments in which lymph node cells removed many months after immunization with KLH or with polymerized HSA were washed and cultured in the absence of further additions of KLH or HSA. They began to synthesize easily detectable amounts of antibody. Data have been obtained to support the proposal that the HSA is localized in the draining lymph node, persists for a short time in medullary macrophages, and remains for many months on the processes of dendritic-type cells (Tew et al., 1973; Tew and Stavitsky, 1974; Stavitsky et al., 1974; Greene et al., 1975). Presumably, persisting immunogen induces the local development of antibody-producing cells as well as of specific T and B memory cells. When the cells are washed to remove antibody, they contain antigen—associated with the dendritic-type cells (Nossal and Ada, 1971)—which with T-B cell collaboration induces antibody synthesis. To explain the persistent antibody synthesis in vivo, it was suggested that the injection polymerized antigen was better localized in the node than monomer (Schmidtke and Unanue, 1971). Depending upon the amount of localized immunogen, the organ will produce a certain amount of antibody and long-lived T and B memory cells (Miller, 1973). Depending upon the relative local concentrations of immunogen and antibody, immunogen will or will not be free to induce antibody and memory cells. Periodically, the antibody level in the node will drop below the critical level for feedback inhibition (Graf and Uhr, 1969); residual immunogen will then be free to induce more antibody and more immunological memory. These cyclical and local activations of memory cells by residual immunogen serve to maintain antibody production. Studies of this type of *in vitro* system with other antigens may provide a useful model of the activation of memory cells by persisting or latent antigens such as viruses. The resulting antibody could provide continued or heightened protection against the virus and/or with residual antigen generate immune complexes which damage the surrounding cells.

D. Nonspecific Induction and Regulation of the Antibody Response

1. Heterologous Antigen

Section IID1 and Table IV presented evidence for the nonspecific induction and regulation of the antibody response to antigen 1 upon addition of antigen 2 to antigen 2-primed cells, presumably T cells (Katz and Benacerraf, 1972; Gershon, 1974). Striking nonspecific enhancement of the IgG, IgM, and IgE antibody responses was reported. Indeed, in at least one system the addition of KLH to KLH- and MB-primed cells induced a manyfold greater IgG antibody response to MB than was induced by stimulation of these cells with MB *per se* (Stavitsky *et al.*, 1975). In several studies it was found that the concentration of antigen (such as KLH) that induces maximal antibody synthesis to the heterologous antigen (such as MB) evoked only a poor response to KLH (Stavitsky and Self, 1972; Gooch *et al.*, 1976). This observation is consistent with the finding by Hunter and Kappler (1975) that the T cells that cooperate specifically with B cells are distinct from those that cooperate nonspecifically to enhance antibody production. The evidence for different soluble factors for the IgG and IgE anti-DNP antibody responses and different factors for nonspecific enhancement and inhibition of these responses also speaks for multiple T-cell populations (Kishimoto and Ishizaka, 1973c). Generally, it appears that the T cell—presumably through its soluble product(s)—acts directly on B cells. Of particular interest was the finding that the nonantigenic MB peptide 1-6 (Atassi, 1964) upon addition to MB-primed rabbit lymph node cells induced antibody synthesis to MB. It is not known with which of the other MB peptides this 1-6-induced antibody combines, but it must be assumed that it does not combine with 1-6. If the specificity of this antibody for peptides other than 1-6 is verified, it would appear most likely that 1-6 is utilized to activate T cells to produce a product that stimulates the response of B cells to other MB peptides; presumably these other determinants are provided by MB persisting from the original priming. Thus 1-6 functions as an immunogen, not as an antigen. Becker *et al.*

(1975) made a similar observation upon immunization of rats and guinea pigs with (4-hydroxy-5-iodo-3-nitrophenyl)acetyl-ε-aminocaproyl-L-tyrosine-azobenzene-p-arsonate [NIP-cap-TYR(ABA)]; antibody formation against NIP-cap but very little against ABA-TYR occurred. Prior immunization with ABA-TYR primed rats for an enhanced anti-NIP response to the entire molecule. Adult thymectomized X-irradiated rats showed a poor anti-NIP response to the bifunctional antigen if reconstituted with T cells from control mice, but a good response if restored with similar cells from ABA-TYR-primed syngeneic rats.

Clagett and Weigle (1974) obtained data to support the hypothesis that rabbit T cells are unresponsive and B cells responsive to autologous thyroglobulin (Tg). They found that unresponsiveness could be terminated and thyroid lesions produced with a mixture of cross-reacting Tg's and reactive T cells. In view of the nonspecific induction of the antibody response by non-cross-reactive antigens (Table IV), it is conceivable that T-cell unresponsiveness to self components can also be circumvented by the stimulation of responsive B cells by products resulting from the reaction of heterologous antigens with specifically reactive T cells.

2. Cyclic Nucleotides

Our studies (Section IID2) show that the *in vitro* anamnestic IgM and IgG antibody responses to KLH are enhanced by the early introduction of agents that raise intracellular cyclic AMP levels but are inhibited by the addition of these agents several days later. The addition of cyclic GMP does not affect these syntheses. This nonspecific enhancement appears to require T cells, but the inhibition is T-cell independent. Teh and Paetkau (1974) and Watson *et al.* (1973) determined the effects of cyclic nucleotides on the *in vitro* IgM antibody responses of mouse spleen cells to SRBC. They also observed that antibody synthesis was enhanced when DBcAMP was present during the early hours of culture and inhibited when this agent was present later. Cyclic GMP could reverse the cAMP-induced inhibition of this IgM antibody response (Watson *et al.*, 1973). Evidence was presented that cyclic GMP could replace T-cell function in the IgM anti-SRBC antibody response of spleen cells from athymic mice.

These *in vitro* experiments may be unphysiological because rather high concentrations of DBcAMP were added compared to the normal intracellular concentrations of cAMP (R. G. Cook and A. B. Stavitsky, unpublished observations). This objection raises two questions: Will the addition of antigen to lymphoid cells induce increases in intracellular cyclic AMP? If that is so, will elevations of this magnitude regulate the antibody response to the same extent as exogenous DBcAMP or other agents that raise the level of this nucleotide? Even if the answer is yes to both questions, it should still be questioned whether an alteration in cellular cyclic AMP level is required for induction of antibody synthesis—or is it just involved in modulating this response? This question is raised because under two circumstances (removal of certain cell populations and calcium deprivation) the anti-KLH antibody response was still induced, but the response was not enhanced by added cholera toxin or DBcAMP (R. G. Cook and A. B. Stavitsky, 1976).

E. Future Outlook

It is clear that, although a vast amount of new information has accumulated in recent years, much of it is unconnected, and we still have only a primitive understanding of the detailed mechanisms of the antibody response. However, the next few years should witness improved understanding with the use of better-defined antigenic and cell systems and newer methods for the genetic, metabolic, biochemical, and immunochemical study of these systems. A better understanding should also emerge of the relations of the cells and molecules in specific and nonspecific induction and regulation of the antibody response and of the interplay of cellular and humoral immunity.

It is hoped that the evidence and questions presented will at least stimulate the search for more basic information. I agree with Mark Twain that "supposing is good, but knowing is better."

ACKNOWLEDGMENTS

The work was supported by USPHS Grants AI-1865, AI-11420, and CA-18648 and Training Grant 5T1-GM-171.

V. References

Adler, F. L., 1964 *Prog. Allergy* **8**:41.
Adler, F. L., Fishman, M., and Dray, S., 1966, *J. Immunol.* **97**:554.
Adler, L. T., Curley, D. M., and Fishman, M., 1973, *J. Immunol.* **110**:811.
Ambrose, C. T., 1969, *J. Exp. Med.* **130**:1003.
Ambrose, C. T., 1973, *J. Exp. Med.* **137**:1369.
Armerding, D., and Katz, D. H., 1974, *J. Exp. Med.* **140**:19.
Armerding, D., and Katz, D. H., 1975, *J. Immunol.* **114**:1248.
Armerding, D., Sachs, D. H., and Katz, D. H., 1974, *J. Exp. Med.* **140**:1717.
Armstrong, W. D., Langman, R. E., and Diener, E., 1974, *J. Immunol.* **113**:251.

Askonas, B. A., and Rhodes, J. M., 1965, *Nature (London)* **205**:470.

Atassi, M. Z., 1964, *Nature (London)* **202**:496.

Atassi, M. Z., 1975, *Immunochemistry* **12**:423.

Atassi, M. Z., and Saplin, B. J., 1968, *Biochemistry* **7**:688.

Becker, M. J., Ray, A., Andersson, L. C., and Makela, O., 1975, *Eur. J. Immunol.* **5**:262.

Bell, C., and Dray, S., 1970, *J. Immunol.* **105**:541.

Bloom, B. R., Jimenz, L., and Marcus, P. I., 1970, *J. Exp. Med.* **132**:16.

Britton, S., and Moller, G. J., 1968, *J. Immunol.* **100**:1326.

Bullock, W. W., and Rittenberg, M. B., 1970, *J. Exp. Med.* **132**:926.

Bustin, M., Tarrab, R., Strausbauch, P. H., Sulica, A., and Sela, M., 1972, *Eur. J. Immunol.* **2**:288.

Calderon, J., and Unanue, E. R., 1974, *J. Immunol.* **112**:1804.

Calderon, J., Kiely, J-M, Lefko, J., and Unanue, E., 1975, *J. Exp. Med.* **142**:151.

Cerottini, J. C., and Trnka, Z., 1970, *Int. Arch. Allergy Appl. Immunol.* **38**:37.

Cheers, C., and Miller, J. F. A. P., 1972, *J. Exp. Med.* **136**:1661.

Cheers, C., Breitner, J. C. S., Little, M., and Miller, J. F. A. P., 1971, *Nature (London)* **232**:248.

Clagett, J. A., and Weigle, W. O., 1974, *J. Exp. Med.* **139**:643.

Claman, H. N., Chaperon, E. A., and Triplett, R. F., 1966, *Proc. Soc. Exp. Biol. Med.* **122**:1167.

Cone, R. E., and Marchalonis, J. J., 1974, *Biochem. J.* **140**:345.

Cook, R. G., and Stavitsky, A. B., 1975, *J. Immunol.* **114**:426.

Cook, R. G., and Stavitsky, A. B., 1976, *Cell. Immunol.,* in press.

Cook, R. G., Stavitsky, A. B., and Schoenberg, M. D., 1975, *J. Immunol.* **114**:426.

Cunningham, A. J., 1969, *Aust. J. Biol. Med. Sci.* **47**:493.

Davies, A. J. S., Leuchars, E., Wallis, V., Marchant, R., and Elliot, E. V., 1967, *Transplantation* **5**:222.

Decker, J. M. Clarke, J., Bradley, L. M., Miller, A., and Sercarz, E. E., 1974a, *J. Immunol.* **113**:1823.

Decker, J. M., Kim, Y. B., and Miller, A., 1974b, *J. Immunol.* **113**:1599.

Delespesse, G., Ishizaka, K., and Kishimoto, T., 1975, *J. Immunol.* **114**:1065.

DeLuca, D., Decker, J., Miller, A., and Sercarz, E., 1974, *Cell. Immunol.* **10**:1.

Diener, E., 1968, *J. Immunol.* **100**:1062.

Diener, E., and Langman, R. E., 1975, *Prog. Allergy* **18**:6.

Diener, E., and Paetkau, V. H., 1972, *Proc. Natl. Acad. Sci. U.S.A.* **69**:2364.

Diener, E., Lee, K.-C., Langman, R. E., Kraft, N., Paetkau, V. H., and Pernis, B., 1974, Regulation of the immune response at the single cell level, *in: Control of Proliferation in Animal Cells* (B. Clarkson and R. Baserga, eds.), pp. 411–422, Cold Spring Harbor Laboratory, Cold Spring Harbor, N.Y.

Dixon, F. J., and McConahey, P. J., 1963, *J. Exp. Med.* **117**:833.

Dresser, D. W., and Mitchison, N. A., 1968, *Adv. Immunol.* **8**:129.

Dutton, R. W., 1961, *Nature (London)* **192**:462.

Dutton, R. W., and Mishell, R. I., 1967, *J. Exp. Med.* **126**:443.

Dutton, R. W., and Pearce, J. D., 1962, *Nature (London)* **194**:93.

Dutton, R. W., Falkoff, R., Hirst, J. A., Hoffmann, M., Kappler, J. W., Kettman, J. R., Lesley, J. F., and Vann, D., 1971, Is there evidence for a nonantigen specific diffusable chemical mediator from the thymus-derived cell in the initiation of the immune response, *in: Progress in Immunology* (B. Amos, ed.), pp. 355–368, Academic Press, New York.

Eisen, H. N., and Siskind, G. W., 1964, *Biochemistry* **3**:996.

Ekpaha-Mensa, A., and Kennedy, J. C., 1971, *Nature (London) New Biol.* **233**:174.

Engers, H. D., and Unanue, E. R., 1973, *J. Immunol.* **110**:465.

Erb, P., and Feldmann, M., 1975a, *Nature (London)* **254**:352.

Erb, P., and Feldmann, M., 1975b, *J. Exp. Med.* **142**:460.

Fanger, M. W., Hart, D. A., Wells, J. V., and Nisonoff, A., 1970, *J. Immunol.* **105**:1484.

Fauci, A. S., and Johnson, J. S., 1971, *J. Immunol.* **107**:1052.

Feldmann, M., 1922*a*, *J. Immunol.* **2**:130.

Feldmann, M., 1972*b*, *J. Exp. Med.* **135**:735.

Feldmann, M., 1972*c*, *J. Exp. Med.* **135**:1049.

Feldmann, M., 1972*d*, *J. Exp. Med.* **136**:737.

Feldmann, M., 1972*e*, *J. Exp. Med.* **136**:532.

Feldmann, M., 1974*a*, *Eur. J. Immunol.* **4**:660.

Feldmann, M., 1974*b*, *Eur. J. Immunol.* **4**:667.

Feldmann, M., and Basten, A., 1972*a*, *J. Exp. Med.* **136**:49.

Feldmann, M., and Basten, A., 1972*b*, *J. Exp. Med.* **136**:722.

Feldmann, M., and Basten, A., 1972*c*, *J. Exp. Med.* **136**:737.

Feldmann, M., and Basten, A., 1972*d*, *Eur. J. Immunol.* **2**:213.

Feldmann, M., and Nossal, G. J. V., 1972, *Q. Rev. Biol.* **47**:269.

Feldmann, M., and Schrader, J. W., 1974, *Cell. Immunol.* **14**:255.

Feldmann, M., Cone, R. E., and Marchalonis, J. J., 1973, *Cell. Immunol.* **9**:1.

Feldmann, M., Greaves, M. F., Parker, D. C., and Rittenberg, M. B., 1974, *Eur. J. Immunol.* **4**:591.

Fisher, D. B., and Mueller, G. C., 1969, *Biochim. Biophys. Acta* **176**:316.

Fishman, M., 1961, *J. Exp. Med.* **114**:837.

Fishman, M., and Adler, F. L., 1963, *J. Exp. Med.* **117**:595.

Friedman, H. (ed.), 1973, RNA in the Immune Response, *Ann. N.Y. Acad. Sci.* **207**:1.

Friedman, H. (ed.), 1975, Thymus Factors in Immunity, *Ann. N. Y. Acad. Sci.* **249**:1.

Friedman, H. P., Stavitsky, A. B., and Solomon, J. M., 1965, *Science* **149**:1106.

Gershon, R. K., 1974, *Contemp. Topics Immunobiol.* **3**:1.

Gisler, R. H., Staber, F., Rude, E., and Dukor, P., 1973, *Eur. J. Immunol.* **3**:650.

Goldstein, A. L., Guha, A., Zak, M. M., Hardy, M., and White, A., 1972, *Proc. Natl. Acad. Sci. U.S.A.* **69**:1800.

Gooch, G. T., Stavitsky, A. B., Atassi, M. Z., Manderino, G., and Harold, W. W., 1976, manuscript in preparation.

Gorczynski, R. M., Miller, R. G., and Phillips, R. I., 1973, *J. Immunol.* **110**:968.

Graf, M. W., and Uhr, J. W., 1969, *J. Exp. Med.* **130**:1175.

Greaves, M. F., and Bauminger, S., 1972, *Nature (London) New Biol.* **235**:67.

Greaves, M. F., and Brown, G., 1974, *J. Immunol.* **112**:420.

Greaves, M. F., and Janossy, G., 1972, *Transplant. Rev.* **11**:89.

Greaves, M. F., Owen, J. T., and Raff, M. C., 1973, *T and B. Lymphocytes,* Excerpta Medica, Amsterdam.

Greenberg, L. J., Gray, E. D., and Yunis, E. J., 1975, *J. Exp. Med.* **141**:935.

Greene, E. J., Tew, J. G., and Stavitsky, A. B., 1975, *Cell. Immunol.* **18**:476.

Grey, H. M., Kubo, R. T., and Cerottini, J. C., 1972, *J. Exp. Med.* **136**:1323.

Heber-Katz, E., and Wilson, D. B., 1975, *J. Exp. Med.* **142**:928.

Herscowitz, H. B., and Stavitsky, A. B., 1970, *J. Immunol.* **105**:1389.

Herscowitz, H. B., Stavitsky, A. B., and Tew, J. G., 1971, *Cell. Immunol.* **2**:259.

Hirst, J. A., and Dutton, R. W., 1970, *Cell. Immunol.* **1**:190.

Hudson, L., Sprent, J., Miller, J. F. A. P., and Playfair, J. H. L., 1974, *Nature (London)* **251**:60.

Hunter, P., and Kappler, J. W., 1975, *J. Immunol.* **114**:1116.

Hunter, P., and Kettman, J. R., 1974, *Proc. Natl. Acad, Sci. U.S.A.* **71**:512.

Hunter, P., and Munro, A. J., 1972, *Immunology* **23**:69.

Hunter, P., Kappler, J. W., and Kettman, J. R., 1974, *J. Immunol.* **113**:830.

Hurme, M., Nakamura, I., Kaartinen, M., and Makela, O., 1975, *Scand. J. Immunol.* **4**:229.

Hyslop, H. E., Dourmashkin, R. R. Green, N. H., and Porter, R. R., 1970, *J. Exp. Med.* **131**:783.

Ingraham, J. S., 1963, *C. R. Acad. Sci.* **256**:5005.

Ishizaka, K., and Kishimoto, T., 1972, *J. Immunol.* **109**:65.

Janeway, C. A., Sharrow, S. O., and Simpson, E., 1975, *Nature (London)* **253**:544.

Jerne, N. K., and Nordin, A. A., 1963, *Science* **140**:405.

Jonard, J., and Panijel, J., 1973, *Eur. J. Immunol.* **3**:245.

Katz, D. H., and Benacerraf, B., 1972, *Adv. Immunol.* **15**:1.

Katz, D. H., and Unanue, E. R., 1973, *J. Exp. Med.* **137**:967.

Katz, D. H., Paul, W. E., Goidl, E. A., and Benacerraf, B., 1970, *Science* **170**:462.

Katz, D. H., Paul, W. E., Goidl, E. A., and Benacerraf, B., 1971, *J. Exp. Med.* **133**:169.

Katz, D. H., Hamaoka, T., and Benacerraf, B., 1973, *J. Exp. Med.* **137**:1405.

Katz, D. H., Dorf, M. E., and Benacerraf, B., 1974a, *J. Exp. Med.* **140**:290.

Katz, D. H., Hamaoka, T., Dorf, M. E., and Benacerraf, B., 1974b, *J. Immunol.* **112**:855.

Kelly, B., Levy, J. G., and Hull, D., 1973, *Eur. J. Immunol.* **3**:574.

Kelly, B., Kaye, B., Yoshizawa, W., Levey, J. G., and Kilburn, D. G., 1974, *Eur. J. Immunol.* **4**:356.

Kettman, J., and Dutton, R. W., 1971, *Proc. Natl. Acad. Sci. U.S.A.* **68**:699.

Kim, K. J., Cooper, R. B., and Herscowitz, H. B., 1975, *Fed. Proc.* **34**:959.

Kishimoto, T., and Ishizaka, K., 1971, *J. Immunol.* **107**:1567.

Kishimoto, T., and Ishizaka, K., 1972, *J. Immunol.* **109**:612.

Kishimoto, T., and Ishizaka, K., 1973a, *J. Immunol.* **111**:1.

Kishimoto, T., and Ishizaka, K., 1973b, *J. Immunol.* **111**:720.

Kishimoto, T., and Ishizaka, K., 1973c, *J. Immunol.* **111**:1194.

Kishimoto, T., and Ishizaka, K., 1974, *J. Immunol.* **112**:1685.

Kishimoto, T., and Ishizaka, K., 1975a, *J. Immunol.* **114**:585.

Kishimoto, T., and Ishizaka, K., 1975b, *J. Immunol.* **114**:1177.

Klinman, N. R., 1971, *J. Exp. Med.* **133**:963.

Klinman, N. R., 1972, *J. Exp. Med.* **136**:241.

Klinman, N. R., and Doughty, R. A., 1973, *J. Exp. Med.* **138**:473.

Klinman, N. R., Long, C. A., and Karush, F., 1969, *J. Immunol.* **99**:1128.

Kreth, H. W., and Williamson, A. R., 1971, *Nature (London)* **234**:454.

Kunin, S., Shearer, G. M., Segal, S., Globerson, A., and Feldman, M., 1971, *Cell Immunol.* **2**:229.

Lamelin, J.-P., Lisowska-Bernstein, B., Matter, A., Ryser, J. E., and Vassali, P., 1972, *J. Exp. Med.* **136**:984

Lazda, V. A., Starr, J. L., and Rachmeler, M., 1968, *J. Immunol.* **101**:349.

Lee, K.-C., Langman, R. E., Diener, E., and Paetkau, V. H., 1973, *Eur. J. Immunol.* **3**:306.

Lefkovits, I., Quintans, J., Munro, A., and Waldmann, H., 1975, *Immunology* **28**:1149.

Levy, J. G., Hull, D., Kelly, B., Kilburn, D. G., and Teather, R. M., 1972, *Cell. Immunol.* **5**:87.

Loor, F. L., Forni, L., and Pernis, B., 1972, *Eur. J. Immunol.* **2**:203.

Macario, A. J. L., and de Macario, E. C., 1974, *J. Immunol.* **113**:756.

Mach, B., and Vassalli, P., 1965a, *Proc. Natl. Acad. Sci. U.S.A.* **54**:975.

Mach, B., and Vassalli, P., 1965b, *Science* **150**:622.

Marbrook, J., 1967, *Lancet* **2**:1279.

McCullagh, P. J., 1970, *J. Exp. Med.* **132**:916.

McDevitt, H. O., and Benacerraf, B., 1969, *Adv. Immunol.* **11**:31.

Mendelsohn, J., Skinner, S. A., and Kornfeld, S., 1971, *J. Clin. Invest.* **50**:818.

Michaelides, M. C., and Coons, A. H., 1963, *J. Exp. Med.* **117**:1035.

Miller, J. F. A. P., and Mitchell, G. F., 1967, *Nature (London)* **216**:659.

Miller, J. F. A. P., Sprent, J., Basten, A., Warner, N. L., Breitner, J. C. S., Rowland, G., Hamilton, J., Silver, H., and Martin, W. J., 1971, *J. Exp. Med.* **134**:1266.

Miller, J. J., III, 1973, *Cell. Immunol.* **8**:413.

Mitchison, N. A., 1969, *Isr. J. Med. Sci.* **5**:230.

Mitchison, N. A., 1971, *Eur. J. Immunol.* **1**:68.

Moorhead, J. W., Walters, C. S., and Claman, H. N., 1973, *J. Exp. Med.* **137**:411.

Muller-Eberhard, H. J., 1968, *Adv. Immunol.* **8**:1.

Munro, A., and Hunter, P., 1970, *Nature (London)* **225**:277.

Munro, A. J., Taussig, M. J., Campbell, R., Williams, H., and Lawson, Y., 1974, *J. Exp.Med.* **140**:1579.

Nakamura, I., Segal, S., Globerson, A., and Feldman, M., 1972, *Cell. Immunol.* **4**:351.

Nossal, G. J. V., and Ada, G. L., 1971, *Antigens, Lymphoid Cells and the Immune Response,* Academic Press, New York.

Nossal, G. J. V., and Makela, O., 1962, *J. Exp. Med.* **115**:209.

O'Brien, T. F., and Coons, A. H., 1963, *J. Exp. Med.* **117**:1063.

Osborne, D. P., and Katz, D. H., 1973a, *J. Immunol.* **111**:1164.

Osborne, D. P., and Katz, D. H., 1973b, *J. Immunol.* **111**:1176.

Pai, R. C., and Atassi, M. Z., 1975, *Immunochemistry* **12**:285.

Panijel, J., Delamette, F., and Leneveu, M,, 1971, *Eur. J. Immunol.* **1**:87.

Pelley, R. P., and Stavitsky, A. B., 1976, manuscript in preparation.

Perkins, W. D., Karnovsky, M. J., and Unanue, E. R., 1972, *J. Exp. Med.* **135**:267.

Peters, J. H., and Hausen, P., 1971, *Eur. J. Biochem.* **19**:509.

Piguet, P. F., and Vassalli, P., 1973, *Eur. J. Immunol.* **3**:477.

Quastel, M. R., and Kaplan, J. G., 1970, *Exp. Cell Res.* **63**:230.

Raff, M. C., and de Petris, S., 1973, *Fed. Proc.* **32**:48.

Raff, M. C., Feldmann, M., and de Petris, S., 1973, *J. Exp. Med.* **137**:1024.

Rittenberg, M. B., and Bullock, W. W., 1972, *Immunochemistry* **9**:491.

Roelants, G. E., and Askonas, B. A., 1971, *Eur. J. Immunol.* **1**:151.

Roelants, G., Forni, L., and Pernis, B., 1973, *J. Exp. Med.* **137**:1060.

Romball, C. G., and Weigle, W. O., 1973, *J. Exp. Med.* **138**:1426.

Rosenthal, A. S., and Shevach, E. M., 1973, *J. Exp. Med.* **138**:1194.

Rubin, A. S., and Coons, A. H., 1972a, *J. Immunol.* **108**:1597.

Rubin, A. S., and Coons, A. H., 1972b, *J. Exp. Med.* **135**:437.

Rubin, A. S., and Coons, A. H., 1972c, *J. Exp. Med.* **136**:1501.

Rubin, A. S., McDonald, A. B., and Coons, A. H., 1973, *J. Immunol.* **111**:1314.

Rubin, A. S., MacDonald, B., and Coons, A H., 1974, *J. Exp. Med.* **139**:439.

Rubin, B., and Wigzell, H., 1974, *J. Exp. Med.* **139**:732.

Schechter, I., Schechter, B., and Sela M., 1966, *Biochem. Biophys. Acta* **127**:438.

Schimpl, A., and Wecker, E., 1972a, *Nature (London)* **237**:15.

Schimpl, A., and Wecker, E., 1972b, *J. Exp. Med.* **137**:547.

Schmidtke, J. R., and Unanue, E. R., 1971, *J. Immunol.* **107**:331.

Schmiege, S. K., and Miller, H. C., 1974, *J. Immunol.* **113**:110.

Schrader, J. W., 1973, *J. Exp. Med.* **138**:1466.

Schrader, J. W., 1975, *J. Exp. Med.* **141**:962.

Schrader, J. W., and Feldmann, M., 1973, *Eur. J. Immunol.* **3**:711.

Schreffler, D. C., and David, C. S., 1975, *Adv. Immunol.* **20**:125.

Segal, S., Globerson, A., and Feldman, M., 1971a, *Cell. Immunol.* **2**:205.

Segal, S., Globerson, A., and Feldman, M., 1971b, *Cell. Immunol.* **2**:222.

Segal, S., Globerson, A., Feldman, M., Haimovich, J., and Sela, M., 1970, *J. Exp. Med.* **131**:93.

Sela, M., 1969, *Science* **166**:1365.

Self, C. H., Tew, J. G., Cook, R. G., and Stavitsky, A. B., 1974, *Immunochemistry* **11**:227.

Senyk, G., Williams, E. B., Nitecki, D. E., and Goodman, J. W., 1971, *J. Exp. Med.* **133**:1294.

Shearer, G. M., Cudcowicz, G., Connel, M.S.J., and Priore, R. L., 1968, *J. Exp. Med.* **128**:437.

Shortman, K., and Palmer, J., 1971, *J. Cell. Immunol.* **2**:399.

Singer, S. J., and Nicolson, G. L., 1972, *Science* **175**:720.

Siskind, G. W., and Thorbecke, G. J., 1971, *Immunology* **20**:151.

Spitler, L., Benjamini, E., Young, J. D., Kaplan, H., and Fudenberg, H. H., 1970, *J. Exp. Med.* **131**:133.

Stavitsky, A. B., 1954, *J. Infect. Dis.* **94**:306.

Stavitsky, A. B., and Cook, R. G., 1974, *J. Immunol.* **112**:583.

Stavitsky, A. B., and Gusdon, J. P., 1966, *Bacteriol. Rev.* **30**:418.

Stavitsky, A. B., and Self, C. H., 1972, *Immunol. Communi.* **1**:491.

Stavitsky, A. B., Tew, J. G., and Harold, W. W., 1974, *J. Immunol.* **113**:2045.

Stavitsky, A. B., Atassi, M. Z., Gooch, G. T., Pelley, R. P., and Harold, W. W., 1975, *Immunochemistry* **12**:959.

Stecher, V. J., and Thorbecke, G. J., 1967, *J. Exp. Med.* **125**:33.

Steiner, L. A., and Eisen, H. N., 1967, *J. Exp. Med.* **126**:1185.

Sterzl, J., 1959, *Nature (London)* **183**:547.

Strausbauch, P. H., Tarrab, R., Sulica, A., and Sela, M., 1972, *J. Immunol.* **108**:236.

Tao, T. W., 1972, *Eur. J. Immunol.* **2**:332.

Tao, T. W., and Leary, P. L., 1969, *Nature (London)* **233**:306.

Tarrab, R., Sulica, A., Haimovich, J., and Sela, M., 1971, *Eur. J. Immunol.* **1**:231.

Taussig, M. J., Munro, A. J., Campbell, R., David, C. S., and Staines, N. A., 1975, *J. Exp. Med.* **142**:694.

Taylor, R. B., Philips, W., Duffus, P. H., Raff, M. C., and de Petris, S., 1971, *Nature (London) New Biol.* **233**:225.

Teh, H. S., and Paetkau, V., 1974, *Nature (London)* **250**:505.

Tew, J. G., and Stavitsky, A. B., 1974, *Cell. Immunol.* **14**:1.

Tew, J. G., Self, C. H., Harold, W. W., and Stavitsky, A. B., 1973, *J. Immunol.* **111**:416.

Thomas, D. W., Roberts, W. K., and Talmage, D. W., 1975, *J. Immunol.* **114**:1616.

Unanue, E. R., 1972, *Adv. Immunol.* **15**:95.

Unanue, E. R., and Calderon, J., 1975, *Fed. Proc.* **34**:1737.

Unanue, E. R., and Cerottini, J.-C., 1970, *J. Exp. Med.* **131**:711.

Unanue, E. R., and Katz, D. H., 1973, *Eur. J. Immunol.* **3**:559.

Unanue, E. R., Perkins, W. D., and Karnovsky, M. J., 1972, *J. Exp. Med.* **136**:885.

Unanue, E. R., Ault, K. A., and Karnovsky, M. J., 1974, *J. Exp. Med.* **139**:295.

Urso, P., and Makinodan, T., 1963, *J. Immunol.* **90**:897.

Vaughan, J. H., Dutton, A. H., Dutton, R. W., George, M., and Marston, R. Q., 1960, *J. Immunol.* **84**:258.

Vitetta, E. S., and Uhr, J. W., 1975a, *Science* **189**:964.

Vitetta, E. S., and Uhr, J. W., 1975b, *Biochim. Biophys. Acta* **415**:253.

Vitetta, E. S., Bianco, C., Nussenzweig, V., and Uhr, J. W., 1972, *J. Exp. Med.* **136**:81.

Waldmann, H., 1975, *Immunology* **28**:497.

Waldmann, H., and Munro, A., 1974, *Immunology* **27**:53.

Waldmann, H., Munro, A., and Hunter, P., 1973, *Eur. J. Immunol.* **3**:167.

Waterfield, D., Levy, J. G., Kilburn, D. G., and Teather, R. M., 1972, *Cell. Immunol.* **3**:253.

Watson, J., Epstein, R., and Cohn, M., 1973, *Nature (London)* **246**:405.

Weigle, W. O., 1966, *Immunology* **10**:377.

Weinbaum, F. I., Butchko, L. S., Thorbecke, G. J., and Nisonoff, A., 1974, *J. Immunol.* **113**:257.

Wilson, G. S., and Miles, A. A., 1964, *Topley and Wilson's Principles of Bacteriology and Immunity*, Vol. 2, 5th ed., pp. 1370–1374. Williams and Wilkins, Baltimore.

Wood, D. D., and Gaul, S. L., 1974, *J. Immunol.* **113**:925.

Wust, C. J., Gall, C. L., and Novelli, G. D., 1964, *Science* **143**:1041.

5

Immunochemistry of Encephalitogenic Protein

Håkan Bergstrand

I. Introduction

A. Characteristics of Experimental Allergic Encephalomyelitis

More than 40 years ago, Hurst (1932), Rivers *et al.* (1933), and Rivers and Schwentker (1935) were among the first to observe that repeated injections of a homogenate of brain tissue into animals could, after a time, induce a kind of disseminated encephalomyelitis in some of the injected animals. The study of this experimental disorder was greatly simplified when Kabat *et al.* (1946, 1947), Morgan (1946, 1947), and Freund *et al.* (1947) found that induction of the disease was markedly facilitated if the brain tissue was emulsified in mineral oil containing mycobacteria—i.e., Freund's complete adjuvant or FCA—one single injection then being sufficient.

Today, this disease is generally known as experimental allergic encephalomyelitis (EAE). It is probably the best-examined disease within the group of experimental disorders that are known as autoimmune (because they are induced by sensitization to an organ-specific antigen, which can even be of autologous origin). EAE is readily produced in most experimental animals. Approximately 2 weeks after a challenge injection, affected animals begin to lose weight and often develop incontinence, ataxia, and an ascending paralysis, the major clinical characteristic of the disease in rodents. The disease often leads to death, but surviving animals tend to

Håkan Bergstrand · Tornblad Institute, University of Lund, and Research Laboratory, AB Draco, Lund Sweden.

show a marked reversibility of clinical symptoms, and they are protected at renewed inoculations of encephalitogenic emulsions.

At microscopic examinations of brains from diseased guinea pigs, a disseminated meningoencephalomyelitis with infiltrations of mononuclear cells around the small veins can be seen. The infiltrating cells show the characteristics of small and medium lymphocytes and macrophages; some plasma cells are also present. Depending on the severity of the lesions, a varying proportion of polymorphonuclear cells can be found in the perivascular cuffs.

A primary demyelination does not seem to be a general feature of EAE in guinea pigs or rats (Adams and Leibowitz, 1969); the degree is apparently dependent partly on the nature of the encephalitogenic challenge (cf. Hoffman et al., 1973; Wisniewski and Bloom, 1975). However, in diseased monkeys, the picture of demyelination can be pronounced. Moreover, the inflammatory lesions seem to be more severe in monkeys than in rodents (see Jackson et al., 1972; Rauch and Einstein, 1974a,b), but the injuries tend to be less concentrated to the spinal cord in the former species than they usually are in rodents. Electron microscopic investigations confirm the essentially inflammatory and vascular nature of the lesions (for references, see Adams and Leibowitz, 1969; Raine et al., 1974; Dal Canto et al., 1975).

Apart from the ordinary type of EAE, other forms of the disease have been characterized in the rat (for a review, see Levine, 1974). They differ from ordinary EAE in manner of induction, location within the target tissue, and histopathological criteria. A recurrent form of the disease was observed in adult Lewis rats (McFarlin et al., 1974; Paterson et al., 1974; Levine and Sowinski, 1975a), and a chronic form of EAE can be induced in young guinea pigs (see Stone et al., 1969; Raine et al., 1974; Lisak and Behan, 1975).

In the postvaccinal rabies encephalomyelitis (which might be the human counterpart of EAE), cuffs of small lymphocytes, plasma cells, and macrophages are generally seen around the small veins. The similarities in histological characteristics constitute one of the reasons why many investigators regard EAE as a fairly good experimental model for some of the human demyelinating diseases (for reviews of these aspects, see Adams and Leibowitz, 1969; Paterson, 1969, 1971, 1972; Ridley, 1971; Field et al., 1972; Nilsson, 1972; Wolfgram et al., 1972; Kies, 1973; Mackay et al., 1973; Rauch and Einstein, 1974b).

B. The Autoimmune Component(s)

The prevailing opinion is that EAE is an autoimmune disorder of the central nervous system. This opinion is based on the following established conditions: The antigen responsible for the induction of the disease is known. It is a strongly basic protein located primarily in central nervous system myelin. It is capable of triggering an immune response of both the humoral and the cell-mediated types when appropriately administered to animals. The disease can be transferred to normal animals with living cells of lymphoid origin from animals with EAE (Paterson, 1960; Stone, 1961; Åström and Waksman, 1962; Paterson, 1968; Rauch and Einstein, 1974b; Driscoll et al., 1975). Indeed, the development of EAE in Lewis rats injected with syngeneic lymphoid cells sensitized to encephalitogenic protein (EP) in vitro has been described (Orgad and Cohen, 1974). Attempts to transfer EAE with immune serum have not been successful. The development of the disease can be prevented, at least partially, by the administration of a variety of immunosuppressive drugs, antilymphocytic serum, l-asparaginase, or even injection of the antigen in a nonencephalitogenic form prior to or after the encephalitogenic challenge (for reviews, see Alvord, 1970; Rauch and Einstein, 1974b; Rosenthale, 1974). Susceptibility to EAE, which differs among inbred strains of a species (see Levine and Wenk, 1965; Kornblum, 1968; Stone et al., 1969; Hughes and Stedronska, 1973; Levine and Sowinski, 1973; Webb et al., 1973a; Kies et al., 1975), was proposed to be controlled, at least in the rat, by a single dominant gene closely linked to but not identical with the major histocompatibility gene locus (Gasser et al., 1973; Williams and Moore, 1973, but cf. Gasser, et al., 1975). The dominance of this gene has recently been questioned (Perlík and Zídek, 1974; Levine and Sowinski, 1975b). The major histocompatibility complex does not solely control susceptibility to EAE in mice (Levine and Sowinski, 1974). Susceptibility for EAE in guinea pigs and in rats has also been correlated to the ability to mount a cell-mediated immune response against the complete or a specified part of the encephalitogenic antigen (see Lisak et al., 1975; McFarlin et al., 1975a,b).

There is an extensive literature which deals with the various etiological and pathological aspects of EAE. For further references to this basic work, the reader is referred to several reviews or symposia on these topics that are available, e.g., Kies and Alvord (1959), Waksman (1959), Pette and Bauer (1964), Scheinberg et al. (1965), Paterson (1966, 1968), Alvord (1968, 1970), Adams and Leibowitz (1969), Burdzy and Kallos (1969), Rowe (1969), Field et al. (1972), Wolfgram et al. (1972), Einstein (1972a), Kies (1973), and Rauch and Einstein (1974b). This chapter will deal with these aspects of EAE only insofar as they are relevant to the issue. Furthermore, most of the reports cited herein contain references to earlier important work on this subject.

For the moment, it is sufficient to say that the pathogenesis of EAE is not completely elucidated. As mentioned above, available evidence points to a major involvement of cell-mediated immunity, whereas humoral autoimmunity is considered by many workers to be less important. Thus, for example, a report by Gonatas and Howard (1974) has clearly demonstrated the obligate role in disease induction played by the thymus-dependent cells. Mononuclear cells, specifically sensitized to the antigen, i.e., the encephalitogenic protein (in the following referred to as EP), are thought to be produced in the lymphoid organs. They may enter their target tissue, the central nervous system, via the bloodstream, and there they may attack it through a direct cytotoxic action and/or a local production of cytopathic humoral antibodies/lymphokines (cf. Paterson, 1968; Alvord, 1970; Rauch and Einstein, 1974b). It is possible that the initial reaction between the sensitized lymphoid cell and the antigen occurs with released and not with tissue-bound EP (Simon and Anzil, 1974; Westall, 1974). There are several reports which indicate that the histopathological changes and the clinical manifestations of EAE can be dissociated, and it has been proposed that tissue injuries could depend primarily on a cell-mediated type of immunity, whereas clinical signs might be connected to a humoral autoimmune response, the full-blown EAE arising from multiple immune responses to neuroantigen (see Richardson and Paterson, 1970; Simon and Simonova, 1971; Hoffman et al., 1973; Lennon and Byrd, 1973; Paterson et al., 1974, 1975). On the other hand, Levine et al. (1975) maintain that significant clinical signs occur in EAE only when inflammatory lesions are, or have been, present. There are also several reports which fail to find any relation between EAE and humoral antibodies to EP (see Alvord, 1970; Alvord et al., 1970; Kies, 1973; Day and Pitts, 1974b; Gonatas et al., 1974a).

The growing realization of the complex nature of the autoimmune response to EP has made it desirable to identify those parts of the protein that are engaged in reactions of humoral and of cell-mediated immunity, respectively—i.e., the antigenic determinants for the two major types of immunity—and to clarify their relation to the disease-inducing site(s) and their relation to the protective effect of the protein. The desirability of such investigations is borne out by several observations which indicate that in human demyelinating diseases (see Field and Caspary, 1972; Bergstrand et al., 1974), and even in malignant neoplasia (Field and Caspary, 1970), an immunological response to EP or to some cross-reacting protein(s) could be present.

Studies on the antigenic determinants of EP and their relation to the disease-inducing part of it are thus of great immunopathological interest. But the results of such investigations are also of considerable interest from a pure immunochemical point of view, since much of the present knowledge regarding localization and characteristics of antigenic determinants for cell-mediated immunity within natural protein molecules stems from work on encephalitogenic protein (cf. Crumpton, 1974).

With these aspects in mind, the present review on the immunochemistry of EP will concentrate on four topics. Since the exact relation between EAE and the various parts of the immune response still remains unsettled, the immunochemistry of regions in the protein inducing EAE or interfering with the induction or expression of the disease will be dealt with separately for each. Regions that are capable of inducing conventionally assayed cell-mediated immunity and/or of reacting in experimental systems thought to reflect this part of the immune response will then be considered, and finally regions capable of inducing or reacting with humoral antibodies will be dealt with. However, before approaching the immunochemical aspects of EP, a short survey of the pertinent biochemical properties of the protein will be given. This topic has been reviewed in detail by Eylar (1971, 1972, 1973), Kies (1973), Eylar *et al.* (1974*b*), and Rauch and Einstein (1974*b*).

II. Nature and Properties of Encephalitogenic Protein

A. Localization and Biochemical Characteristics

1. Location in Vivo

Many investigators have contributed to the identification and characterization of the substance of CNS tissue that induces EAE. Indications that a water-soluble basic protein was responsible for the activity were afforded by Kies *et al.* (1961) and Einstein *et al.* (1962). Robertson *et al.* (1962) provided evidence that the active principle was of polypeptide nature. The connection between encephalitogenic activity and myelin was shown by Laatsch *et al.* (1962), Rauch and Raffel (1964), and Kornguth and Anderson (1965).

Today, it is well established that a basic protein of some 170 residues (the actual number depends upon the species of origin) and constituting some 30% of the total protein content of CNS myelin (Eng *et al.*, 1968; Eylar *et al.*, 1969; Gonzalez-Sastre, 1970) is the major and probably the sole obligate encephalitogenic agent. However, the immunologic activity of this protein is affected by other constituents of the CNS tissue (Hoffman *et al.*, 1973; Levine and Sowinski, 1975*b*; Kies *et al.*, 1975). Some rodent species have two basic myelin proteins (Cotman and Mahler, 1967; Eng *et al.*, 1968; Martenson *et al.*, 1970*a*, 1971*a,b*; Mehl and Halaris, 1970); the "larger" one is comparable to EPs from other species whereas the "smaller" one lacks a fragment comprising 40 amino acids that normally is situated in the C-terminal part of the larger EP (Martenson *et al.*, 1972*a*; Dunkley and Carnegie, 1974*a*). EP has been localized to the intraperiod line of lamellar myelin (Dickinson *et al.*, 1970), to the major dense line of the myelin sheet (Wolman, 1971; Herndon *et al.*, 1973; Poduslo and Braun, 1975), and partly even to the synaptosomal membrane fraction (Whittingham *et al.*, 1972). There is increasing evidence that when EP is part of the intact tissue the antigenic sites of the protein are masked, at least in regard to reactivity to humoral antibodies (for references, see Herndon *et al.*, 1973; Guarnieri *et al.*, 1974; Cohen *et al.*, 1975; Wood *et al.*, 1975).

Peripheral nerve tissue contains, among other basic proteins, a component which seems to be similar or identical to the EP of the central nervous system (Bencina *et al.*, 1969; Uyemura *et al.*, 1970; Brostoff and Eylar, 1972; Kiyota and Egami, 1972; *cf.* Brostoff *et al.*, 1974*b*, 1975; Abramsky *et al.*, 1975; Kitamura *et al.*, 1975). But within intact peripheral myelin the encephalitogenic activity of the protein seems to be partially inaccessible (Brostoff and Eylar, 1972; Dal Canto *et al.*, 1974).

2. Chemistry

The amino acid sequences of the bovine, the human, and the smaller rat EP and parts of the rabbit, guinea pig, pig, and monkey proteins have been determined (Kibler *et al.*, 1969; Eylar, 1970; Carnegie, 1971*a,b*; Eylar *et al.*, 1971*a,b*, 1974*a*; Shapira *et al.*, 1971*a*; Kornguth *et al.*, 1972; Martenson *et al.*, 1972*a*; Brostoff *et al.*, 1974*a*; Dunkley and Carnegie, 1974*a*; the earlier studies were reviewed by Kies, 1973), and sequences for the complete rabbit (Brostoff and Eylar, 1972) and chimpanzee (Westall *et al.*, 1975) proteins have been proposed. Figure 1 shows the sequences of the bovine, human, and smaller rat proteins and some essential parts of the guinea pig, rabbit, and monkey proteins. In order to obtain uniformity between the proteins of various species in the numbering of amino acid residues, this review follows the numbering of Dunkley and Carnegie (1974*a*), who achieved maximum homology between sequences by introduction of gaps.

The mammalian EPs contain a single tryptophan situated in position 118, two methionines (one near each end of the molecule—positions 22 and 170), four tyrosines (in positions 15, 70, 129, and 136, respectively), but no cysteine residue. The N-terminal alanine is N-acetylated (Carnegie, 1969; Hashim and Eylar, 1969*b,c*). The basic amino acids are rather randomly distributed over most of the polypeptide chain, but five regions exist where basic residues are absent over spans of eight to ten units (Eylar, 1970). Most of the glutamic acid residues, but only a few of the aspartic ones, are amidated. Region 92–118 has a number of interesting features. An arginine residue in position 109 has been shown to be partially mono- or dimethylated (Baldwin and Carnegie, 1971*a,b*; Brostoff and Eylar, 1971; Brostoff *et al.*, 1972; Martenson and Deibler, 1975; *cf.* Miyake, 1975). A threonine residue in position 100 is a receptor *in vitro* for the N-acetylgalactosaminyltransferase of the submaxillary gland (Hagopian *et al.*, 1971). Region 98–103 contains no less than four proline residues. The region surrounding the tryptophan residue has been proposed to serve as a receptor for serotonin (Carnegie, 1971*a*; *cf.* Smythies *et al.*, 1972). The functional implications of these properties of region 92–118 is not known—not

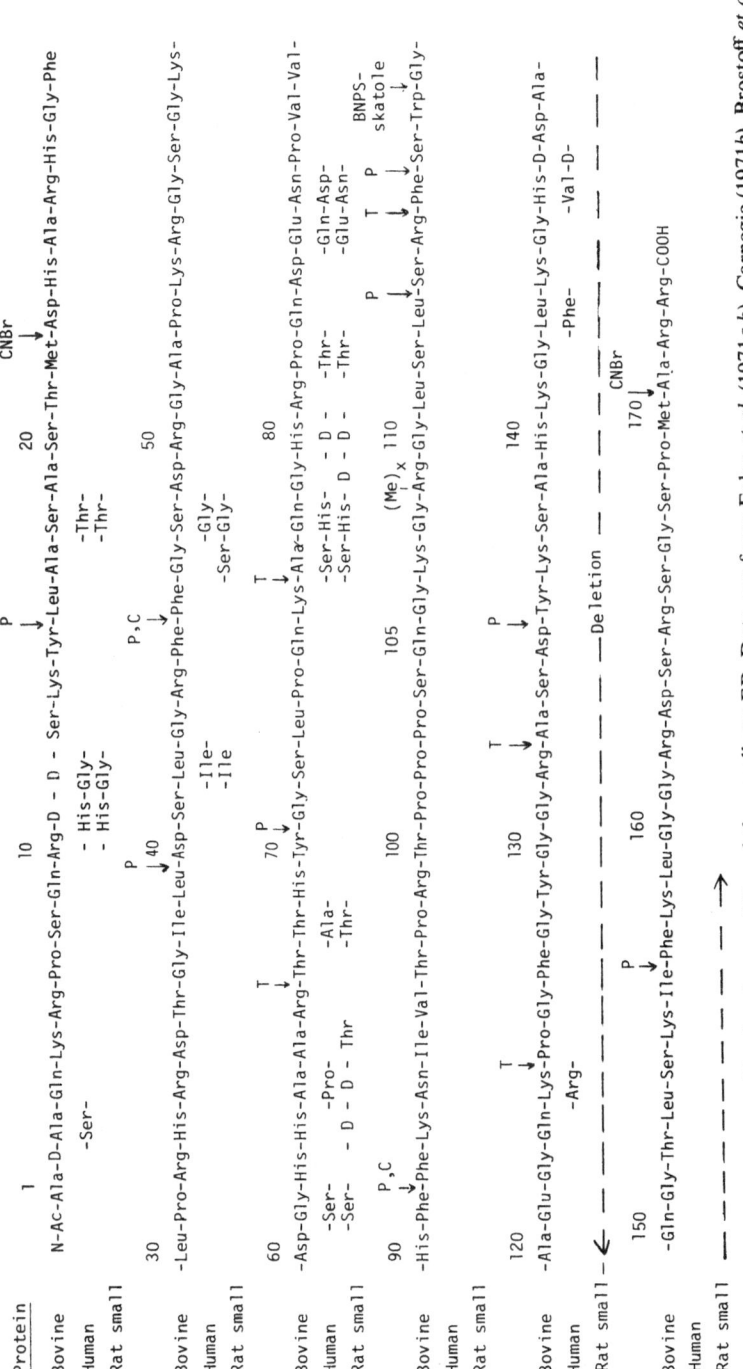

Figure 1. Amino acid sequences of bovine, human EP, and the small rat EP. Data are from Eylar *et al.* (1971*a*,*b*), Carnegie (1971*b*), Brostoff *et al.* (1974*a*), and Dunkley and Carnegie (1974*a*), and the numbering is that introduced by the last-mentioned authors. For the human and the small rat protein, the sequence is identical to that of the bovine EP except for the residues indicated in the figure. The sequences of the guinea pig and rabbit proteins are identical to that of bovine EP within region 67–76 (Shapira *et al.*, 1971*a*) and region 116–132 (Eylar *et al.*, 1974*a*). D stands for a deletion. The figure also indicates some linkages susceptible to cleavage by various agents: CNBr, cyanogen bromide; P, pepsin; C, cathepsin D of brain; T, trypsin; BNPS-skatole, the bromide adduct of 2-(2-nitrophenyl)-3-methylindole. For a complete delineation of bonds susceptible to peptic and tryptic hydrolysis, see Eylar *et al.* (1971*a*,*b*), Carnegie (1971*b*), and Martenson *et al.* (1975*c*); for further information regarding partial sequences of EPs from other species, see Dunkley and Carnegie (1974*a*).

even the biological function of the protein has yet been delineated (see Eylar *et al.*, 1974*b*)—but they may have profound effects on the immunochemical characteristics of the protein. A soluble protein kinase, purified from bovine brain and stimulated by cyclic AMP, and an endogenous myelin protein kinase (see Miyamoto, 1975) both phosphorylate EP *in vitro*, with a maximum amount of 3.8 moles phosphate being incorporated per mole of protein (Miyamoto *et al.*, 1974; Miyamoto and Kakiuchi, 1974). Phosphorylation of EP also occurs *in vivo*; native EP isolated from bovine tissue was reported to contain 0.07 mole of phosphoserine and 0.09 mole of phosphothreonine per mole of protein. Steck and Appel (1974) found serine to be the major phosphorylated amino acid when examining phosphorylation of rat EPs; the small and the large EP appeared to be equally good substrates for endogenous or added protein kinases. The cyclic AMP-stimulated protein kinase from rabbit muscle phosphorylates primarily serine residues 13 and 112 and threonine residue 36 (Carnegie *et al.*, 1973; Daile *et al.*, 1975); when EP is part of the myelin structure, a substantial phosphorylation by this protein kinase occurs only at residue 112 (Carnegie *et al.*, 1974). The major site phosphorylated by the endogenous myelin protein kinase apparently is serine residue 57 (Carnegie *et al.*, 1974).

A microheterogeneity of the protein has been observed in gel electrophoretic examinations at alkaline pH (Martenson and Gaitonde, 1969*a,b*; Martenson *et al.*, 1969*a,b*, 1970*b*). Five components purified by carboxymethylcellulose chromatography of guinea pig EP at alkaline pH were each identified with one of the electrophoretically observed components. These fractions did not differ in size, amino acid composition, or content of methylated arginine residues (Deibler and Martenson, 1973; Martenson and Deibler, 1975). The reason for the microheterogeneity is not fully elucidated, although deamidation of glutamine residues (Eylar, 1970; Eylar *et al.*, 1974*b*; Chou *et al.*, 1976), the presence of the phosphorylated serine (or threonine) residue(s) (Dunkley and Carnegie, 1974*a*; Miyamoto and Kakiuchi, 1974; Chou *et al.*, 1976; Martenson *et al.*, 1976), and the limited proteolytic degradation at the C-terminal end (Bergstrand, 1971; Martenson and Deibler, 1975; Martenson *et al.*, 1975*c*; Martenson *et al.*, 1976) possibly contribute to the pattern of heterogeneity.

In a purified state, the EP seems to be free from lipids and carbohydrates (Eylar and Thompson, 1969). However, various specific lipids, e.g., cerebroside sulfate and triphosphoinositide, have been observed to readily form complexes with the protein (Palmer and Dawson, 1969*a*; Demel *et al.*, 1973); in some instances changing its conformation (Palmer and Dawson, 1969*a*; Anthony and Moscarello, 1971; London and Vossenberg, 1973) or its susceptibility to different proteolytic enzymes (London and Vossenberg, 1973; London *et al.*, 1973; *cf.* Banik and Davidson, 1974).

Early studies indicated that EP exists in aqueous solutions primarily as a random coil lacking α-helical or β-form elements (Eylar and Thompson,

1969; Palmer and Dawson, 1969b; Chao and Einstein, 1970a; Anthony and Moscarello, 1971; cf. Krigbaum and Hsu, 1975). Encephalitogenic activity can, for example, withstand prolonged boiling or treatment with 8 M urea solution. The presence of a highly proline-rich region in the middle part of the molecule led Brostoff and Eylar (1971) to propose an open, double-chain, hairpinlike structure for it, which London et al. (1973) found to be in agreement with data on the interaction of EP with lipids. Epand et al. (1974) and Moscarello et al. (1974) observed that the protein, in fact, is folded in a specific compact conformation, compatible with an asymmetrical, prolate ellipsoid structure model. Finally, it should be mentioned that EPs of submammalian origin have also been characterized to some extent (Brostoff et al., 1974a; Martenson and Deibler, 1975; Martenson et al., 1975d).

3. Isolation of Native Protein and Preparation of Defined Derivatives of It

Procedures for isolation of the encephalitogenic antigen from whole brain tissue, spinal cord, or purified myelin have been described by several investigators, e.g., Einstein et al. (1962), Caspary and Field (1965), Kies (1965), Wolfgram (1965), Lowden et al. (1966), Martenson and LeBaron (1966), Nakao et al. (1966a,b), Carnegie et al. (1967), Tomasi and Kornguth (1967), Eng et al. (1968), Eylar et al. (1969), Martenson et al. (1969a), Gonzalez-Sastre (1970), Hirschfeld et al. (1970), Oshiro and Eylar (1970a), Uyemura et al. (1970), Bergstrand (1971), Sammeck et al. (1971), Barton et al. (1972a), Saito et al. (1972), Vepreková et al. (1972), Banik and Davison (1973), Hegstrand and Kornguth (1973), and Quelin et al. (1975). Comprehensive reviews of these procedures were given by Dunkley and Carnegie (1974b) and Eylar et al. (1974b). A large-scale preparation procedure without chromatographic moments has been developed by Deibler et al. (1972), and these authors have also pointed out pitfalls present when purifying EP for immunological work (cf. Martenson et al., 1971a; Kies, 1972). The preparation of smaller encephalitogenic antigens (which are probably fragments derived during isolation from native protein) has also been described by several of the abovementioned authors and by others, e.g., Robertson et al. (1962), Kibler et al. (1964, 1972), Nakao and Einstein (1965), Carnegie and Lumsden (1966, 1967), Lumsden et al. (1966), Chao and Einstein (1968), Kibler and Shapira (1968), and Eylar et al. (1971a). In most of these reports, isolation of the encephalitogenic products from brain or spinal cord tissue has been performed by employing the following basic procedure outlined by Kies (1965) and Nakao et al. (1966a): An initial simultaneous defatting and homogenization of the tissue, either with a chloroform–methanol (2 : 1) mixture [this solvent mixture inactivates the brain proteolytic enzyme(s) that would otherwise have a profound degradative effect on EP at acid extraction (Nakao et al., 1966a,b; cf. Chao and Einstein, 1968; Einstein *et al.*, 1968*b*, 1969; Rauch *et al.*, 1973)] or with acetone, is followed by an extraction of the residue with an acidified buffer or dilute mineral acid. Neutralization of this extract gives a precipitate which contains a minor part of the EP. The remaining soluble proteins are usually precipitated with ammonium sulfate and/or acidified acetone and then chromatographed on a cationic exchanger. To obtain a highly purified preparation of the protein, it is sometimes necessary to perform several ion exchange chromatographic and gel filtration procedures. The yield is in the order of 0.1–1 % of the tissue wet weight (*cf.* Eylar *et al.*, 1969, 1974*b*; Oshiro and Eylar, 1970*a*; Dunkley and Carnegie, 1974*b*).

EP is sensitive to proteolytic degradation either *in situ* (Eylar *et al.*, 1969; Sammeck and Brady, 1972; *cf.* Wood and King, 1971) or during isolation (*cf.* work of Einstein *et al.*, 1968*b*, referred to above). Autolytic changes *in situ* of bovine EP apparently occur in frozen and thawed tissue only (Ansari *et al.*, 1975). Only a few of the smaller encephalitogénic antigens, prepared in a more or less purified form, that were referred to above have been clearly identified and related to the native EP. The antigenic moiety isolated by Kibler and Shapira (1968; *cf.* Kibler *et al.*, 1972) was later shown to represent region 46–90 (Shapira *et al.*, 1971*a*). This fragment can also be prepared by digestion with pepsin or cathepsin D of purified EP (Eylar *et al.*, 1971*a*; Bergstrand, 1972*b*, 1973*a*; Benuck *et al.*, 1975; Martenson *et al.*, 1975*c*; McFarlin *et al.*, 1975*b*; Swanborg, 1975*a*; Whitaker *et al.*, 1975). Chao and Einstein (1968) described the preparation of a fragment corresponding to the *C*-terminal half of EP and Bergstrand (1971) the isolation of fragments 1–45, 46–173, and 92–173 directly from central nervous tissue extracts. Data from the reports of Nakao *et al.* (1966*a*,*b*) can, in retrospect, be interpreted to show the purification of regions 1–45, 1–39, 92–173, 46–91, and 46–173, and the complete protein (fractions A–D, F, and G, respectively). These observations point out the extreme lability for proteolytic degradation of the two Phe–Phe linkages of the protein *in vivo* (*cf.* Eylar, 1970), the brain cathepsin D most probably being the responsible enzyme (Einstein *et al.*, 1968*b*, 1969; Marks *et al.*, 1974; Benuck *et al.*, 1975). The corresponding enzyme from liver attacks only the linkage in position 45–46 but not that in position 91–92 (Brostoff *et al.*, 1974*a*). Limited digestion of EP during isolation from the tissue or *in vitro* with pepsin also produces peptides 1–39 (Driscoll *et al.*, 1974*a*; Bergstrand and Källén, 1975; Martenson *et al.*, 1975*c*; *cf.* Nakao *et al.*, 1966*a*), 1–91, 40–91, 92–156, 114–173, and 117–173 (Martenson *et al.*, 1975*c*), and 136–173 (Eylar *et al.*, 1971*b*). Oxidative cleavage of the protein can be performed at the tryptophanyl bond with either *N*-bromosuccinimide or, even better, the bromide adduct of 2-(2-nitrophenylsulfenyl)-3-methylindole (BNPS-skatole) (Eylar and Hashim, 1969; Bergstrand, 1971; Burnett and Eylar, 1971; Eylar *et al.*, 1974*a*; Martenson and Deibler, 1975; Martenson *et al.*, 1975*a*; Swanborg 1975*b*; Whitaker *et al.*, 1975), resulting in peptides 1–118 and 119–173 with or without oxidized tyrosine residues. Cyanogen bromide cleavage is readily performed at the two methionine residues in positions 22 and 170 (Carnegie, 1969; Hashim and Eyler, 1969*b,c*; Palmer and Dawson, 1969*b*; Carnegie *et al.*, 1970; Chao and Einstein, 1970*b*; Bergstrand, 1971, 1972*a*; Martenson *et al.*, 1972*a*, 1975*a*; Martenson and Deibler, 1975; Whitaker *et al.*, 1975).

Smaller, defined peptide derivatives of EP have been prepared by tryptic, peptic, or chymotryptic digestion of the native EP or larger peptide parts of it (e.g., Hashim and Eylar, 1969*a,d*; Lennon *et al.*, 1970; Carnegie, 1971*b*; Eylar *et al.*, 1971*a,b*; Shapira *et al.*, 1971*a*; Bergstrand, 1972*b*, 1973*a*; Bergstrand and Källén, 1973*a*; Hashim *et al.*, 1973; Karkhanis *et al.*, 1975). The main sites for tryptic and peptic cleavage are depicted in Fig. 1.

Conventional protein/peptide purification methods, such as ion exchange chromatography, gel filtration, and paper electrophoresis/chromatography (peptide mapping) have been successfully applied for the isolation of these peptide derivatives. However, the basic nature of EP demands that gel filtration procedures, at least with Sephadex gels, are performed with suitable eluents to avoid unspecific adsorption to the gel; 0.01 M hydrochloric acid (see Dunkley and Carnegie, 1974*b*) and 0.25 M ammonium acetate (Bergstrand, 1971) have been used with success. Estimation of the molecular weight of EP or derivatives of it by gel filtration should be performed with suitably chosen reference polypeptides or under denaturating conditions (Chao and Einstein, 1969; Deibler *et al.*, 1970; Bergstrand, 1971; Martenson *et al.*, 1975*c*).

A thorough examination of protein/peptide purity is, of course, of utmost importance before immunochemical examinations are performed or their results interpreted. Amino acid analysis, gel electrophoresis, and paper electrophoresis are currently preferred methods (*cf.* Kies, 1973; Dunkley and Carnegie, 1974*b*). But it should also be kept in mind, as has repeatedly been stressed, that physicochemical purity in no way implies immunological purity (e.g., Martenson *et al.*, 1975*a*).

Specifically modified derivatives of EP have also been prepared. 2-Hydroxy-5-nitrobenzylation (or similar modifications) of the tryptophan residue has been accomplished and the derivatives have been extensively examined (*cf.* Chao and Einstein, 1970*b*; Eylar *et al.*, 1970; Swanborg, 1970; Eylar, 1971). The tyrosine residues have been oxidized, which leads to an immunologically altered product (see Bergstrand and Källén, 1972). Diazotization of the protein, the final product containing both arsanilic and sulfanilic acid residues, acetylation of the lysine residues, and modification of the arginine residues by reaction with 2,3-butane-dione have been performed (Swanborg, 1969, 1970). Fragment 1–45 has been modified by succinylation of the lysine residues in positions 5 and 14, by nitration of tyrosine residue 15, and by carboxymethylation at methionine-22 (Bergstrand and Källén, 1973*a*). Histidine residues within region 62–69 have been carboxymethylated (Bergstrand, 1973a). Finally, synthetic derivatives and analogues of the tryptophan region (Eylar *et al.*, 1970; Westall *et al.*, 1971; Lamoureux *et al.*, 1972; Westall, 1972; Suzuki *et al.*, 1973; Hashim and Sharpe, 1974, 1975; Suzuki and Sasaki, 1974), region 67–76 (Shapira *et al.*, 1971b; Hashim and Sharpe, 1974), parts of the N-terminal region (Barton *et al.*, 1972b; Hashim *et al.*, 1973), and region 136–149 (see Karkhanis *et al.*, 1975) have been prepared and examined immunologically.

B. General Immunological Aspects

The early observations on the conformation of EP led most investigators of the immunochemistry of the protein to assume (1) that the major part of it is probably accessible to an immune response and (2) that its antigenic determinants can be expected to conform to the type that Sela (1969a,b) has named "sequential." These assumptions permit the investigator to degrade the protein to smaller fragments when searching for the determinants without any serious risk of losing the reactivity, since the antigenic sites might be expected to be conserved in relatively small peptides.

It is clear that combinations of the degradative procedures mentioned above will ultimately lead to a set of peptide fragments which is highly suitable for a thorough immunochemical investigation of EP, although a precise localization and characterization of each immunologically reactive region inevitably demand a painstaking examination of a set of suitable synthetic peptide derivatives covering that region. In fact, most, if not all, immunochemical data regarding EP have been obtained following this strategy and they turn out to fit the two assumptions mentioned above very well. But it must be clearly pointed out that in no case has the conformation of a peptide fragment (reactive or not) been examined and compared to that of the pertinent region in the native protein. Such examinations are highly desirable (especially with the nonreactive sequences encountered) now that Epand *et al.* (1974) have shown that the protein exhibits a certain degree of order.

III. Antigenic Determinants with Disease-Inducing Properties

During recent years, a number of distinct parts of EP have been identified, all of which have the ability to induce EAE. A pronounced species variability in the responses to these different sites has become obvious; a region that is highly encephalitogenic in one animal species can be virtually inactive in another species and *vice versa*. The present part of the discussion will be devoted to such determinants of EP, operationally defined solely by their capacity to induce EAE when appropriately injected.

Sometimes, two or more laboratories have reported different activities for certain specified encephalitogenic antigens. There are several conceivable explanations for such discrepancies which we feel should be mentioned collectively here as space does not permit scrutinizing the details of each particular report (see also Kies, 1973).

1. When the results from two laboratories diverge, different doses could have been used. Contrary to what might be expected, it could be that injection of a higher dose of an encephalitogenic antigen does not inevitably lead to a higher degree of response. Thus when testing a synthetic nonapeptide with high encephalitogenic activity in guinea pigs, Young et al. (1974) and McDermott and Caspary (1975) observed a critical dose above which the response was claimed to decrease. On the other hand, the native EP showed a normally increasing dose–response relation.

2. The route of injection is clearly very important, but the number of injection sites also seems to determine the outcome. Robson et al. (1971) found guinea pigs showed higher incidence of disease if the same dose of antigen was given in two injection sites instead of one.

3. The amount of mycobacteria used for preparing the adjuvant, the proportion of mycobacteria to antigen, and the stability of the emulsion seem to be very important (see, e.g., Lee and Schneider, 1962; Shaw et al., 1962, 1964; Alvord et al., 1964; Jackson et al., 1972; Behan et al., 1973; Rauch and Einstein, 1974a; Simon and Anzil, 1974). In rats and monkeys, pertussis vaccine has a potentiating effect which must be considered; in fact, it can replace the mycobacterial adjuvant (see Paterson, 1968; Behan et al., 1973; Levine, 1974). The recently published observation that the degree of encephalitogenicity evidently depends on the choice of adjuvant (Levine and Sowinski, 1975b) does not need to be emphasized. Furthermore, encephalomyelitic lesions obtained by injections of synthetic polynucleotide, pertussis, or mycobacterial adjuvants without nervous tissue antigens have been described (e.g., Kantchourine and Kapitanova, 1969; Paterson and Drobish, 1974; Lindh and Bergstrand, 1975) which question the specificity of very weak encephalitogenic effects.

4. The possibility that the encephalitogenic activity ascribed to a certain peptide in fact depends on a highly active contaminant has repeatedly been stressed by many authors; this objection cannot be rejected completely until synthetic derivatives analogous to the pertinent active site have been shown to induce disease. On the other hand, low activity of a normally highly active sequence can possibly depend on deamination of an essential glutamine or asparagine residue within the active region (see Westall et al., 1971; Westall,

1972, 1973). According to Dunkley and Carnegie (1974a), glutamine residue 105, which is part of a region that hitherto has been ascribed no clear-cut encephalitogenic activity in guinea pigs, is the residue most prone to deamidation, but other regions, including the one containing tryptophan, have also been implicated in deamination (Eylar et al., 1971b; Chou et al., 1976).

5. The genetic constitution of the experimental animal also deter-mines the response (see Section IB); divergent data on the sus-ceptibility to EAE of an inbred strain might depend on genetic drift (see Levine and Sowinski, 1973).

6. Although the encephalitogenic activity within one species can vary with the source of EP, it should become clear that there is no general trend pointing to either a higher or a lower response when heter-ologous as compared to homologous EP is employed for sensiti-zation.

7. Deprivation of vitamin C in guinea pigs (Mueller et al., 1962) or a general malnutrition of young Lewis rats (Gonatas et al., 1974b) markedly reduces the effect of an encephalitogenic challenge, and irradiation of recipients alters the disease pattern at transfer within Lewis rats (Paterson et al., 1975).

A. The Tryptophan-Containing Region

Eylar and Hashim (1968) and Hashim and Eylar (1969a) first pointed out the importance of the tryptophan-containing region of EP when guinea pigs are used for tests of encephalitogenicity. They isolated two small over-lapping peptides derived from this part of the protein by peptic hydrolysis, and found these peptides responsible for the overwhelming part of the encephalitogenic activity of the protein. Their finding was confirmed by Lennon et al. (1970; cf. Carnegie, 1971a), and indirectly by observations that the activity of EP specifically modified at the tryptophan residue in different ways was greatly impaired (Chao and Einstein, 1970b; Eylar et al., 1970; Swanborg, 1970; Eylar, 1971; Einstein et al., 1972a; Swanborg et al., 1974; Lindh and Bergstrand, 1975). However, weak oxidation of the tryptophan residue converting it to an oxindole derivative did not alter the encephalitogenicity (Burnett and Eylar, 1971), nor did acetylation of part of the lysine residues or modification of the majority of arginine residues with 2,3-butane-dione alter the encephalitogenicity (Swanborg, 1970). Since a complete modification of neither the lysine nor the arginine residues was reached, the interpretation of the last-mentioned results is equivocal. Modification of the lysine residues of procine EP with imidates did not eliminate its disease-inducing activity (Westall and Thompson, 1975). The biochemical requirements for induction of EAE in guinea pigs with this part of the protein were then clarified by synthesis and tests of a variety of peptides analogous to the native tryptophan-containing sequence (Eylar *et al.*, 1970; Westall *et al.*, 1971). It was found that a nonapeptide with the sequence

Phe–Ser–Trp–Gly–Ala–Glu–Gly–Gln–Lys

and constituting region 116–124 of bovine EP was the smallest peptide retaining activity, and initially the identity and spatial relationship between the three indicated residues

X–X–Trp–X–X–X–X–Gln–Lys

were reported to be the essential features of an encephalitogenic determinant. Arginine could substitute for lysine in the *C*-terminal position; in fact arginine occupies this place in native human protein. The report of Westall (1972) pointed to some further essential characteristics of the determinant. Replacement either of Gly-119 with Ala or of Phe-116 with Gly reduced the activity markedly, and deamidation of Gln-123 practically abolished it. Peptides having an extra glycine residue between residues 122 and 123 or between 123 and 124 showed a reduced activity.

Reports from other laboratories have confirmed the encephalitogenicity of synthetic peptide 116–124 and the inability of peptide 118–124 to induce disease (Suzuki *et al.*, 1973; Hashim *et al.*, 1973; Hashim and Sharpe, 1974, 1975). The report of Suzuki and Sasaki (1974) indicates that the integrity of residue Ala-120 is also essential for activity, whereas Ser-117 and Glu-121 can be replaced by glycine without substantial loss of activity. Asn can possibly replace Gln-123 (Sasaki, 1974).

Lamoureux *et al.* (1972) have reached a slightly different conclusion regarding the extension of the encephalitogenic tryptophan-containing determinant. They synthesized peptides of increasing chain length starting with Gly-128 and going toward Ser-114. In this way, 15 peptides were prepared containing from one to 15 residues. They found all peptides that were lacking the tryptophan residue incapable of inducing EAE. However, the addition of a single tryptophan residue to synthetic peptide 119–128 converted this molecule to a highly encephalitogenic compound. This suggests that the sequence Ser–Arg–Phe–Ser (residues 114–117) is not implicated in the encephalitogenic determinant, at least not if the molecule extends beyond residue 124, where Westall's peptides ended. In fact, Lamoureux *et al.* (1972) found that addition of these extra residues lowered the activity. However, if the molecule is not long enough, deletion of residues 114–117 abolishes activity even at high doses (Hashim and Sharpe, 1974). Together these reports might be interpreted to mean that the encephalitogenicity of this region is determined only by a short sequence of residues, but in order to express the activity the molecule must probably contain a minimum number of residues, either on the *N*-terminal or on the *C*-terminal side of the determinants, e.g., in order to make the molecule "immunogenic" or to impose a suitable conformation on it. A similar situation was encountered with region 40–45 when tested in Lewis rats (Martenson *et al.*, 1975*b*). Carnegie *et al.* (1970), Lennon *et al.* (1970), and Eylar (1972) reported results that diverge somewhat from those of Lamoureux *et al.* (1972). They isolated peptides 114–128, 114–135, 117–127, and 117–135 from tryptic and peptic digests of human EP and could find no clinical signs of EAE in animals that had received peptides 117–127 or 117–135, whereas full effect was obtained with comparable doses of the two other peptides (114–128 and 114–135). These authors used lower doses of the peptides than did Lamoureux *et al.* (1972). Lennon *et al.* (1970) also found histological signs of EAE with peptide 117–135. Furthermore, Lamoureux *et al.* (1972) performed a supplemental injection with pertussis vaccine at sensitization.

An investigation of the primary structure of tryptophan-containing tryptic peptides derived from EPs of a variety of different species (Eylar *et al.*, 1974*a*) showed that those EPs which had a substantial encephalitogenic activity in guinea pigs were all apparently identical to the human or bovine proteins as regards the sequence of tryptophan region, whereas EPs differing from the mammalian ones in primary sequence within this region were those showing only minimal activity (chicken EP) or no activity (turtle EP). The low activity of the chicken EP was ascribed to the replacement of Glu-123 with His, but Suzuki and Sasaki (1974) observed that replacement of Ala-120 with Gly inactivates a synthetic peptide analogue, which makes the former conclusion premature. Similar results in the study of the encephalitogenicity of various EPs were reported by Martenson *et al.* (1972*b*). These observations further strengthen the importance of the tryptophan region for induction of EAE in guinea pigs.

Lennon and Carnegie (1974) examined the dose–response curve of synthetic peptide 114–124, Arg-124, and found that the lowest dose inducing clinical disease was approximately 0.1 μg, maximal response occurring at approximately a five- to tenfold higher dose. A similar conclusion was reached by Young *et al.* (1974) and McDermott and Caspary (1975) employing the synthetic peptide 116–124, Arg-124, but, as mentioned above, these authors also claimed that still higher doses led to decreased responses in regards to both clinical and histopathological criteria of the disease. Figure 2 summarizes the hitherto delineated structural requirements within the tryptophan-containing region for expression of encephalitogenicity in guinea pigs.

There are only two reports directly examining the disease-inducing activity of the tryptophan region in rabbits. Eylar *et al.* (1971*a*) sensitized the animals with 100 μg of the tryptically derived nonapeptide (116–124, Lys-124); five out of six were diseased, four showing clinical EAE. Hashim and Sharpe (1974) used synthetic peptide 116–125 (Lys-124, Gly-125) at a

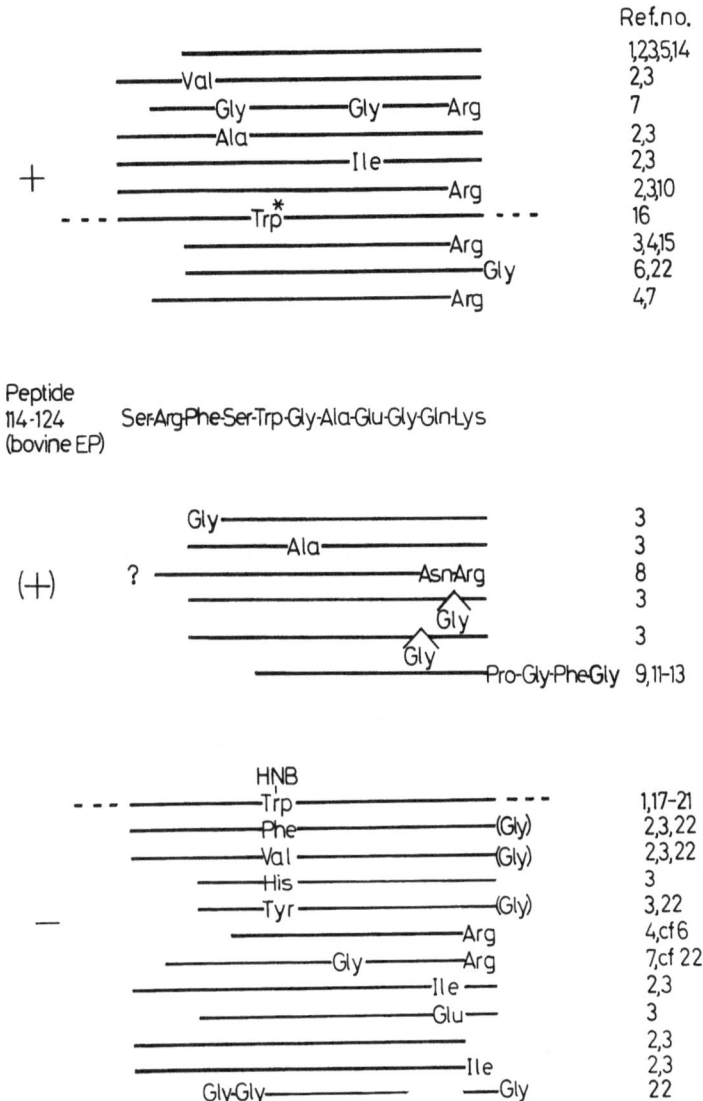

Figure 2. Schematic summary of the structural requirements for encephalitogenicity of the tryptophan region in guinea pigs. Data are from (1) Eylar *et al.* (1970), (2) Westall *et al.* (1971), (3) Westall (1972), (4) Suzuki *et al.* (1973), (5) Hashim *et al.* (1973), (6) Hashim and Sharpe (1974), (7) Suzuki and Sasaki (1974), (8) Sasaki (1974), (9) Lamoureux *et al.* (1972), (10) Lennon and Carnegie (1974), (11) Lennon *et al.* (1970), (12) Carnegie *et al.* (1970), (13) Eylar (1972), (14) Young *et al.* (1974), (15) Swanborg (1975), (16) Burnett and Eylar (1971), (17) Chao and Einstein (1970*b*), (18) Swanborg (1970), (19) Einstein *et al.* (1972*a*), (20) Swanborg *et al.* (1974), (21) Lindh and Bergstrand (1975), (22) Hashim and Sharpe (1975). Symbols: +, amino acid replacements that do not change the activity; (+), residue replacements that apparently reduce but do not abolish activity; −, nonpermissible replacements. Trp* stands for an oxindole derivative of tryptophan and ∧ for insertion between indicated residues.

comparable dose without substantial effect, whereas another synthetic peptide (region 67–77, Gly-77) was highly encephalitogenic at that dose. Indirect evidence, also pointing to a low or moderate activity (in rabbits) of this region as compared to other parts of the protein, has been obtained by Chao and Einstein (1970b) and Einstein et al. (1972a). EP modified in the tryptophan region was found to retain high activity, although the development of the disease with some modified preparations was delayed.

Nor does the tryptophan region seem to be a major disease-inducing site when tested in rats. Guinea pig, bovine, and rat EP, blocked at the tryptophan residue by hydroxynitrobenzylation, show an unimpaired encephalitogenicity in the Lewis rat (Swanborg and Amesse, 1971; Swanborg et al., 1974). The smaller rat protein—where an essential part of the tryptophan determinant is deleted—is also highly active (Swanborg and Amesse, 1971; Martenson et al., 1972b; Dunkley et al., 1973; Swanborg et al., 1974). Lennon and Dunkley (cited by Dunkley et al., 1973) in fact found a 15-residue tryptophan-containing fragment from human EP (peptide 114–128?) to be inactive in the rat, although it was highly active in guinea pigs. A similar conclusion was reached by Hashim and Sharpe (1974) when they tested their synthetic preparation of peptide 116–125, Lys-124, Gly-125, at the 100 µg level. However, supplemental adjuvant injection of pertussis vaccine was not performed by the last-mentioned authors.

Monkeys, finally, seem to be resistant to induction of EAE with the tryptophan region (Eylar et al., 1972b; Jackson et al., 1972; Rauch and Einstein, 1974a).

B. Region 46–91

Another disease-inducing region of EP, identified by its high activity when tested in rabbits, was initially described by Kibler and Shapira (1968). It proved to be localized in the second fourth of the intact protein, constituting residues 46–90 (91) (Shapira et al., 1971a; Eylar et al., 1971a). A synthetic decapeptide analogous to sequence 67–76 of the bovine EP was then synthesized and shown to have a clear-cut effect in the rabbit (Shapira et al., 1971b; Hashim and Sharpe, 1974). The latter workers found peptide 70–77, Gly-77, inactive, thus implicating the N-terminal residues as essential parts of this encephalitogenic determinant. Peptide 67–76 has a striking similarity to the tryptophan region (Shapira et al., 1971b), the tyrosine corresponding to the tryptophan and the glutamine-lysine sequence five to six residues C-terminal to the aromatic one being conserved:

```
          116                                 124
     –Phe–Ser–Trp–Gly–Ala–Glu–Gly–Gln–Lys–
     –Thr–Thr–His–Tyr–Gly–Ser–Leu–Pro–Gln–Lys–
      67                                   76
```

However, region 67–76 is perhaps not the only encephalitogenic site for rabbits within fragment 46–90. Bergstrand (1973b) isolated peptide 46–70 and found a moderate activity connected to it when tested at a dose of 50 μg; peptide 71–91 was found inactive at a comparable dose. The possibility cannot yet be dismissed that region 67–70, which is common to both of the active peptides, constitutes the encephalitogenic principle which expresses its activity only when part of a larger peptide (cf. analogous reasoning for the tryptophan region above).

Region 46–91 is also capable of inducing EAE in monkeys (Shapira et al., 1971b; Kibler et al., 1972), although Eylar et al. (1971a, 1972a) maintain that it does not encompass the major encephalitogenic site for this species. According to Kies (1973), both regions 1–118 and 119–173 are highly encephalitogenic.

Although there is no doubt that the tryptophan region is by far the major encephalitogenic site in guinea pigs, it is suspected that other parts of the protein can also induce the disease in this species. Most of the workers examining EPs modified at the tryptophan residue found a slight residual activity connected to the derivative, and Hoffman et al. (1973) observed differences in histopathology between animals injected with whole CNS tissue, with native EP, or with a synthetic nonapeptide, which indicated that the last antigen could not account for all the effects exerted by the two former ones. Martenson et al. (1972b) and Swanborg (1973) found the small rat EP, which does not contain an intact tryptophan determinant, to be weakly active.

Furthermore, besides the activity ascribed to peptide 1–22 (see below) there is evidence that some part of region 46–91 has a slight disease-inducing effect in guinea pigs (Lennon et al., 1970; Carnegie 1971a; Shapira et al., 1971b; Lindh and Bergstrand, 1975; Swanborg, 1975a). However, others have been unable to confirm this proposal (Eylar et al., 1971a). Hashim and Schilling (1973a) reported on histological EAE without clinical signs of the disease in 15 out of 40 guinea pigs injected with synthetic peptide 67–76 at a dose of 20 μg; a similar finding was reached by Hashim et al. (1973), with 18 out of 25 injected at the same dosage. However, the same laboratory (Hashim and Sharpe, 1974) found the synthetic peptide 67–77, Gly-77, to be inactive at a dose of 0.1 μM (approximately 100 μg) since none of the ten animals tested was affected. The same group also reported that peptide 71–86 of bovine EP is completely inactive in guinea pigs (Hashim et al., 1973; Hashim and Schilling, 1973a). These discrepancies are apt to be because of the variables mentioned in the introduction to this section, but it is clear that this region is only of minor importance for disease induction in the guinea pig.

On the other hand, region 46–91 seems to be the most interesting part of EP when EAE in rats is considered. Thus Swanborg and Amesse (1971) and Swanborg *et al.* (1974) found that 2-hydroxy-5-nitrobenzylation of the tryptophan residue in bovine, guinea pig, or either of the two rat EPs did not alter the activity when tested in the Lewis strain, and, moreover, the disease-inducing effect was retained in fragment 23–170 of bovine EP. Martenson *et al.* (1972*b*), who investigated the encephalitogenicity of myelin basic proteins from a variety of species, showed that the activities of the large and the small rat proteins were of comparable degree. Together these results indicated that rats respond to an encephalitogenic sequence that is different from the tryptophan-containing one and this sequence does not reside in the *N*-terminal part of the protein. Martenson *et al.* (1972*b*) furthermore observed that the activity of the guinea pig EP was higher than that of the other mammalian proteins (rat, bovine, rabbit, and human EP); similar conclusions were reached by McFarlin *et al.* (1973) and by Vandenbark and Hinrichs (1974). Lennon and Dunkley (1974) examined dose–response curves of rat and human EP and observed an apparently higher encephalitogenic potency with human than with rat EP; the opposite results were reported by Martenson *et al.* (1972*b*). Dau and Peterson (1969) found that human EP injected without pertussis vaccine was inactive. McFarlin *et al.* (1973) furthermore directly implicated fragment 46–90 as the sequence encompassing the major encephalitogenic site for rats; that region isolated from either guinea pig or rat EP was as active as the corresponding native protein, whereas bovine peptide 46–90 had only slight activity and then at very high doses. These results were confirmed by Martenson *et al.* (1975*b*). Dunkley *et al.* (1973) found fragment 46–91 of the small rat EP highly encephalitogenic in the Lewis rat, and so were regions 1–118 and 23–118 of guinea pig EP (Martenson *et al.*, 1975*a*). However, both the natural and the synthetic peptide 67–76 were found completely inactive (Dunkley *et al.*, 1973; McFarlin *et al.*, 1973), an observation confirmed by Hashim and Sharpe (1974). According to preliminary data, the activity, or at least a part of it, can apparently be traced to a peptide encompassing residues 68–91 (see McFarlin *et al.*, 1974).

Recently, the induction with EP of EAE in SJL/J mice was described (Bernard and Carnegie, 1975), and preliminary experiments suggested that fragment 46–91 is an encephalitogenic principle for this species.

C. The *N*-Terminal Region

The *N*-terminal part of EP (residues 1–45) has also been ascribed encephalitogenic activity by various authors. Carnegie (1969), while working with peptide 1–22 of human EP, first observed this site, but it was found to be of minor importance for disease induction in guinea pigs

(Carnegie *et al.*, 1970; Robson *et al.*, 1971; Swanborg *et al.*, 1974; Lindh and Bergstrand, 1975). Indeed, other investigators have been unable to confirm the encephalitogenicity of this region, especially when working with bovine EP (Hashim and Eylar, 1969*b*,*c*; Palmer and Dawson, 1969*b*; Chao and Einstein, 1970*b*). However, the probability of the presence of disease-inducing sequences within this part of the protein was shown by Barton *et al.* (1972*b*), who prepared synthetic peptides corresponding to regions 8–12, 12–21, and 13–21 of human EP. All three peptides occasionally induced mild clinical signs of EAE, and peptide 13–21 in five out of 40 animals caused even severe disease. No histopathological signs were encountered with any of the peptides, an observation which is interesting since Carnegie *et al.* (1970) originally reported "severe histological lesions unaccompanied by clinical disease" in some animals injected with peptide 1–22. A synthetic derivative, thought to correspond to region 1–5, and the *N*-terminal tryptic peptide of bovine EP were tested by Hashim *et al.* (1973) and by Hashim and Schilling (1973*a*) without apparent encephalitogenicity. However, the relevance of this observation is not quite clear, since the primary sequence of the *N*-terminal part of bovine EP has been revised (Brostoff *et al.*, 1974*a*).

Region 1–22 apparently also induces EAE in rabbits, although the potency is of moderate degree (Shapira *et al.*, 1971*b*). Bergstrand and Källén (1973*b*) and Berg and Bergstrand (1974) employed the natural fragment 1–45 of bovine EP for tests and encountered a rather high encephalitogenic potency. Results by the latter authors corroborated by unpublished studies indicate that peptides 23–44 and 17–37 might encompass a disease-inducing site for this species. Thus it is possible, but not yet proved, that region 1–45 contains two sites with encephalitogenic activity in rabbits.

Region 1–45 has been ascribed disease-inducing activity also in monkeys (Brostoff *et al.*, 1974*a*), and for this species, too, the relative potency seems to be low.

Peptide 1–22, slightly active in guinea pigs, completely lacked encephalitogenicity when tested in Lewis rats (Swanborg *et al.*, 1974; Martenson *et al.*, 1975*a*). On the other hand, region 40–45 of bovine EP was recently found to express moderate encephalitogenicity in the Lewis rat (Martenson *et al.*, 1975*b*).

D. The *C*-Terminal Region

The remaining part of EP to be discussed, the *C*-terminal region, has also been claimed to show encephalitogenic activity. This was initially proposed by Bergstrand and Berg (1971), who tested peptide 119–173,

Tyr,* obtained by BNPS-skatole oxidation of bovine EP, in rabbits. Eylar *et al.* (1972*a*) reported that peptide 136–173 encompasses the major site for induction of EAE in monkeys. Bergstrand (1972*a*) further delineated the activity of that region in rabbits to peptides 136–153 and 157–173. He showed that both peptides had moderate disease-inducing effects when tested at the 20 and 100 μg levels. A recent report by Karkhanis *et al.* (1975) suggested that the latter peptide is responsible for the activity in monkeys, whereas a synthetic peptide corresponding to residues 136–149 was found inactive.

The C-terminal region may also be slightly active when tested in guinea pigs, as indicated by the results obtained with peptide 119–173 (Burnett and Eylar, 1971, but *cf.* Swanborg 1975*b*) and with peptide HNB 92–173 (Lindh and Bergstrand, 1975). The last-mentioned authors reported that a 2-hydroxy-5-nitrobenzylated fragment., 92–173, at a dose level of 15 μg per animal, induced clinical signs in six out of 20 animals and histological EAE in the majority of the guinea pigs. Martenson *et al.* (1975*a*) and Swanborg (1975*b*) observed a very weak encephalitogenic activity of region 119–173 in Lewis rats, but could not dismiss the possiblility that it was dependent on highly active contaminants. On the other hand, according to Martenson and Deibler (1975) and Martenson *et al.* (1975*b*), peptides 92–173 and 92–153 but not 114–173 of bovine EP are encephalitogenic in the Lewis rat, which suggests the presence of another encephalitogenic site for this species near the polypeptide chain bend. The reported difference in activity between bovine peptides 23–118 (Martenson *et al.*, 1975*a*) and 46–90 (McFarlin *et al.*, 1973) agrees with this proposal, but the enhancement of the encephalitogenicity of bovine EP or fragment 23–118 by BNPS-skatole oxidation, which was described by Martenson *et al.* (1975*b*), could also explain this difference. It should also be mentioned that the activity of EP in rats is abolished if the protein is conjugated to horseradish peroxidase with the glutaraldehyde method be mentioned that the activity of EP in rats is abolished if the protein is conjugated to horseradish peroxidase with the glutaraldehyde method (Gonatas *et al.*, 1974*a*); this reagent reacts with the ε-amino groups of lysine.

The encephalitogenic activity ascribed to the C-terminal half of EP— which, at least in regards to the rabbit and the monkey, seems unequivocal— is especially interesting because the amino acid sequence does not contain any sequence where an aromatic residue is positioned five to six residues N-terminal to a Gln–Lys (Arg) grouping. Thus encephalitogenicity is not restricted to regions showing such structural properties (*cf.* Bergstrand, 1972*a*; Sasaki, 1974).

Figure 3 schematically summarizes the localization of the various encephalitogenic sites hitherto described.

---

* The appended "Tyr" used in the nomenclature for some peptides indicates that the peptide during preparation has been treated with a high excess of BNPS-skatole, causing oxidation of its tyrosine residues.

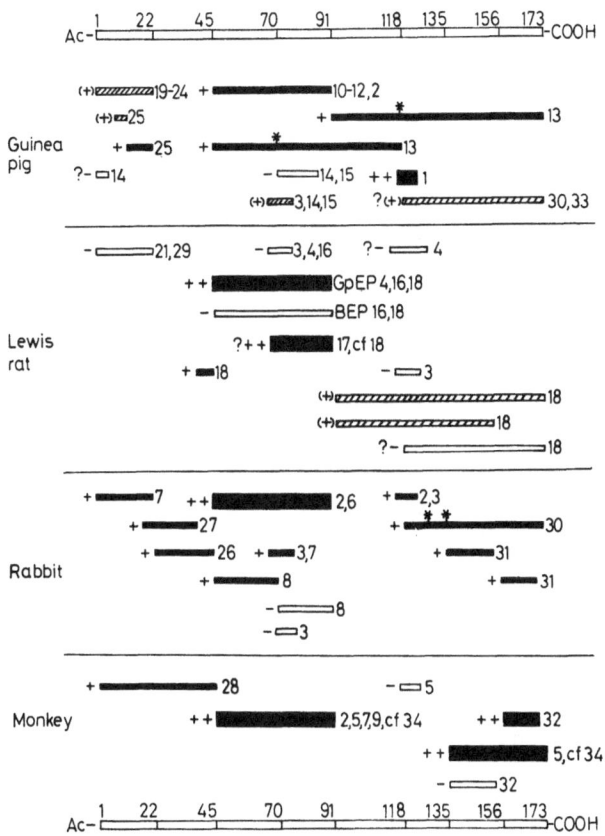

Figure 3. Schematic representation of the location within EP of various disease-inducing regions. Regions that have been ascribed encephalitogenic activity are represented by black bars and regions that in tests even with rather high doses have failed to induce EAE are shown by open bars. On the basis of the published data (the references used are shown to the right of each peptide), the present author has tried to group the potency of each active region as slight to medium (+) or medium to high (++). It is emphasized that this grouping is very rough and only serves the purpose of fitting the schematic representation. Reference key: (1) see Fig. 2, (2) Eylar *et al.* (1971*a*), (3) Hashim and Sharpe (1974), (4) Dunkley *et al.* (1973), (5) Eylar *et al.* (1972*a*), (6) Shapira *et al.* (1971*a*), (7) Shapira *et al.* (1971*b*), (8) Bergstrand (1973*b*), (9) Kibler *et al.* (1972), (10) Lennon *et al.* (1970), (11) Carnegie (1971*a*), (12) Swanborg (1975), (13) Lindh and Bergstrand (1975), (14) Hashim and Schilling (1973*a,b*), (15) Hashim *et al.* (1973), (16) McFarlin *et al.* (1973), (17) McFarlin *et al.* (1974), (18) Martenson *et al.* (1975*b*), (19) Carnegie *et al.* (1970), (20) Robson *et al.* (1971), (21) Swanborg *et al.* (1974), (22) Hashim and Eylar (1969*b,c*), (23) Palmer and Dawson (1969*b*), (24) Chao and Einstein (1970*b*), (25) Barton *et al.* (1972*b*), (26) Berg and Bergstrand (1974), (27) Bergstrand (unpublished), (28) Brostoff *et al.* (1974*a*), (29) Martenson *et al.* (1975*a*), (30) Bergstrand and Berg (1971), (31) Bergstrand (1972*a*), (32) Karkhanis *et al.* (1975), (33) Burnett and Eylar (1971), (34) Kies (1973). Further references supporting the location of encephalitogenicity shown mainly by indirect means are given in the text.

IV. Antigenic Determinants Connected with Protection against Disease

The pathological events induced by an encephalitogenic sensitization or the passive transfer of sensitized lymphoid cells can be diminished or even abrogated by administration of heterologous or homologous EP in a nonencephalitogenic form, either prior to or after the challenge injection (see, e.g., Field and Caspary, 1964; Alvord et al., 1965; Einstein et al., 1968a; Paterson, 1968; Alvord, 1970; Ellison and Waksman, 1970; Levine et al., 1970, 1972; Eylar et al., 1972b; Swanborg, 1972, 1973; Kies, 1973; Driscoll et al., 1974b, 1975; Rauch and Einstein, 1974a,b). But, in contrast to the diseased state, the protected state cannot be transferred passively to un-protected guinea pigs with lymphoid cells (Falk et al., 1969). A variety of plausible explanations can be put forth to explain these findings, and certainly more than one process must be considered to account for all aspects of the protective effect of EP treatment (see Alvord et al., 1965; Falk et al., 1969; Levine et al., 1970; Day and Pitts, 1974b). Depending on the time chosen for administration of the nonencephalitogenic form of EP in relation to challenge, a protective effect is defined as either preventive, suppressive, or therapeutic (Alvord et al., 1965).

It has not been ascertained that different sites within EP account for the disease-inducing or protective effects of the protein. Indeed, Alvord (1970) maintained that the protective effect exerted by any antigen prepa-ration is proportional to its encephalitogenic activity, and Martenson et al. (1975b) found only the highly encephalitogenic region 46–91 of guinea pig EP to inhibit the passive transfer of EAE in Lewis rats. But some recent findings indicate that under certain circumstances the disease-inducing and protective properties might be differentiated (cf. Rauch and Einstein, 1974b). Thus protective effects were obtained in guinea pigs with a nonenceph-alitogenic basic protein derived from CNS tissue (Einstein et al., 1968a)— the amino acid sequence of this protein is indeed similar to that of fragment 1–39 (cf. Nakao et al., 1966a)—and with EP specifically modified at the tryptophan residue (Eylar, 1971; Einstein, 1972b; Einstein et al., 1972b; Spitler et al., 1972; Swanborg, 1972). Spitler et al. (1972) observed that guinea pigs which had received protective immunization with HNB-modi-fied EP did not show delayed dermal reactivity to EP. However, after the challenge injection of EP in FCA they displayed normal responses of cell-mediated immunity but still did not develop the disease. The argument that an encephalitogenic contaminant present in low concentrations could account for this kind of protection has been put forward (Coates et al., 1974), and this objection is difficult to reject. However, there are several observations which make such a situation unlikely:

1.   In guinea pigs the protective activity of homologous EP has been estimated to be 5 times as high as that of bovine EP (Alvord *et al.*, 1965), but according to recent sequence data the primary structure of the major disease-inducing determinant, the tryptophan region, of these two proteins is the same (Eylar *et al.*, 1974a).

2.   A marked diminishing effect on disease induction in guinea pigs and in rabbits was obtained by Teitelbaum *et al.* (1971, 1973) employing a random copolymer of tyrosine, alanine, glutamic acid, and lysine. Although clear-cut prevention could not be attained, a suppressive intravenous injection schedule, starting from 1 to 5 days after sensitization, was efficient. The polyamino acid, which had a molecular weight of some 23,000, was found to be without encephalitogenic or general immunosuppressive activity. A few synthetic copolymers and the basic proteins lysozyme, RNase, and cytochrome *c* were also tested for suppressive activity; only two closely similar copolymers showed substantial effect. Similarly Einstein *et al.* (1968a) and Eylar *et al.* (1972b) found histone preparations without suppressing activity. However, the development of delayed skin reactivity to the bovine EP in the guinea pigs was unaffected by the suppressive treatment. Moreover, prevention could be obtained with the copolymer if the injection schedule was initiated with a single injection of a minute amount of EP [which in itself produces only a limited degree of protection (Teitelbaum *et al.*, 1972)]. As mentioned above, the major encephalitogenic determinant for guinea pigs contains a glutamine–lysine grouping whose integrity is essential for activity. Deamination of the glutamine residue produces an inactive peptide (Westall, 1972) whose preventive/suppressive effect unfortunately has not been examined directly. Westall (1973) has speculated on the possibility that deamination might convert the peptide to a form which might be tolerogenic from a disease-inducing point of view. The possibility then exists that there are, by chance, some regions in the above-mentioned synthetic copolymer which are sufficiently "similar" to such a deaminated tolerogenic determinant that they are able to mimic its action. However, Swanborg (1975a) tested a commercial preparation of peptide 116–124 which was possibly partially deaminated since its encephalitogenic activity was low. It had no protective effect. The copolymer is evidently also active in suppressing clinically manifest EAE in monkeys (Teitelbaum *et al.*, 1974), which further argues against the initially mentioned interpretation since the main encephalitogenic determinants for guinea pigs, rabbits, and monkeys differ. In any case, a cross-reactivity on the cellular level between the active copolymers and the bovine EP has been established in the delayed skin test and in the lymphoid cell transformation test *in vitro* (Webb *et al.* 1973b). The cross-reactivity observed at the humoral level was of a limited extent. Recently, Hashim (1975; see also Hashim *et al.*, 1976) reported that another nonencephalitogenic synthetic peptide with the

sequence H–(Phe–Ser–Trp–Gln–Lys)$_4$–Gly–OH is capable of inhibiting the development of EAE and reversing a full blown stage of the disease and Webb et al. (1976) found another copolymer containing tryptophan to possess suppressive activity.

3. A report by Coates et al. (1974) indicates that immunological tolerance in the sense of abrogation of humoral and/or in vitro demonstrable cell-mediated immunity (tested by macrophage migration inhibition) is not involved. These authors obtained protection against EAE in guinea pigs by injection of peptide 114–124, Arg-124, in incomplete Freund's adjuvant (FIA) if challenge was performed with the same peptide. The protection was less evident in the case of challenge with native EP. Protected animals did not differ from diseased ones in tests in vitro for cell-mediated immunity against either EP or the synthetic peptide. These results substantiate the findings of Spitler et al. (1972) which indicate a dissociation between in vitro observed cell-mediated immunity and protection. Coates et al. (1974) found the most probable explanation for their own findings to be induction of a class of "suppressor lymphocytes" capable of overriding the disease-inducing cells. Whether these two kinds of cells should be considered as sensitized to the same or to different parts of the peptide is an open question. Suppressor cells were recently suggested to control unresponsiveness to EAE also in Lewis rat (Swierkosz and Swanborg, 1975).

4. Eylar et al. (1972a) reported that two monkeys which were sensitized with peptide 116–124 but which failed to develop the disease—this region is not encephalitogenic in monkeys—when injected with an encephalitogenic dose of the complete protein 45 days later both developed encephalomyelitis within 14 days, suggesting that prevention had not been induced by peptide 116–124. According to this reasoning, the complete human EP should lack preventive effects in monkeys, because an analogous situation was reported for two monkeys initially challenged with that protein that failed to develop the disease (Jackson et al., 1972; see also Eylar et al., 1974b). They suffered from EAE within 14 days after rechallenge.

5. The reports by Yo and MacPherson (1972) and MacPherson and Yo (1973) are highly interesting. A basic protein, SCP, in physicochemical aspects apparently similar to EP, was obtained from bovine spinal cord by extraction at neutrality. However, the protein did exhibit an amino acid composition markedly different from that of EP, and it was reported not to be encephalitogenic in guinea pigs even when tested at high doses (300 μg per animal). When administered in FIA, this protein had a marked protective activity. Although the authors suggest that a critical level of antibodies must be present to prevent the development of EAE, a cross-reactivity with EP at the cellular level is another conceivable explanation for the protection afforded by SCP, but it is not yet tested.

6. Barton et al. (1972b) found that synthetic peptides corresponding to regions 8–12, 12–21, and 13–21 (human EP) were capable of inducing

weak signs of clinical EAE in a few of the examined guinea pigs without histopathological criteria of the disease being observed. Moreover, they reported that peptide 13–21, given in FCA, could protect animals from developing histological EAE if they were later challenged with native human EP. A puzzling and yet unexplained finding was that the N-terminal addition of a single glycine residue to peptide 13–21, which converted it to peptide 12–21, seemed to markedly reduce its protective activity.

7. Swanborg (1973) has reported that protection against encephalitogenic challenge was obtained in guinea pigs by treating the animals with the small rat EP. This protein was not quite as effective as the encephalitogenic large rat EP in respect to its ability to induce protection, but it is (as mentioned in Section III) less encephalitogenic in that species. The protective activity was then ascribed to peptide 46–91 (Swanborg, 1975a). Animals treated with peptide 119–173 were not rendered unresponsive to EAE (Swanborg 1975b).

8. Hashim and Schilling (1973b) digested bovine EP with chymotrypsin and found that the encephalitogenic activity was completely destroyed (cf. Hashim and Eylar, 1969a). The tryptophan residue was liberated as part of a dipeptide which was separated from the rest of the digest by gel filtration. A mixture of the other chymotryptic peptides, nonencephalitogenic at the 10, 25, and 500 μg dose levels, did induce a high degree of protection when injected in mg doses in FIA.

9. Employing the passive transfer system in Lewis rats, Levine et al. (1970) found that basic protein from rat and guinea pig CNS inhibited transfer of EAE with lymphoid cells from donors sensitized with rat or guinea pig spinal cord or basic protein, whereas monkey basic protein inhibited transfer from donors sensitized with monkey or human CNS. There was only a partial cross-inhibition between the rodent and primate groups (see Levine et al., 1972; Martenson et al., 1975b).

10. Pretreatment of guinea pigs with an injection of FCA before the encephalitogenic challenge has been observed to induce a certain degree of protection against the disease (Kies and Alvord, 1958; Svet-Moldavsky et al., 1959; Caspary and Field, 1963; Cunningham and Field, 1965; Lisak and Zweiman, 1974b; but cf. Hashim and Schilling, 1973b) accompanied by a diminished cell-mediated immune response to homologous EP in vivo (Lisak and Kies, 1968; Lisak and Zweiman, 1974b) and in vitro (Lisak and Zweiman, 1974b). In view of these findings, those of Einstein et al. (1968a) and Barton et al. (1972b) suggesting protective activity connected to parts of region 1–45, and those of Bergstrand and Källén (1973a) suggesting cross-reactivity between this region and some mycobacterial antigen in the macrophage migration inhibition (MMI) test (cf. Section VB1), it is highly desirable that the immunochemical relationship, if any, between the mycobacterial antigens, e.g., PPD, and EP be clarified.

Taken together, the reports cited clearly suggest the existence either of different encephalitogenic and protective sites within EP or of different disease-inducing and protective cell populations (suppressor cells?) potentially reactive with EP (possibly a combination of both alternatives is more likely). It could be that the seemingly paradoxical finding that a tryptic digest of EP shows only a slight disease-inducing activity (Kies *et al.*, 1965; Hashim and Eylar, 1969a; *cf.* Eylar *et al.*, 1974a), whereas the isolated tryptic peptide 116–124 is highly encephalitogenic, can be explained by such a balance between disease-inducing and protective sites on EP (*cf.* Alvord, 1970; Eylar *et al.*, 1970).

V. Antigenic Determinants Connected with Cell-Mediated Immunity

Studies on the nature and properties of antigenically reactive regions connected with the cell-mediated form of the immune response have attracted substantial attention for only a short time. To some extent this is due to a prolonged lack of convenient and reliable *in vitro* methods for evaluating this form of immunity, only partly overcome during the past decade. Because of the immunopathological interest in EP, this protein is probably the best characterized of all in regard to antigenic determinants for cell-mediated immunity. When such determinants are considered, it is desirable from the immunopathological point of view that special significance be paid to the question of species specificity, i.e., whether a reaction is obtained only when heterologous antigen is employed or whether the reaction is a true autoimmune response obtained also with homologous antigen (*cf.* Alvord, 1970). Most of the available data have been recorded in heterologous systems, and the complete amino acid sequences of all pertinent EPs have not yet been elucidated. The investigations that have been performed with homologous systems show that a cell-mediated immune response can indeed be induced with homologous EP, but hitherto only a few attempts at localizations of pure autoimmune antigenic determinants have been reported. Thus some of the determinants dealt with below might be autoimmune, while others might turn out to reflect species differences in the sequences of various EPs.

A. Delayed-Type Hypersensitivity *in Vivo*

It is well known that EP concomitantly to EAE induces a delayed type of dermal hypersensitivity (DTH) when injected in FCA emulsions (*cf.* Shaw *et al.*, 1965; Paterson, 1966; Alvord, 1970). In guinea pigs the magnitude of the response to homologous EP in skin tests 10 days after sensitization is correlated to the temporal appearance and the severity of the ensuing disease (Shaw *et al.*, 1965; Lisak and Zweiman, 1974*a*). A similar situation occurs in the case of passively transferred EAE in guinea pigs (Falk *et al.*, 1968*a*). Further evidence for a correlation between encephalitogenicity and the capacity to induce a DTH response was provided by Carnegie *et al.* (1967), who prepared a disease-inducing peptide fraction from bovine EP, which was subsequently shown to mount a positive delayed dermal reaction (Lamoureux *et al.*, 1967*a*). However, the location of the peptide within the protein was not identified. The same group suggested that the capacity of this polypeptide fraction to evoke a DTH response could be reduced without affecting its encephalitogenic activity by heavy iodination (Lamoureux *et al.*, 1967*b*). Swanborg (1969) observed the reciprocal condition, that an EP (in this case rabbit EP) could be stripped of the major part of its encephalitogenic activity but still retain the capacity to give rise to a DTH response. Swanborg performed this partial dissociation of antigenic properties by diazotization with arsanilic and sulfanilic acid groups. These findings were subsequently borne out by Eylar *et al.* (1970), who found that a modification of the tryptophan residue in bovine EP with HNB-Br greatly affected the encephalitogenicity of bovine EP but not its ability to produce a delayed dermal reaction in guinea pigs sensitized to native EP. On the contrary, none of the highly encephalitogenic peptides 114–124 (synthetic), 116–124, or 114–127 did react in the DTH test. A gross location of the active sites in the skin test was afforded by Burnett and Eylar (1971), who examined peptides 1–118 and 119–173 (obtained by BNPS-skatole degradation of bovine EP), and they found both peptides capable of inducing a DTH response and provoking such tests in guinea pigs, sensitized with the native EP or an oxidized derivative of it. The two parts of the protein did not cross-react. On the other hand, human and bovine EP have been found to cross-react extensively (August *et al.*, 1967; Oshiro and Eylar, 1970*b*).

Spitler *et al.* (1972) investigated synthetic peptide derivatives of the tryptophan region; some were highly encephalitogenic, whereas others were inactive. From the present point of view concerning the DTH response, the main findings were the following: Peptide 116–124, Lys-124, i.e., the homologous tryptophan region (Eylar *et al.*, 1974*a*), could sensitize guinea pigs to a positive dermal response in tests with native bovine EP. The reaction obtained with EP modified at the tryptophan residue was minimal. However, if the animals were sensitized with a closely similar encephalitogenic peptide, 114–124 with Ser-117 replaced by Ala, no DTH response was obtained with EP or modified EP. Peptide 114–123 did sensitize animals for a positive DTH response to EP, but it was not encephalitogenic whereas peptide 114–124 with Glu-121 replaced by Ile could do so only when high sensitizing doses were used. If the animals were sensitized with bovine EP, a positive skin test could be found neither with peptide 114–124, Ala-117, nor with 114–124, Arg-124. Similar results were obtained when human EP and the corresponding synthetic peptide 116–124, Arg-124, were examined (Spitler et al., 1975). These findings, corroborated by the work of Hashim and coworkers (see below), are significant because they imply that the disease-inducing properties of a peptide can be dissociated from its ability to induce or evoke a delayed skin test reaction even in a *strictly homologous* system where the possible interferences of species-specific determinants are eliminated. This apparently applies both to the guinea pig and the rabbit (Hashim and Sharpe, 1974).

Lamoureux et al. (1972) also investigated synthetic peptides analogous to the tryptophan region. Their peptides were prepared by serially adding the naturally occurring amino acid residue (according to the human EP sequence) to Gly-128. Significant reactivity was not encountered until the peptide length reached ten amino acids (sequence 119–128) but clearly before addition of the tryptophan residue which was essential for encephalitogenicity.

Hashim and coworkers have addressed themselves primarily to the reactivity of three specified regions of bovine EP in guinea pigs. From a chymotryptic digest of bovine EP they isolated, among other peptides, fragments 119–127, 71–76, 71–86, 77–86, and peptide 1–5 (Hashim et al., 1973). The analytical data given for the last-mentioned peptide do not conform to the primary sequence of bovine EP (Brostoff et al., 1974a), making the relevance of the immunochemical findings with this peptide unclear. In short, the authors claimed that all these peptides, except 77–86, were capable of inducing cell-mediated immunity as manifested by positive DTH responses in tests with the pertinent peptide or with the intact protein (Hashim et al., 1973; Hashim and Schilling, 1973a). The ability of peptide 77–86 to elicit a positive skin test was minimal. Their data indicate that region 71–86 is more efficient than region 71–76 in animals sensitized to intact BEP or peptide 71–86 but not in animals sensitized to peptide 71–76, thus suggesting the existence of two sites within this region. Contrary to the findings of Eylar et al. (1970) and Spitler et al. (1975) with peptide 116–124, peptide 119–124 (synthetic) evoked a positive DTH reaction in animals sensitized to EP. Comparatively high doses were used by Hashim et al. (1973) in the skin test (on a molar basis several hundred times higher than the dose of native protein which produced a strong DTH reaction). It is notable that all three regions examined by Hashim et al. (1973), i.e., the N-terminal, the mid-region, and the tryptophan region, showed substantial cross-reactivity which was ascribed to a common X–X–X–Gln–Lys sequence. The results were corroborated and extended with other synthetic derivatives of these regions (Hashim and Sharpe, 1974). In short, guinea pigs were found to mount a better DTH response than rabbits when peptide 116–125, Gly-125, was used for sensitization and skin tests, whereas the opposite situation occurred when peptide 67–77, Gly-77, was employed. Interestingly, serial deletion of residues from the N-terminal end of peptide 116–125, Gly-125, produced peptides which showed a serially decreased ability to evoke DTH responses in guinea pigs immunized with the complete peptide 116–125, Gly-125. Even peptide Gln–Lys–Gly–OH was claimed to give a significant dermal reaction which was substantially increased by the N-terminal addition of a tryptophan residue. Similar results were obtained in the rabbit with derivatives of peptide 67–77, Gly-77. Neither peptide 116–125, Gly-125, nor 67–77, Gly-77, was found to induce a DTH reaction in the Lewis rat. According to a recent report by Hashim and Sharpe (1975), a number of nonencephalitogenic synthetic analogues of the tryptophan region retain the capacity to induce and elicit DTH responses in guinea pigs.

The results of the three last-mentioned groups seem to deviate significantly in certain respects, those of Spitler et al. (1972) and Lamoureux et al. (1972) suggesting a higher degree of specificity in the DTH response than the results of Hashim et al. (1973) implicate. It might be that the doses used for sensitization and in the tests are of critical importance. This possibility is seen in the report by Spitler et al. (1972). When sensitized with

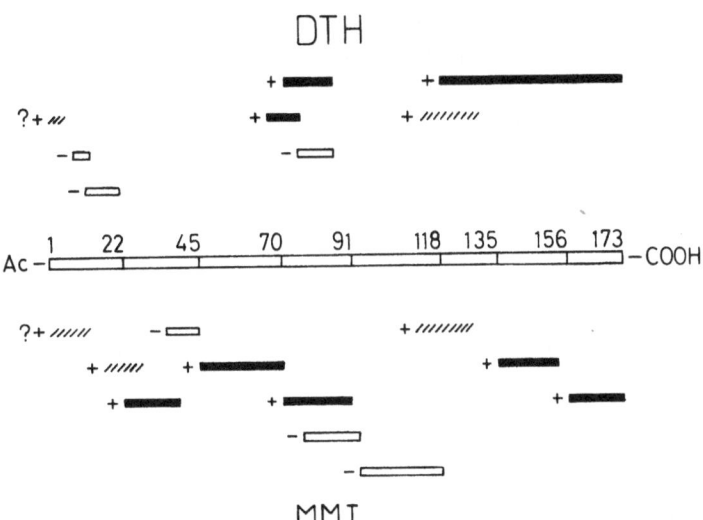

Figure 4. Schematic representation of regions of bovine EP reacting in vivo (DTH) or in vitro (MMI) in tests for cell-mediated immunity in guinea pigs. Regions represented by black bars have been ascribed significant activity, hatched bars indicate that either the very presence or the limits for the determinant are equivocal. The outer limits for each reactive peptide are given; the essential sequences might be much smaller. Regions failing to react are shown by open bars. Further information regarding the sites active in the MMI test is given in Table I. For references, see text (DTH, Section VA; MMI, Section VB1).

20 µg of peptide 114–124, Ile-121, the animals failed to show at DTH response to EP; if the sensitizing dose was raised to 100 µg, the protein did provoke a positive dermal response. Moreover, some of the dermal reactions claimed by Hashim *et al.* (1973) to be significant are of a magnitude which many other workers regard as negative. For the moment, these considerations invalidate efforts to reduce the antigenic activities described by the three groups to a common denominator.

Barton *et al.* (1972b) examined their synthetic derivatives, mimicking regions 8–12, 12–21, and 13–21 of human EP, respectively, for capability of sensitizing guinea pigs for a DTH response. None was found active if tests were performed with the sensitizing peptide or with native EP.

In summary, it is now definitely established that at least two regions of bovine EP (which do not incorporate the tryptophan residue) are capable of inducing and provoking a DTH response in guinea pigs, and the evidence clearly favors the existence of other such sites. Whether these responses are genuinely autoimmune or whether some reflect sensitization to species-specific determinants of heterologous EPs remains to be established. Present knowledge regarding the location of antigenic regions within EP discernible with the delayed skin test procedure in guinea pigs is schematically summarized in Fig. 4.

Delayed dermal reactivity to EP has also been demonstrated in Lewis rats (susceptible to EAE) and in Brown Norway rats (normally considered to be resistent to EAE, but *cf.* Levine and Sowinski, 1975b) but only the first-mentioned strain shows reactivity to the encephalitogenic region 46–90 (McFarlin *et al.*, 1975a,b). Guinea pig EP was utilized as antigen.

B. Tests *in Vitro*

There are a number of *in vitro* techniques available which are thought mainly to reflect the cell-mediated part of the immune response. Some of these test systems have been utilized in studies on EAE and EP.

1. Macrophage Migration Inhibition Tests

Using probably the best-characterized *in vitro* correlate of DTH, the macrophage migration inhibition (MMI) technique (see Bloom, 1971; David and David, 1971, 1972; Lamelin, 1971) with peritoneal cells from guinea pigs, several authors have demonstrated reactivity to CNS tissue or EP in guinea pigs sensitized to develop EAE (e.g., David and Paterson, 1965; Hughes and Field, 1968; Hughes and Newman, 1968; Brockman *et al.*, 1968; Rauch *et al.*, 1969; Hughes *et al.*, 1970; Lennon *et al.*, 1970; Bergstrand and Källén, 1972; Lamoureux *et al.*, 1972; Spitler *et al.*, 1972,

1975; Lisak *et al.*, 1975). Lennon and Dunkley (1974) reached the same conclusion employing Lewis rats and homologous EP; furthermore, a positive test was statistically associated with the occurrence of histological EAE (Lennon and Byrd, 1973). With a slightly modified test system, similar results were reported by McFarlin *et al.* (1975a), and the observations were extended to mice by Bernard and Carnegie (1975). Lennon *et al.* (1970) provided the first data regarding specified fragments of EP that showed reactivity in the test. Animals sensitized with human EP, peptide 114–135, or 114–128 provided cells which were inhibited in their migration by peptide 114–135. This finding was corroborated by Lamoureux *et al.* (1972) and by Bernard and Lamoureux (1975), who examined the synthetic peptide 114–128 (of human EP). Spitler *et al.* (1972) also tested synthetic derivatives of the tryptophan region with the MMI technique. As mentioned above, their results pointed to a dissociation between the disease-inducing properties of this region and its ability to react in the *in vitro* test. As could be expected, cells from animals sensitized with peptide 116–124, Lys-124 (i.e., the homologous sequence), reacted to native bovine EP (identical sequence of tryptophan region) but not to EP modified at the tryptophan residue. Similar observations were made by Lennon and Carnegie (1974) and Bailey (1972) with cells from guinea pigs sensitized to peptide 114–124 (human EP) or peptide 116–124 upon exposure to the native EPs. However, Spitler *et al.* (1972) observed no reaction to EP with cells from animals sensitized to peptide 116–124, Ala-117, or peptide 114–123, although the former peptide was highly encephalitogenic and the latter one induced a positive DTH reaction in tests with EP. Only at a high immunizing dose could peptide 114–124, Ile-121 (encephalitogenic), sensitize the animals to reactivity against EP. Neither peptide 114–124, Ala-117 (encephalitogenic), nor peptide 114–124, Arg-124 (i.e., the native tryptophan region of human EP), nor peptide 116–124, Lys-124 (Bailey 1972), nor 116–124, Arg-124 (Spitler *et al.*, 1975), reacted with cells from animals sensitized to the EPs used (bovine or human). These results indicate a high degree of specificity for the pertinent immune response and substantiate the findings with the DTH test (see above) that the antigenic determinant(s) reacting in conventional assays of cell-mediated immunity can be dissociated from the disease-inducing sites even in homologous systems.

Studies in our laboratory have also been concerned with the intramolecular localization of regions within EP capable of reacting in the MMI test in guinea pigs. The sensitizing antigens used—either native bovine EP or some of its main fragments—were shown to inhibit the migration of specifically sensitized cells but not significantly that of cells from animals sensitized only to FCA. The reactivity of various fragments of EP with cells from a suitably sensitized group of animals could then be compared to that of the immunizing antigen using a kind of multiple regression

Table I. Effects of Various Fragments of Bovine EP on Migration
of Cells from Guinea Pigs Immunized with the Native Protein, the
HNB-Blocked Derivative, or Either of the Two BNPS-Digested
Fragments[a]

Antigen tested	Antigen used for immunization			
	1–173	HNB-1–173	1–118, Tyr	119–173, Tyr
1–173	—	0.62	0.83	0.36
46–173	0.94	—	0.75	—
92–173	0.76	0.48	0.61	0.27
HNB-1–173	0.79	—	0.68	0.30
1–45	0.45	0.33	0.45	0.00
1–118, Tyr	0.69	0.56	—	0.88
119–173, Tyr	0.58	0.50	0.78	—
46–118, Tyr	0.56	0.57	0.98	0.53

[a] The effects are expressed as A values, i.e., the mean ratio of migration inhibition relative
to that obtained with the fragment used for immunization. For details, see Bergstrand
and Källén (1972).

analysis (Bergstrand and Källén, 1973c), the effect of a certain peptide being
described by an A value* which reflects the fractional effect of that peptide
compared to that of the immunizing antigen. The significance of deviations
from the theoretically expected limits $A = 0$ (i.e., no significant migration
inhibition) and $A = 1$ (i.e., effect comparable to that of sensitizing antigen)
can be statistically evaluated using t tests. It should be pointed out that
throughout this work the experimental peptides have always been tested
at concentrations equimolar to those employed for the test of the immunizing antigen.

In our first report we tested the reactivity of a set of extensively purified
polypeptides covering various parts of EP with cells from animals injected
with the intact protein (Bergstrand and Källén, 1972). The effects observed,
shown in Table I, in most cases significantly differed from $A = 0$. On the
other hand, the effect of peptides 46–173 and 92–173 did not differ from that
of the intact protein. The high reactivity of all main regions of the protein
was corroborated when testing these fragments on cells derived from
animals immunized with peptides HNB-1–173, 1–118, Tyr, or 119–173, Tyr
(see Table I). Viewed as a whole, the results clearly implicated the existence
within EP of at least four different antigenic determinants, one each within
regions 1–45, 46–118, and 119–173, and the fourth connected to the tryptophan region. A high reactivity was obtained with peptide 92–173 when
tested on cells from animals sensitized with region 1–118, Tyr; it was ten-

* In earlier reports we described the effects by an a value. The relation between A and a is
simply $A = 1 - a$.

tatively interpreted to reflect the existence of an antigenic site within the region common to these two peptides, i.e., sequence 92–118. Similarly, a high degree of cross-reactivity was observed between peptides 1–118, Tyr, and 119–173, Tyr; at that time it was ascribed to the presence of oxidized tyrosine residues within each of these two fragments. In later reports (Bergstrand, 1972b, 1973a) a couple of smaller peptides derived from region 46–173 were examined. Significant reactivity with cells from animals sensitized with EP could be ascribed to the following peptides: 46–70 ($A = 0.18$), 46–91, Tyr ($A = 0.18$), 136–153 ($A = 0.23$), and 157–173 ($A = 0.19$). A direct comparison between 46–91, Tyr, and 46–70 revealed that the former peptide reacted more strongly than the latter one, in close agreement with the attribution of significant activity to peptide 71–91 (Bergstrand, 1973a). On the other hand, at least one of the histidine residues 62, 63, and 69 or tyrosine residue 70 seemed not to be involved in reactive sites and no significant effect was observed with peptides 77–93 ($A = -0.02$), 95–118 ($A = 0.06$), or notably 116–132 ($A = 0.065$). However, when cells from animals sensitized to peptide 92–173 were employed, peptides 114–128, 114–135, and 117–135 all showed clear-cut activity (Bergstrand, 1973a). Furthermore, cells from animals sensitized to peptide 92–173 showed migration inhibition when tested with peptide 46–70 or 71–91 and cells from animals sensitized to peptide 46–91 reacted to peptides 136–153 and 157–173. The last-mentioned data indicated the existence of a substantial degree of cross-reactivity between several parts of the molecule. Further evidence for such a situation, indicating the involvement in addition of region 1–45, was subsequently described (Bergstrand and Källén, 1973d, 1975). The purity of the peptide fragments employed is of course of utmost importance for the interpretation of these results; however, for several reasons peptide contamination was considered an unlikely explanation for the cross-reactivity (cf. Bergstrand and Källén, 1973d, 1975).

The N-terminal region of the protein was also examined in some detail (Bergstrand and Källén, 1973a). The presence of at least two but probably three antigenic determinants was revealed when cells from animals sensitized to peptide 1–45 were employed. A major determinant of this peptide was localized to its C-terminal half (within residues 23–39), one site seemed to encompass the methionine residue in position 22, and the presence of a third reactive sequence within region 1–21 was found probable. Peptide 35–44 was considered unreactive.

Considered as a whole, the data indicate at least seven, but probably more, separated sequences within bovine EP encompassing antigenic determinants discernible in the MMI test. The tentative location of these determinants is depicted in Fig. 4.

The picture that emerges from the results with the MMI technique agrees well with those obtained employing skin tests (as discussed above).

Thus, for example, also with the MMI test there is ambiguity regarding the reactivity connected to the tryptophan region. It is clear that this region does contain at least one antigenic determinant demonstrable both by the DTH and by the MMI test. But the actual number and the precise localization of the reactive site(s) have not been unequivocally determined with either test (*cf.* Bergstrand, 1973a; Spitler *et al.*, 1975). It might be that different parts of this region do react (or fail to react) depending on the dose and the size of the antigen used for sensitization and/or the test; i.e., the nature of the environment might be of importance for the expression of a determinant.

Interesting results pertinent to the cross-reactivity issue have recently been described by Vandenbark and Hinricks (1974). They sensitized Lewis rats for EAE with either guinea pig or bovine EP. The development of cell-mediated immunity was monitored *in vitro* with the MMI test. Clear-cut inhibitory effects were obtained with the sensitizing EP, regardless of whether it was of rat or bovine origin, but the degree of cross-reactivity between the two proteins was considered very low. The reason for this could be that rats respond to different determinants than guinea pigs do within these two EPs, a situation that seems to exist also for encephalitogenic determinants (see Fig. 3).

Peptide 1–45 of bovine EP was found to have another interesting effect on the migration of guinea pig peritoneal cells (Bergstrand and Källén, 1973a). When these cells were obtained from animals sensitized to FCA only (without admixture of any EP antigen)—but not when normal cells were employed—and when tests were performed in the presence of 50 μg/ml of peptide 1–45, the migration of the cells was often enhanced. A similar observation has been made by Lisak and Zweiman (1974a) employing homologous EP in guinea pigs. The migration stimulating activity of peptide 1–45 was further delineated to some of the smaller peptides employed, which suggests the presence of at least three reactive regions. Their location does not completely coincide with the location of the sites reacting with cells from animals sensitized to peptide 1–45 in FCA. These data were tentatively interpreted as evidence for an immunological cross-reactivity between region 1–45 of bovine EP and some antigenic component of the mycobacteria used at sensitization. Several other reports have also proposed the existence of some kind of cross-reactivity between EP and mycobacterial antigens/PPD (Field *et al.*, 1963; Cunningham and Field, 1965; Hughes *et al.*, 1970; McDermott *et al.*, 1974b; Vandenbark *et al.*, 1975) but, as mentioned above, the issue is far from clear (*cf.* Day and Pitts, 1974b).

Since human leukocyte migration enhancing factors have gained growing interest (*cf.* Weisbart *et al.*, 1974; Bergstrand *et al.*, 1975), the above-mentioned experimental system might also find application as a suitable model for studies of this new interesting lymphokine.

2. Tests with Human Peripheral Leukocytes

The possibility that some of the human demyelinating diseases might depend on autoimmunity to EP has led to an extensive search within this group of disorders for leukocytes specifically reacting to the protein in various tests *in vitro*. Most of the work has been devoted to questions of whether reactive cells exist or not, if their presence is specifically connected to a certain disorder or not, and so on, and thus fall outside the scope of the present review. But a few observations are pertinent to the issue. Sensitivity to human EP has been claimed for cells from patients suffering from a number of diseases when these cells are tested in the macrophage electrophoretic mobility test (Caspary and Field, 1971; for further references, see Preece and Light, 1974). This test is based on the principle that sensitized lymphocytes—whose nature has not yet been ascertained (*cf.* McDermott *et al.*, 1974*b*)—upon stimulation with specific antigen release/ produce a factor which has the property of slowing down the movement of guinea pig macrophages in an electric field. The test has been apprehended as a manifestation of a cell-mediated immune response, but a closer methodological examination would certainly be welcome. Using this test, McDermott *et al.* (1974*a*) concluded that human EP cross-reacts with measles virus antigen, because filtration of cells from an individual showing sensitization to EP through a column of Biorad to which measles antigen had been covalently linked removed the reactivity to EP. The capability of the measles antigen–Biorad column to remove the cells sensitized to EP could be blocked by pretreatment of the column with antimeasles antibodies. A similar approach also indicated the existence of cross-reactivity between EP and PPD (see also Field *et al.*, 1971) but not between EP and a calf thymus histone preparation (McDermott *et al.*, 1974*b*). Cross-reactivity with another basic protein, a common tumor-specific antigen (Dickinson *et al.*, 1974), was also claimed (see also Coats and Carnegie, 1975).

Cells showing sensitization to EP also reacted to the synthetic encephalitogenic peptide 114–124 (Field *et al.*, 1971). This reactivity could be blocked by pretreating the EP or the peptide with serotonin. The specificity of the reaction, as regards both the antigen and the neuropharmacological agent, was shown by the failure of serotonin to influence the reaction between sensitized cells and the relevant antigen in two other cases, and by the failure of other agents, with the exception of lysergic acid diethylamide (LSD), to block the reaction between the sensitized cell and EP (Carnegie *et al.*, 1972). The results were interpreted to support the concept that the encephalitogenic determinant is a binding site for serotonin (see Carnegie, 1971*a*).

Another migration test, which estimates the inhibition or enhancement of migration in an agarose gel of antigen-treated leukocytes was utilized by Bergstrand *et al.* (1974, 1975) to show reactivity to human or bovine EP for cells from some patients with multiple sclerosis and carcinoma. Reactivity to all three main regions of the EP molecule (i.e., to regions 1–45, 46–91, and 92–173, and especially to the tryptophan region; see Berg *et al.*, 1975) was observed.

Kibler *et al.* (1971) used peptide 46–90 of bovine origin and the transformation test (see below) with peripheral·leukocytes, but could find no evidence for sensitivity to this part of EP with cells from patients with multiple sclerosis. (In fact, there is disagreement whether positive reactions to EP occur with this test with MS or not; see Frick *et al.*, 1974; Offner *et al.*, 1974; Webb *et al.*, 1974.)

3. Lymphoid Cell Transformation Tests

Another widely used technique for demonstrating lymphocyte reactivity to specific antigen *in vitro* is the transformation test (see reviews by Bloom, 1971; Valentine, 1971). It has been utilized for studies on reactivity to EP with cells from appropriately sensitized animals. Dau and Peterson (1969) showed that lymphoid cells from rats and guinea pigs, immunized with human EP so as to develop EAE, transform when stimulated with the antigen. Spleen cells and, to a lesser extent, peripheral blood leukocytes were examined. Bergstrand and Källén (1971) observed that the degree of transformation of rabbit peripheral leukocytes was most significant about 11 days after sensitization; clinically diseased animals often failed to react (Fowler, 1972). Webb *et al.* (1973b) obtained a clear-cut transformation of lymph node cells from strain 2, strain 13, and randombred DH guinea pigs immunized with bovine EP and stimulated with the same antigen. A cross-reactivity to some synthetic copolymers, capable of suppressing EAE when appropriately administered (see Section IV), was demonstrated. Interestingly, the cross-reactivity could be directly demonstrated with cells from strain 2 guinea pigs, which are rather resistant to EAE, but only indirectly (by inhibition of transformation) with cells from strain 13 and DH animals, which are susceptible to EAE. A direct cross-reactivity could also be demonstrated when sensitized rabbit lymph node cells were examined. Lisak and Zweiman (1973; *cf.* Lisak *et al.*, 1975) have experienced difficulties with the LT test in guinea pigs using peripheral blood cells. However, if peritoneal cells were utilized, a high degree of reactivity was observed.

With respect to the intramolecular localization of antigenic determinants reactive in this test, the tryptophan region has received most interest. Bailey (1972) and Spitler *et al.* (1972, 1975) did not find significant stimulation with peptide 116–124 tested on cells from animals sensitized to intact protein, but the peptide was found capable of inducing reactivity to itself or to the native EP. Furthermore, Spitler *et al.* (1972) found no significant transformation of lymph node cells from guinea pigs sensitized with either of the peptides 114–124, Ala-117, or 114–124, Ile-121, on tests with native bovine EP. Lamoureux *et al.* (1972) claimed that peptide 119–128 was the smallest one of their synthetic derivatives of the tryptophan region capable of inducing lymphoid cells to reactivity in tests with the peptide used for sensitization or with the intact protein. Lennon and Carnegie (1974) recorded mean stimulation indices for spleen cell cultures in response to human EP which did not differ between guinea pigs injected with the native protein and those injected with peptide 114–124, Arg-124. Kibler *et al.* (1971), who used rabbits sensitized to a fragment of bovine EP (residues 46–90), found that most of the animals had peripheral blood cells that transformed upon stimulation with the fragment. However, no consistent correlation was found between disease and degree of transformation. Finally, lymph node cells from Lewis rats sensitized to guinea pig EP also show reactivity to the encephalitogenic fragment (residues 46–90), whereas cells from Brown Norway rats similarly sensitized show only a marginal response to intact protein and none to the peptide (McFarlin *et al.*, 1975a).

Studies in our laboratory have utilized the LT technique to localize antigenic determinants within bovine EP which show reactivity with cells from sensitized rabbits. In our first study (Bergstrand, 1972c), blood leukocytes were employed and reactivity was evaluated with a regression method analogous to that used in the MMI experiments. All of the three main fragments of EP were considered reactive, whereas the effect of the HNB-modified EP did not differ significantly from that of native EP (in contrast to the findings with the MMI technique in guinea pig). A further delineation of reactive regions was obtained (Bergstrand and Källén, 1973e); in that study lymph node cells were utilized instead of blood leukocytes. The findings of these and other studies (Bergstrand and Källén, 1973b, 1974) are summarized in Fig. 5. We found it likely that most parts of the protein contain sequences that react in the test; for example, region 1–45 was tentatively ascribed four different antigenic sites (Bergstrand and Källén, 1973b). The only more extended region that failed to react seemed to be the bend in the hairpin model, residues 92–118. However, none of the reactive sequences has been closely delineated. Furthermore, it was considered likely that the major reactive sequence of the C-terminal part of the protein has not yet been identified. The tryptophan region was found to have a very slight reactivity. In close agreement with the results obtained using the MMI test in guinea pigs, an almost complete cross-reactivity between the three main parts of the protein was observed (Bergstrand and Källén, 1975). And in agreement with their findings with the MMI test in Lewis rats, Vandenbark and Hinrichs (1974) have reported that lymph

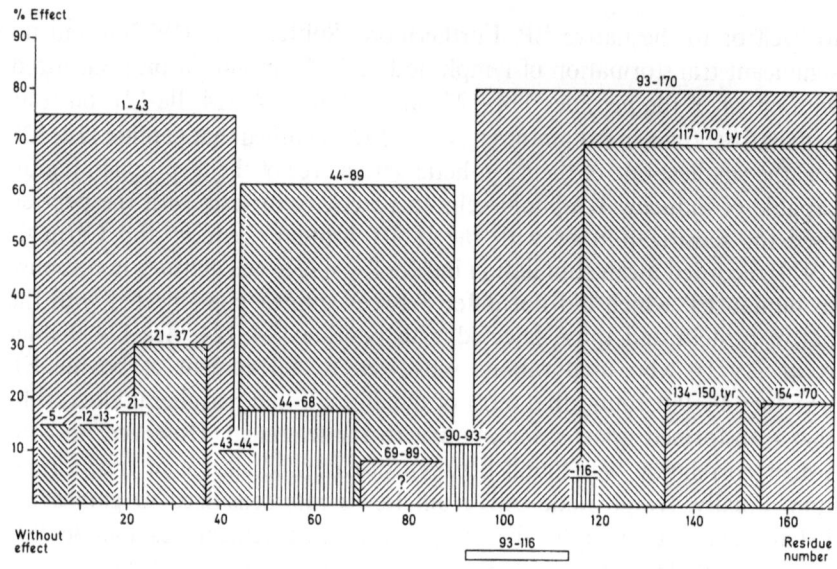

Figure 5. Schematic summary of the localization of antigenic determinants on bovine en-cephalitogenic protein with the lymph node cell transformation test in rabbits. The efficiency values, *approximate* estimates of efficiency compared with EP, are based on results from Bergstrand and Källen (1973b,e, 1974). Smaller peptides failing to show effect have not been indicated. In this figure, which is reproduced from Bergstrand and Källén (1974) with the per-mission of the editor of *Neurobiology*, numbering of amino acid residues follows the originally proposed sequence of bovine EP (see Eylar *et al.* 1971a,b).

node cells from such animals, sensitized to either guinea pig or bovine EP and showing only a limited degree of response to the antigen employed for sensitization, did not reveal more than a minimal extent of cross-reactivity when tested with the other EP. As discussed above (Section VB), the reason for these apparently deviating results might be the different species employed for the test.

VI. Antigenic Determinants for the Humoral Immune Response

Contrary to the situation encountered with most other protein anti-gens, studies on the immunochemical characteristics of EP have been more concerned with cell-mediated immune reactions than with humoral ones. Hitherto, a limited number of experiments have been described which have aimed at the localization of antigenic sites for humoral immunity within EP. Although EP, as most other basic proteins, is a weak antigen (see

Alvord, 1970), it can be administered so as to induce the production of comparatively high titers of antibodies (see Webb *et al.*, 1973*a*; Driscoll *et al.*, 1974*a*,*b*; Whitaker 1975). A detailed examination of the parameters of importance for antibody induction in the Lewis rat has been provided by Day and Pitts (1974*b*) and Pitts *et al.* (1975). Even in homologous systems it is possible to induce antibodies to EP (Falk *et al.*, 1968*b*; Dunkley *et al.*, 1973; Lebar and Voisin, 1973; McFarlin *et al.*, 1973; Driscoll *et all.*, 1974*a*,*b*; Lennon and Dunkley, 1974; Pitts *et al.*, 1976). Serum from guinea pigs sensitized to homologous EP reacted equally well with guinea pig and bovine EP; however, if bovine EP was used for sensitization, a species-specific antigenic determinant(s) was revealed (Falk *et al.*, 1968*b*). The physicochemical characteristics of the antibodies that are induced by injection of EP apparently depend on the route of sensitization and the nature of the sensitizing injection (see Alvord, 1970; Alvord *et al.*, 1970; Kies, 1973; Lebar and Voisin, 1973; Driscoll *et al.*, 1974*a*). Obviously it is even possible to obtain the cytophilic (Gibbs *et al.*, 1970; Coates and Lennon, 1973) and the reaginic (Moore *et al.*, 1974) type of antibodies to EP. Complement fixation (Caspary *et al.*, 1966; Lebar and Voisin, 1973; Whitaker 1975), various hemagglutination techniques (Field *et al.*, 1963; Alvord *et al.*, 1965; Eylar *et al.*, 1969; Hruby *et al.*, 1969; Amesse and Swanborg, 1972), passive cutaneous anaphylaxis (Nakao and Einstein, 1965; Nakao *et al.*, 1966*b*; Falk *et al.*, 1968*b*; Lebar and Voisin, 1973; Webb *et al.*, 1973*a*), precipitation or gel diffusion (*cf.* Alvord *et al.*, 1965; Eylar *et al.*, 1969; Hruby *et al.*, 1969; Kies and Bump, 1972; Hashim and Schilling, 1973; Webb *et al.*, 1973*b*; Martenson and Deibler, 1975), and immunofluorescence (McFarland, 1970; Lennon *et al.*, 1971) are methods that have been employed for demonstrating humoral antibodies to EP. But most authors have utilized radioimmunoassays of varying design. The technique developed by McPherson and Carnegie (1968; *cf.* Lennon *et al.*, 1970, 1971) utilizes gel filtration for the separation of bound and unbound ^{125}I-labeled EP. The method used by Kies and co-workers (Lisak *et al.*, 1970; Driscoll *et al.*, 1974*a*), by Webb *et al.* (1973), and by McFarlin *et al.* (1975) employs coprecipitation of antigen–antibody complexes with antiglobulin antiserum for the same purpose, whereas the methods of Kibler and Barnes (1962), Caspary (1966), Brostoff *et al.* (1974*a*), Day and Pitts (1974*a*,*b*), and Cohen *et al.* (1975) are based on the selective precipitation of the complexes with inorganic salts or ethanol. Schmid *et al.* (1974*a*) have described separation of bound and free EP by treatment of the mixture with dextran-coated charcoal. The precision in the method developed by Day and co-workers seems to permit even meaningful day-to-day single-point measurements (Day and Wexler, 1974).

Cells producing/possessing antibodies (or otherwise binding EP) have been identified by immunofluorescence (Rauch and Raffel, 1965), by the demonstration of plaque-forming cells to EP-coated erythrocytes (Lennon and Feldmann, 1972; Lennon *et al.*, 1972), by histochemical identification of reactive cells with horseradish peroxidase conjugated EP (Johnson *et al.*, 1971; Gonatas *et al.*, 1974*a*), by binding of iodine-labeled EP (Coates and Lennon, 1973; Liburd and McPherson, 1973; Yung *et al.*, 1973), and by affinity chromatography (Webb *et al.*, 1975).

As far as the location of antigenic sites is concerned, all available evidence indicates that in guinea pigs and rats the tryptophan region neither induces antibody production nor reacts with antibodies with specificity for EP (e.g., Lamoureux *et al.*, 1967*a*, 1970, 1972; Lennon *et al.*, 1970, 1971; Eylar, 1971; Coates and Lennon, 1973; Lennon and Carnegie, 1974), the only hint at an antigenic site encompassing this part of EP being a report by Lennon *et al.* (1972), who observed that peptide 114–124, although with slight activity, was capable of inducing antibody production in guinea pigs.

On the other hand, positive results have been obtained in attempts to localize the antigenic sites to other regions. Bovine EP seems to carry a main determinant (at least in heterologous systems) in its N-terminal part. Thus with the aid of an antiserum raised in sheep and the passive hemagglutination inhibition technique, Burnett and Eylar (1971), Eylar (1971) and Eylar *et al.* (1971*a*) showed that the HNB-substituted protein and peptide 1–118 but not region 119–173 or 46–91 reacted with the antisera. This indicated the presence of a dominant antigenic determinant either within the N-terminal fourth of the protein or within sequence 92–118. Moreover, Hashim and Eylar (1969*c*) observed that cyanogen bromide cleavage of the protein at the methionine residues (No. 22 and 170) destroyed its antibody-combining activity, which further pointed to the involvement of sequence 1–45. Chymotryptic digestion of the protein did not affect its antigenic properties (Hashim and Eylar, 1969*d*; Hashim and Schilling, 1973*b*), but it has not yet been possible to evaluate this observation properly, because the pattern of peptide bonds within EP cleaved by chymotrypsin has not yet been reported. Brostoff *et al.* (1974*a*) used an antiserum prepared in rabbits, and again they found that most of the antibody-combining activity of bovine EP was connected to peptide 1–45. This region was also shown to be responsible for the induction in rabbits of a complement-dependent gliotoxic factor, presumably of antibody nature (Berg and Bergstrand, 1974). A further clear-cut delineation of the reactivity of peptide 1–45 has not yet been accomplished, but most authors agree that peptide 1–22 or synthetic derivatives of it have no or only a very faint antigenic reactivity (Carnegie *et al.*, 1970; Barton *et al.*, 1972*b*; Swierkocz and Swanborg, 1974; but *cf.* Whitaker *et al.*, 1975), whereas preliminary results with the gliotoxicity test suggest localization of a site to region 23–45 (Berg and Bergstrand, 1974).

In homologous situations it has been observed that the smaller of the rat EPs induces factors, probably antibodies, which bind ^{125}I-labeled protein, but fragment 46–91 prepared from either bovine or small rat EP could not induce the production of such factors in the Lewis rats (Dunkley et al., 1973; McFarlin et al., 1973). Similarly, intact guinea pig EP induces production of antibodies which, however, do not react with peptide 46–90 (McFarlin et al., 1975a). However, small amounts of antibody against this portion of EP can be produced on Lewis rats by hyperimmunization (McFarlin et al. 1975b). In a similar system, Swierkosz and Swanborg (1974) obtained antibodies capable of passively hemagglutinating erythrocytes coated with guinea pig EP. Inhibition of the hemagglutination could be performed with guinea pig, bovine, and the large rat EP, but not with the small rat EP, suggesting the presence of a reactive site within region 119–159. The data reported by Nakao et al. (1966a,b) may, in retrospect, be interpreted similarly; their fragments C and F (probably constituting regions 92–173 and 46–173, respectively) did react in PCA tests with a rabbit antiserum against the "far-cathodic" fraction containing bovine EP, whereas fragments D (region 46–91?), B (region 1–39?), and A (region 1–45?) failed to react. Acetylation of bovine EP did not alter its properties in this test system when examined with a rabbit anti-bovine EP (Amesse and Swanborg, 1972). However, incomplete antigenic derivation makes the relevance of this finding equivocal.

The most extensive localization of antigenic sites within EP has been reached with guinea pig antisera raised by immunization with either homologous or the small rat EP (Driscoll et al., 1974a). Interestingly, both of these proteins induce antisera with an individual type of specific reactivity for various parts of these proteins depending on the conditions at sensitization. With the aid of these antisera, three separate parts of the protein were shown to contain antigenic determinants; regions 1–91, 92–118, and 119–173. Some antisera reacted only to one or two of these sites. The finding that region 92–118 encompasses a strong antigenic determinant is significant; this is the part of the protein that contains the bend in the polypeptide chain and the peculiar amino acid substitutions (see Section II). It has so far not been ascribed clear-cut encephalitogenic activity in guinea pigs; neither has it been found to react in tests for cell-mediated immunity (see Bergstrand and Källén, 1974). A preliminary communication by Alvord et al. (1974) also suggests the existence of at least three antigenic sites within EP; some of these could be cross-reacting. Rabbits were used for production of antibodies, but the origin of the EP was not specified. The data of Driscoll et al. (1974a) did not reveal any evidence of a cross-reactivity between the various regions. Finally, another recent report ascribes the antigenic reactivity of bovine EP, tested in rabbits, to regions 1–45 and 92–173, whereas region 46–91 was found to be nonreactive (Whitaker et al., 1975). Figure 6 gives a highly simplified and schematic summary of the localization of antibody-combining regions within EP.

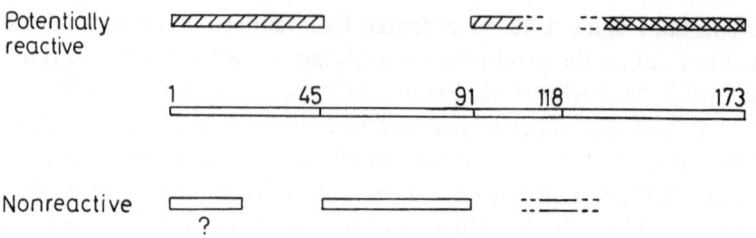

Figure 6. Rough compilation of the localization of antigenic sites reacting with antibodies against EP. Regions represented by hatched bars have been ascribed antibody combining activity; the open end of the bars represents high uncertainty of limits for determinants. The figure gives the outer limit for each reactive peptide; the essential sequences might turn out to be much smaller. Regions failing to react are shown by open bars. For details regarding the origin of EP, the species used for immunization, and the technique employed, see text.

Based on results in some different experimental systems, a cross-reactivity between EP and various histone fractions has been suggested by some authors (Lennon *et al.*, 1971; Whittingham *et al.*, 1972; Johns *et al.*, 1973; Liburd and McPherson, 1973; *cf.* Kornguth *et al.*, 1972). However, a thorough investigation of this issue did not sustain the suggestion, at least not with respect to humoral immunity (Schmid *et al.*, 1974*b*; Bustin *et al.*, 1975; Whitaker, 1975; *cf.* Eylar, 1971). One possible explanation for the observed cross-reactivity could be impurity of the EP employed; the F1-histone fraction is a plausible contaminant (see Kies, 1972). On the other hand, cross-reactivity between histone F2A1 and EP was observed on the cellular level *in vitro* and *in vivo* (Bustin *et al.*, 1975). Cross-reactivity between EP and mycobacterial antigens have also been claimed (see Section VB1). Day and Pitts (1974*b*) observed induction of anti-EP antibody formation in Lewis rats sensitized with FCA only. However, these antibodies failed to cross-react with mycobacterial constituents in adsorption tests. On the other hand, a complete serological cross-reactivity between bovine and human EP has been described by Oshiro and Eylar (1970*b*), Lennon and Dunkley (1974), and Schmid *et al.* (1974*b*). With a rabbit antiserum against chicken EP, reactions of identity in diffusion tests were observed between bovine, human, rabbit, chicken, turtle, and frog EPs (Martenson and Deibler, 1975).*

Finally, it should be mentioned that to our knowledge there is no report clearly showing the existence of antibodies to EP in serum or CSF from human beings (*cf.* Lisak *et al.*, 1968; Lennon and Mackay, 1972), although binding of EP to peripheral blood leukocytes was observed (Yung *et al.*, 1973).

---

* Recently, similar results were obtained with syngeneic rat-anti-EP antisera (Pitts *et al.*, 1976).

VII. Concluding Remarks

It should have become clear that investigations of the immunochemical characteristics of EP have been intimately connected to the pathological aspects of EAE. This is quite natural, but it could unfortunately lead to lack of attention to observations significant from other points of view. Therefore, it has been one of the aims of the present review to emphasize the interesting implications for immunochemistry in general that emerge from the studies on EP. Although still incomplete, they indicate that numerous distinct parts of EP are immunologically reactive in one way or the other. The antigenic/immunogenic properties of these regions have been examined not only by their capacity to induce humoral or cell-mediated immunity or to react in a variety of immunochemical tests *in vitro* but also by their capacity to induce EAE or protection against this disease. The following are among the main findings:

The identification of at least four encephalitogenic regions seems established and in addition the existence of four or five other disease-inducing determinants has been proposed. The potency of most of these encephalitogenic sites is clearly dependent on the species employed for testing. Thus the capacity to induce disease in the Lewis rat has hitherto been connected mainly to one, apparently highly species-specific, part of guinea pig and rat but not bovine EP. The guinea pig and the monkey primarily respond to yet other, more or less species-specific, regions but also to some minor more common determinants, whereas the rabbit seems to be susceptible to disease induction with several different parts of EP.

In regards to the antigenic determinants reacting in conventional assays of cell-mediated immunity, the situation seems to be similar. Tests performed *in vitro* or *in vivo* suggest that the ultimate number of antigenic sites, irrespective of the species employed for preparation of EP or for testing immunochemical reactivity, will probably exceed a dozen. Many of these sites have been encountered in heterologous systems; their relevance in a true autoimmune situation is not yet known.

Although there are divergent observations, a number of reports have proposed a dissociation of the disease-inducing properties of EP and its capacity to induce or elicit a cell-mediated immune response as demonstrated by DTH, MMI, or LT tests. There is evidence that regions exist which can induce a cell-mediated immune response—in the abovementioned respect—without concomitant disease even in homologous situations. The opposite situation, i.e., disease induction without conventional cell-mediated immune response, has also been claimed to exist. A similar dissociation between regions capable of inducing disease and those inducing protection against it has been proposed by some workers. A logical interpretation of these observations would be to propose, as Spitler et al. (1972) have done, the existence of different antigenic/immunogenic sites within EP capable of triggering different lymphoid cell populations. Thus the encephalitogenic (or the protective) activity of a certain region might be connected to its capacity to induce an immune response in one specific disease-promoting (or suppressing) lymphoid cell population; which would not necessarily be expected to react in tests monitoring the activity of cells participating in other parts of the total cell-mediated immune response. This could be a manifestation of the dissociation of various T-cell functions that has been proposed by several authors (see, e.g., Elliott and Haskill, 1974; Silver and Benacerraf, 1974; Bullock et al. 1975; Cantor and Boyse, 1975; Dennert, 1975; Janeway et al., 1975; Scavulli and Dutton, 1975). Dissociation of the antigenic regions of an immunogen has also been observed previously (for references, see Senyk et al., 1971; Spitler et al., 1972; Crumpton, 1974). It seems that EP could be the most extensively examined immunogen in the last-mentioned respect.

One could imagine another level of dissociation between antigenic determinants of EP. Those reacting with humoral antibodies seem to be more restricted in number than those concerned with cell-mediated immunity. Furthermore, one of the major antigenic sites for humoral immunity has been localized in the "corner" of the protein, i.e., in region 92–118, a sequence where no antigenic site for cell-mediated immunity or disease induction hitherto has been clearly localized. The cross-reactivity between the humoral sites does not seem to be important, whereas evidence for an internal and external cross-reactivity with respect to cell-mediated immunity has been presented. These findings are also in agreement with observations made in some other systems and could háve relevance to the controversial issue of T-cell receptor specificity (for references, see Chapter 4 in this volume; Crumpton, 1974; Hämmerling and McDevitt, 1974; Rajewsky and Mohr, 1974; Weinbaum et al., 1974). One might speculate that the humoral immune response is directed primarily to regions within EP showing some degree of ordered structure or being "corners" in the molecule, whereas cell-mediated immunity is directed primarily to antigenic sites whose properties are determined mainly by the primary structure of the sequence.

Finally, one impression obtained upon scrutinizing the numerous reported studies on the tryptophan region is that the expression of a potential antigenic/immunogenic determinant in regards to cell-mediated immunity could depend not only on the immunizing and test doses used but also on the presence and nature of the surrounding sequences. This speculation is mentioned only to stimulate further studies aimed at examining the possible existence of a kind of fluent intramolecular antigenic competition in the cell-mediated type of immune response.

VIII. References

Abramsky, O., Teitelbaum, D., Webb, C., and Arnon, R., 1975, *J. Neuropathol. Exp. Neurol.* **34**:36.

Adams, C. W. M., and Leibowitz, S., 1969, The general pathology of demyelinating diseases, in: *The Structure and Function of Nervous Tissue*, Vol. III (G. Bourne, ed.), pp. 309–382, Academic Press, New York.

Alvord, E. C., Jr., 1968, The etiology and pathogenesis of experimental allergic encephalomyelitis, in: *The Central Nervous System: Some Experimental Models of Neurological Diseases* (O. T. Bailey and D. E. Smith, eds.), pp. 52–70, The Williams and Wilkins Co., Baltimore.

Alvord, E. C., Jr., 1970, Acute disseminated encephalomyelitis and "Allergic" neuroencephalopathies, in: *Handbook of Clinical Neurology*, Vol. 9 (P. J. Vinken and G. W. Bruyn, eds.), pp. 500–571, North-Holland, Amsterdam.

Alvord, E. C., Jr., Shaw, Ch-M., Fahlberg, W. J., and Kies, M. W., 1964, *Z. Immun. Allergieforsch.* **126**:193.

Alvord, E. C., Jr., Shaw, C. M., Hruby, S., and Kies, M. W., 1965, *Ann. N.Y. Acad. Sci.* **122**:333.

Alvord, E. C., Jr., Shaw, C. M., Lisak, R. P., Falk, G. A., and Kies, M. W., 1970, *Int. Arch. Allergy* **38**:403.

Alvord, E. C., Jr., Hruby, S., Petersen, R., Barker, W. C., and Dayhoff, M. O., 1974, *Fed. Proc.* **33**:786 (abst. 3268).

Amesse, L. S., and Swanborg, R. H., 1972, *Proc. Soc. Exp. Biol. Med.* **140**:1082.

Ansari, K. A., Hendrickson, H., Sinha, A. A., and Rand, A., 1975, *J. Neurochem.* **25**:193.

Anthony, J. S., and Moscarello, M. A., 1971, *Biochim. Biophys. Acta* **243**:429.

Åström, K. E., and Waksman, B. H., 1962, *J. Pathol. Bacteriol.* **83**:89.

August, C. S., Kies, M. W., and Alvord, E. C., Jr., 1967, *Nature (London)* **214**:1021.

Bailey, P. J., 1972, *Fed. Proc.* **31**:462 (abst. 1389).

Baldwin, G. S., and Carnegie, P. R., 1971*a*, *Science* **171**:579.

Baldwin, G. S., and Carnegie, P. R., 1971*b*, *Biochem. J.* **123**:69.

Banik, N. L., and Davison, A. N., 1973, *J. Neurochem.* **21**:489.

Banik, N. L., and Davison, A. N., 1974, *Biochem. J.* **143**:39.

Barton, M. A., McPherson, T. A., and Martin, J. K., 1972*a*, *Can. J. Biochem.* **50**:684.

Barton, M. A., McPherson, T. A., Lemieux, R. U., and Bain, G. O., 1972*b*, *Can. J. Biochem* **50**:689.

Behan, P. O., Kies, M. W., Lisak, R. P., Sheremata, W., and Lamarche, J. B., 1973, *Arch. Neurol. (Chicago)* **29**:4.

Bencina, B., Carnegie, P. R., McPherson, T. A., and Robson, G., 1969, *FEBS Lett.* **4**:9.

Benuck, M., Marks, N., and Hashim, G. A., 1975, *Eur. J. Biochem.* **52**:615.

Bernard, C. C., and Carnegie, P. R., 1975, *J. Immunol.* **114**:1537.

Bernard, C. C., and Lamoureux, G., 1975, *Cell. Immunol.* **16**:182.

Berg, O., and Bergstrand H., 1974, *Neurobiology* **4**:191.

Berg, O., Bergstrand, H., Källén, B., and Nilsson, O., 1975, *Acta Neurol. Scand.* **52**:303.

Bergstrand, H., 1971, *Eur. J. Biochem.* **21**:116.

Bergstrand, H., 1972*a*, *FEBS Lett.* **23**:195.

Bergstrand, H., 1972*b*, *Eur. J. Biochem.* **27**:126.

Bergstrand, H., 1972*c*, *Eur. J. Immunol.* **2**:266.

Bergstrand, H., 1973*a*, *Immunochemistry* **10**:611.

Bergstrand, H., 1973*b*, *Neurobiology* **3**:124.

Bergstrand, H., and Berg, O., 1971, *Eur. J. Immunol.* **1**:499.

Bergstrand, H., and Källén, B., 1971, *Acta Pathol. Microbiol. Scand. Sect. B.* **79**:551.

Bergstrand, H., and Källén, B., 1972, *Cell Immunol.* **3**:660.

Bergstrand, H., and Källén, B., 1973*a, Immunochem.* **10**:229.

Bergstrand, H., and Källén, B., 1973*b, Neurobiology* **3**:246.

Bergstrand, H., and Källén, B., 1973*c, Scand. J. Immunol.* **2**:173.

Bergstrand, H., and Källén, B., 1973*d, Immunochemistry* **10**:471.

Bergstrand, H., and Källén, B., 1973*e, Eur. J. Immunol.* **3**:287.

Bergstrand, H., and Källén, B., 1974, *Neurobiology* **4**:328.

Bergstrand, H., and Källén, B., 1975, *Acta Pathol. Microbiol. Scand. Sect. C* **83**:165.

Bergstrand, H., Källén, B., and Nilsson, O., 1974, *Acta Neurol. Scand.* **50**:227.

Bergstrand, H., Källén, B., and Nilsson, O., 1975, *Acta Allergol.* **30**:150.

Bloom, B. R., 1971, *Adv. Immunol.* **13**:102.

Brockman, J. A., Stiffey, A. V., and Tesar, W. C., 1968, *J. Immunol.* **100**:1230.

Brostoff, S., and Eylar, E. H., 1971, *Proc. Natl. Acad. Sci. U.S.A.* **68**:765.

Brostoff, S. W., and Eylar, E. H., 1972, *Arch. Biochem. Biophys.* **153**:590.

Brostoff, S. W., Rosegay, A., and Vandenheuvel, W. J. A., 1972, *Arch. Biochem. Biophys.* **148**:156.

Brostoff, S. W., Reuter, W., Hichens, M., and Eylar, E. H., 1974*a, J. Biol. Chem.* **249**:559.

Brostoff, S. W., Sacks, H., Dal Canto, M., Johnson, A. B., Raine, C. S., and Wisniewski, H., 1974*b, J. Neurochem.* **23**:1037.

Brostoff, S. W., Karkhanis, Y. D., Carlo, D. J., Reuter, W., and Eylar, E. H., 1975, *Brain Res.* **86**:449.

Bullock, W. W., Katz, D. H., and Benacerraf, B., 1975, *J. Exp. Med.* **142**:275.

Burdzy, K., and Kallos, P. (eds.), 1969, Pathogenesis and etiology of demyelinating diseases, in: *Int. Arch. Allergy* **36**:1.

Burnett, P. R., and Eylar, E. H., 1971, *J. Biol. Chem.* **246**:3425.

Bustin, M., Teitelbaum, D., and Webb, C., 1975, *Eur. J. Biochem.* **53**:615.

Cantor, H., and Boyse, E. A., 1975, *J. Exp. Med.* **141**:1376.

Carnegie, P. R., 1969, *Biochem. J.* **111**:240.

Carnegie, P. R., 1971*a, Nature (London)* **229**:25.

Carnegie, P. R., 1971*b, Biochem. J.* **123**:57.

Carnegie, P. R., and Lumsden, C. E., 1966, *Nature (London)* **209**:1354.

Carnegie, P. R., and Lumsden, C. E., 1967, *Immunology* **12**:133.

Carnegie, P. R., Bencina, B., and Lamoureux, G., 1967, *Biochem. J.* **105**:559.

Carnegie, P. R., McPherson, T. A., and Robson, G. S. M., 1970, *Immunology* **19**:55.

Carnegie, P. R., Caspary, E. A., Smythies, J. R., and Field, E. J., 1972, *Nature (London)* **240**:561.

Carnegie, P. R., Kemp, B. E., Dunkley, P. R., and Murray, A. W., 1973, *Biochem. J.* **135**:569.

Carnegie, P. R., Dunkley, P. R., Kemp, B. E., and Murray, A. W., 1974, *Nature (London)* **249**:147.

Caspary, E. A., 1966, *J. Neurol. Neurosurg. Psychiatry* **29**:103.

Caspary, E. A., and Field, E. J., 1963, *Nature (London)* **197**:1218.

Caspary, E. A., and Field, E. J., 1965, *Ann. N.Y. Acad. Sci.* **122**:182.

Caspary, E. A., and Field, E. J., 1971, *Br. Med. J.* **2**:613.

Caspary, E. A., Sinden, R. E., and Field, E. J., 1966, *Z. Immun. Allegieforsch.* **130**:454.

Chao, L.-P., and Einstein, E. R., 1968, *J. Biol. Chem.* **243**:6050.

Chao, L.-P., and Einstein, E. R., 1969, *J. Chromatogr.* **42**:485.

Chao, L.-P., and Einstein, E. R., 1970*a, J. Neurochem.* **17**:1121.

Chao, L.-P., and Einstein, E. R., 1970*b, J. Biol. Chem.* **245**:6397.

Chou, F. C-H., Chou, C-H. J., Shapira, R., and Kibler, R. F., 1976, *J. Biol. Chem.* **251**:2671.

Coates, A. S., and Carnegie, P. R., 1975, *Clin. Exp. Immunol.* **22**:16.

Coates, A. S., and Lennon, V. A., 1973, *Immunology* **24**:425.

Coates, A., Mackay, I. R., and Crawford, M., 1974, *Cell. Immunol.* **12**:370.

Cohen, S. R., McKhann, G. M., and Guarnieri, M., 1975, *J. Neurochem.* **25**:371.

Cotman, C. W., and Mahler, H. R., 1967, *Arch. Biochem. Biophys.* **120**:384.

Crumpton, M. J., 1974, Protein antigens: The molecular bases of antigenicity and immunogenicity, in: *The Antigens*, Vol. II, (M. Sela, ed.), pp. 1–78, Acad. Press, New York.

Cunningham, V. R., and Field, E. J., 1965, *Ann. N.Y. Acad. Sci.* **122**:346.

Daile, P., Carnegie, P. R., and Young, J. D., 1975, *Nature (London)* **257**:416.

Dal Canto, M. C., Johnson, A. B., Raine, C. S., Wisniewski, H. M., and Brostoff, S. W., 1974, *J. Immunol.* **113**:387.

Dal Canto, M. C., Wisniewski, H. M., Johnson, A. B., Brostoff, S. W., and Raine, C. S., 1975, *J. Neurol. Sci.* **24**:313.

Dau, P. C., and Peterson, R. D. A., 1969, *Int. Arch. Allergy* **35**:353.

David, J. R., and David, R., 1971, Assay for inhibition of macrophage migration, in: *In Vitro Methods in Cell Mediated Immunity* (B. R. Bloom, and P. R. Glade, eds.), pp. 249–258, Academic Press, New York.

David, J. R., and David, R. A., 1972, *Prog. Allergy* **16**:300.

David, J. R., and Paterson, P. Y., 1965, *J. Exp. Med.* **122**:1161.

Day, E. D., and Pitts, O. M., 1974a, *Immunochemistry* **11**:651.

Day, E. D., and Pitts, O. M., 1974b, *J. Immunol.* **113**:1958.

Day, E. D., and Wexler, M. A., 1974, *J. Immunol.* **113**:1952.

Deibler, G. E., and Martenson, R. E., 1973, *J. Biol. Chem.* **248**:2392.

Deibler, G. E., Martenson, R. E., and Kies, M. W., 1970, *Biochim. Biophys. Acta* **200**:342.

Deibler, G. E., Martenson, R. E., and Kies, M. W., 1972, *Prep. Biochem.* **2**:139.

Demel, R. A., London, Y., Geurts van Kessel, W. S. M., Vossenberg, F. G. A., and van Deenen, L. L. M., 1973, *Biochim. Biophys. Acta* **311**:507.

Dennert, G., 1975, *J. Immunol.* **114**:1570.

Dickinson, J. P., Jones, K. M., Aparicio, S. R., and Lumsden, C. E., 1970, *Nature (London)* **227**:1133.

Dickinson, J. P., McDermott, J. R., Smith, J. K., and Caspary, E. A., 1974, *Br. J. Cancer* **29**:425.

Driscoll, B. F., Kramer, A. J., and Kies, M. W., 1974a, *Science* **184**:73.

Driscoll, B. F., Kies, M. W., and Alvord, E. C., Jr., 1974b, *J. Immunol.* **112**:392.

Driscoll, B. F., Kies, M. W., and Alvord, E. C., Jr., 1975, *J. Immunol.* **114**:291.

Dunkley, P. R., and Carnegie, P. R., 1974a, *Biochem. J.* **141**:243.

Dunkley, P. R., and Carnegie, P. R., 1974b, Isolation of myelin basic proteins, in: *Research Methods in Neurochemistry*, Vol. 2, (N. Marks and R. Rodnight, eds.), pp. 219–245, Plenum Press, New York.

Dunkley, P. R., Coates, A. S., and Carnegie, P. R., 1973, *J. Immunol.* **110**:1699.

Einstein, E. R., 1972a, Basic protein of myelin and its role in experimental allergic encephalomyelitis and multiple sclerosis, in: *Handbook of Neurochemistry*, Vol. 7, (A. Lajtha, ed.), pp. 107–128, Plenum Press, New York.

Einstein, E. R., 1972b, Suppression of experimental allergic encephalomyelitis with encephalitogen modified through tryptophan, in: *Multiple Sclerosis: Progress in Research* (E. J. Field, T. M. Bell, and P. R. Carnegie, eds.), (Clinical Studies, Vol. 3), pp. 121–128, North-Holland, Amsterdam.

Einstein, E. R., Roberstson, D. M., DiCaprio, J. M., and Moore, W., 1962, *J. Neurochem.* **9**:353.

Einstein, E. R., Csejtey, J., Davis, W. J., and Rauch, H. C., 1968a, *Immunochemistry* **5**:567.

Einstein, E. R., Csejtey, J., and Marks, N., 1968b, *FEBS Lett.* **1**:191.

Einstein, E. R., Csejtey, J., Davis, W. J., Lajtha, A., and Marks, N., 1969, *Int. Arch. Allergy* **36**:363.

Einstein, E. R., Chao, L.-P., Csejtey, J., Kibler, R. F., and Shapira, R., 1972a, *Immunochemistry* **9**:73.

Einstein, E. R., Chao, L.-P., and Csejtey, J., 1972b, *Immunochemistry* **9**:1013.

Elliott, B. E., and Haskill, J. S., 1974, *Nature (London)* **252**:608.

Ellison, G. W., and Waksman, B. H., 1970, *J. Immunol.* **105**:322.

Eng, L. F., Chao, F-C., Gerstl, B., Pratt, D., and Tavaststjerna, M. G., 1968, *Biochemistry* **7**:4455.

Epand, R. M., Moscarello, M. A., Zierenberg, B., and Vail, W. J., 1974, *Biochemistry* **13**:1264.

Eylar, E. H., 1970, *Proc. Natl. Acad. Sci. U.S.A.* **67**:1425.

Eylar, E. H., 1971, Basic A1 protein of myelin: Relationship to experimental allergic encephalomyelitis, in: *Immunological Disorders of the Nervous System,* (P. Rowland, ed.), pp. 50–75, Williams and Wilkins, Baltimore.

Eylar, E. H., 1972, *Ann. N.Y. Acad. Sci.* **195**:481.

Eylar, E. H., 1973, Myelin-specific proteins, in: *Proteins of the Nervous System,* (D. Johnson Schneider, R. H. Angeletti, R. A. Bradshaw, A. Grasso, and B. W. Moore, eds.), pp. 27–44, Raven Press, New York.

Eylar, E. H., and Hashim, G. A., 1968, *Proc. Natl. Acad. Sci. U.S.A.* **61**:644.

Eylar, E. H., and Hashim, G. A., 1969, *Arch. Biochem. Biophys.* **131**:215.

Eylar, E. H., and Thompson, M., 1969, *Arch. Biochem. Biophys.* **129**:468.

Eylar, E. H., Salk, J., Beveridge, G. C., and Brown, L. V., 1969, *Arch. Biochem. Biophys.* **132**:34.

Eylar, E. H., Caccam, J., Jackson, J. J., Westall, F. C., and Robinson, A. B., 1970, *Science* **168**:1220.

Eylar, E. H., Westall, F. C., and Brostoff, S. W., 1971a, *J. Biol. Chem.* **246**:3418.

Eylar, E. H., Brostoff, S. W., Hashim, G., Caccam, J., and Burnett, P., 1971b, *J. Biol. Chem.* **246**:5770.

Eylar, E. H., Brostoff, S. W., Jackson, J., and Carter, H., 1972a, *Proc. Natl. Acad. Sci. U.S.A.* **69**:617.

Eylar, E. H., Jackson, J., Rothenberg, B., and Brostoff, S. W., 1972b, *Nature (London)* **236**:74.

Eylar, E. H., Jackson, J. J., Bennett, C. D., Kniskern, P. J., and Brostoff, S. W., 1974a, *J. Biol. Chem.* **249**:3710.

Eylar, E. H., Kniskern, P. J., and Jackson, J. J., 1974b, Myelin Basic Proteins, in: *Methods in Enzymology,* Vol. XXXII, Part B, (S. P. Colowick, and N. O. Kaplan, eds.), pp. 323–341, Acad. Press, New York.

Falk, G. A., Kies, M. W., and Alvord, E. C., Jr., 1968a, *J. Immunol.* **101**:638.

Falk, G. A., Heinze, R. G., Kies, M. W., and Alvord, E. C., Jr., 1968b, *J. Immunol.* **100**:321.

Falk, G. A., Kies, M. W., and Alvord, E. C., Jr., 1969, *J. Immunol.* **103**:1248.

Field, E. J., and Caspary, E. A., 1964, *Nature (London)* **201**:936.

Field, E. J., and Caspary, E. A., 1970, *Lancet* II:1337.

Field, E. J., and Caspary, E. A., 1972, Cellular sensitization studies in Multiple Sclerosis: Application of macrophage electrophoresis method, in: *Multiple Sclerosis: Progress in Research* (E. J. Field, T. M. Bell, and P. R. Carnegie, eds.), (Clinical Studies, Vol. 3), pp. 51–62, North-Holland, Amsterdam.

Field, E. J., Caspary, E. A., and Ball, E. J., 1963, *Lancet* II:11.

Field, E. J., Caspary, E. A., and Carnegie, P. R., 1971, *Nature* **233**:284.

Field, E. J., Bell, T. M., and Carnegie, P. R., (eds.), 1972, *Multiple Sclerosis, Progress in Research* (Clinical Studies, Vol. 3), pp. 1–273, North-Holland, Amsterdam.

Fowler, I., 1972, *J. Immunol.* **108**:903.

Freund, J., Stern, E. R., and Pisani, T. M., 1947, *J. Immunol.* **57**:179.

Frick, E., Stickl, H., and Zinn, K.-H., 1974, *Klin. Wochenschr.* **52**:238.

Gasser, D. L., Newlin, C. M., Palm, J., and Gonatas, N. K., 1973, *Science* **181**:872.

Gasser, D. L., Palm, J., and Gonatas, N. K., 1975, *J. Immunol.* **115**:431.

Gibbs, N., Hruby, S., Alvord, E. C., Jr., and Shaw, C.-M., 1970, *Int. Arch. Allergy* **38**:394.

Gonatas, N. K., and Howard, J. C., 1974, *Science* **186**:839.

Gonatas, N. K., Gonatas, J. O., Stieber, A., Lisak, R., Suzuki, K., and Martenson, R. E., 1974a, *Am. J. Pathol.* **76**:529.

Gonatas, N. K., Gonatas, J. O., Pfaff, L., and Stieber, A., 1974*b*, *Brain Res.* **76**:133.

Gonzalez-Sastre, F., 1970, *J. Neurochem.* **17**:1049.

Guarnieri, M., Himmelstein, J., and McKhann, G. M., 1974, *Brain Res.* **72**:172.

Hagopian, A., Westall, F. C., Whitehead, J. S., and Eylar, E. H., 1971, *J. Biol. Chem.* **246**:2519.

Hämmerling, G. J., and McDevitt, H. O., 1974, *J. Immunol.* **112**:1726.

Hashim, G. A., 1975, *Nature (London)* **256**:593.

Hashim, G. A., and Eylar, E. H., 1969*a*, *Arch. Biochem. Biophys.* **129**:645.

Hashim, G. A., and Eylar, E. H., 1969*b*, *Biochem. Biophys. Res. Commun.* **34**:770.

Hashim, G. A., and Eylar, E. H., 1969*c*, *Arch. Biochem. Biophys.* **135**:324.

Hashim, G. A., and Eylar, E. H., 1969*d*, *Arch. Biochem. Biophys.* **129**:635.

Hashim, G. A., and Schilling, F. J., 1973*a*, *Biochem. Biophys. Res. Commun.* **50**:589.

Hashim, G. A., and Schilling, F. J., 1973*b*, *Arch. Biochem. Biophys.* **156**:287.

Hashim, G. A., and Sharpe, R. D., 1974, *Immunochemistry* **11**:633.

Hashim, G. A., and Sharpe, R. D., 1975, *Nature (London)* **255**:484.

Hashim, G. A., Hwang, F., and Schilling, F. J., 1973, *Arch. Biochem. Biophys.* **156**:298.

Hashim, G. A., Sharpe, R. D., Carvalho, E. F., and Stevens, L. F., 1976, *J. Immunol.* **116**:126.

Hegstrand, L. R., and Kornguth, S. E., 1973, *Biochim. Biophys. Acta* **317**:380.

Herndon, R. M., Rauch, H. C., and Einstein, E. R., 1973, *Immunol. Commun.* **2**:163.

Hirschfeld, H., Teitelbaum, D., Arnon, R., and Sela, M., 1970, *FEBS Lett.* **7**:317.

Hoffman, P. M., Gaston, D. D., and Spitler, L. E., 1973, *Clin. Immunol. Immunopathol.* **1**:364.

Hruby, S., Alvord, E. C., and Shaw, C.-M., 1969, *Int. Arch. Allergy* **36**:599.

Hughes, D., and Field, E. J., 1968, *Int. Arch. Allergy* **33**:45.

Hughes, D., and Newman, S. E., 1968, *Int. Arch. Allergy* **34**:237.

Hughes, D., Caspary, E. A., and Field, E. J., 1970, *Z. Immun. Allergieforsch.* **141**:14.

Hughes, R. A. C., and Stedronska, J., 1973, *Immunology* **24**:879.

Hurst, E. W., 1932, *J. Hyg.* **32**:33.

Jackson, J. J., Brostoff, S. W., Lampert, P., and Eylar, E. H., 1972, *Neurobiology* **2**:83.

Janeway, C. A., Jr., Sharrow, S. O., and Simpson, E., 1975, *Nature (London)* **253**:546.

Johns, E. W., Pritchard, J. V. A., Moore, J. L., Sutherland, W. H., Joslin, C. A. F., Forrester, J. A., Davies, A. J. S., Neville, A. M., and Fish, R. G., 1973, *Nature (London)* **254**:98.

Johnson, A. B., Wisniewski, H. M., Raine, C. S., Eylar, E. H., and Terry, R. D., 1971, *Proc. Natl. Acad. Sci. U.S.A.* **68**:2694.

Kabat, E. A., Wolf, A., and Bezer, A. E., 1946, *Science* **104**:362.

Kabat, E. A., Wolf, A., and Bezer, A. E., 1947, *J. Exp. Med.* **85**:117.

Kantchourine, A. Kh., and Kapitonova, M. E., 1969, *Ann. Inst. Pasteur Paris* **177**:378.

Karkhanis, Y. D., Carlo, D. J., Brostoff, S. W., Eylar, E. H., 1975, *J. Biol. Chem.* **250**:1718.

Kibler, R. F., and Barnes, A. E., 1962, *J. Exp. Med.* **116**:807.

Kibler, R. F., and Shapira, R., 1968, *J. Biol. Chem.* **243**:281.

Kibler, R. F., Fox, R. H., and Shapira, R., 1964, *Nature (London)* **204**:1273.

Kibler, R. F., Shapira, R., McKneally, S., Jenkins, J., Selden, P., and Chou, F., 1969, *Science* **164**:577.

Kibler, R. F., Paty, D. W., and Sherr, V., 1971, Immunology of multiple sclerosis, in: *Immunological Disorders of the Nervous System* (P. Rowland, ed.), pp. 95–105, Williams and Wilkins, Baltimore.

Kibler, R. F., Ré, P. K., McKneally, S., Shapira, R., and Keeling, M. E., 1972, *J. Biol. Chem.* **247**:969.

Kies, M. W., 1965, *Ann. N.Y. Acad. Sci.* **122**:161.

Kies, M. W., 1972, Use of myelin basic protein for immunological studies, in: *Multiple Sclerosis: Progress in Research* (E. J. Field, T. M. Bell and P. R. Carnegie, eds.), (Clinical Studies, Vol. 3), pp. 80–89, North-Holland, Amsterdam.

Kies, M. W., 1973, Experimental Allergic Encephalomyelitis, in: *Biology of Brain Dysfunction,* Vol. 2, (G. E. Gaull, ed.), pp. 185–224, Plenum Press, New York.

Kies, M. W., and Alvord, E. C., Jr., 1958, *Nature (London)* **182**:1106.
Kies, M. W., and Alvord, E. C., Jr., (eds.), 1959, *Allergic Encephalomyelitis*, pp. 1–576. Charles C. Thomas, Springfield, Illinois.
Kies, M. W., and Bump, E. A., 1972, *Res. Comm. Chem. Path. Pharm.* **4**:569.
Kies, M. W., Murphy, J. B., and Alvord, E. C., Jr., 1961, Studies on the encephalitogenic factor in guinea pig central nervous system, in: *Chemical Pathology of the Nervous System*, (J. Folch-Pi, ed.), pp. 197–204, Pergamon Press, New York.
Kies, M. W., Thompson, B. E., and Alvord, E. C., Jr., 1965, *Ann. N.Y. Acad. Sci.* **122**:148.
Kies, M. W., Driscoll, B. F., Lisak, R. P., and Alvord, E. C., Jr., 1975, *J. Immunol.* **115**:75.
Kitamura, K., Yamanaka, T., and Uyemura, K., 1975, *Biochim. Biophys. Acta* **379**:582.
Kiyota, K., and Egami, S., 1972, *J. Neurochem.* **19**:857.
Kornblum, J., 1968, *J. Immunol.* **101**:702.
Kornguth, S. E., and Anderson, J. W., 1965, *J. Cell Biol.* **26**:157.
Kornguth, S. E., Kozel, L. R., and Smithies, O., 1972, *Nature (London)* **237**:49.
Krigbaum, W. R., and Hsu, T. S., 1975, *Biochemistry* **14**:2542.
Laatsch, R. H., Kies, M. W., Gordon, S., and Alvord, E. C., Jr., 1962, *J. Exp. Med.* **115**:777.
Lamelin, J.-P., 1971, Inhibition of Macrophage Migration, in: *Cell Mediated Immunity, In Vitro Correlates* (J. P. Revillard, ed.), pp. 75–102, S. Karger, Basel.
Lamoureux, G., Carnegie, P. R., McPherson, T. A., and Johnston, D., 1967*a, Clin. Exp. Immunol.* **2**:601.
Lamoureux, G., Carnegie, P. R., and McPherson, T. A., 1967*b, Immunochemistry* **4**:273.
Lamoureux, G., Carnegie, P. R., McPherson, T. A., Mackay, I. R., and Bernard, C., 1970, *Ann. Inst. Pasteur Paris* **118**:562.
Lamoureux, G., Thibeault, G., Richer, G., and Bernard, C., 1972, *Union Med. Can.* **101**:674.
Lebar, R., and Voisin, G. A., 1973, *Int. Arch. Allergy* **46**:82.
Lee, J. M., and Schneider, H. A., 1962, *J. Exp. Med.* **115**:157.
Lennon, V. A., and Byrd, W. J., 1973, *Eur. J. Immunol.* **3**:243.
Lennon, V. A., and Carnegie, P. R., 1974, *Eur. J. Immunol.* **4**:60.
Lennon, V. A., and Dunkley, P. R., 1974, *Int. Arch. Allergy* **47**:598.
Lennon, V. A., and Feldmann, M., 1972, *Int. Arch. Allergy* **42**:627.
Lennon, V., and Mackay, I. R., 1972, *Clin. Exp. Immunol.* **11**:595.
Lennon, V. A., Wilks, A. V., and Carnegie, P. R., 1970, *J. Immunol.* **105**:1223.
Lennon, V. A., Whittingham, S., Carnegie, P. R., McPherson, T. A., and Mackay, I. R., 1971, *J. Immunol.* **107**:56.
Lennon, V., Feldmann, M., and Crawford, M., 1972, *Int. Arch. Allergy* **43**:749.
Levine, S., 1974, *Acta Neuropathol.* **28**:179.
Levine, S., and Sowinski, R., 1973, *J. Immunol.* **110**:139.
Levine, S., and Sowinski, R., 1974, *Immunogenetics* **1**:352.
Levine, S., and Sowinski, R., 1975*a, Proc. Soc. Exp. Biol. Med.* **149**:1032.
Levine, S., and Sowinski, R., 1975*b, J. Immunol.* **114**:597.
Levine, S., and Wenk, E. J., 1965, *Ann. N.Y. Acad. Sci.* **122**:209.
Levine, S., Hoenig, E. M., and Kies, M. W., 1970, *Clin. Exp. Immunol.* **6**:503.
Levine, S., Sowinski, R., and Kies, M. W., 1972, *Proc. Soc. Exptl. Biol. Med.* **139**:506.
Levine, S., Sowinski, R., Shaw, C.-M., and Alvord, E. C., Jr., 1975, *J. Neuropathol. Exp. Neurol.* **34**:501.
Liburd, E. M., and McPherson, T. A., 1973, *J. Immunol. Methods* **3**:79.
Lindh, J., and Bergstrand, H., 1975, *Neurobiology* **5**:137.
Lisak, P. R., and Behan, P. O., 1975, *Biomedicine* **22**:81.
Lisak, R. P., and Kies, M. W., 1968, *Proc. Soc. Exp. Biol. Med.* **128**:214.
Lisak, R. P., and Zweiman, B., 1973, *Res. Commun. Chem. Pathol. Pharmacol.* **6**:221.
Lisak, R. P., and Zweiman, B., 1974*a, Cell. Immunol.* **11**:212.
Lisak, R. P., and Zweiman, B., 1974*b, Cell. Immunol.* **14**:242.

Lisak, R. P., Heinze, R. G., Falk, G. A., and Kies, M. W., 1968, *Neurology* **18**:122.

Lisak, R. P., Heinze, R. G., and Kies, M. W., 1970, *Int. Arch. Allergy* **37**:621.

Lisak, R. P., Zweiman, B., Kies, M. W., and Driscoll, B., 1975, *J. Immunol.* **114**:546.

London, Y., and Vossenberg, F. G. A., 1973, *Biochim. Biophys. Acta* **307**:478.

London, Y., Demel, R. A., Geurts van Kessel, W. S. M., Vossenberg, F. G. A., and van Deenen, L. L. M., 1973, *Biochim. Biophys. Acta* **311**:520.

Lowden, J. A., Moscarello, M. A., and Morecki, R., 1966, *Can. J. Biochem.* **44**:567.

Lumsden, C. E., Robertson, D. M., and Blight, R., 1966, *J. Neurochem.* **13**:127.

Mackay, I. R., Carnegie, P. R., and Coates, A. S., 1973, *Clin. Exp. Immunol.* **15**:471.

MacPherson, C. F. C., and Yo, S.-L., 1973, *J. Immunol.* **110**:1371.

Marks, N., Benuck, M., and Hashim, G., 1974, *Biochem. Biophys. Res. Commun.* **56**:68.

Martenson, R. E., and Deibler, G. E., 1975, *J. Neurochem.* **24**:79.

Martenson, R. E., and Gaitonde, M. K., 1969a, *J. Neurochem.* **16**:333.

Martenson, R. E., and Gaitonde, M. K., 1969b, *J. Neurochem.* **16**:889.

Martenson, R. E., and LeBaron, F. N., 1966, *J. Neurochem.* **13**:1469.

Martenson, R. E., Deibler, G. E., and Kies, M. W., 1969a, *J. Biol. Chem.* **244**:4261.

Martenson, R. E., Deibler, G. E., and Kies, M. W., 1969b, *J. Biol. Chem.* **244**:4268.

Martenson, R. E., Deibler, G. E., and Kies, M. W., 1970a, *Biochim. Biophys. Acta* **200**:353.

Martenson, R. E., Deibler, G. E., and Kies, M. W., 1970b, *J. Neurochem.* **17**:1329.

Martenson, R. E., Deibler, G. E., and Kies, M. W., 1971a, *J. Neurochem.* **18**:2417.

Martenson, R. E., Deibler, G. E., and Kies, M. W., 1971b, *J. Neurochem.* **18**:2427.

Martenson, R. E., Deibler, G. E., Kies, M. W., McKneally, S. S., Shapira, R., and Kibler, R. F., 1972a, *Biochim. Biophys. Acta* **263**:193.

Martenson, R. E., Deibler, G. E., Kies, M. W., Levine, S., and Alvord, E. C., Jr., 1972b, *J. Immunol.* **109**:262.

Martenson, R. E., Deibler, G. E., Kramer, A. J., and Levine, S., 1975a, *J. Neurochem.* **24**:173.

Martenson, R. E., Levine, S., and Sowinski, R., 1975b, *J. Immunol.* **114**:592.

Martenson, R. E., Kramer, A. J., and Deibler, G. E., 1975c, *Biochemistry* **14**:1067.

Martenson, R. E., Deibler, G. E., and Kramer, A. J., 1975d, *J. Neurochem.* **24**:959.

Martenson, R. E., Kramer, A. J., and Deibler, G. E., 1976, *J. Neurochem.* **26**:733.

McDermott, J. R., and Caspary, E. A., 1975, *J. Neurochem.* **25**:711.

McDermott, J. R., Field, E. J., and Caspary, E. A., 1974a, *J. Neurol. Neurosurg. Psychiatry* **37**:282.

McDermott, J. R., Caspary, E. A., and Dickinson, J. P., 1974b, *Clin. Exp. Immunol.* **17**:103.

McFarland, H. F., 1970, *Proc. Soc. Exp. Biol. Med.* **133**:1195.

McFarlin, D. E., Blank, S. E., Kibler, R. F., McKneally, S., and Shapira, R., 1973, *Science* **179**:478.

McFarlin, D. E., Blank, S. E., and Kibler, R. F., 1974, *J. Immunol.* **113**:712.

McFarlin, D. E., Hsu, S. C-L., Slemenda, S. B., Chou, F. C-H., and Kibler, R. F., 1975a, *J. Exp. Med.* **141**:72.

McFarlin, D. E., Hsu, S. C-L., Slemenda, S. B., Chou, F. C-H., and Kibler, R. F., 1975b, *J. Immunol.* **115**:1456.

McPherson, T. A., and Carnegie, P. R., 1968, *J. Lab. Clin. Med.* **72**:824.

Mehl, E., and Halaris, A., 1970, *J. Neurochem.* **17**:659.

Miyake, M., 1975, *J. Neurochem.* **24**:909.

Miyamoto, E., 1975, *J. Neurochem.* **24**:503.

Miyamoto, E., and Kakiuchi, S., 1974, *J. Biol. Chem.* **249**:2769.

Miyamoto, E., Kakiuchi, S., and Kakimoto, Y., 1974, *Nature (London)* **249**:150.

Moore, M. J., Behan, P. O., Kies, M. W., and Matthews, J. M., 1974, *Res. Commun. Chem. Pathol. Pharmacol.* **9**:119.

Morgan, I. M., 1946, *J. Bacteriol.* **51**:614.

Morgan, I. M., 1947, *J. Exp. Med.* **85**:131.

Moscarello, M. A., Katona, E., Neumann, A. W., and Epand, R. M., 1974, *Biophys. Chem.* **2**:290.

Mueller, P. S., Kies, M. W., Alvord, E. C., Jr., and Shaw, C-M., 1962, *J. Exp. Med.* **115**:329.

Nakao, A., and Einstein, E. R., 1965, *Ann. N.Y. Acad. Sci.* **122**:171.

Nakao, A., Davis, W. J., and Einstein, E. R., 1966*a, Biochim. Biophys. Acta* **130**:163.

Nakao, A., Davis, W. J., and Einstein, E. R., 1966*b, Biochim. Biophys. Acta* **130**:171.

Nilsson, O., 1972, *Acta Neurol. Scand.* 48, suppl. **51**:321.

Offner, H., Ammitzbøll, T., Clausen, J., Fog, T., Hyllested, K., and Einstein, E., 1974, *Acta Neurol. Scand.* **50**:373.

Orgad, S., and Cohen, I., 1974, *Science* **183**:1083.

Oshiro, Y., and Eylar, E. H., 1970*a, Arch. Biochem. Biophys.* **138**:392.

Oshiro, Y., and Eylar, E. H., 1970*b, Arch. Biochem. Biophys.* **138**:606.

Palmer, F. B., and Dawson, R. M. C., 1969*a, Biochem. J.* **111**:637.

Palmer, F. B., and Dawson, R. M. C., 1969*b, Biochem. J.* **111**:629.

Paterson, P. Y., 1960, *J. Exp. Med.* **111**:119.

Paterson, P. Y., 1966, *Adv. Immunol.* **5**:131.

Paterson, P. Y., 1968, Experimental autoimmune (allergic) encephalomyelitis, in: *Textbook of Immunopathology,* Vol. 1, (P. A. Miescher and H. J. Muller-Eberhard, eds.), pp. 132–149, Grune & Stratton, New York.

Paterson, P. Y., 1969, *Annu. Rev. Med.* **20**:75.

Paterson, P. Y., 1971, The demyelinating diseases: Clinical and experimental correlates, in: *Immunological diseases* (M. Samter, ed.), Chapter 78, pp. 1269–1299, Little, Brown, and Co., Boston.

Paterson, P. Y., 1972, Experimental allergic encephalomyelitis and multiple sclerosis as immunological diseases: a critique, in: *Multiple Sclerosis—Immunology, Virology, and Ultrastructure* (F. Wolfgram, G. W. Ellison, J. G. Stevens, and J. M. Andrews, eds.), pp. 539–568, Academic Press, New York.

Paterson, P. Y., and Drobish, D. G., 1974, *J. Immunol.* **113**:1942.

Paterson, P. Y., Drobish, D. G., and Ginsberg, M. M., 1974, *Clin. Immunol. Immunopathol.* **2**:456.

Paterson, P. Y., Richardson, W. P., and Drobish, D. G., 1975, *Cell. Immunol.* **16**:48.

Perlík, F., and Zídek, Z., 1974, *Z. Immun. Allergieforsch.* **147**:191.

Pette, E., and Bauer, H. (eds.), 1964, *Z. Immun. Allergieforsch.* **126**:1.

Pitts, O. M., Varitek, V. A., and Day, E. D., 1975, *J. Immunol.* **115**:1114.

Pitts, O. M., Varitek, V. A., and Day, E. D., 1976, *Immunochemistry* **13**:307.

Poduslo, J. F., and Braun, P. E., 1975, *J. Biol. Chem.* **250**:1099.

Preece, A. W., and Light, P. A., 1974, *Clin. Exp. Immunol.* **18**:543.

Quelin, S., Martinez, G., and Brahic, M., 1975, *Biochimie* **57**:247.

Raine, C. S., Snyder, D. H., Valsamis, M. P., and Stone, S. H., 1974, *Lab. Invest.* **31**:369.

Rajewsky, K., and Mohr, R., 1974, *Eur. J. Immunol.* **4**:111.

Rauch, H. C., and Einstein, E. R., 1974*a, J. Neurol. Sci.* **23**:99.

Rauch, H. C., and Einstein, E. R., 1974*b,* Specific brain proteins: A biochemical and immunological review, in: *Review of Neurosciences* (S. Ehrenpreis and I. J. Kopen, eds.), pp. 283–343, Raven Press, New York.

Rauch, H. C., and Raffel, S., 1964, *J. Immunol.* **92**:452.

Rauch, H. C., and Raffel, S., 1965, *Ann. N.Y. Acad. Sci.* **122**:297.

Rauch, H. C., Ferraresi, R. W., Raffel, S., and Einstein, E. R., 1969, *J. Immunol.* **102**:1431.

Rauch, H. C., Einstein, E. R., and Csejtey, J., 1973, *Neurobiology* **3**:195.

Richardson, W. P., and Paterson, P. Y., 1970, *J. Immunol.* **105**:1563.

Ridley, A., 1971, *Clin. Allergy* **1**:311.

Rivers, T. M., and Schwentker, F. F., 1935, *J. Exp. Med.* **61**:689.

Rivers, T. M., Sprunt, D. H., and Berry, G. P., 1933, *J. Exp. Med.* **58**:39.

Robertson, D. M., Blight, R., and Lumsden, C. E., 1962, *Nature (London)* **196**:1005.

Robson, G. S. M., McPherson, T. A., and Mackay, I. R., 1971, *Brit. J. Exp. Path.* **52**:338.

Rosenthale, M. E., 1974, Evaluation of immunosuppressive and antiallergic activity, in: *Antiinflammatory Agents. Chemistry, and Pharmacology*, Vol. II (R. A. Sherrer, and M. W. Whitehouse, eds.), pp. 123–192, Academic Press, New York.

Rowe, M. J., 1969, *Bull. Los Angeles Neurol. Soc.* **34**:55.

Saito, M., Nagai, J., and Tsumita, T., 1972, *Jpn. J. Exp. Med.* **42**:473.

Sammeck, R., and Brady, R. O., 1972, *Brain Res.* **42**:441.

Sammeck, R., Martenson, R. E., and Brady, R. O., 1971, *Brain Res.* **34**:241.

Sasaki, Y., 1974, *Chem. Pharm. Bull.* **22**:2188.

Scavulli, J., and Dutton, R. W., 1975, *J. Exp. Med.* **141**:524.

Scheinberg, L. C., Kies, M. W., and Alvord, E. C., Jr., (eds.), 1965, *Ann. N.Y. Acad. Sci.* **122**:1.

Schmid, G., Thomas, G., Hempel, K., and Grüninger, W., 1974a, *Eur. Neurol.* **12**:173.

Schmid, G., Thomas, G., Lange, H. W., and Hempel, K., 1974b, *Int. Arch. Allergy* **47**:161.

Sela, M., 1969a, *Science* **166**:1365.

Sela, M., 1969b, *Naturwissenschaften* **56**:206.

Senyk, G., Williams, E. B., Nitecki, D. E., and Goodman, J. W., 1971, *J. Exp. Med.* **133**:1294.

Shapira, R., McKneally, S. S., Chou, F., and Kibler, R. F., 1971a, *J. Biol. Chem.* **246**:4630.

Shapira, R., Chou, F. C.-H., McKneally, S., Urban, E., and Kibler, R. F., 1971b, *Science* **173**:736.

Shaw, C. M., Alvord, E. C., Jr., Fahlberg, W. J., and Kies, M. W., 1962, *J. Exp. Med.* **115**:169.

Shaw, C. M., Alvord, E. C., Jr., Fahlberg, W. J., and Kies, M. W., 1964, *J. Immunol.* **92**:28.

Shaw, C. M., Alvord, E. C., Jr., Kaku, J., and Kies, M. W., 1965, *Ann. N.Y. Acad. Sci.* **122**:318.

Silver, J., and Benacerraf, B., 1974, *J. Immunol.* **113**:1872.

Simon, J., and Anzil, A. P., 1974, *Acta Neuropathol.* **27**:33.

Simon, J., and Simonova, O., 1971, *Z. Neurol.* **200**:105.

Smythies, J. R., Benington, F., and Morin, R. D., 1972, *Experientia* **28**:23.

Spitler, L. E., von Muller, C. M., Fudenberg, H. H., and Eylar, E. H., 1972, *J. Exp. Med.* **136**:156.

Spitler, L. E., von Muller, C., and Young, J. D., 1975, *Cell. Immunol.* **15**:143.

Steck, A. J., and Appel, S. H., 1974, *J. Biol. Chem.* **249**:5416.

Stone, S. H., 1961, *Science* **134**:619.

Stone, S. H., Lerner, II, E. M., Goode, J. H., 1969, *Proc. Soc. Exp. Biol. Med.* **132**:341.

Suzuki, K., and Sasaki, Y., 1974, *Chem. Pharm. Bull.* **22**:2181.

Suzuki, K., Abiko, T., Endo, N., Sasaki, Y., and Arisue, J., 1973, *Chem. Pharm. Bull.* **21**:2627.

Svet-Moldavsky, G. J., Svet-Moldavskaya, I. A., and Raffkina, L. I., 1959, *Nature (London)* **184**:1552.

Swanborg, R. H., 1969, *J. Immunol.* **102**:381.

Swanborg, R. H., 1970, *J. Immunol.* **105**:865.

Swanborg, R. H., 1972, *J. Immunol.* **109**:540.

Swanborg, R. H., 1973, *J. Immunol.* **111**:1067.

Swanborg, R. H., 1975a, *J. Immunol.* **114**:191.

Swanborg, R. H., 1975b, *Immunol. Commun.* **4**:387.

Swanborg, R. H., and Amesse, L. S., 1971, *J. Immunol.* **107**:281.

Swanborg, R. H., Swierkosz, J. E., and Saieg, R. G., 1974, *J. Immunol.* **112**:594.

Swierkosz, J. E., and Swanborg, R. H., 1974, *Fed. Proc.* **33**:814 (abst. 3432).

Swierkosz, J. E., and Swanborg, R. H., 1975, *J. Immunol.* **115**:631.

Teitelbaum, D., Meshorer, A., Hirschfeld, T., Arnon, R., and Sela, M., 1971, *Eur. J. Immunol.* **1**:242.

Teitelbaum, D., Webb, C., Meshorer, A., Arnon, R., Sela, M., 1972, *Nature (London)* **240**:564.

Teitelbaum, D., Webb, C., Meshorer, A., Arnon, R., and Sela, M., 1973, *Eur. J. Immunol.* **3**:273.

Teitelbaum, D., Webb, C., Bree, M., Meshorer, A., Arnon, R., and Sela, M., 1974, *Clin. Immunol. Immunopathol.* **3**:256.

Tomasi, L. G., and Kornguth, S. E., 1967, *J. Biol. Chem.* **242**:4933.

Uyemura, K., Tobari, C., and Hirano, S., 1970, *Biochim. Biophys. Acta* **214**:190.

Valentine, F. T., 1971, The transformation and proliferation of lymphocytes *in vitro*, in: *Cell Mediated Immunity: In Vitro Correlates* (J.-P. Revillard, ed.), pp. 6–50, S. Karger, Basel.

Vandenbark, A. A., and Hinrichs, D. J., 1974, *Cell. Immunol.* **12**:85.

Vandenbark, A. A., Burger, D. R., and Vetto, R. M., 1975, *Proc. Soc. Exp. Biol. Med.* **148**:1233.

Vepřeková, A., Pekárek, J., Doutlík, S., Pavlík, V., and Jedlička, P., 1972, *Z. Immun. Allergieforsch.* **142**:448.

Waksman, B. H., 1959, *Int. Arch. Allergy Suppl.* **14**:1.

Webb, C., Teitelbaum, D., Arnon, R., and Sela, M., 1973a, *Immunol. Comm.* **2**:185.

Webb, C., Teitelbaum, D., Arnon, R., and Sela, M., 1973b, *Eur. J. Immunol.* **3**:279.

Webb, C., Teitelbaum, D., Abramsky, O., Arnon, R., and Sela, M., 1974, *Lancet* **II**:66.

Webb, C., Teitelbaum, D., Rauch, H., Maoz, A., Arnon, R., and Fuchs, S., 1975, *J. Immunol.* **114**:1469.

Webb, C., Teitelbaum, D., Herz, A., Arnon, R., and Sela, M., 1976, *Immunochemistry* **13**:333.

Weinbaum, F. I., Butchko, G. M., Lerman, S., Thorbecke, G. J., and Nisonoff, A., 1974, *J. Immunol.* **113**:257.

Weisbart, R. H., Bluestone, R., Goldberg, L. S., and Pearson, C. M., 1974, *Proc. Natl. Acad. Sci. U.S.A.* **71**:875.

Westall, F. C., 1972, Solid phase peptide synthesis as applied to experimental allergic encephalomyelitis, in: *Multiple Sclerosis: Progress in Research* (E. J. Field, T. M. Bell, and P. R. Carnegie, eds.), (Clinical Studies, Vol. 3), pp. 72–79, North-Holland, Amsterdam.

Westall, F. C., 1973, *J. Theor. Biol.* **38**:139.

Westall, F. C., 1974, *Immunochemistry* **11**:513.

Westall, F. C., and Thompson, M., 1975, *Immunol. Commun.* **4**:187.

Westall, F. C., Robinson, A. B., Caccam, J., Jackson, J., and Eylar, E. H., 1971, *Nature (London)* **229**:22.

Westall, F. C., Thompson, M., and Kalter, S. S., 1975, *Life Sci.* **17**:219.

Whitaker, J. N., 1975, *J. Immunol.* **114**:823.

Whitaker, J. N., Chou, C.-H. J., Chou, F. C.-H., and Kibler, R. F., 1975, *J. Biol. Chem.* **250**:9106.

Whittingham, S., Bencina, B., Carnegie, P. R., and McPherson, T. A., 1972, *Int. Arch. Allergy* **42**:250.

Williams, R. M., and Moore, M. J., 1973, *J. Exp. Med.* **138**:775.

Wisniewski, H. M., and Bloom, B. R., 1975, *J. Exp. Med.* **141**:346.

Wolfgram, F., 1965, *Ann. N.Y. Acad. Sci.* **122**:104.

Wolfgram, F., Ellison, G. W., Stevens, J. G., and Andrews, J. M. (eds.), 1972, in: *Multiple Sclerosis—Immunity, Virology, and Ultrastructure*, pp. 1–597, Academic Press, New York.

Wolman, M., 1971, *Exp. Neurol.* **30**:309.

Wood, D. D., Vail, W. J., and Moscarello, M. A., 1975, *Brain Res.* **93**:463.

Wood, J. G., and King, N., 1971, *Nature (London)* **229**:56.

Yo, S.-L., and MacPherson, C. F. C., 1972, *J. Immunol.* **109**:1009.

Young, J. D., Tsuchiya, D., Geier, M., Geier, S., Westall, F. C., Thompson, M., Cyr, R., Ward, E., and Yurochko, F., 1974, *Immunol. Commun.* **3**:219.

Yung, L. L. L., Diener, E., McPherson, T. A., Barton, M. A., and Hyde, H. A., 1973, *J. Immunol.* **110**:1383.

6

Immunochemistry of Collagen

Dov Michaeli

I. Chemical and Structural Considerations of Collagen

Vertebrate collagen (Fig. 1B) is made up of three polypetide chains (designated α-chains), each of about 1000 amino acid residues and having a molecular weight of about 95,000. Each chain is coiled in a left-handed helix, and the three chains are coiled in a right-handed superhelix. The triple-stranded, coiled-coil structure is rod shaped, having the dimensions of 3000 × 15 Å. Chemical studies established that the three component polypeptide chains extend in parallel the full length of the molecule.

Determination of amino acid composition of the α-chains showed that glycine makes up about 33 % of the total number of residues. Sequence studies of α-chains have revealed a repeating pattern of the triplet Gly–X–Y through most of the chain. The glycine residues, which have no side chains, are positioned inside the triple helix. The following two residues, X and Y, could be almost any amino acid residue, and the bulky ring structures (in the case of proline and hydroxyproline) and side chains are all on the outside. The triple helix structure is maintained by hydrogen bonds, and probably by the high proportion of imino acids, whose rigid structure restricts rotation of the chains.

Determination of the amino acid sequence was greatly facilitated by cleavage of the α-chains with CNBr into smaller peptides, and by ascertaining their respective location in the chain from which they originated

Dov Michaeli · Departments of Biochemistry and Biophysics and Surgery, University of California School of Medicine, San Francisco, California 94143.

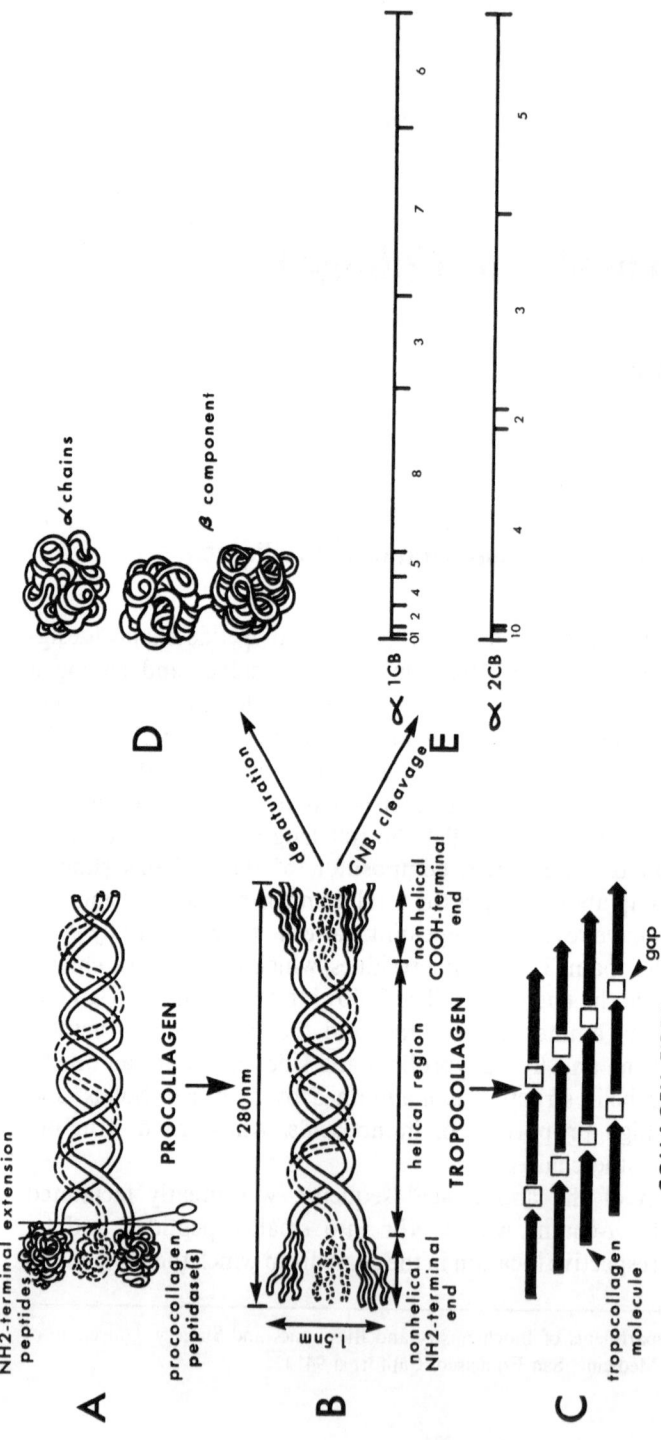

Figure 1. Schematic diagram of collagen biosynthesis and structure. (A) Procollagen is the biosynthetic precursor of collagen. It is made up of three polypeptide chains having a rodlike conformation, with globular extensions at their NH$_2$-terminal ends. Specific procollagen peptidases cleave off the NH$_2$-terminal extension sequences. (B) Tropocollagen is made up of three polypeptide chains coiled about each other in a left-handed helix, and the three chains are coiled in a right-handed superhelix. The NH$_2$- and the COOH-terminal ends of the molecule are nonhelical. (C) The collagen fibril is organized by tropocollagen molecules arranged in a quarter stagger. A gap exists between the COOH-terminal end of one molecule and the amino-terminal end of the following molecule. (D) Following denaturation of the molecule, the α-chains separate, lose their helical structure, and assume a random conformation. (E) CNBr cleavage of the molecule results in the formation of eight α$_1$-peptides and five α$_2$-peptides. The location of these peptides in their respective chains has been determined.

(Fig. 1E). (The nomenclature of the peptides, however, does not reflect their position in the chain, but rather the order of their elution off an ion exchange column.) From the amino acid sequence studies it became evident that the α-chain contains a central helical region, 1011 residues long, and short (nine to 25 residues) nonhelical regions at both ends of the α-chain. The helical region contains a glycine in every third position, as mentioned above, whereas the nonhelical sequences at the NH_2- and COOH-terminal ends of the chain do not contain the repetitive glycine structure.

The native molecule can be denatured by heating a short time at mildly elevated temperatures (45°C, 10 min) (Fig. 1D). The α-chains separate, lose their helical structure, and assume an extended conformation. This process is reversible, and renaturation of the molecule can be effected by incubation at a lowered temperature (25°C).

Separation of the chains, following denaturation of collagen, on CM-cellulose columns, reveals that a certain proportion of the α-chain formed crosslinks, resulting in dimers (β-components) and trimers (γ-components) of α-chains. The formation of crosslinks is part of the normal process of collagen maturation, and both intramolecular and intermolecular crosslinks can form. As a result of this process, the fibrils become insoluble and acquire increased mechanical strength. It was shown that in rat skin collagen each chain contains a lysine residue in position 5. These lysine residues undergo oxidative deamination, catalyzed by lysyl oxidase, to form the δ-semialdehyde of α-aminoadipic acid. The bond between the two aldehydes then forms by an aldol-type condensation, followed by dehydrogenation.

It has been recently demonstrated that different types of collagen can be obtained from different tissues and by using different extraction procedures. Thus collagen obtained from skin, tendon, and bone comprises two identical $α_1$-chains, and a third chain which is homologous but not identical to $α_1$, called $α_2$. This collagen is called type I, and its molecular formula is $[α_1(I)]_2α_2$. So far, three other types of collagen have been discovered, each of which is made up of three identical chains. Thus the molecular formula of collagen type II is $[α_1(II)]_3$, that of collagen type III is $[α_1(III)]_3$, and that of collagen type IV is $[α_1(IV)]_3$. Table I summarizes the information on the sources of the various types of collagen, and some of their distinctive features.

The biosynthetic precursor of collagen is procollagen, made up of three pro-α-chains with additional NH_2-terminal extensions (Fig. 1A). The extension sequences differ in their amino acid sequence from collagen, and they have a globular conformation, rather than the rodlike conformation of collagen. These peptides are linked together by an interchain disulfide bond and they probably serve a function in chain aggregation

Table I. Types of Collagen [a]

Type	Source	Chain composition	Distinctive features
I	Skin, bone, tendon	$[\alpha_1(I)]_2\alpha_2$	α_2, < 10 Hyl/chain, low carbohydrate
II	Cartilage	$[\alpha_1(II)]_3$	> 10 Hyl/chain, 10% carbohydrate
III	Fetal skin, blood vessels	$[\alpha_1(III)]_3$	Cys, high Hyp and Gly, low carbohydrate
IV	Basement membrane	$[\alpha_1(IV)]_3$	High 3-Hyp, > 20 Hyl/chain, low Ala

[a] Based on Martin et al. (1975). With the publisher's permission.

and generation of a triple helix. Finally, specific procollagen peptidases cleave off the NH_2-terminal extension sequences, resulting in the conversion of procollagen to collagen.

For a more extensive treatment of structural and functional aspects of collagen, the reader is referred to a number of recent reviews (Kühn, 1969; Traub and Piez, 1971; Gallop et al., 1972; Fietzek and Kühn, 1975). A review dealing with the biosynthesis of collagen has recently been published (Bornstein, 1974).

Also, several reviews of various aspects of the immunology of collagen have been published (O'Dell, 1968; Kirrane and Glynn, 1968; Timpl et al., 1973a; Furthmayr and Timpl, 1975).

II. Immunochemistry of Collagen

A. Rat Collagen

One of the earliest reports of an attempt to locate the antigenic determinants of rat skin collagen was published in 1967 by Davison et al. Although techniques for detailed study of collagen molecular structure were only beginning to appear at the time, these investigators described the broad outline of the distribution of antigenic determinants in human, calf, carp, and rat tropocollagens (type I). Using a microcomplement fixation technique, they established the species specificity of collagen from various sources. The antigenic activity resided in both the α_1- and α_2-chains and depended on maintenance of the triple-helical native conformation. Moreover, pepsin-treated rat collagen resulted in loss of some complement-fixing activity, and pronase treatment abolished almost completely the antigenicity of this collagen. Thus the authors concluded that the major antigenic determinants were probably located in the "telopeptides," namely, the nonhelical amino- and carboxyl-terminal peptides.

Michaeli et al. (1970) have reported that, as in guinea pig skin collagen, the major antigenic determinant of rat skin collagen resided in the α_2-chain. However, no attempt was made to further define the location of the antigenic activity in this chain.

Using CNBr cleavage to obtain smaller fragments derived from rat collagen, Lindsley et al. (1971) determined by radioimmunoassay the antigenic activity of these peptides. They found that α_1- and α_2-chains were immunologically distinct and failed to show any significant cross-reactivity. The major antigenic determinant of the α_1-chain was located in α_1 CB6, which is at the carboxy-terminal end of the chain. The α_2-chain had two non-cross-reacting determinants: α_2 CB1 at the amino-terminal end and α_2 CB5 at the carboxy-terminal end of the chain. These findings were confirmed by Timpl et al. (1971) and by Furthmayr et al. (1972). Moreover, these investigators have shown (Timpl et al., 1972) that antibodies in early antisera were directed primarily against α_1 CB6 and α_2 CB5, namely, the carboxy-terminal regions of α_1 and α_2, respectively. With continued immunization, antibodies directed to the amino-terminal end of α_2 appeared; this was accompanied by reduction in the titer of antibodies against the carboxy-terminal end of the molecule. Using eight rabbit antisera, Furthmayr and Timpl (1972) defined three overlapping antigenic determinants in the amino-terminal end of α_2 (Fig. 2). These determinants had several common features. Their minimal size was four to six residues, all three determinants included [5]Lys–Gly and two included a tyrosyl residue in position 2. Oxidation of the ε-amino group of [5]Lys to an aldehyde resulted in a marked reduction in antigenic activity. The most common determinant (six out of eight rabbits) had the sequence

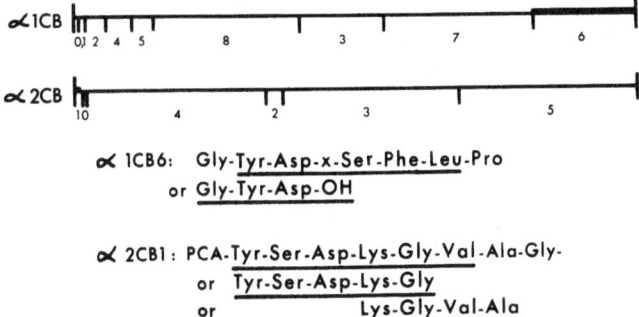

Figure 2. Major antigenic determinants of rat collagen type I. The bold bars indicate the CNBr peptides that contain the major antigenic determinants. The peptide sequences which constitute the antigenic determinants are underlined. Based on data from Timpl et al. (1973a), Stoltz et al. (1973), and Furthmayr and Timpl (1972).

of [2]Tyr–Ser–Asp–Lys–Gly–Val; antibodies from one rabbit recognized the same sequences minus Val, and antibodies from another recognized the sequence [5]Lys–Gly–Val–Ser.

Additional evidence that the lysyl residue in position 5 (CB1) is part of the rat collagen antigenic determinant was provided by Bailey and his co-workers (Chidlow et al., 1974). They prepared immunoadsorbent columns from sheep and rat tropocollagen which were then used to absorb labeled peptides from CNBr digests of rat tail tendons reduced with tritiated borohydrides. Such treatment resulted in the reduction of the crosslinks between the collagen chains and incorporation of a tritium label into the reduced products. They found four antigenic peptides, all containing reducible crosslinks. One of the peptides was most likely the amino-terminal end (CB1) of α_1 and/or α_2. Another peptide had an amino acid composition consistent with that of α_1 CB6.

A major problem in the immunochemical analysis of proteins is the question of structural alteration from the native state of the antigen. This problem was highlighted by the Munich group. They observed that the α_1-chain of neutral salt-extracted rat skin collagen was shortened during the extraction procedure at the COOH-terminus by tissue proteases (Stoltz et al., 1972). Based on this observation, they reexamined the antigenicity of α_1 CB6 obtained both from collagen extracted under denaturing conditions and from a neutral salt extract (Stoltz et al., 1973). The former procedure presumably yields the intact peptide, whereas the latter procedure yields a peptide shortened by 20 amino acid residues from the COOH-terminal nonhelical end (designated α_1 CB6[b]). Their results indicated that α_1 CB6 was essentially devoid of antigenic activity, whereas α_1 CB6[b] was strongly antigenic, with the penultimate tyrosyl and the COOH-terminal aspartic acid constituting part of the antigenic determinant (Fig. 2). This observation then suggests that the antigenic determinant at the COOH-terminus of rat collagen may be an artifact and that the major determinant of this protein resides at the NH_2-terminal end.

Timpl et al. (1971) have demonstrated that about 20% of rabbit antibodies to rat collagen cross-reacted with denatured rabbit collagen. These antibodies were specific for a variety of CNBr peptides derived from the helical regions of the α_1- or α_2-chains of rat collagen. The determinants were conformation independent, since their binding with antibodies was not significantly altered by denaturation of the molecule. Since these determinants are antigenically active in the denatured state and they show structural similarity to denatured helical regions of rabbit collagen (as shown by antigenic cross-reactivity), they may be inaccessible in the native molecule, and may become exposed following denaturation during the extraction procedure and/or during the metabolic turnover process of this protein.

B. Calf Collagen

Schmitt *et al.* (1964) and Davison *et al.* (1967) have demonstrated by a complement fixation assay that the antigenic determinants of calf skin collagen reside in the "telopeptides," namely, in the nonhelical portion of the molecule. The antigenic determinants were present in the α_1- and in the α_2-chains. The complement-fixing activity was lost upon heat denaturation of tropocollagen and was recovered following renaturation by cooling. No specificity with respect to tissue of origin or with respect to individual animals of the same or different strains could be demonstrated in these experiments.

A more definitive determination of the location of antigenic determinants was accomplished by the Max-Planck group (Pontz *et al.*, 1970; Rauterberg *et al.*, 1972; Becker *et al.*, 1972). Using peptides obtained from CNBr cleavage of collagen, it was found that the major determinants are located at the NH_2-terminal end of the α_1-chain (Rauterberg *et al.*, 1972) and at the COOH-terminal end of the α_1-chain (Pontz *et al.*, 1970). The latter determinant was later defined more precisely and was assigned to a hexapeptide in the nonhelical region of α_1-CB6 (Becker *et al.*, 1972), (Fig. 3). However, it has been reported that neutral salt or acid extraction of calf skin collagen results in the loss of 19 amino acid residues from the nonhelical end of α_1 CB6 which originally is made up of 25 residues (Stark *et al.*, 1971). It was postulated that tissue proteases are responsible for this phenomenon when collagen is extracted under nondenaturing conditions. A number of antisera raised against such collagen indeed recognized an antigenic determinant on the truncated COOH-terminal peptide, designated α_1 CB6[b] (Becker *et al.*, 1972). The new artifactual determinant comprises Tyr–Asp–Leu–OH which is part of the original determinant Tyr–Asp–Leu–Ser–Phe–Leu (Fig. 3).

As in the case of rat collagen (Chidlow *et al.*, 1974), the occurence

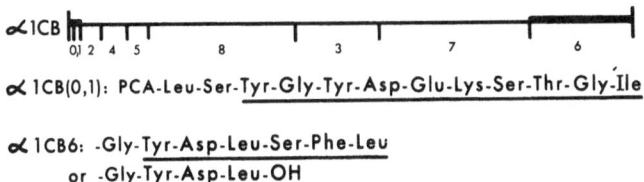

α 1CB(0,1): PCA-Leu-Ser-Tyr-Gly-Tyr-Asp-Glu-Lys-Ser-Thr-Gly-Ile

α 1CB6: -Gly-Tyr-Asp-Leu-Ser-Phe-Leu
or -Gly-Tyr-Asp-Leu-OH

Figure 3. Major antigenic determinants of calf collagen type I. The bold bars indicate the CNBr peptides that contain the major antigenic determinants. The peptide sequences which constitute the antigenic determinants are underlined. Based on data from Rauterberg *et al.* (1972) and Becker *et al.* (1972).

of the major antigenic determinants at the nonhelical ends of the α-chains of calf skin collagen makes the immunochemical analysis of insoluble collagen a potentially powerful tool for elucidating the peptides that participate in crosslinking. Becker *et al.* (1975) used gel filtration chromatography to separate peptides obtained by tryptic digestion of denatured insoluble calf skin collagen. The peptides were analyzed for their amino acid composition, their molecular weight, and their immunochemical characteristics. Five peptides with a high tyrosine content (indicating that they contained nonhelical sequences) and comprising between 87 and 142 amino acid residues were purified. Four of these peptides contained antigenic determinants of the NH_2-terminal or COOH-terminal nonhelical regions. On the basis of terminal amino acid determinations, it was concluded that these peptides are composed of two or three crosslinked chains. The fact that different peptides contained the same antigenic marker indicated crosslinking with different peptides on the adjacent chain, which is consistent with the quarter-stagger arrangement of the collagen fibril. An additional crosslink, between the helical regions of α_1 CB6 and α_1 CB5, was identified. This site for crosslinking, like the ones involving nonhelical regions, is compatible with the quarter-stagger packing of collagen molecules in a fibril. One can conclude from these studies that the ε-amino group of a lysyl residue (e.g., in position 5) probably does not play a major role in the binding with antibody. In this connection, the studies of Timpl *et al.* (1970) should be mentioned. They showed that modification of acid-soluble calf collagen by succinylation, methylation, or deamination little changed its serological activities. These experiments lend support to the conclusion drawn from the studies of Becker *et al.* (1975) with respect to the role of the ε-amino group of lysine.

About 20% of the antibodies in rabbit antisera to native calf collagen is directed to conformation-independent determinants in the helical region of the molecule (Timpl *et al.*, 1971). Most of the CNBr peptides, when coated on tanned red blood cells, could be agglutinated by antibodies against collagen. Furthermore, hemagglutination-inhibition studies with these peptides indicate widespread distribution of these determinants in the helical region (the authors estimated a minimum number of nine), in both α_1- and α_2-chains. Although the location in the helical region and the cross-reactivity with rabbit collagen could indicate a Gly–Pro–X structure for these determinants, evidence was presented that this is probably not the case. For instance, the NH_2-terminal half of α_1 CB6 contains the typical Gly–Pro–X triplets in long apolar sequences (von der Mark *et al.*, 1970), yet it was devoid of antigenic activity. Also, the synthetic polypeptides $(Gly–Pro–Pro)_n$, $(Gly–Pro–Ala)_n$, and $(Gly–Pro–Gly)_n$ failed to inhibit antibodies with affinities to rabbit collagen.

C. Human Collagen

The immunochemical study of human collagen has been carried out in several laboratories. Furthmayr *et al.* (1971) immunized rabbits with collagen from human dura mater and measured their specificity by passive hemagglutination, coating tanned red cells with either denatured collagen, α-chains, or isolated CB-peptides. By immunoadsorption techniques, they separated the antisera into two fractions: a minor one with cross-reactivity with rabbit collagen, and another containing most of the antibodies and showing no cross-reactivity with rabbit collagen. The latter antibody fraction had its major antigenic activity in the α_1-chain, whereas the α_2-chain contained only minor activity. In the antibodies with affinity for rabbit collagen, the antigenic specificity was directed to both α-chains, although the α_1-chain exhibited stronger activity than α_2. The major determinant of the α_1-chain was shown to reside in the COOH-terminal peptide, α_1 CB6, and probably at the COOH-terminal end of this peptide, since activity was abolished by pronase digestion. The antibodies with affinity for rabbit collagen also reacted with α_1 CB6, but, in addition, could react with α_1 CB3, α_1 CB7, and α_1 CB8, all originating from the helical portion of the molecule (Fig. 4). Confirmation that the major antigenic activity of human collagen resides in the α_1-chain was provided by the Ouchterlony double-diffusion technique (Lindsley *et al.*, 1969).

Michaeli and Epstein (1971) investigated the same problem but obtained different results. According to these authors, the major activity resided in the α_2-chain and the determinants were located within the helical portion of the molecule (α_2 CB3, α_2 CB4, α_2 CB5), as well as the NH_2-terminal end of the chain (α_2 CB1 and α_2 CB0,1[a]). The antigenic activity of α_1 was much weaker and was confined to its NH_2-terminal end (α_1 CB0,1 and α_1 CB0,1[A]) (Fig. 4). This discrepancy in results between two laboratories in spite of similar immunization procedures and assay techniques is puzzling. As has been discussed above, the NH_2-terminal end of the molecule was found to be antigenically important in rat, calf,

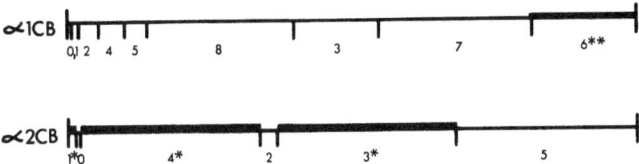

Figure 4. Major antigenic determinants of human collagen type I. The bold bars indicate the CNBr peptides that contain the major antigenic determinants. Symbols: *, based on data from Furthmayr *et al.* (1971); **, based on data from Michaeli and Epstein (1971).

and guinea pig collagens. Timpl's *et al.* (1972) observation that the antigenicity of rat skin collagen shifts from the COOH-terminal end to the NH$_2$-terminal end with continued immunization might account for this discrepancy.

D. Guinea Pig Skin Collagen

The immunochemistry of guinea pig skin collagen was investigated by Michaeli and his co-workers (Michaeli *et al.*, 1968, 1969, 1971; Timpl *et al.*, 1971). In a study of the precipitin reaction, it was shown (Michaeli *et al.*, 1968) that the amount of immune precipitate was inversely related to the ionic strength of the buffer and to the temperature in which the reaction took place. Rather than reflecting on the antigen–antibody interaction, these observations probably reflect the increased fibril formation that occurs under these conditions.

An interesting observation was the complete inhibition of the precipitation of collagen by preincubation of the antiserum with denatured collagen. This was interpreted at the time, probably erroneously, as "suggesting that the quaternary and tertiary structures of collagen played little or no role in the recognition and binding with the anti-collagen sera used." An alternative interpretation could be that most, or all, of the *precipitating* antibodies were directed against conformation-independent determinants in the helical portion of the molecule. Indeed, further work on this subject provided evidence to support such an interpretation. For instance, it was shown (Michaeli *et al.*, 1969) that both collagen chains and β-components precipitated with anticollagen antisera, although α_2 and β_{12} were more active than α_1 and β_{11}. Yet by the hemagglutination inhibition assay only the α_2- and β_{12}-chains showed activity when tested against native collagen. However, when the red blood cells were coated with denatured collagen, both α-chains and the β-components exhibited inhibitory activity.

When antigenic activity of the individual CNBr peptides was tested by the hemagglutination technique, only α_2 CB1 could inhibit the agglutination collagen-coated red blood cells (Michaeli *et al.*, 1971).

It can therefore be concluded that, as in the cases of rat, calf, and human collagens, the major determinants are in the nonhelical portion of the molecule, whereas weaker determinants are present in the helical region (Fig. 5). The latter determinants were shown in the case of guinea pig collagen to contribute significantly to the precipitin reaction with anticollagen antisera.

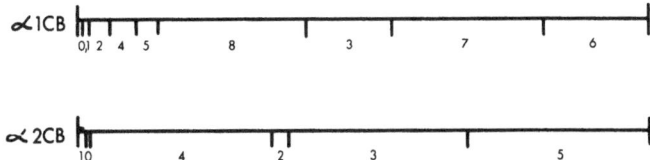

Figure 5. Major antigenic determinants of guinea pig collagen type I. The bold bar indicates the CNBr peptide that contains the major antigenic determinant(s). Based on data from Michaeli *et al.* (1969).

E. Fish Collagen

Rabbit antibodies against carp swim bladder collagen were fractionated into two fractions, one with and one without affinity for a rabbit collagen immunoadsorbent. The major fraction showed no cross-reactivity with rabbit collagen, reacted strongly with the homologous collagen, and showed decreased cross-reactivity with collagens of increasing phylogenetic distance. The fraction with affinity for rabbit collagen showed strong cross-reactivity with other fish species, as well as with collagen obtained from invertebrates. The antigenic determinants of this collagen were shown to be present in both α_1- and α_2-chains, but further localization, using CNBr peptides, has not been attempted (Meigel *et al.*, 1971).

F. Invertebrate Collagens

Meigel *et al.* (1971) immunized rabbits with liver fluke collagen and with sea anemone collagen. Both types of antisera were fractionated on a rabbit collagen immunoadsorbent column and the fractions were assayed with homologous and heterologous collagens. The same pattern as with other collagens emerged. There was high species specificity in the major fraction, which lacked affinity for rabbit collagen, and extensive cross-reactivity with collagens of other species in the minor fraction, which possessed affinity for rabbit collagen.

A more detailed immunochemical study of sea anemone collagen has been reported (Nowack *et al.*, 1974). This collagen is composed of three identical α-chains (Nordwig *et al.*, 1973) rather than the $\alpha_1(I)\alpha_2$ structure of vertebrate collagen type I. Rabbit antibodies against sea anemone collagen reacted with random-coiled α-chains. Removal of the terminal, nonhelical, portion of the molecule by proteolytic digestion did not affect its antigenic activity. Hence, unlike mammalian collagens that have been studied in detail, the major antigenic activity seemed to reside in sites other than the NH_2- or COOH-terminal portions. Indeed, a peptide obtained from the helical region of the molecule (CB6, not to be confused with α_1 CB6 of type I collagen, which is located at the COOH-terminal end) possessed strong antigenic activity. This peptide was the only one to contain tyrosine residues in its structure, a fact which might be important in determining its antigenic character.

Ascaris cuticle collagen probably has a peculiar tertiary and quaternary structure, which in turn may be responsible for its unusual immunochemical characteristics. McBride and Harrington (1967) suggested that in native *Ascaris* collagen each subunit is a single polypeptide chain of molecular weight 62,000 back-folded to form a three-stranded, hydrogen-bonded superhelix. Chromatography on CM-Sephadex suggested the presence of two nonidentical polypeptide subunits. The collagen subunits are held together through disulfide bridges to form a polymer of 900,000 molecular weight.

Fuchs and Harrington (1970) immunized rabbits with *Ascaris* cuticle collagen and showed that the antibodies reacted with the RCM subunits but did not cross-react with native or denatured earthworm cuticle collagen, calf skin collagen, or rat skin collagen. On the other hand, anti-RCM *Ascaris* collagen did not cross-react with *Ascaris* collagen (Maoz *et al.*, 1971) and also failed to react with rat tail tendon collagen. It is possible that reduction and carboxymethylation of the disulfide bridges resulted in the expression of some new determinants in the RCM molecule which were immunologically inactive in the native collagen. Both antisera, however, reacted equally well with both subunits comprising the RCM *Ascaris* collagen.

Of a variety of collagens tested, only RCM *Ascaris* cuticle collagen precipitated with anti (Pro–Gly–Pro–)$_n$ antibodies and, conversely, anti-RCM collagen precipitated (Pro–Gly–Pro)$_n$-conjugated proteins. *Ascaris* collagen could also inhibit the inactivation of (Pro–Gly–Pro)$_n$-coated T4 bacteriophage by anti (Pro–Gly–Pro)$_n$-ovalbumin serum. In addition, out of a variety of anticollagen sera, only anti-*Ascaris* collagen could inactivate the modified bacteriophage (Fuchs *et al.*, 1974).

These interesting observations may indicate that *Ascaris* collagen contains sequences of ordered (Pro–Gly–Pro)$_n$ in its primary structure, whereas other collagens do not. Alternatively, (Pro–Gly–Pro)$_n$ or a similar structure may be common to all collagens, but it becomes immunologically potent in *Ascaris* collagen due to the unique folding of its polypeptide chains.

Michaeli *et al.* (1972) showed that native and RCM *Ascaris* collagen exhibited complete cellular and humoral cross-reactivity. Their data indicated that reduction and alkylation of native *Ascaris* collagen did not alter the antigenic determinants of this protein.

G. Collagens of Types II, III, and IV

The recent discovery of collagen type II (Miller, 1971) and the even more recent discovery of collagen type III (Chung et al., 1974; Epstein, 1974) and satisfactory purification of type IV (Kefalides, 1974; Daniels and Chu, 1975) have not permitted sufficient time for the detailed elucidation of structure that collagen type I has undergone. Nevertheless, some progress in understanding the immunochemistry of collagen type II has been made. It was shown (Hahn et al., 1975) that collagen type II is immunogenic in rabbits, and that the antibodies are type specific. Only weak cross-reaction with collagen type I of the same or other species was exhibited. On the other hand, antisera to chick collagen type II cross-reacted strongly with bovine collagen type II, and vice versa.

A major determinant of α_1(II) resides in the CB11 peptide. This peptide is derived from the helical portion of the molecule, and is homologous to α_1(I) CB8 (Miller et al., 1973). It is noteworthy that α_1(I) CB8 possessed no significant antigenic activity when rat collagen type I was used as an immunogen.

The complete immunochemical analysis of collagen type II is still pending. In particular, it would be of great interest to establish the role of the nonhelical regions of the molecule in determination of its immunogenicity.

The information on collagen type III is even scantier than that available for type II. Gay et al. (1975) have demonstrated, by immunofluorescence, the immunogenicity of collagen type III. Their data also suggest that, like anti-$[\alpha_1(\text{II})]_3$, antibodies to $[\alpha_1(\text{III})]_3$ display type specificity; i.e., they do not cross-react with other collagen types to any significant degree. Work on the immunochemical analysis of this molecule has not yet been published.

Virtually no immunochemical information on collagen type IV is currently available. Kefalides (1970) showed that one of the antigenic components of glomerular basement membrane and of anterior lens capsule contained hydroxyproline and hydroxylysine. However, detailed immunochemical analysis of collagen type IV is still lacking, although the recent report by Daniels and Chu (1975) on the purification of collagen type IV from glomerular basement membrane promises to provide a good basis for such studies.

It should be noted that collagen type IV was defined primarily on the basis of studies on collagen derived from glomerular basement membrane. This basement membrane is made up of components of both epithelial and endothelial origin. There is no certainty that these cell types make identical basement membrane collagen. Analysis of collagen from epithelial basement membrane (Bowman's capsule, kidney tubules, respiratory, intestinal and glandular epithelium, etc.) and from endothelial basement membrane should be carried out. An additional approach would be the isolation of collagen synthesized by pure epithelial and endothelial cells in culture, respectively. In any event, immunochemical characterization of the isolated collagens should prove of great help in resolving this problem, especially in view of the emerging evidence that type-specific antibodies can be produced.

H. Modified Collagens and Collagenlike Synthetic Peptides

In a series of classical papers, Sela and Arnon used modified gelatins (i.e., heat-denatured collagen) to study the chemical basis of the antigenicity of proteins (Sela and Arnon, 1960a,b; Arnon and Sela, 1960). Enrichment of gelatin with tyrosine to the extent of 2.4% enhanced the immunogenicity of the protein, whereas greater enrichment (11%) resulted in production of antisera with antityrosine specificity but with poor reactivity with gelatin (Arnon and Sela, 1960). Enhancement of antigenicity of gelatin could also be effected by enrichment with other aromatic amino acids (phenylalanine, tryptophan). Attachment of cysteine residues to gelatin contributed to an increase in antigenicity, although to a much lower extent than the aromatic amino acids. The authors raise the possibility that this could be due to the formation of disulfide bonds, which increase the rigidity of the protein (Sela and Arnon, 1960a). To test the hypothesis that aromatic amino acids (and to a lesser extent disulfide bonds) increased the antigenicity of gelatin by introducing rigidity into the molecule, Sela and Arnon (1960b) tested the effect of coupling poly-L-cyclohexylalanine to gelatin. As predicted by their hypothesis, this molecule converted gelatin to a powerful antigen. On the other hand, the nonaromatic amino acid serine failed to confer enhanced antigenicity on the gelatin. Also, the following polymers and copolymers were tested for their capacity to inhibit the precipitin reaction of gelatin with antibodies: poly-L-proline, poly-L-hydroxyproline, random copolymers of L-proline and glycine, L-proline and sarcosine, L-hydroxyproline and glycine, L-proline glutamine acid and glycine, and a low molecular weight polymer of Pro–Gly–Gly. None of these synthetic peptides exhibited any inhibitory effect.

Jasin and Glynn (1965a) studied the antigenic properties of synthetic polyimino acids. These polymers, which were weak immunogens, were assayed by active cutaneous anaphylaxis, passive cutaneous anaphylaxis, delayed skin hypersensitivity, and hemagglutination. By these methods, the antigenicity of poly-L-proline was demonstrated in guinea pigs. This homopolymer is of special immunochemical interest since it exists in two forms: form I having a right-handed helix and form II having a left-handed helix. Both forms were antigenic but non-cross-reactive. The antisera against both forms also failed to cross-react with collagen, as well as with a random copolymer of proline and glycine. Examination of the antigenic relationships between synthetic polymers containing hydroxyproline and acetylhydroxyproline collagen and acetylated collagen revealed cross-reactivity between the acetylated synthetic polymer and acetylated collagen. However, no cross-reactivity could be demonstrated between either poly-hydroxyproline or poly-acetylhydroxyproline and native collagen (Jasin and Glynn, 1965b). Thus these studies further extend and confirm Sela and Arnon's observation (1960b) that antigelatin failed to react with poly-L-proline, poly-L-hydroxyproline, and random copolymers of proline or hydroxyproline and glycine, sarcosine, or glutamic acid.

Following the failure of antisera to homopolymers and to random copolymers that include proline and hydroxyproline to react with native or denatured collagen, and *vice versa*, the next logical step was to test ordered copolymers whose structure more closely resembles collagen. Engl *et al.* (1966) synthesized the ordered copolymer (L–Pro–Gly–L–Pro)$_n$ which probably exists in solution as a triple-stranded helix of the collagen type. Traub and Yonath (1966) studied this peptide by X-ray diffraction and showed that it gives a pattern which has all the main features of the collagen pattern. Borek *et al.* (1969) reported that this peptide was immunogenic (albeit poorly) in guinea pigs and rabbits and was weakly cross-reactive with fish, rat, and guinea pig collagens. In order to increase the antibody response, rabbits were immunized with (Pro–Gly–Pro)$_n$ conjugated to ovalbumin (Maoz *et al.*, 1973a,b). The antiserum precipitated the ordered polymer conjugated to an unrelated carrier (RNase), and was inhibited by the unconjugated ordered copolymer. However, the monomeric tripeptide Pro–Gly–Pro failed to inhibit the precipitin reaction, and the tripeptide conjugated to ovalbumin failed to react with antibodies against the polymer. On the other hand, the reaction of anti Pro–Gly–Pro–ovalbumin with Pro–Gly–Pro–RNase could be inhibited by (Pro–Gly–Pro)$_n$–RNase T4 by anti (Gly–Pro–Gly)$_n$ serum. It was observed that the ordered copolymers were more efficient inhibitors than random copolymers of similar molecular weights, by about 2 orders of magnitude. Inhibition was strongly dependent on the size of the polymer at the lower range of molecular weights (up to molecular weight of approximately 1000–2000) and became largely independent of size at molecular weights over 2000. These observations may indicate dependence of inhibitory capacity on the conformation of the polymer. Random copolymers and ordered copolymers of low molecular weight probably do not assume the collagenlike conformation that may be required for binding with anti (Pro–Gly–Pro)$_n$ at significant levels of binding energy.

Anti $(Pro-Gly-Pro)_n$ (molecular weights 6300 and 6800) gave both delayed and immediate skin reactions when tested in guinea pigs with $(Pro-Gly-Pro)_n$, $(Pro-66, Gly-34)_n$, guinea pig skin collagen, RCM *Ascaris* collagen, and rat tail tendon collagen (Fuchs *et al.*, 1974*a*). In the rabbit, however, only RCM *Ascaris* collagen cross-reacted with anti $(Pro-Gly-Pro)_n$, and, conversely, out of several anticollagen sera, only anti RCM *Ascaris* collagen reacted with anti $(Pro-Gly-Pro)_n$, as tested by the bacteriophage inactivation technique (Haimovich and Sela, 1966). The possible interpretations of this phenomenon were discussed above.

A different approach to the study of collagen antigenicity through synthetic peptides was taken by Kettman *et al.* (1967). Rationalizing that antibodies to collagen may recognize a determinant composed of a certain combination of glycine (33% of the collagen residues) and an imino acid (about 20% of the collagen residues), the following octapeptide was synthesized: Gly-Pro-Gly-Pro-Pro-Gly-Ala-Lys. This peptide exhibited specific precipitin reactions with rabbit anti-guinea pig collagen serum, which could be inhibited by an immunologically active tryptic digest of guinea pig collagen. Rabbit antiserum against the octapeptide was raised by immunization with the peptide conjugated to succinyl-BSA (Benjamini *et al.*, 1973). This antiserum was tested against the octapeptide and against the following derivatives:

Gly-Pro-Gly-Pro-Pro-Gly-Ala-Lys
Pro-Gly-Pro-Pro-Gly-Ala-Lys
Gly-Pro-Pro-Gly-Ala-Lys
Pro-Pro-Gly-Ala-Lys
Pro-Gly-Ala-Lys

It was shown that the antigenic specificity of the octapeptide resided in the COOH-terminal pentapeptide having the amino acid sequence Pro-Pro-Gly-Ala-Lys. The ordered polymer $(Pro-Gly-Pro)_n$ of molecular weight 1910 could also inhibit the precipitin reaction. Hence, it was concluded that the antigenic specificity of the octapeptide was probably dependent on the sequence Pro-Pro-Gly.

I. General Considerations

1. Antigenic Determinants in the NH_2- and COOH-Terminal Regions

The above discussion of the immunochemistry of collagens of different mammalian species has brought out a common feature: rabbit antibodies against these collagens are directed primarily against the NH_2-terminal and COOH-terminal, nonhelical sequences of the molecule. Several conclusions can be drawn from this observation:

1. The nonhelical, terminal portions may have undergone mutational changes at such a rate that the interspecific divergence became pronounced enough to create new antigenic determinants at these portions. Alternatively, the nonhelical sequences of rabbit collagen may have undergone a mutational change that rendered the homologous sequences in other mammalian collagens immunogenic in this species.

2. The relatively low immunogenicity of helical sequences when rabbits were immunized with collagens of other mammalian species could be explained in terms of an extreme degree of evolutionary conversation of the helical portion of collagen on the one hand and antigenic competition of the strong determinants in the nonhelical sequences on the other hand.

Examination of the primary structures of the NH_2-terminal end, nonhelical sequences of rabbit and other mammalian collagens provides us with a structural basis for understanding the immunogenicity of collagen in rabbits (Bornstein and Nesse, 1970). Figures 6 and 7 summarize the NH_2-terminal end sequences of α_1- and α_2-chains of collagen from various species and tissues.

Examination of the sequences in Fig. 6 and Fig. 7 brings out several salient features:

1. Much greater variability exists between NH_2-terminal sequences of the α_2-chain than between those of the α_1-chain.

2. From comparing the NH_2-terminal sequence of rabbit α_1 with those of other species, it is evident that they are either identical (rat) or vary by up to three residues (calf, human).

3. A great deal of variability is evident by comparing the NH_2-terminal sequences of rat, human, calf, and chicken α_2-chains with that of the rabbit. For instance, the rat sequence differs from that of rabbit in six positions out of the ten, and the human sequence differs from rabbit in five out of the first ten residues.

4. Rat, human, and chicken α_2-chains have a tyrosyl residue in position 2; rabbit and calf have a phenylalanyl residue in this position. It has been demonstrated that tyrosine residues can enhance the immunogenicity of collagen (Arnon and Sela, 1960; Kirrane and Van B. Robertson, 1968), possibly by introducing sites of increased rigidity into the molecule. Indeed, the correlation of the presence of tyrosine in position 2 with the location of the antigenic determinants is striking. Rat antisera have been shown to possess antibodies with specificity toward tyrosine in position 2 and several of the following residues (Furthmayr and Timpl, 1972). One laboratory also found human α_2 CB1 to possess strong antigenic activity

SPECIES AND TISSUE — RESIDUE NO.

	1	2	3	4	5	6	7	8	9	10	11	12	13	14	15	16	17	18	19	20
Rat skin					Gly	Tyr	Asp	Glu	Lys	Ser	Ala	Gly	Val	Ser	Val		Pro	Gly	Pro	Met
Rat tendon	PCA	Met	Ser	Tyr	Gly	Tyr	Asp	Glu	Lys	Ser	Ala	Gly	Val	Ser	Val		Pro	Gly	Pro	Met
Calf skin	PCA	Leu	Ser	Tyr	Gly	Tyr	Asp	Glu	Lys	Ser	Thr	Gly		Ile	Val		Pro	Gly	Pro	Met
Human, Baboon skin	PCA	Leu	Ser	Tyr	Gly	Tyr	Asp	Glu	Lys	Ser	Thr	Gly	Ile	Val	Leu		Pro	Gly	Pro	Met
Chicken skin	PCA	Met	Ser	Tyr	Gly	Tyr	Asp	Gly	Lys	Ser	Ala	Gly	Val	Ala	Val		Pro	Gly	Pro	Met
Rabbit skin	PCA	Met	Ser	Tyr	Gly	Tyr	Asp	Glu	Lys	Ser	Ala	Gly	Val	Ser	Val		Pro	Gly	Pro	Met

Figure 6. Comparison of the NH_2-terminal end (CB0,1) of α_1(I)-chains of collagen from rat, calf, human, and chicken with that of rabbit collagen. Sequences are aligned for maximum homology. Amino acid residues that differ from those of rabbit in the homologous position are underlined.

SPECIES AND TISSUE — RESIDUE NO.

	1	2	3	4	5	6	7	8	9	10	11	12	13	14	15
Rat Skin	PCA	Tyr		Ser	Asp	Lys	Gly	Val		Ala	Gly	Pro	Gly	Pro	Met
Human, Baboon skin	PCA	Tyr		Gly	Asp	Lys	Gly	Val	Gly	Leu	Gly	Pro	Gly	Pro	Met
Calf skin	PCA	Phe	Asp		Ala	Lys	Gly	Gly					Gly	Pro	
Chicken skin	PCA	Tyr	Asp	Pro	Ser	Lys	Ala	Ala	Asp	Phe	Gly	Pro	Gly	Pro	Met
Rabbit skin	PCA	Phe		Asp	Gly	Lys	Gly	Gly	Glu	Gly	Pro	Gly	Pro	Met	

Figure 7. Comparison of the NH_2-terminal end (CB1) of α_2-chains from rat, human, calf, and chicken collagen with that of rabbit collagen. Amino acid residues that differ from those of rabbit in the homologous position are underlined.

(Michaeli and Epstein, 1971), although another group failed to confirm this observation (Furthmayr *et al.*, 1971). On the other hand, calf α_2 CB1, which has phenylalanine in position 2, is devoid of antigenic activity.

5. The complexity of the factors that determine immunogenicity of certain sequences is highlighted by a comparison of human and calf NH_2-terminal sequences. Both are essentially identical except that human α_1 contains an extra glycine residue. They differ from rabbit in positions 2, 11, and 14. Yet different sequences comprise the antigenic determinants in α_1 CB0,1 of the two species. The antigenic determinant in human collagen comprises residues 2–5, with [2]Leu probably being the major determining structural factor in creating this determinant. On the other hand, the major antigenic determinant in calf α_1 CB0,1 comprises residues 4–13, with residues 11 (Phe) and/or 13 (Leu) determining the recognition of this area as foreign to the rabbit.

The structural basis for immunogenicity of calf and rat α_1 CB6 sequences becomes apparent when compared with the homologous sequence of rabbit α_1 CB6 (Fig. 8). Within the first ten nonhelical residues of rat and calf α_1 CB6 there are four or five substitutions. Moreover, phenylalanine in position 4 is substituted with tyrosine. This is similar to the situation of the α_2 CB1 peptide, where substitution of phenylalanine for tyrosine in position 2 was probably a major factor in the creation of an antigenic determinant in that area.

2. Antigenic Determinants in the Central Portion

Several workers have concluded, on the basis of indirect evidence, that the central portion of the collagen molecule possesses some, albeit minor, antigenic activity (Steffen *et al.*, 1968a; Timpl *et al.*, 1968a). Some of these determinants were probably immunologically inactive in the native state, but became potent following denaturation of the molecule (Steffen *et al.*,

SPECIES AND TISSUE	RESIDUE NO.							
	3	4	5	6	7	8	9	10
Calf skin	Gly-	<u>Tyr</u>-	Asp-	<u>Leu</u>-	Ser-	Phe-	<u>Leu</u>-	Pro
Rat skin	Gly-	<u>Tyr</u>-	Asp-	X	-Ser-	Phe-	<u>Leu</u>-	Pro
Rabbit skin	Gly-	Phe-	Asp-	Phe-		-Ile-	Met-	Pro

Figure 8. Comparison of α_1(1) CB6 nonhelical sequences from rat and calf collagen with that of rabbit collagen. Amino acid residues that differ from those of rabbit in the homologous position are underlined.

1967*a*; Beil *et al.*, 1973). The first direct and quantitative evidence for rabbit antibodies to antigenic determinants in the central portions of calf and rat collagens was provided by Timpl *et al.* (1971), using rabbit α-chains immunoadsorbent columns to isolate these antibodies. The rationale for this approach rests on the observation that there is a structural identity in the helical portions of mammalian collagens that may reach as high as 97 % in certain regions (Bornstein, 1968; Traub and Piez, 1971). Thus the likelihood of cross-reactivity between these regions in the immunogen and the homologous region in rabbit collagen is high. Indeed, about 20 % of rabbit antibodies to calf or rat collagen was directed to such determinants (Timpl *et al.*, 1971). The cross-reactivity of these determinants is high with all mammalian collagen α-chains tested (Timpl *et al.*, 1968*a*; Steffen *et al.*, 1971, Furthmayr *et al.*, 1972*a*), but decreases with increasing phylogenetic distance (i.e., fish collagen) and becomes marginal with invertebrate collagens (Timpl *et al.*, 1968*b*; Wolff *et al.*, 1970; Meigel *et al.*, 1971).

Examination of Figs. 6, 7, and 8 reveals that the interspecific differences between chicken, calf, rat, and human NH_2- and COOH-terminal sequences are much smaller than between these species and the homologous rabbit sequences. Indeed, this is probably the reason for the immunodominance of these regions when injected into rabbits. Immunological theory would predict that immunizing a mammalian species other than rabbit would result in decreased or nonexistent immunodominance of the terminal sequence, which in turn would allow enhanced expression of potential determinant in the central region. Beil *et al.* (1972) demonstrated high levels of chicken antibodies to central region determinants. These determinants could elicit antibodies in high titers even when injected in the denatured state (Beil *et al.*, 1973). A similar shift in specificity from terminal to the central portion of collagen was demonstrated in rat antibodies to calf collagen (Beil *et al.*, 1973; Hahn and Timpl, 1973; Hahn *et al.*, 1974) and mouse antibodies to calf collagen (Nowack *et al.*, 1975*a*).

3. *Antigenic Determinants Dependent on Native Molecular Conformation*

The observation that rats immunized with native calf collagen reacted only with the native or the renatured molecules but failed to react with the denatured protein (Beil *et al.*, 1973) provides evidence that certain antibodies require for recognition the existence of antigenic determinants in their native conformation. The existence of antigenic determinants, the structure of which involves contributions from more than one polypeptide chain, has been elegantly demonstrated by Hahn and Timpl (1973). It has been observed that renaturation to a triple helical molecule can be effected not only with a chain composition of $(\alpha_1)_2\alpha_2$ but also with $(\alpha_1)_3$ or $(\alpha_2)_3$ (Tkocz and Kühn, 1969). Such a set of molecules possesses, therefore, the unique property of having a common conformation but distinct differences in amino acid sequence. Assay of such molecules with rat antibodies to native calf collagen revealed that renaturation of an α-chains mixture having the ratio of $(\alpha_1)_2\alpha_2$ resulted in complete recovery of antigenic activity. On the other hand, $(\alpha_2)_3$ showed a markedly reduced antigenic activity by hemagglutination inhibition assay, and $(\alpha_1)_3$ was essentially devoid of activity. One must conclude, therefore, that both chains, α_1 and α_2, contribute to the formation of calf collagen antigenic determinants as recognized by the rat.

III. Cell-Mediated Immunity to Collagen

In comparison to the relative wealth of information on the humoral response to collagen, the information on cell-mediated immunity to collagen is meager indeed.

Senyk and Michaeli (1973) showed that normal guinea pigs exhibit no preexisting cellular immunity against homologous and heterologous (mouse, human) collagens. However, when guinea pigs were immunized with human collagen, they developed cellular immunity not only to it but also to their own collagen. Moreover, guinea pigs could be immunized with their own collagen in Freund's complete adjuvant and develop cellular immune responses against this autoantigen. By injecting normal guinea pigs with cyclophosphamide and autologous collagen they could be rendered tolerant of their own collagen. This unresponsive state was maintained after immunization with a cross-reacting heterologous (human) collagen. Thus the implications of this study are that the immune response to collagen is mediated by both T and B cells, and that antigen-reactive cells with specificity to autologous collagen exist in the normal, unimmunized animal.

Timpl et al. (1973a) showed that congenitally athymic "nude" mice had a markedly reduced immune response to calf collagen. This experiment suggests that the immune response to calf collagen in mice is thymus dependent. Nowack, Hahn, and Timpl (cited in Furthmayr and Timpl, 1975) used the technique of cell transfer into irradiated thymectomized mice to study the question of cell-mediated immunity to collagen. They also found that reconstitution with B cells only did not result in a measurable antibody response to collagen. Transfer of T cells to either irradiated thymectomized mice or athymic "nude" mice resulted in high antibody response to collagen.

The above results are in apparent conflict with the observations of Fuchs et al. (1974). They evaluated the role of the thymus in the immune response to the ordered polymer (Pro–Gly–Pro)$_n$, to the random polymer (Pro-66, Gly-34)$_n$, to native and denatured rat tail tendon collagen, and to

RCM *Ascaris* collagen. They found a strong immune response to (Pro–Gly–Pro)$_n$, to native rat tail tendon, and to RCM *Ascaris* collagens in the absence of transferred thymocytes. In contrast, the immune response to (Pro-66, Gly-34)$_n$ and to denatured collagen required the cooperation of thymocytes and bone marrow cells. These findings were interpreted as indicating that the unique conformation of the immunogens and the repetitive nature of the primary structure play a role in determining the requirement for cell-to-cell interaction in order to elicit an antibody response.

A possible resolution of the conflicting data may be offered by Nowack *et al.* (1975a). They showed that, unlike rabbit, mouse antibodies to soluble calf skin collagen react with determinants located in the rigid triple-helical portion of the molecule. These determinants are conformation dependent and are lost upon denaturation of the molecule. Pepsin treatment, which removes the terminal nonhelical sequences, had no effect on antigenicity and immunogenicity of collagen. Hahn and Timpl (1973) showed that the helical determinants along the axis of the molecule are unique and are not repetitive. Thus collagen does not fulfill a requirement for T-cell independence, namely, repetitiveness of the antigenic determinant (Feldmann and Basten, 1971).

IV. Genetic Control of the Immune Response to Collagen

Hahn *et al.* (1975) measured the immune response to collagen in various strains of inbred mice. The results of their experiments can be summarized as follows: (1) High responder and low responder strains of mice were identified. (2) Strains congenic to C57BL/10 provided evidence for an association of the gene(s) controlling immune responsiveness to collagen with the H-2 locus. (3) The H-2 haplotypes b, f, and s (Nowack *et al.*, 1975a) were associated with high response; the H-2 haplotypes d, k, m, and r were associated with a low response. (4) Injection of procollagen instead of collagen into low responder mice resulted in the formation of a strong antibody response against antigenic determinants in the collagen molecule. Since procollagen contains a globular extension attached to the NH_2-terminal end of the collagen molecule, it is conceivable that circumvention of the "T-cell gap" was accomplished by providing a carrier moiety for which a T-cell receptor was present in the low responders, thus allowing the cell to cell interaction to occur.

Nowack *et al.* (1975a), using various congenic recombinant lines, further localized the Ir gene which controls immune responsiveness to calf collagen in mice to the Ir-1A subregion of the H-2 complex. Also, based on the occurrence of intermediate responders and of significant differences between low responder strains of the same H-2 haplotype, it was suggested that additional control of the immune response is exerted by non-H-2-linked gene(s). Such control might be mediated via a T cell, or possibly via the B cell. However, data to support such a hypothesis are still lacking.

V. Antibodies to Procollagen

Several groups have used procollagen from a variety of sources to obtain antibodies to the protein. Timpl *et al.* (1973*b*) immunized rabbits with dermatosparactic bovine collagen. Sherr and Goldberg (1973) prepared antiserum against serum-free medium from human fibroblast cultures, which reacted specifically with procollagen. von der Mark *et al.* (1973) used pro-α_1-chain of acid-extracted chick bone procollagen to immunize rabbits. Dehm *et al.* (1974) prepared antibodies to procollagen synthesized by chick tendon cells. Some immunochemical differences were noted between the various procollagens; dermatosparactic collagen had antigenic determinants both in NH_2-terminal extensions and in the collagen molecule (α_1 CB6 at the *C*-terminal end and α_1 CB7,8 in the middle) (Timpl *et al.*, 1973*a*), whereas chick (von der Mark *et al.*, 1973) and human (Sherr and Goldberg, 1973) procollagen determinants were restricted to the NH_2-terminal extensions of the precursor chains. This difference could at least partially be accounted for by the fact that dermatosparactic collagen is presumably a partially degraded procollagen in which the region containing the interchain disulfide bonds is missing (Lenaers *et al.*, 1971; Schofield and Prockop, 1973). This could result in the removal of immunodominant determinants which in turn could allow the immunogenic expression of weaker determinants that are immunosilent in intact procollagen.

Hemagglutination-inhibition data suggest that the determinants in the NH_2-terminal extensions of pro-α_1 and pro-α_2 of dermatosparactic bovine collagen are closely related, but are not identical (Timpl *et al.*, 1973*a*). On the other hand, data on the antigenicity of chick fibroblast procollagen (Dehm *et al.*, 1974) suggest that the antigenic determinant(s) of this protein are restricted to the NH_2-terminal extension of the pro-α_1-chain. This could reflect a species difference, or could result from the removal of an immunodominant determinant in dermatosparactic collagen.

Another antigenic difference was observed when antibodies were prepared against the isolated chick bone pro-α_1-chains (von der Mark *et al.*, 1973) as compared to antibodies prepared against chick fibroblasts intact collagen (Dehm *et al.*, 1974). In the former, reduction of the intrachain bonds in the pro-α_1-chains increased their antigenic activity, presumably by increasing the accessibility of the antigenic determinants. In the latter case, reduction of intrachain disulfide bonds resulted in complete loss of antigenic activity. This indicates that antibodies made against intact procollagen probably recognize a different determinant(s) from those prepared against the isolated pro-α_1-chain.

The strong antigenicity of the NH$_2$-terminal extensions of the pro-α_1- and pro-α_2-chains may reflect a large degree of "foreignness," or inter-specific structural differences. Alternatively, their antigenicity may reflect some inherent structural characteristics that render them highly immunogenic (von der Mark et al., 1973). Evidence for species specificity of the extensions was obtained from inhibition studies of a radioimmunoassay of human procollagen (Taubman et al., 1974). Regardless of the basis for the immunogenicity of the extension peptides, this property can be utilized for the study of collagen biosynthesis and fibrogenesis, and possibly for the diagnosis of diseases affecting collagen metabolism (Taubman et al., 1974). Indeed, Olsen and Prockop (1974) used this approach to demonstrate that procollagen was found in the cisternae of the endoplasmic reticulum of embryonic chick tendon fibroblasts, indicating that the protein passes into this compartment early in its biosynthesis.

VI. Applications of Collagen Immunochemistry to Medical Research

Collagen is the most abundant protein in the body and as such commanded the attention and research interests of medical scientists for many years. Based on morphological changes that occur in collagen bundles at the site of autoimmune reactions, pathologists and clinicians classified diseases such as rheumatoid arthritis, systemic lupus erythematosus, dermatomyositis, and polyarteritis nodosa as "collagen diseases." Better understanding of the pathogenesis of these diseases rendered this classification obsolete. However, with increased sophistication in collagen chemistry and immunochemistry came renewed interest in investigation collagen in health and disease, utilizing specific antibodies as a potent tool. This field of investigation is still in its early stages but is gathering momentum quite rapidly. A detailed account of these investigations is somewhat beyond the scope of this review. However, an account of collagen immunochemistry would be incomplete without a brief review of this new and exciting line of investigations.

Rothbard and Watson (1961, 1965, 1967; Watson et al., 1954) showed by immunofluorescence that antibodies against various mammalian collagens became fixed in the basement membranes of renal glomeruli and tubules. The reaction was shown to be collagen specific and species specific. These early studies were plagued, however, with impure preparations of collagen that resulted in the formation of antibodies to serum proteins (Steffan et al., 1967a) or to acidic connective tissue proteins that resolve from collagen by ion exchange chromatography (LeRoy, 1968, 1969).

Using appropriate immunoadsorption for purification of antibodies to collagen and to procollagen, Wick et al. (1975) studied sections of skin by indirect immunofluorescence. Anticollagen sera stained the whole dermis, whereas antiprocollagen sera stained only the uppermost subepithelial layer of dermis (stratum papillare). These antisera also stained the interstitium in kidney sections; however, both skin and glomerular basement membrane remained unstained. Glomerular basement membrane could be stained if unpurified antisera were used.

Gay and Adelman (1974) showed the feasibility of differentiating between collagen type I- and type II-producing cells using type-specific antisera. Both immunofluorescence and selective complement-dependent cytolysis were employed.

Anti-rat collagen and anti (Pro–Gly–Pro)$_n$ are cytotoxic when added to primary cultures of rat muscle cells or rat embryo fibroblasts (Maoz et al., 1973a). The cytotoxicity was shown to be complement dependent, as well as time and antibody-concentration dependent (Maoz et al., 1973a; Fuchs et al., 1974).

Perhaps the greatest volume of publications on antibodies to collagen concerns rheumatoid arthritis. Steffen (1970) suggested that rheumatoid arthritis is a collagen autoimmune disease. He and his co-workers (Steffen et al., 1968b, 1973) and Michaeli and Fudenberg (1974a) have demonstrated antibodies to collagen in sera from patients with rheumatoid arthritis. The same groups (Steffen et al., 1973; Cracchiolo et al., 1975) demonstrated the occurrence of collagen immune complexes in synovial fluid of patients with rheumatoid arthritis. Both α_1- and α_2-chains were recognized by anticollagen in rheumatoid sera (Michaeli and Fudenberg, 1974a). Assays of five sera showed that the major determinants resided in α_1 CB0,1 and α_2 CB3, although some antigenic activity could be demonstrated in other CNBr peptides. The fact that the antibodies were specific to denatured collagen may indicate that their induction was secondary to denaturation of the molecule in the inflammatory reaction (Michaeli and Fudenberg, 1974a) rather than a primary etiological event in the pathogenesis of rheumatoid arthritis (Steffen, 1970).

A related problem is the phagocytosis of collagen and collagen immune complexes by phagocytic cells. It was shown that macrophages phagocytized particulate collagen and soluble collagen–anticollagen complexes (Knapp et al., 1974). Macrophages could not differentiate between collagens from various species, but did differentiate between conformations, favoring the uptake of denatured collagen. On the other hand, native collagen was phagocytized faster than the denatured protein. Specific antibodies increased fifty-fold the rate of uptake of native collagen (Hopper *et al.*, 1974).

Antibodies to denatured collagen were also detected in patients with pulmonary emphysema (Michaeli and Fudenberg, 1974*b*). A major specificity of these antibodies was α_2 CB3, the same as was found for anti-collagen in rheumatoid arthritis patients (Michaeli and Fudenberg, 1974*a*). These antibodies probably reflect the destruction of pulmonary connective tissue and constitute, therefore, a secondary reaction to the main pathogenetic process of pulmonary emphysema. Wells *et al.* (1973, 1975) have demonstrated antibodies to collagen in patients with selective IgA deficiency. This is quite a common form of human immunodeficiency, and several autoantibodies, in addition to anticollagen, have been reported (Wells *et al.*, 1975).

A report of potentially great importance (Gay *et al.*, 1975) described the collagens from cirrhotic liver. Type III collagen was identified by means of fluorescent type-specific antibodies and by electron microscopy. Another fraction, which had the appearance of type I collagen electron microscopically, did not have the biochemical and immunochemical criteria of this type. It is likely that this protein probably represents a new type of collagen, as yet undescribed.

ACKNOWLEDGMENTS

This work was supported in part by Contract N01 HB 4–2984 and Grants HL 17525 and GM 18470 from the National Institutes of Health, Bethesda, Maryland, and Grant 961 from the Council of Tobacco Research—U.S.A. Inc., New York. Dr. Michaeli is the recipient of Research Career Development Award 5 KO4 AM 50205 from the National Institute of Arthritis, Metabolism, and Digestive Diseases, National Institutes of Health, Bethesda, Maryland.

VII. References

Arnon, R., and Sela, M., 1960, *Biochem. J.* **75**:103.
Becker, U., Timpl, R., and Kühn, K., 1972, *Eur. J. Biochem.* **28**:221.
Becker, U., Furthmayr, H., and Timpl, R., 1975, *Hoppe-Seyler's Z. Physiol. Chem.* **356**:21.
Beil, W., Furthmayr, H., and Timpl, R., 1972, *Immunochemistry* **9**:779.
Beil, W., Timpl, R., and Furthmayr, H., 1973, *Immunology* **24**:13.

Benjamini, E., Michaeli, D., Leung, C. Y. K., Wong, K., and Scheuenstuhl, H., 1973, *Immunochemistry* **10**:629.

Borek, F., Kurtz, J., and Sela, M., 1969, *Biochim. Biophys. Acta* **188**:314.

Bornstein, P., 1968, *Science* **161**:592.

Bornstein, P., 1969, *Biochemistry* **8**:63.

Bornstein, P., 1974, The biosynthesis of collagen, in: *Annual Review of Biochemistry* (E. E. Snell, P. D. Boyer, A. Meister, and R. L. Sinsheimer, eds.), pp. 567–603, Annual Reviews Inc., Palo Alto, Calif.

Bornstein, P., and Nesse, R., 1970, *Arch. Biochem. Biophys.* **138**:443.

Chidlow, J. W., Bourne, F. J., and Bailey, A. J., 1974, *Immunology* **27**:665.

Chung, E., Keele, E. M., and Miller, E. J., 1974, *Biochemistry* **13**:3459.

Click, E. M., and Bornstein, P., 1970, *Biochemistry* **9**:4699.

Cracchiolo, A., Michaeli, D., Goldberg, L. S., and Fudenberg, H. H., 1975, *Clin. Immunol. Immunopathol.* **3**:567.

Daniels, J. R., and Chu, G. H., 1975, *J. Biol. Chem.* **250**:3531.

Davison, P. F., Levine, L., Drake, M. P., Rubin, A., and Bump, S., 1967, *J. Exp. Med.* **126**:331.

Dehm, P., Olsen, B., and Prockop, D., 1974, *Eur. J. Biochem.* **46**:107.

Engl, J., Kurtz, J., Katchalski, E., and Berger, A., 1966, *J. Mol. Biol.* **17**:255.

Epstein, E. H., Jr., 1974, *J. Biol. Chem.* **249**:3225.

Epstein, E. H., Jr., Scott, R. D., Miller, E. J., and Piez, K. A., 1971, *J. Biol. Chem.* **246**:1718.

Feldmann, M., and Basten, A., 1971, *J. Exp. Med.* **134**:103.

Fietzek, P. P., and Kühn, K., 1976, The primary structure of collagen, in: *International Review of Connective Tissue Research,* Vol. 7, Academic Press, New York, pp. 1–60.

Fuchs, S., and Harrington, W. F., 1970, *Biochim. Biophys. Acta* **221**:119.

Fuchs, S., Maoz, A., and Sela, M., 1974a, *Isr. J. Chem.* **12**:681.

Fuchs, S., Mozes, E., Maoz, A., and Sela, M., 1974b, *J. Exp. Med.* **139**:148.

Furthmayr, H., and Timpl, R., 1972, *Biochem. Biophys. Res. Commun.* **47**:944.

Furthmayr, H., and Timpl, R., 1975, Immunochemistry of collagens and procollagens, in: *International Review of Connective Tissue Research,* Vol. 7, Academic Press, New York, 1976, pp. 61–99.

Furthmayr, H., Beil, W., and Timpl, R., 1971, *FEBS Lett.* **12**:341.

Furthmayr, H., Stoltz, M., Becker, U., Beil, W., and Timpl, R., 1972, *Immunochemistry* **9**:789.

Gallop, P. M., Blumenfeld, O. O., and Seifter, S., 1972, Structure and metabolism of connective tissue proteins, in: *Annual Review of Biochemistry* (E. E. Snell, P. D. Boyer, A. Meister, and C. C. Richardson, eds.), pp. 617–672, Annual Reviews Inc., Palo Alto, Calif.

Gay, S., and Adelmann, B. C., 1974, *Z. Immun. Allergieforsch.* **147**:315.

Gay, S., Fietzek, R. P., Remberger, K., Eder, M., and Kühn, K., 1975, *Klin. Wochenschr.* **53**:205.

Hahn, E., and Timpl, R., 1973, *Eur. J. Immunol.* **3**:442.

Hahn, E., Timpl, R., and Miller E. J., 1974, *J. Immunol.* **113**:421.

Hahn, E., Timpl, R., and Miller, E. J., 1975a, *Immunology* **28**:561.

Hahn, E., Nowack, H., Götze, D., and Timpl, R., 1975b, *Eur. J. Immunol.* **5**:288.

Haimovich, J., and Sela, M., 1966, *J. Immunol.* **94**:388.

Hopper, K., Adelmann, B. C., Gentner, G., and Gay, S., 1974, *Z. Immun. Allergieforsch.* **147**:316.

Jasin, H. E., and Glynn, L. E., 1965a, *Immunology* **8**:95.

Jasin, H. E., and Glynn, L. E., 1965b, *Immunology* **8**:260.

Kang, A. H., Bornstein, P., and Piez, K. A., 1967, *Biochemistry* **6**:788.

Kang, A. H., and Gross, J., 1970, *Biochemistry* **9**:796.

Kefalides, N. A., 1970, Comparative biochemistry of mammalian basement membranes, in:

Chemistry and Molecular Biology of the Intercellular Matrix (E. A. Balazs, ed.), pp. 535–573, Academic Press, New York.

Kefalides, N. A., 1974, *J. Clin. Invest.* **53**:403.

Kettman, J. R., Benjamini, E., Michaeli, D., and Leung, D. Y. K., 1967, *Biochem. Biophys. Res. Commun.* **29**:623.

Kirrane, J. A., and Glynn, L. E., 1968, Immunology of collagen, in: *International Review of Connective Tissue Research* (D. A. Hall, ed.), pp. 1–31, Vol. 4, Academic Press, New York.

Kirrane, J. A., and Van B. Robertson, W., 1968, *Immunology* **14**:139.

Knapp, W., Menzel, J., Brunner, H., and Steffen, C., 1974, *Z. Immun. Allergieforsch.* **146**:283.

Kühn, K., 1969, The structure of collagen, in: *Essays in Biochemistry,* Vol. 5 (P. N. Campbell, and G. D. Greville, eds.), pp. 59–87, Academic Press, New York.

Lenaers, A., Ansay, M., Nusgens, B. V., and Lapière, C. M., 1971, *Eur. J. Biochem.* **23**:533.

LeRoy, C. E., 1968, *Proc. Soc. Exp. Biol. Med.* **128**:341.

LeRoy, C. E., 1969, *J. Immunol.* **102**:919.

Lindsley, H. B., Mannik, M., and Bornstein, P., 1969, *Arthritis Rheum.* **12**:676.

Lindsley, H., Mannik, M., and Bornstein, P., 1971, *J. Exp. Med.* **133**:1309.

Maoz, A., Fuchs, S., and Michaeli, D., 1971, *Biochim. Biophys. Acta* **243**:106.

Maoz, A., Fuchs, S., and Michaeli, D., 1971, *Biochim. Biophys. Acta* **243**:106.

Maoz, A., Dym, H., Fuchs, S., and Sela, M., 1973a, *Eur. J. Immunol.* **3**:839.

Maoz, A., Fuchs, S., and Sela, M., 1973b, *Biochemistry* **12**:4238.

Maoz, A., Fuchs, S., and Sela M., 1973c, *Biochemistry* **12**:4246.

Martin, G. R., Byers, P. H., and Piez, K. A., 1975, *Advan. Enzymol.* **42**:167.

McBride, O. W., and Harrington, W. F., 1967, *Biochemistry* **6**:1484.

Meigel, W., Pontz, B., Timpl, R., Hieber, E., Nordwig, A., Steffen, C., and Kühn, K., 1971, *J. Immunol.* **107**:1146.

Michaeli, D., and Epstein, E. H., 1971, *Isr. J. Med. Sci.* **7**:462.

Michaeli, D., and Fudenberg, H. H., 1974a, *Clin. Immunol. Immunopathol.* **2**:153.

Michaeli, D., and Fudenberg, H. H., 1974b, *Clin. Immunol. Immunopathol.* **3**:187.

Michaeli, D., Kamenecka, H., Benjamini, E., Kettman, J. R., Leung, D. Y. K., and Miner, R. C., 1968, *Immunochemistry* **5**:433.

Michaeli, D., Martin, G. R., Kettman, J., Benjamini, E., Leung, D. Y. K., and Blatt, B. A., 1969, *Science* **166**:1522.

Michaeli, D., Martin, G. R., and Benjamini, E., 1970, Localization of the antigenic determinants of collagen, in: *Chemistry and Molecular Biology of the Intercellular Matrix,* Vol. 1 (E. A. Balazs, ed.), pp. 275–278, Academic Press, New York.

Michaeli, D., Benjamini, E., and Leung, D. Y. K., 1971, *Immunochemistry* **8**:1.

Michaeli, D., Senyk, G., Maoz, A., and Fuchs, S., 1972, *J. Immunol.* **109**:103.

Miller, E. J., 1971, *Biochemistry* **10**:1652.

Miller, E. J., Woodall, D. L., and Vail, M. S., 1973, *J. Biol. Chem.* **248**:1666.

Nordwig, A., Nowack, H., and Hieber-Rogall, E., 1973, *J. Mol. Evol.* **2**:175.

Nowack, H., Timpl, R., and Nordwig, A., 1974, *Eur. J. Immunol.* **4**:698.

Nowack, H., Hahn, E., David, C. S., Timpl, R., and Götze, D., 1975a, *Immunogenetics* **2**:331.

Nowack, H., Hahn, E., and Timpl, R., 1975b, *Immunology* **29**:621.

O'Dell, D. S., 1968, Immunology of collagen and related materials, in: *Treatise on Collagen,* Vol. 2 (B. S. Gould, ed.), pp. 311–322, Part A, Academic Press, New York.

Olsen, B. R., and Prockop, D. J., 1974, *Proc. Natl. Acad. Sci. U.S.A.* **71**:2033.

Pontz, B., Meigel, W., Rauterberg, J., and Kühn, K., 1970, *Eur. J. Biochem.* **16**:50.

Rauterberg, J., and Kuhn., 1971, *Eur. J. Biochem.* **19**:398.

Rauterberg, J., Timpl, R., and Furthmayr, H., 1972, *Eur. J. Biochem.* **27**:231.

Rothbard, S., and Watson, R. F., 1961, *J. Exp. Med.* **113**:1041.

Rothbard, S., and Watson, R. F., 1965, *J. Exp. Med.* **122**:441.

Rothbard, S., and Watson, R. F., 1967, *J. Exp. Med.* **125**:595.

Schmitt, F. O., Levine, L., Drake, M. P., Rubin, A. L., Pfahl, D., and Davison, P. F., 1964, *Proc. Natl. Acad. Sci. U.S.A.* **51**:493.

Schofeld, J. D., and Prockop, D. J., 1973, *Clin. Orthop. Related Res.* **93**:175.

Sela, M., and Arnon, R., 1960a, *Biochem. J.* **75**:91.

Sela, M., and Arnon, R., 1960b, *Biochem. J.* **77**:394.

Senyk, G., and Michaeli, D., 1973, *J. Immunol.* **111**:1381.

Sherr, C. J., and Goldberg, B., 1973, *Science* **180**:1190.

Stark, M., Rauterberg, J., and Kühn, K., 1971, *FEBS Lett.* **13**:101.

Steffen, C., 1970, *Z. Immun. Allergieforsch.* **139**:219.

Steffen, C., Timpl, R., and Wolff, I., 1967a, *Z. Immunitaetsforsch.* **134**:91.

Steffen, C., Timpl, R., and Wolff, I., 1967a, *Z. Immunitaetsforsch.* **134**:91.

Steffen, C., Timpl, R., and Wolff, I., 1967b, *Z. Immunitaetsforsch.* **134**:205.

Steffen, C., Timpl, R., and Wolff, I., 1968a, *Immunology* **51**:135.

Steffen, C., Schuster, F., Tausch, G., and Pecker, I., 1968b, *Klin. Wochenschr.* **46**:976.

Steffen, C., Dichtl, M., Knapp, W., and Brunner, H., 1971, *Immunology* **21**:649.

Steffen, C., Ludwig, H., Thumb, N., Frank, O., Eberl, R., and Tausch, F., 1973, *Klin. Wochenschr.* **51**:222.

Steffen, C., Ludwig, H., and Knapp, W., 1974, *Z. Immun. Allergieforsch.* **147**:229.

Stoltz, M., Timpl, R., and Kühn, K., 1972, *FEBS Lett.* **26**:61.

Stoltz, M., Timpl, R., Furthmayr, H., and Kühn, K., 1973, *Eur. J. Biochem.* **37**:287.

Taubman, M. B., Goldberg, B., and Sherr, C. J., 1974, *Science* **186**:1115.

Timpl, R., Wolff, I., Furthmayr, H., and Steffen, C., 1968a, *Immunology* **15**:145.

Timpl, R., Wolff, I., Wick, G., Furthmayr, H., and Steffen, C., 1968b, *J. Immunol.* **101**:725.

Timpl, R., Wolff, I., Meigel, W., Pontz, B., Steffen, C., and Kühn, K., 1970, *J. Immunol.* **105**:1131.

Timpl, R., Beil, W., Furthmayr, H., Meigel, W., and Pontz, B., 1971, *Immunology* **21**:1017.

Timpl, R., Furthmayr, H., and Beil, W., 1972, *J. Immunol.* **108**:119.

Timpl, R., Furthmayr, H., Hahn, E., Becker, V., and Stoltz, M., 1973a, *Behring Inst. Mitt.* **53**:66.

Timpl, R., Wick, G., Furthmayr, H., Lapière, C. M., and Kühn, K., 1973b, *Eur. J. Biochem.* **32**:584.

Tkocz, C., and Kühn, K., 1969, *Eur. J. Biochem.* **7**:454.

Traub, W., and Piez, K. A., 1971, The chemistry and structure of collagen, in: *Advances in Protein Chemistry*, Vol. 25 (C. B. Anfinsen, Jr., J. T. Edsall, and F. M. Richards, eds.), pp. 243–352, Academic Press, New York.

Traub, W., and Yonath, A., 1966, *J. Mol. Biol.* **16**:404.

von der Mark, K., Wendt, P., Rexrodt, F., and Kuhn, K., 1970, *FEBS Lett.* **11**:105.

von der Mark, K., Click, E. M., and Bornstein, P., 1973, *Arch. Biochem. Biophys.* **156**:356.

Watson, R. F., Rothbard, S., and Vanamee, P., 1954, *J. Exp. Med.* **99**:535.

Wells, J. V., Michaeli, D., and Fudenberg, H. H., 1973, *Clin. Exp. Immunol.* **13**:203.

Wells, J. V., Michaeli, D., and Fudenberg, H. H., 1975, Auto-immunity in selective IgA deficiency, in: *Birth Defects: Original Article Series* (D. Bergsma and R. A. Good, eds.), Sinauer Associates, New York, Vol. 6, No. 1, pp. 144–146.

Wick, G., Furthmayr, H., and Timpl, R., 1975, *Int. Arch Allergy Appl. Immunol.* **48**:664.

Wolff, I., Wick, G., Furthmayr, H., Timpl. R., and Steffen, C., 1970, *Immunology* **18**:843.

7

Histocompatibility Antigens

Raymond N. Hiramoto and Vithal K. Ghanta

I. The HL-A System of Man

Human leukocyte antigens (HL-A) can be used to type an individual just as he can be typed by the ABO antigens on his erythrocytes. HL-A antigens are determined by the genes on a single pair of chromosomes (chromosome 6) that occupy a region defined as the HL-A complex. The HL-A gene complex can be divided into two regions, as is true of the genetic loci for the H-2 system in the mouse (Fig. 1). Each sublocus of human HL-A carries a series of alternative alleles that appear to be codominant. Within a family, a given sublocus 1 (LA) determinant will always travel with the same sublocus II (Four) determinant. An individual can have only two to four specificities, each of which is controlled by many alleles. To date, 14 LA and 26 Four antigens and their corresponding alleles have been identified. Table I lists some of these antigens and alleles; a more extensive listing is given by Kissmeyer-Nielsen *et al.* (1972). Examples of the possible inheritance patterns of HL-A antigens are shown in Fig. 2.

The presence of HL-A antigens on the surface of lymphocytes can be detected and defined by the use of cytotoxic antisera, which are capable of damaging lymphoid cells that carry these antigens, or by leukoagglutination. Serologically defined antigens (SD) are coded by the SD loci; lymphocyte-defined determinants (LD) are coded by the LD loci and detected by the mixed lymphocyte reaction (MLR) (Fig. 1). Since it is impossible to establish congenic resistant lines in humans, it has been difficult to control the

Raymond N. Hiramoto and Vithal K. Ghanta · Department of Microbiology, University of Alabama in Birmingham, Birmingham, Alabama 35294.

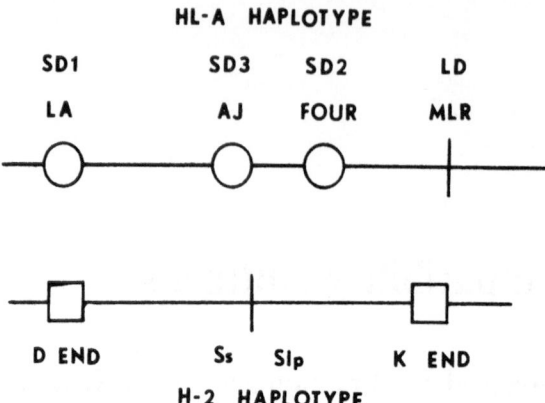

Figure 1. Human and mouse histocompatibility gene complex.

specificities of the antisera used to evaluate HL-A antigens. Most reagents for HL-A typing are obtained either from multiply transfused individuals or from multiparous women immunized by the white cells (from the fetus) that express the HL-A haplotype of the father. Other sera are obtained by active immunization of volunteers who have white blood cells of the

Table I. Serologically Defined (SD) Specificities of the LA, AJ, and Four Series

LA (SD$_1$)[a]	AJ (SD$_3$)	Four (SD$_2$)[a]
HL-A1	T1	HL-A5
HL-A2	T2	W-5
W-28	T3	W-18
HL-A3	T4	HL-A7
HL-A11	T5	HL-A8
HL-A9 . 1 (W-23)		HL-A12
HL-A9 . 2 (W-24)		HL-A13
HL-A10 . 1 (W-25)		W-10
HL-A10 . 2 (W-26)		W-27
W19 . 1 (W-29)		W-15
W19 . 3 (W-30)		W-22
W19 . 4 (W-31)		HL-A14
W19 . 5 (W-32)		W-21
W19 . 6		HL-A17
		W-16

[a] From Miller (1974).

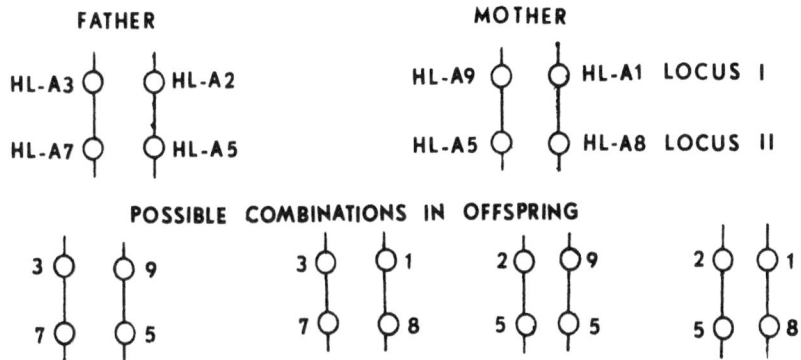

Figure 2. Segregation of HL-A in the siblings. Each line of chromosome (with two subloci) represents a haplotype. The specificities determined by the haplotype are inherited together so that only four possible combinations of specificities can result. The father's phenotype is HL-A2, HL-A5, HL-A3, and HL-A7. His genotype would be the same designation. His haplotype would be HL-A3, HL-A7 for one chromosome and HL-A2, HL-A5 for the other.

desired specificities. Since many of these antisera contain multiple specificities, confusion has arisen as to the number of alloantigens detected.

The HL-A literature also contributes to the confusion because various investigators have given different labels to similar specificities. These discrepancies will be erased when the WHO nomenclature committee assigns official HL-A designations. Unfortunately, the HL-A designations do not identify the subloci to which the alloantigen belongs. The various designations used by different laboratories, the workshop numbers given to the specificities (Fourth Workshop), and WHO nomenclature are tabulated by Kissmeyer-Nielsen and Thorsby (1970).

A third sublocus (AJ) has been postulated but, at present, seems to have no defined or detectable transplantation activity. Table 1 lists specificities of the LA, AJ, and Four loci. The inclusion of the AJ locus into the HL-A system would increase individual HL-A specificities to six or less. However, the HL-A system presently is defined by two segregating series of alleles.

It was formerly believed that the MLR predicted the serological identity at the two HL-A loci and that allografts would survive if the MLR between two individuals was negative. This theory is now challenged by the finding, in certain instances, that individuals who were identical at the HL-A locus have displayed a positive MLR and, on the other hand, that individuals who were not identical at the HL-A locus did not display an MLR. Analyses of MLR reactivities suggest that the separate loci (Fig. 1) that occur on chromosome 6 control the degree of MLR (Eijsvoogel et al., 1972, 1973; Eijsvoogel, 1974) (Fig. 1).

II. Alloantigens of the Mouse

A. H-2 Complex of the Mouse

Histocompatibility alloantigens (isoantigens) are the products of histocompatibility genes and are involved in tissue transplant rejection (Amos, 1964; Snell and Stimpfling, 1964; Shreffler, 1967). In the mouse, more than 20 histocompatibility systems are described; one of these, identified as the major histocompatibility complex (MHC), is located on chromosome 17 (linkage group IX). This system, which was found to be polymorphic, gives rise to many distinct specificities.

In H-2 nomenclature, mice of different genotypes are given superscript letters a, b, c (e.g., H-2^a, H-2^b, H-2^c), and individual specificities that are determined by an allele are given arabic numbers (e. g., H-2 specificity 1 as H-2.1 and H-2 specificity 33 as H-2.33). Identification of such specificities can be made by developing alloantisera in congenic strains (Snell and Stimpfling, 1964; Shreffler, 1967; Nathenson, 1970).

In early 1950 the multiple-loci hypothesis was in vogue, and meant that an H-2 allele represented a series of adjacent histocompatibility loci, each of which resulted in the appearance on the cell surface of one or more serologically detectable antigen specificities (Neauport-Sautes et al., 1973; Stimpfling and Snell, 1972; Stimpfling and Richardson, 1965). There were many such alleles and each determined a different number of H-2 specificities; many of these individual specificities were cross-reactive for different alleles. Subsequently, it became clear that certain other genes, unrelated to the H-2 locus, were interspersed among the H-2 determinants so that the H-2 loci could no longer be said to lie adjacent to each other (Klein and Shreffler, 1971). From these observations, it became more feasible to simplify the multiple-loci hypothesis to a two-gene concept (Fig. 1). Since, in a few cases, a single H-2 specificity can map in either of two places within the H-2 region, it was possible to develop an H-2 map consisting of only two, rather than several, antigen-determining subloci. The two genes, H-2K and H-2D, appear adequate to account for all the serologically detectable antigen determinants (Klein and Shreffler, 1972). Thus the H-2^b haplotype is equivalent to the phenotype specificities of the H-2K^b allele and to the closely linked phenotype specificities for the H-2D^b allele. Additional support for the two-gene concept is provided by the observation that the major antigens governed by the H-2K and the H-2D alleles are separable on the cell surface (Boyse et al., 1968; Neauport-Sautes et al., 1973) and are coded on different molecules. For example, in heterozygotes (H-2^b/H-2^d) where the two H-2K alleles and the two H-2D alleles carried different specificities on the cell surface, it was possible, by using specific antisera, to isolate four different molecules (Cullen *et al.*, 1972*b*). Since much more is known about the H-2 regions (Fig. 3) than about those of HL-A, the mouse genetic model will serve as the prototype for the HL-A system.

The H-2 complex can be divided into several regions that are designated as K, I, S, X (unknown), and D. The construction of a genetic map that will represent genes located at particular intervals in these regions is described by Shreffler (1974) and by Srb and Owen (1953); Ivanyi (1970) and Klein (1972) have also given detailed accounts of these regions. The H-2 genes are separable by a recombination frequency of about 0.5% and within the interval that separates these genes are found the determinants of the I (McDevitt *et al.*, 1972), S (Passmore and Shreffler, 1970), and X regions.

The K region consists of a single gene (*H-2K*) or a cluster of genes, products of which are detectable by serological and transplantation methods.

The I region is believed to consist of numerous genes. Some products of these genes have recently been identified and are known to control immune response to a wide variety of thymus-dependent antigens (Benacerraf and McDevitt, 1972; McDevitt and Benacerraf, 1969) as well as to I-region-associated (Ia) antigens that are present only in certain tissues (Hauptfeld *et al.*, 1973; David *et al.*, 1973). A current hypothesis suggests that products of the immune response (*Ir*) gene are actually cell surface receptors for the different antigens (Benacerraf and McDevitt, 1972), and that various gene products from the I region serve as cell recognition molecules, which promote cooperation between T and B cells in the immune response (Katz *et al.*, 1973).

The S region probably consists of at least two genes, *Ss* and *Slp*. The *Ss* gene controls a serum antigen that is found in high concentration (Ss^h) in some mouse strains and low concentration (Ss^l) in others (Shreffler, 1965). The *Slp* gene controls a sex-linked protein that is present in the serum of males of some inbred strains (Passmore and Shreffler, 1970).

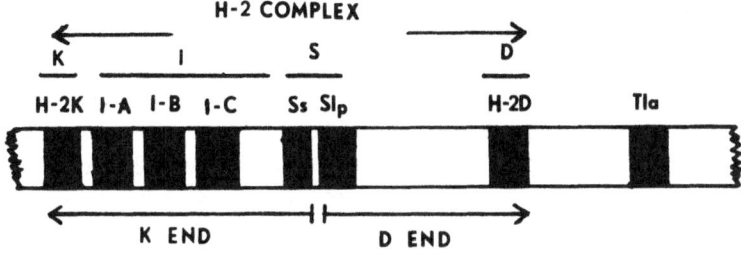

Figure 3. Major histocompatibility complex (MHC) of the mouse. Adapted from Klein and Park (1973).

Thus far, *Ss* and *Slp* traits have not been separated by genetic recombination. The S region appears to be functionally unrelated to the rest of the H-2 complex.

An X region is located between the S and D regions. Of the 34 mapped intra-H-2 recombinants, 21 occur in the X region. The function of this region and its relationship to the rest of the H-2 complex is not known (Klein and Park, 1973), although it is likely that it contains numerous genes.

The D region consists of a gene cluster (*H-2D*) that codes for serologically detectable, transplantation antigens similar to the alloantigens controlled by the *H-2K* region.

The TL region has not yet been considered a part of the H-2 complex, though the *Tla* gene is about one map unit away from the *H-2D* gene (Boyse *et al.*, 1966). It codes for membrane alloantigens that can be detected serologically on thymocytes and certain leukemic cells, but not on other cell types. It has been shown that a difference in the TL region can lead to skin graft rejection (Boyse *et al.*, 1972).

Testing of the different H-2 regions is made possible by the availability of H-2 recombinant strains, which are defined as progeny that received the *H-2K* gene from one chromosome and the *H-2D* gene from another chromosome of the H-2 heterozygote parent by crossing over.

Table II shows some of the alleles responsible for the various specificities determined at the loci of the *H-2K* and *H-2D* genes. Klein and Shreffler (1971) provide a more detailed chart. Alloantisera of various specificities are prepared (Table III) from mouse strains that carry different alleles (Table IV).

H-2 antigens coded by the *H-2K* and *H-2D* regions are the major barriers to skin grafting. However, graft rejection has also occurred because of incompatibility in the I region (Klein *et al.*, 1974). The S and X regions appear not to be involved in rejection of skin grafts (Shreffler, 1974).

A single chromosome that bears the two H-2 subloci, *H-2K* and *H-2D*, is a haplotype. Many forms (alleles) of the *H-2K* and *H-2D* exist; in the mouse alone, about 41 haplotypes have been distinguished (Klein, 1972); each of these is responsible for two H-2 gene products of more than one specificity. These specificities include private and public specificities confined to a single gene product (Table II). Private specificities are restricted to a few haplotypes, whereas public specificities are shared by many haplotypes. For example, the H-2.5 public specificity occurs with $H-2K^a$, $H-2K^b$, and $H-2K^k$. Figure 4 shows that the haplotype H-2^b produces gene products on the cell surface that stem from the $H-2K^b$ gene and the $H-2D^b$ gene. These individual entities on the cell surface (Boyse *et al.*, 1968; Neauport-Sautes *et al.*, 1973) represent separate molecules (Cullen *et al.*, 1972b). Specificities assumed to be direct gene products of the *H-2D* and *H-2K* ends

Table II. Public and Private Specificities Associated with H-2 Haplotypes[a]

H-2K region

H-2 chromosome symbol	H-2 region symbol	Private											Public						
		20	21	19	25	17	16	23	15	31	33	11	36	35	34	8	5	3	1
b	b	—	—	—	—	—	—	—	—	—	33	—	36	35	—	—	—	—	—
d	d	—	—	—	—	—	—	—	—	31	—	—	—	—	34	8	—	—	—
f	f	—	—	—	—	—	—	—	15	—	—	—	—	—	—	8	—	—	—
j	j	—	—	—	25	—	—	—	—	—	—	—	—	—	·	—	—	—	—
k	k	—	—	—	—	—	—	23	—	—	—	11	—	—	·	8	—	3	1
p	p	—	—	—	—	—	16	—	—	—	—	—	—	—	·	8	5	—	—
q	q	—	—	—	—	17	—	—	—	—	—	—	—	—	34	—	5	—	—
r	r	—	—	—	25	—	—	—	—	—	—	11	—	—	·	8	5	—	—
s	s	—	—	19	—	—	—	—	—	—	—	11	—	—	—	—	5	—	—
v	v	—	21	—	—	—	—	—	—	—	—	—	—	—	·	—	5	—	—

H-2D region

H-2 region symbol	Public														Private					
	1	3	5	6	7	13	27	28	29	35	36	41	42	43	2	4	9	32	30	18
b	—	—	5	6	—	—	—	28	29	—	—	—	—	—	2	—	—	—	—	—
d	—	3	—	6	—	13	27	28	29	35	36	41	42	43	—	4	—	—	—	—
f	—	—	—	6	7	—	27	—	29	—	—	—	—	—	—	—	9	—	—	—
j	1*	3*	5*	6	7	—	27	28	—	—	—	—	—	—	—	—	—	—	—	—
k	1*	3*	5*	6	7	—	—	—	—	—	—	—	—	—	2	—	—	32	—	—
p	1*	3*	5*	6	7	c	—	28	—	35	—	41	—	—	—	—	—	—	—	—
q	1*	3*	·	6	—	13	27	—	29	c	c	c	c	c	—	—	—	—	30	—
r	1*	3*	·	6	7	c	—	28	—	—	c	c	c	—	—	—	—	—	—	—
s	1*	3*	·	6	7	c	—	—	—	c	36	c	42	—	—	—	—	—	—	18
v	1*	3*	·	·	·	c	—?	28?	·	—	—	—	42	—	—	—	—	—	30*	—

[a] Part of table from Klein and Shreffler (1971). —, Absence of an antigen; ·, not tested; *, modified form of an antigen; c, weak cross-reactivity; ?, questionable results.

Table III. Preparation of Alloantisera

	H-2K specificities		*H-2D* specificities	
	Private	Public	Private	Public
Recipient (H-2^b)	33	36,35	2	5, 6, 27, 28, 29
Donor (H-2^d)	31	34,8	4	3, 6, 13, 27, 28, 29 35, 36, 41, 42, 43
H-2^b anti-H-2^d	31	34,8	4	3, 13, 35, 36, 41, 42, 43

are expressed on different molecules. Multiple public specificities can be located on the same molecule with private specificities (Davies, 1969, 1970; Cullen *et al.*, 1972*a*). The *H-2K^b* gene has the private specificity H-2.33 and public specificities H-2.5 and H-2.35. The *H-2D^b* gene product, which has H-2.2 private specificity, also has 6, 27, 28, and 29 public specificities (Brown *et al.*, 1974; Nathenson and Cullen, 1974; Demant, 1973). Public specificities have been found to map in the *K* or *D* genes, and, in some strains, they map in both genes. Furthermore, the gene products of different genetic loci often produce different amounts of alloantigens in different tissues. Nathenson (1970) isolated two classes of alloantigens. Class I proteins (mol. wt. 58,000–65,000) from H-2^b and H-2^d strains carried several specifi-

Table IV. H-2 Alleles of Different Strains of Mice

H-2 type	Inbred lines	Congenic resistant line[a]
H-2^u	A/J; A/HeJ	B10·A
H-2^b	C57BL/6J	B10
H-2^d	Balb/c; NZB; DBA/2J	B10·D2
H-2^f	A/Sn	
H-2^h		B10·A (2R)
H-2^i		B10·A (5R)
H-2^k	AKR/J; C3H/HeJ; CBA	B10·BR
H-2^m	AKR/M	
H-2^p	BDP	
H-2^q	DBA/1J	
H-2^s	SJL/J	

[a] "Congenic resistant lines" implies that all strains have the same genetic background of B10 (C57BL/10Sn), from which they differ only in the H-2 complex.

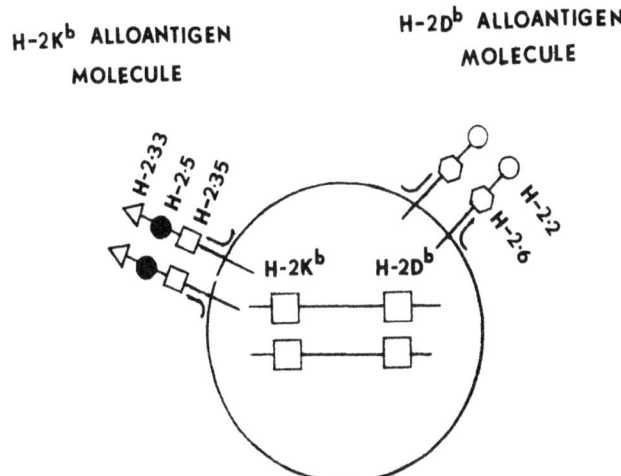

Figure 4. Schematic representation of alloantigens on the surface of a cell produced by haplotype H-2ᵇ. Each alloantigen molecule is shown to carry both private and public specificities coded by the *H-2Kᵇ* and *H-2Dᵇ* loci.

cities for the H-2ᵇ and H-2ᵈ genotypes, whereas, the Class II proteins (mol. wt. 33,000–37,000) carried only a single specificity.

B. Other Antigen-Determining Loci of the Mouse H-2 Complex

The foregoing presentation has described genes of the H-2 region and the antigenic specificities expressed on their cell surfaces. Other antigen-determining loci have been identified, and, in the mouse, some of these loci are within, as well as outside, the H-2 complex of chromosome 17.

Cytotoxicity tests were used for the detection of non-H-2 lymphocyte alloantigens, which include Ia, Thy-1 (θ), Tla (TL), Ly-1, Ly-2, Ly-4, plasma cell, skin and antigens associated with the T (Brachury) locus. Other antigenic systems are the erythrocyte antigens and immunoglobulin allotypes. All of these loci are essentially distinct from each other.

The number of possible antigenic specificities that involve different alleles and different loci and can be expressed on the cell surface indicate the range of individual diversity in the animal world in even a single species (mouse). It has been estimated that within the interval between *H-2K* and *Tla* enough DNA would be present to account for some 500–1000 genes of 1000 base pairs each (Shreffler and Klein, 1970); this would indicate that sufficient DNA exists along these stretches of chromosomes for genetic diversity.

C. Ia Antigens and *Ir* Genes

The Ia antigens represent a new group of alloantigens determined by the H-2 complex, but not by the K or D ends. Recombinant analysis places the responsible locus in the I region, which is subdivided into I-A, I-B, and I-C. As stated previously, the H-2 complex consists of numerous loci concentrated into essentially four regions: K, I, S, and D. Identification of I-region determinants became possible only with the availability of congenic mice that have identical specificities in K and D regions but different ones in the I region. Immunization across the congenic strains ATL and ATH allowed identification of Ia cellular antigens (Hammerling *et al.*, 1974; David *et al.*, 1973) (Table V). Many currently used anti-H-2 sera are contaminated with anti-Ia specificities because they were produced in strains that had both H-2 and I-region differences (Sachs and Cone, 1973). For example, B10.A (4R) anti-B10 sera contain antibodies to *H-2K* and to I-A regions.

Individual Ia specificities are under the genetic control of different I subregions. Genes in the I region are believed to control cellular recognition, specific immune responses, and cell surface antigens on T and B cells. The genetic control by I-A and I-B subregions of specific immune responses to distinct antigens was related to T-cell carrier recognition functions, which allowed T and B cell interactions (McDevitt *et al.*, 1974; Katz and Benacerraf, 1975). Ia antigens coded in these subregions are 1, 2, 8, 9, and 11 in I-A and 3 in I-B. The I-C region was found to have no immune response functions, but it is believed to code the Ia surface antigens 5, 6, and 7 on lymphoid cells (McDevitt *et al.*, 1974; Shreffler, 1975). Ia antigens are expressed on both T and B cells. Ia-6 is expressed exclusively on T cells. Ia-1, 7, 9, 11, 12, 13, and 15 have been found on both cell types, and

Table V. H-2 Recombinant Strains with the Identical and Nonidentical Loci within the H-2 Complex

Congenic strains	H-2 regions (origins)					
	K	I-A	I-B	I-C	S	D
ATH	s	s	s	s	s	d
ATL	s	k	k	k	k	d
B10·A (7R)	s	s	k	k	k	d
B10	b	b	b	b	b	b
B10·A (5R)	b	b	b	d	d	d
B10·A (4R)	k	k	b	b	b	b
B10·A (2R)	k	k	k	d	d	b

Ia-2, 3, 4, 5, 8, 10, and 14 were found on B cells, but their presence on T cells was inconclusive. Native Ia that is not detectable on resting T cells can be detected if the cells are stimulated to transform. The reaction of T-blast cells with the anti-Ia eluted from B cells is evidence of the close similarity of the T and B Ia (David *et al.*, 1975). The Ia surface antigens found primarily on mature B cells (Hammerling *et al.*, 1974) might allow T-cell recognition. Genes that code for cell interaction (CI) molecules are located in the I region (Katz *et al.*, 1974; Katz and Benacerraf, 1975). If genes are identical in the I region, cells from such animals are capable of developing cooperative T and B immune response even when they differ in the K, S, and D region. Gene differences in the I-A subregion prevent development of T- and B-cell cooperation even when gene identities exist in the I-C subregion and in the H-2 complex (Katz, 1975).

Alloantigen-stimulated T cells produce a nonantigen specific, allogeneic effect factor (AEF) that can stimulate B-cell differentiation in the presence of antigen (Armerding and Katz, 1974). AEF from T cells with H-2^d haplotype can be specifically removed by anti-H-2^d antibody or by anti-Ia serum that is reactive with I-region specificities of H-2^d haplotype (Armerding *et al.*, 1974). Analysis of AEF indicates a bimolecular complex comprised of a heavy molecule (35,000) and a lighter molecule (12,000); the latter suggests the participation of a β_2-microglobulinlike component (Armerding and Katz, 1975). It is likely that AEF and CI molecules are similar in nature. Taussig (1975), using (TG)AL, has shown an antigen-specific, nonimmunoglobulin (50,000 mol. wt.) protein synthesized by the T cell and coded by the I-A subregion. *In vivo* this factor replaces the T cells in promoting response of allogeneic bone marrow cells. The factor can bind (TG)AL and adsorb to high- but not to low-responder B cells. High-responder B cells will adsorb the factor whether (TG)AL is present or not, but such cells do not respond with antibody production; in the presence of antigen, an antibody response is induced. Low-responder B cells neither adsorb the factor nor react with antibody response even in the presence of (TG)AL (Taussig *et al.*, 1974; Taussig and Munro, 1974).

In a study of the immune response of guinea pig strains 2 and 13 to antigens controlled by the immune response gene, Paul *et al.*, (1974) identified a 25,000 dalton product that was smaller than the H-2 antigens of the D and K series (Schwartz *et al.*, 1973a). This product is present in a limited number of tissues and appears to be analogous to the Ia antigen of mice (Hauptfeld *et al.*, 1973; Sachs and Cone, 1973; David *et al.*, 1973). These investigators postulated that the product of the immune response gene exists as a molecular complex with the 2/13 histocompatibility antigen and is responsible for the specific recognition functions of the complex and for biological functions such as the histocompatibility-dependent cellular interactions, which are mediated by alloantigens.

With respect to T-cell functions, cytotoxicity, and blast transformation, the interrelated role of the H-2 locus (K and D regions) and the I-region locus are now being delineated in congenic strains (Bach, 1975). Immune response is controlled by the I rather than the H-2 locus. Using thymidine uptake and lymphocyte cytotoxicity as an index of immune recognition, it was found that a proliferation response, but little cytotoxicity, was initiated in effector cells by differences found only at loci in the I region, that differences found only at the H-2 loci caused neither proliferation nor cytotoxicity, and that differences at loci of both regions caused blast transformation, as well as development of cytotoxic killer cells. Based on the interrelated role of the I and the H-2 regions, the apparent dissociation of T-cell activity is extremely important. Whether these differences in the H-2 complex direct other cellular mediated correlates such as MIF, DTH, and graft rejection obviously should be investigated.

Ia and H-2 antigens display the following similarities and differences:

1. Similarities: Both antigens (a) appear to be glycoproteins (Cullen and Nathenson, 1974), (b) serve as allontigens (Klein *et al.*, 1974), (c) are present on the cell surface and, presumably, act as recognition molecules (Paul *et al.*, 1974; Taussig and Munro, 1974; Katz, 1975), (d) may have possible β_2-microglobulinlike components (Katz, 1975), and (e) are polymorphic in nature and can be determined by a single haplotype (Cullen and Nathenson, 1974).
2. Differences: (a) The two antigens are coded by different genetic regions, as shown by recombination studies (Hauptfeld *et al.*, 1973; David *et al.*, 1973). (b) Serological studies reveal that H-2 antigens are found on all cells, whereas Ia appears to be primarily located on T and B cells, and in lesser quantities on sperm, epidermal cells, and macrophages (McDevitt *et al.*, 1974). (c) The molecular weights of Ia antigens range between 30,000 and 35,000; those of HL-A and H-2 are closer to 45,000. (d) The mode of releasing the molecules is different. H-2 is not secreted in detectable amounts, but Ia molecules appear to be released from the cell surface (Vitetta *et al.*, 1974).

Since the products of the immune response gene, like AEF from T cells and Ia antigens from B cells, are secreted by both T and B cells, one can speculate that these products might act as specific signals between different subpopulations of lymphocytes by mediating helper functions, suppressor functions, and lymphokinelike activities. Whatever the case, the assignment of biological activities to the soluble directive molecules and the firm unifying genetic basis provided by the current studies will afford new insights into the roles of histocompatibility antigens and the I region.

III. Purification Methods for H-2 and HL-A Alloantigens

The functions of histocompatibility antigens, as well as their structure and their mode of integration into the cell membrane, is not known. Purification and characterization of the molecule may help to supply answers to some of these questions, but further clarification of the structure of the alloantigen can be achieved only if the technology of isolation is improved. It is hoped that the procedures and results described in this chapter will promote this improvement.

Histocompatibility antigens are localized on the membrane surface, but they comprise less than 1% of the membrane components. To obtain a sufficient quantity of antigens for analysis, many procedures have been developed to extract them from surface membranes (Nathenson, 1970; Reisfeld and Kahan, 1970; Mann and Fahey, 1971). Most of the procedures are nonselective and tend to solubilize large amounts of complex materials from the cell membrane, but alloantigens make up a relatively small quantity of these materials. Moreover, minor differences in essentially similar approaches of isolation (e.g., papain digestion) yield end products of the alloantigen that differ in molecular size.

With some procedures, it is possible to obtain active fragments, mol. wt. 31,000, that are without carbohydrate moieties; in other cases, a fragment of about 45,000 mol. wt. can be reduced to a fragment of 30,000 mol. wt. only under conditions of denaturation. Attention is directed to the details of the various procedures used and to the experimental results obtained. In most instances, the HL-A type being isolated and the nature of the starting materials, such as viable cells, crude membrane extracts, and hypotonically lysed preparations, are indicated.

In the process of isolating alloantigens, attention should also be given to the cell state. Strominger et al. (1974) used transformed, tissue-cultured, lymphoid cells to obtain an increased yield of HL-A antigens (20–50×) as compared with that obtained from peripheral blood lymphocytes. This increase occurs at the membrane, and although a greater quantity of alloantigen was recovered, 5'-nucleotidase activity was not increased in the transformed fraction. As much as 40 mg of purified HL-A antigen was obtained from 1 kg of lymphocyte culture. Therefore, during transformation, 1–2% of the HL-A antigen is represented on the surface of the cultured lymphocyte.

A. Cell Disruption

H-2 antigens are believed to be present on all tissues. In general, these antigens are highly concentrated in lymphoid tissue (e.g., spleen and lymph node) and liver; however, H-2 is present on thymocytes in lesser amounts than on lymphocytes. Intermediate amounts are present in lung, adrenal gland, and the gastrointestinal tract; only small amounts are found in the heart, skeletal muscle, brain, and red blood cells (Snell and Stimpfling, 1964). Alloantigens are known to be present on cell surfaces, but distribution in subcellular locations cannot be completely ruled out. A method for isolation of surface and subcellular antigens includes cell breakage or fractionation of components that may contain alloantigens and the subsequent solubilization of these alloantigens. Cell disruption methods require careful antigenic and enzymatic analyses of subcellular fractions to establish which of these subcellular fractions is involved (Wilson and Amos, 1972).

Nitrogen decompression, which appears to be the preferred technique for cell disruption methods (Hunter and Commerford, 1961), entails subjecting cell suspension to 100–1200 psi nitrogen for 15–20 min at 4°C. The suspension is passed through a small orifice beyond which an instantaneous drop to atmospheric pressure is allowed. Microbubbles of nitrogen, dissolved under pressure, expand within each cell and cause the cell to explode. This method causes a minimal loss of antigenicity and a maximum efficiency in breakage of individual cells. Large quantities of cells can be readily processed, and unwanted heating is prevented by the rapid cooling that results from the drop in pressure. Since breakage occurs under inert conditions, inactivation of sensitive sulfhydryl groups is minimized. Nuclei are not disrupted at 100–1200 psi pressure, which is sufficient to rupture most cells (Avis, 1972).

Protocols (Fig. 5) have been devised to isolate membranes and subcellular fractions by centrifugation in sucrose density gradients (Allan and Crumpton, 1970). The membrane and ribosome pellets are suspended in 5 mM Tris-HCl in 40% sucrose and overlaid with 60% sucrose. During centrifugation, membranes migrate to the discontinuous interface. Possible loss of membrane can occur during centrifugation. For example, when the cell homogenate is centrifuged to pellet the nuclei or various subcellular fractions, a loss of membrane fragments to these fractions must be considered (Manson et al., 1968). Although significant losses occur during initial purification, these losses can, upon reprocessing of the various fractions, be reclaimed with only a small loss of activity. By electron microscopy, purified membranes can be monitored for homogeneity and then solubilized by various methods. With deoxycholate (2%), it has been possible to solubilize 95% of pig lymphocyte plasma membrane (Allan and Crumpton, 1971). In addition to protein concentration and activity, enzymatic activities that serve as markers (Table VI) for the various subcellular fractions should be followed.

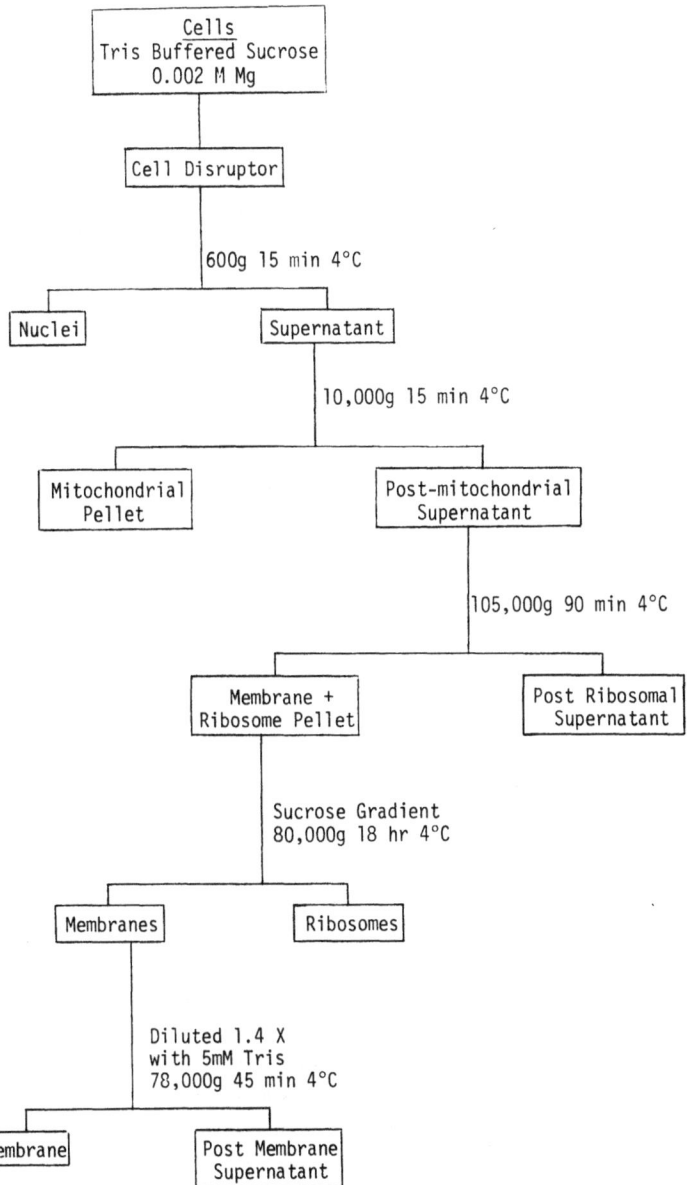

Figure 5. Scheme for isolation of plasma membrane and subcellular fractions. Data from Acton *et al.* (unpublished results).

Table VI. Methods for Monitoring Various Subcellular Fractions during Fractionation[a]

Subcellular fraction	Marker	Method of determination	Described by
Nuclei	DNA	Colorimetrically	Burton (1956)
Mitochondria	Succinic dehydrogenase	Decrease in the color intensity of 2, 6-dichlorophenolindophenol	Green et al. (1955)
Lysosomes	Acid RNase	Spectrophotometric measurement of liberated nucleosides	Kochakian and Williams (1973)
Microsomes	RNA	Spectrophotometrically	DeDeken-Grensen and DeDeken (1959)
Endoplasmic reticulum	DPNH diaphorase	Oxidation of NADP is measured by decrease of absorbance at 340 nm	Wallach and Kamat (1966)
Plasma membranes	5'-Nucleotidase	Inorganic P released from AMP	Tousler et al. (1970)
Plasma membranes	Na^+-K^+-dependent ATPase	Inorganic P released from ATP	Wallach and Kamat (1966)

[a] From Acton et al. (unpublished results).

B. Papain Solubilization

Figure 6 outlines the papain solubilization procedure (Shimada and Nathenson, 1969; Yamane and Nathenson, 1970), which compares the separation of specificities from two genotypes, H-2^b and H-2^d. In this procedure, Table VII shows the wide range of molecular sizes encountered during purification and the degree of complexity to be expected in isolating alloantigens, which is, of course, contigent on the allotype being used. The activities recovered at various stages are given in detail in the original studies.

The material obtained autolytically is separable into two major fractions: the first was excluded from the Sephadex G-200 gel volume with a molecular weight of 10^6 and can be further digested by papain to yield a fraction of 66,000 mol. wt.; the second fraction has a molecular weight of 66,000 and was included in the gel volume.

The source of antigens (H-2^b or H-2^d) is among the many variables on which papain effects depend. In these studies, crystalline papain was efficient in releasing H-2.2 and H-2.31. H-2.2 from H-2^b was a 39,000 mol. wt. substance (class II), and H-2.31 from H-2^d was a 76,000 mol. wt. substance (class I). On the other hand, crude papain on H-2^d type cells produced H-2.31 of 40,000 daltons. At a high concentration of crystalline

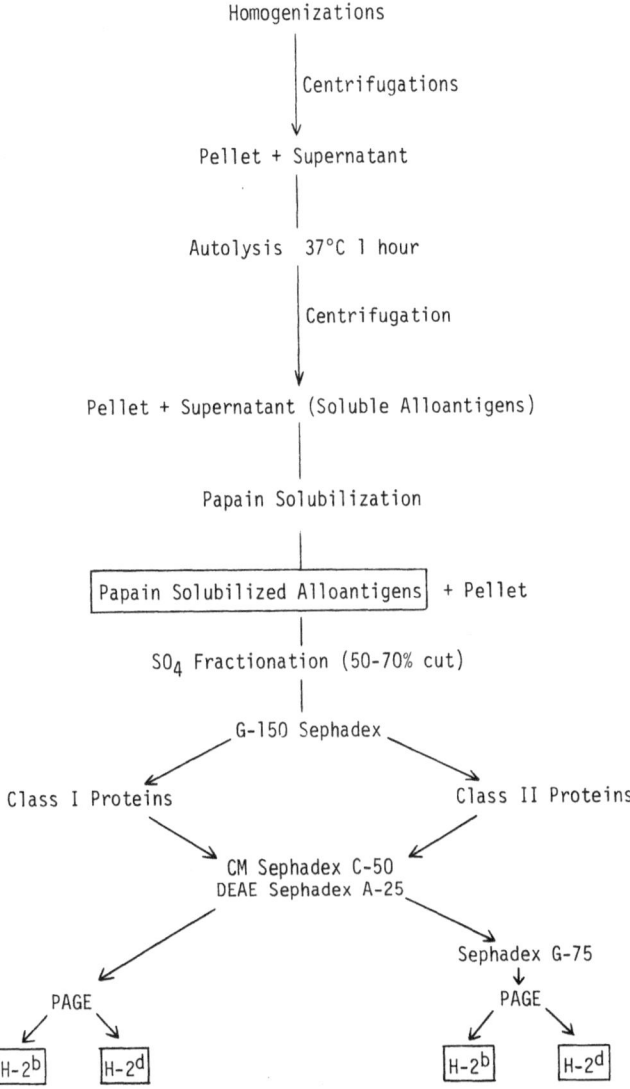

Figure 6. Purification of class I and class II proteins (alloantigens) from 450 g of mouse spleen tissue. Data from Shimada and Nathenson (1969) and Yamane and Nathenson (1970).

papain, H-2.31 could also be reduced to 40,000 mol. wt. Papain also solubilizes different specificities at different efficiencies. During the same interval, 18% of the H-2.5 specificity as opposed to only 5% of the H-2.2 was solubilized from the H-2^b cell type. With autolysis both specificities were solubilized in equivalent amounts. Therefore, the source and concentration of papain and the time required for digestion, as well as the substrate involved, play a major role in the size and amount of the product

Table VII. Range of Molecular Sizes Encountered during H-2[b] and
H-2[d] Alloantigen Isolation by Autocatalysis and Papain Digestion[a]

	Molecular size			
Autocatalysis	1,000,000	66,000		
Papain digestion				
H-2.5		65,000 ± 3000		
H-2.2			39,000 ± 2000	
H-2.4, 10, 13		65,000 ± 3000		
H-2.31 (large)		76,000 ± 4000		
H-2.31 (small)			40,000 ± 2000	
H-2.2				33,000
H-2.31				34,000

[a] Data from Shimada and Nathenson (1969) and Yamane and Nathenson (1970).

obtained. It should be remembered that papain treatment can also in-activate alloantigens differentially. Papain destroyed 62% of H-2.4 but only 14% of H-2.31 (Hess and Davies, 1974; Hartree, 1972).

A papain (crude) isolation procedure somewhat similar in protocol to the one described has been used by Mann and Nathenson (1969) and Mann et al. (1969) to isolate HL-A antigens from RPMI 4265 (LA 2, LA 4, 4d, 6b, 7c) and from Raji (LA 3, 4c, 4d, 6b). The active fraction was a glyco-protein with a molecular weight of 50,000 (Davies et al., 1968; Sanderson and Batchelor, 1968). When tested for stability, the activities of LA 2. LA 4, 4d, 6b, and 7c were largely inactivated by heating at 56°C and 37°C for 60 min. Standing at room temperature (24°C) caused a 50% loss of activity in these antigens over a period of 24 hr. The products were stable at − 10°C or at 4°C for only 24 hr. The rapid inactivation at various tem-peratures indicates possible contamination with proteolytic enzymes. Extreme pH changes caused inactivation; at pH 12.0 a 25% loss of activity occurred, but pH 6–10 afforded good recovery of activity. The papain procedure gave 0.025–0.030 mg purified antigens from 10^9 cultured cells and achieved a 25-fold increase in specific activity (Reisfeld and Pellegrino, 1972).

1. Plasma

From plasma, Miyakawa et al. (1973) purified alloantigens of different molecular sizes. These investigators showed that all papain-soluble activity isolated from lymphoid cell membrane is present in plasma components that have a molecular weight of 48,000 and $2–8 × 10^5$ daltons. When treated with papain, the large fragment consistently yielded fragments of 48,000 mol. wt. all of which had a common HL-A (β_2-microglobulin) component. Approximately 10% of the total HL-A2 activity of whole blood was present in soluble form in the plasma; the remaining 90% presumably represented alloantigens on cellular elements. Prolonged storage in the refrigerator did not change the HL-A activity in plasma, which provided evidence that HL-A products were not being leached from the cells. The presence of HL-A specificities on the different molecular species that were noted in blood may, to some extent, represent autolytic processes.

2. Spleen Membranes

Peterson *et al.* (1974) used crystalline papain digestion of spleen membranes for the isolation of 40,000–50,000 mol. wt. fragments composed of polypeptide chains of 33,000 and 12,000 mol. wt. These workers obtained HL-A preparations with specificities HL-A1, 2, W-10, W-15 at 80–90 % purity. The β_2-microglobulin (β_2-M), which carries no HL-A specificity, was present in the HL-A antigen of both the LA and Four series.

Large quantities of alloantigens from human, mouse, and rat were separated by hypotonic lysis in conjunction with papain treatment (Sanderson and Welsh, 1972). Table VIII compares alloantigens and proteins recovered from the three species at various stages of the experiment. The method provides a means of obtaining certain H-2 or HL-A specificities by DE-52, DEAE-Sephadex, or PAGE separation without dissociating them from specific immunoprecipitates. HL-A2 can usually be separated completely from HL-A1, 5, 7, 10, and 12 (Sanderson and Welsh, 1972). The PAGE migration pattern of antigenic materials affords a means of predetermining the elution position of these materials from DE-52 cellulose. On PAGE, the faster the mobility of the antigen the later it will emerge from a DE-52 column.

3. Tissue-Cultured Cells

HL-A2 and HL-A7 specificities were isolated on a large scale from starting material of 50 g tissue-cultured cells (Sanderson *et al.*, 1971; Sanderson and Welsh, 1972; Cresswell *et al.*, 1973). The overall yield of 16% was based on activity measurements from 50 g cells. This activity was equivalent to 490 μg HL-A2 and 560 μg HL-A7. The purified HL-A2 and HL-A7 on SDS-PAGE showed two bands with 34,000 and 11,000 mol. wt.

External labeling of HL-A antigens by ^{125}I or ^{131}I and internal labeling of alloantigens and their subsequent purification have been described. Labeling of alloantigens with either [14C] or [3H] amino acids or with either [3H]glucosamine or [3H]mannose makes it possible to follow

Table VIII. Results of Isolation of Alloantigens from Three Species: Comparison of Protein Recovery and Specific Activities at Various Stages of Preparation[a]

	Human		Mouse		Rat	
	Protein (mg)	Specific activity (units/mg)	Protein (mg)	Specific activity (units/mg)	Protein (mg)	Specific activity (units/mg)
Spleen	100,000	ND[b]	100,000	ND	100,000	ND
Membrane						
lipoprotein	3,000	ND	3,000	600	10,000	ND
Papain	1,000	400	1,200	75	4,000	400
$(NH_4)_2SO_4$	ND	ND	100	700	ND	ND
Sephadex	300	1,000	20	1,200	2,000	250
Cation exchange	150	2,000	8	2,000	500	400
Anion exchange	5	25,000	1.6	5,000	25	5,000
Disk						
electrophoresis	<0.05[c]	>100,000	0.05	40,000	0.5	25,000

[a] This table is intended only as a guide to the expected recoveries at each purification step; several points are worth nothing: (1) Sephadex and disc electrophoresis give up to 100% recovery of inhibitory units if distilled water is used for elution. (2) Antigen seems to bind strongly to anion exchange resin, and slow elution is necessary for optimal separation and recovery of inhibitory units (3) The purification at any stage is dependent on the foregoing procedure. (4) For large-scale preparations or for separation of a single specificity, anion exchange can be carried out before Sephadex chromatography. The rationale for this is that DE-52, for example, in quite small columns can handle large quantities of protein in high dilution without recourse to concentration. This is not so for Sephadex separations, where loading volumes of material must be small compared with the gel column bed volume. From Sanderson and Welsh (1972).
[b] Not done.
[c] Protein estimations at this most purified stage are inaccurate because of the necessity to conserve material.

the HL-A fragments that contain carbohydrate as well as the non-carbohydrate-containing β_2-M. This labeling was performed at 37°C over a period of 16 hr because cells stripped by papain digestion can reexpress 40–60% of their HL-A antigens at this temperature in this length of time (Cresswell et al., 1972). The papain treatment was capable of removing 60% of the activity of H-2^d alloantigens on tumor cell membranes; with such cells, resynthesis of the antigens occurred in 60 min and recovery was 100% after 6 hr (Schwartz and Nathenson, 1971a). Turnover rates of such membrane antigens can be studied and the $T_{1/2}$ of the radiolabeled surface antigens can be established (Schwartz et al., 1973b). Turner et al. (1972) conducted similar studies for the regeneration of HL-A antigens.

Separation of pure products by the procedure of Cresswell et al. (1973) yielded peptides of relatively constant molecular weights; those obtained through use of Sephadex G-200 in SDS were 32,000 and 13,000, through agarose filtration in 6 M guanidine were 29,000 and 11,000, and through SDS-PAGE were 34,000 and 11,000. The fragments were separated either with or without mercaptoethanol reduction of the complexes, which shows that the two peptide fragments are not linked by disulfide bonds. When either [³H]glucosamine or [³H]mannose was used as a label, only the larger of the two alloantigen fragments was labeled. Since β_2-M contains no carbohydrate, neither glucosamine nor mannose was incorporated. Identical results were obtained with HL-A2 and HL-A7. The large peptide fragments of HL-A2 and HL-A7 can be electrophoretically separated, but the small fragment β_2-M cannot. At pH 8.7 the HL-A7 glycopeptide had greater mobility. At pH 4.5 the HL-A2 glycopeptide had greater mobility. However, the small peptide fragment displayed identical mobilities at either pH value. Radioactive amino acids were used in measuring the two fragments, which had a 2.6:1 ratio of molecular weight and 1.9:1 ratio of radioactivity. The similarity of both ratios suggests that the fragments are present in a 1:1 molar ratio. The discrepancy in the two ratios is probably due to the unlabeled carbohydrates in the large molecular weight fragments.

The use of rabbit anti-β_2 sera provides a mild means of dissociating a 33,000 mol. wt. HL-A fragment from the β_2-M. By this method, the released fragment remains fully antigenic rather than having its antigenic activity reduced or eliminated as is the case when the fragments are dissociated by using NaI, NaSCN, SDS, urea, or guanidine-HCl (Nakamuro et al., 1975).

C. Lectin Affinity Column

Considerable progress has been made in the isolation of human and mouse histocompatibility antigens. Methods are being devised to allow quantitative yields of the HL-A and H-2 alloantigens with a minimum loss of activity and fewer experimental steps. Hayman et al. (1972, 1973) and Snary et al. (1974) used the specific binding of glycoproteins to plant lectins (Lens culinaris phytohemagglutinin, LCH) for isolating alloantigens. LCH has antibodylike activity for glucose, mannose, and related sugar residues and is superior to concanavalin A (Con A) for the purification of glycoproteins. Because of strong binding, the Con A column separation gave poor yields and also incomplete removal of the glycoprotein from the column.

LCH was coupled to Sepharose 4B that had been activated with cyanogen bromide in the presence of methyl-α-D-glucopyranoside. Detergent-solubilized plasma membrane proteins were passed through this column. The column-bound glycoproteins were eluted with methyl α-D-glucopyranoside. The eluted fraction contained most of the added HL-A activity. Snary et al. (1974) gives a detailed description of this procedure.

D. Detergent Solubilization

The primary purpose for using detergent extraction procedures is to avoid enzymatic or autolytic breakdown of alloantigens in order to procure, as nearly as possible, the entire lipoglycoprotein molecule in its native form. Nonionic detergents were used to solubilize mouse and human histocompatibility antigens (Schwartz and Nathenson, 1971b; Schwartz et al., 1973a; Springer and Strominger, 1973), as well as components from purified membranes of various cell types (Allan and Crumpton, 1971; Helenius and Simons, 1972; Meunier et al., 1972; Helenius and Sönderlund, 1973; Hayman et al., 1973).

Detergent-solubilized alloantigens can be monitored by a radioimmune binding assay. Briefly, target cells are fixed with 0.25% glutaraldehyde, which does not destroy antigenicity and permits binding assays to be carried out in nonionic detergents at concentrations of 1–2% (Williams, 1973; Acton et al., 1974).

To assay a particular alloantigen, mouse antiserum is titrated to determine an appropriate dilution that gives about 30,000 cpm when reacted with $[^{125}I]F(ab')_2$ rabbit anti-mouse IgG. Standard absorption curves can be established by using the antiserum dilution and absorbing with increasing amounts of target cells. Determination of the effective range of cells required to provide an absorption curve will allow a comparison with the absorptive capacity of detergent-solubilized antigen relative to the number of cells from which it was extracted. The yield and specific activity can be determined at each step during solubilization and purification.

These approaches have been used by Acton et al. (unpublished results) in extracting rat histocompatibility antigen (H-1) from rat thymocytes with the nonionic detergent Lubrol PX. Rat red blood cells that express H-1 served as glutaraldehyde-fixed target cells. Nonionic detergents show variable efficiency in extracting rat H-1 and Thy-1.1 alloantigens from thymocytes (Table IX). Several detergents were effective in solubilizing 100% of the H-1. With Lubrol PX, Triton X-67, and Tween-40 it was possible to extract Thy-1.1 into a 2500g particulate fraction, but not a 200,000g soluble fraction. On leukemic cells that derived from a rat thymoma, Lubrol PX and Triton X-67 proved ineffective. These experiments show that, although detergents can be effectively utilized to solubilize membrane components, each new component to be studied must be reevaluated with a group of nonionic detergents for each given cell type.

The NP-40 nonionic detergent extraction of HL-A antigens was used in conjunction with electrofocusing to isolate active fragments of 200,000 and 15,000–30,000 mol. wt. In certain instances, the HL-A specificities were separable, based on their isoelectric point (Dautigny et al.,

Table IX. Detergent Solubilization of Rat Thymocyte Membrane Components[a]

Detergent 2% at 10⁸ cells/ml	Percent Thy-1.1 in solution		Percent H-1 in solution	
	30 min 2500g	30 min 200,000g	30 min 2500g	30 min 200,000g
Thymocytes				
NP-40	20	10	100	100
Triton X-100	34	12	100	100
Triton X-67	100	25	100	100
Lubrol PX	100	65	100	100
Brij-35	50	10	—	—
Tween-40	100	20	—	—
Leukemic cells				
Lubrol PX	25	10		
Triton X-67	50	0		

[a] Data from Letarte-Muirhead *et al.* (1974) and Acton (unpublished results).

1973). Strominger *et al.* (1974) showed HL-A specificities migrating as a single species on PAGE, but microheterogeneity caused by differences in sialic acid content was evident by electrofocusing. The soluble HL-A antigens extracted by NP-40 produced high yields of activity from platelets and did not sediment at 165,000g even after 90 min. The preparation remained soluble even after 90% of the detergent was removed. The molecular sizes of active fragments were determined by the detergent protein ratio (D/P) used: 20 mg protein in 0.5% NP-40 v/v yielded a 200,000 mol. wt. active fragment, whereas 5 mg protein in 0.5% NP-40 v/v yielded a 15,000–30,000 mol. wt. active fragment. The characteristics of the purified extract preparations are given in Table X. Soluble antigen from platelets extracted by detergent was believed to be 10 times more active than that from papain digestion (Weydert *et al.*, 1971). Storage of platelets before extraction did not influence the activity of the extract.

E. Solubilization by Sonication

Sonication provides a means of obtaining water-soluble alloantigens. Low molecular weight fragments (15,000 daltons for guinea pigs and 34,000 daltons for HL-A) were antigenically active proteins without lipid or carbohydrate residues (Kahan and Reisfeld, 1968a,b; Reisfeld and Kahan, 1970). Purified guinea pig alloantigen (1–3 μg) induced accelerated rejection of skin allograft; 0.1 μg caused DTH in a sensitized host (Kahan and

Table X. Characteristics of NP-40 Isolated HL-A Alloantigens[a]

	Molecular weight	Electrofocusing	Isoelectric point
At low detergent/protein ratio			
Platelets (HL-A2, HL-A5)[b]	200,000	HL-A2, HL-A5 in same fraction	6.2
Platelets (HL-A2, HL-A9)	200,000	HL-A2, HL-A9 in same fraction	5.5
At high detergent/protein ratio			
Platelets (HL-A2, HL-A7)	15,000–30,000	HL-A specificities separated	
		HL-A7	5
		HL-A2	7

[a] Data from Dautigny et al. (1973).
[b] PAGE of this preparation at pH 7.5, 7.5% gel showed a single protein band with R_f of 0.42.

Reisfeld, 1967; Kahan, 1967) and evoked blast transformation of sensitized leukocytes *in vitro* (Kahan *et al.*, 1967). A 10,000-fold increase in specific activity of the antigen liberated by ultrasound was obtained after PAGE. The guinea pig alloantigen was strain specific and could be obtained from lung, spleen, kidney, and liver (kidney and liver components were heterogeneous). In PAGE of varying porosity in the presence of 8 M urea, spleen and lung gave homogeneous components.

With respect to HL-A antigens from lymphocytes, the sonic method produced yields that were, at best, 22% of the total absorptive capacity of the cell membrane. The amount of lipoprotein released from the lymphocytes was excessive in comparison with that released from other tissue sources; this was a disadvantage. The sonic method does not permit large-scale manipulations; i.e., 30 g (3×10^{10} cells) required 100 separate sonic treatments (Reisfeld and Kahan, 1972). The purified HL-A material contained no lipid or carbohydrate and was stable for several months at $-20°C$. In PAGE, the isolated homogeneous alloantigen ranged in RF from 0.78–0.80. Ultracentrifugal analysis (Yphantis sedimentation equilibrium) revealed that 94% was monodisperse and had a molecular weight of 34,600, and 6% aggregated material with a molecular weight of 150,000. A flow diagram of this method is given in Fig. 7.

F. 3 M KCl Extraction

The 3 M KCl (chaotropic ions) extraction method is one of the most reliable for isolating various alloantigens from viable cells. It has been claimed

```
Spleens and Lungs
        | 75 guinea pigs (strain 2 or 13)
        | Single cell suspension prepared by pressing
        |    tissues through sequential series of cyto-sieves
        | Erythrocytes lysed with 2% acetic acid in
        |    Tris-sucrose buffer '

50 ml (4 x 10⁶ cells/ml)
Expose 5 min 10 KC/sec sound generated by a Raytheon
model DF 101 magnetostriction apparatus

        | Centrifuge
        |

         Pellet + Supernatant
(Cellular debris       |Ultracentrifuge (130,000 g)
 discarded)            |

         Pellet + Supernatant
(Cell membranes        |Concentrate by dialysis vs Aquacide I
 discarded)            | C grade (Calbiochem., Los Angeles, Calif.)

    Sephadex G-200 (2.5 x 100 cm)
        |Equilibrated with 0.5 M glycine, 0.2 M Tris,
        | 0.5% mannitol, pH 8.0 at 25°C
        |

    Sephadex Fraction I
            (Antigenic activity eluted at the front
            of the inner volume)
    Desalt over Sephadex G-25, equilibrate with
     0.05% mannitol and lyophilize
    Reconstitute in distilled water (Dis. H₂0)
        |

    PAGE (Polyacrylamide gel electrophoresis)
        | 7.5% gel
        | 17 components identified
        | Component 15 RF 0.73 to 0.74 active
        | Slice component 15, elute, shake in 0.5 ml
        |  Dis. H₂0 5 days 4°C
        |

  Re-PAGE
            Elute, dialyze 4 changes (2000 ml)
            Dis. H₂0, Lyophilize
```

Figure 7. Isolation of water-soluble alloantigens solubilized by sonication. Data from Kahan and Reisfeld (1968a) and Reisfeld and Kahan (1970).

to give antigenically active HL-A fragments of 31,000 mol. wt. (Fig. 8) in relatively high yields. In the process of isolation, the β_2-M was apparently dissociated from the HL-A specificities (Reisfeld et al., 1971; Reisfeld and Pellegrino, 1972). The excellent recovery of 35–80% of the HL-A2 and HL-A7 activity was realized by this procedure. High cell viability was important for optimal yields. With starting cell preparations of low (23%) viability, yields of only 9% with poor specific activity were obtained.

RPMI 1788 peripheral lymphocyte line or
        WI-L2 spleen cell line
                |
                |
    50 x 10^9 dispersed lymphoid cells
        10^9 cells/20 ml phosphate buffered saline with 3 M KCl, pH 7.4
        Agitate 16 hr, 4°C Eberbach shaker
                    |
                    | Centrifuge 163,000g (average speed) 1 hr
                    |
        Pellet + Supernatant
    (Discard)   Dialysis, 200 ml saline, 3 changes in 24 hr
                        Gelatinous material (mostly DNA)
                            |
                            | Centrifuge 1500g, 20 min
                            |
        Pellet + Supernatant (crude antigen preparation)
(Gelatinous material, | DNA negative by diphenylamine of a
    discard) | hot TCA extract or by isotope studies
                         | Dialyze, Tris-phosphate buffer, pH 6.7
                         | (0.045 M Tris, 0.032 M H$_3$PO$_4$)
                         |
        PAGE (Electrophoresis)
        50-70 mg protein sample
        Applied to Buchler polyprep 100 column
        0°C in system "B", pH 9.6, 7.5% gel
        Constant current 35 ma
        Collect 8 ml fractions, flow rate 0.8 ml/min with
            Tris-HCl elution buffer (0.13 M Tris, 0.18 M HCl,
            pH 8.2, 10% W/V sucrose)
                |
                |
        Antigenic activity in fractions eluting at RF 0.78 to 0.80
                |
                |
        Re-electrophoresis (7.5% gel, 0°C, pH 9.6)
            |
            |
        Single component similar to sonic preparation

Figure 8. High yield KCl extraction. Data from Reisfeld et al. (1971).

Extraction of freeze-thawed cells by KCl, hypotonic elution, or decompression (Hunter and Comerford, 1961) yielded only 3–8% HL-A antigens.

KCl probably dissociates hydrogen bonds and salt linkages in releasing alloantigens in soluble form. The soluble antigens did not sediment at 163,000 g, but passed through a 0.45 Millipore filter. Electron microscopy showed no cellular ultrastructure. The 3 M KCl method extracted more antigen than 0.3 M or 1.0 M KCl. The 16-hr extraction gave maximum yields; repeated extraction was not practical. This KCl extraction procedure caused extensive disruption of intracellular structures and released more nucleoproteins and nuclear DNA, but less lipoprotein from the cell surface than did sonication. KCl has a distinct advantage over the sonication method since lipoproteins interfere with purification by causing aggregation and trapping of antigenically active fragments. The use of 3 M KCl at 40°C rather than at 4°C reduced activity.

Because it is mild, the KCl method may be preferable to other procedures such as papain digestion (which breaks peptide linkages and is difficult to control) or extraction with complex salts and detergents (which are difficult to remove from the antigen product). However, Snary *et al.* (1974) reported that KCl extraction and Na-deoxycholate solubilization yielded 12 and 16% alloantigens, respectively. This was considerably lower than reported earlier (30–80%). In the final purified alloantigen obtained by the KCl method, the lack of carbohydrate suggests that the alloantigen had undergone partial degradation.

Archibald sedimentation equilibrium analysis showed HL-A antigens of 31,000 mol. wt. that were obtained from RPMI 1788 sediment at 2.3S. The HL-A antigen appeared to be a single polypeptide chain with two intrachain disulfide bonds (Reisfeld and Kahan, 1972).

G. Molecular Sizes Encountered in Isolation

A summary of the different molecular sizes encountered by various investigators is presented in Table XI. Schwartz *et al.* (1973a) reported that the molecular fragments (in monomer form) that were solubilized by NP-40 were slightly larger than the corresponding glycoprotein that was solubilized by papain. The NP-40 and papain products displayed a difference in molecular weight of about 5000 (range 2500–6000). Papain treatment of an NP-40 solubilized molecule produces a fragment that is the same size as the papain fragment prepared directly from cell membranes without detergent solubilization and includes the major portion of the molecule, i.e., 75–85% of the native 43,000 mol. wt. H-2 subunit. As described earlier, the H-2 antigens are composed of glycoprotein subunits of 43,000–47,000 daltons depending on the genetic determinant to be isolated. At least some of these antigens may exist as dimers that are linked by disulfide bonds. By noncovalent binding, the dimers and possibly a variable portion of monomers may form an aggregate that has a mol. wt. of 400,000. The properties of different detergents may influence the micelle size, and the extent to which the detergent binds to the functional isolated alloantigen can cause differences in observed molecular weight. Little or no binding occurs between deoxycholate and water soluble proteins (Helenius and Simons, 1972). HL-A glycoproteins solubilized in deoxycholate were of smaller molecular size (Snary *et al.*, 1974) than the NP-40 solubilized 200,000 HL-A (Dautigny *et al.*, 1973) and the 380,000 H-2 alloantigen

Table XI. Molecular Sizes Encountered with Selected Number of Solubilization Procedures

Histocompatibilities	HL-A	H-2	H-2	HL-A	HL-A	HL-A	HL-A
Authors	Dautigny	Schwartz	Nathenson	Pressman	Others[a]	Reisfeld	Reisfeld and Kahan
Tissue source	Platelets	Cells	Cells	Plasma	Cells	Cells	Cells
Method	NP-40 (low D/P[b] high D/P)	NP-40, 0.5%	Autolysis, papain	Papain	Papain	Sonication	3 M KCl
Molecular sizes detected							
> 100,000	200,000	380,000	> 1,000,000	800,000; 200,000			
~ > 50,000		SDS → 88,000 (dimer) → 47,000 H-2K[d]	Papain → 66,000 / 57,000 (Class I)	Papain → 48,000	50,000		
~ > 40,000		SDS + ME → 43,000 H-2D[d] (monomer)	Papain → 40,000 (Class II)		43,000		
~ > 30,000	30,000; 15,000 (active)		33,000	SDS → 34,000 +11,000	SDS → 33,000 +11,000	33,000 (active); 15,000 (guinea pig; active)	34,000
Chemical nature	Glycoprotein	Glycoprotein	Glycoprotein	Glycoprotein	Glycoprotein	Protein	Protein

[a] Data from Miyakawa et al. (1973), Cresswell et al. (1973), Peterson et al. (1974), Mann et al. (1971).

[b] Detergent to protein ratio.

(Schwartz *et al.*, 1973*a*). It is conceivable that an 88,000 dimer may appear two- to fourfold larger if large amounts of nonionic detergents are bound to the alloantigen as suggested by Snary *et al.* (1974).

Because the physical properties of HL-A and H-2 are highly similar, it was postulated that a fragment comparable to β_2-M will be discovered for H-2 antigens. Silver and Hood (1974) used Triton X-100 detergent to solubilize an H-2 alloantigen containing two polypeptides which were noncovalently linked with mol. wt. of 47,000 and 11,500. The 11,500 mol. wt. polypeptide appears to be equivalent to a mouse β_2-M. Antiserum to human β_2-M cross-reacts with such a mouse fragment. Peptide mapping experiments revealed close homology between the mouse protein and human β_2-M (Rask *et al.*, 1974).

Table XI shows that active HL-A fragments of low molecular weight (33,000) can be directly obtained by the methods of Dautigny *et al.* (1973) and Reisfeld and Kahan (1970). Broadly speaking, active molecules can be isolated in sizes from > 30,000 to > 1,000,000. Notably, in most of the isolation procedures the size of the monomer subunit ranges from 40,000 to 70,000 mol. wt.

Probably the 88,000 mol. wt. fragment that was solubilized in detergent and isolated by Schwartz and Nathenson (1971*a*) represents a dimer of heavy chains. Monomers that range from 48,000 to 65,000 mol. wt. and are associated with β_2-M can be isolated with papain digestion. Strominger *et al.* (1974) showed that in detergent and ME an approximately 56,000 mol. wt. HL-A antigen dissociates into two polypeptide chains of 44,000 and 12,000 mol. wt.; the larger protein was hydrolyzed by papain, in two steps, to an intermediate, 39,000 mol. wt. fragment and a final, 34,000 mol. wt. fragment.

In detergent without ME, it was possible to demonstrate an 82,000 mol. wt., polypeptide chain dimer that was not associated with β_2-M. In the presence of ME, this dimer dissociates into a 44,000 mol. wt. monomer. The heavy chains are linked by disulfide bridges located in a portion of the molecule that is probably embedded in the cell membrane and can be removed by papain proteolysis. This indicates that an additional protein fragment of approximately 10,000 mol. wt. for each monomer exists, that this fragment is susceptible to papain digestion, and that it plays some role in holding the heavy chain dimer together. The probable function of the additional protein fragment is to integrate the HL-A determinant into the cell membrane. It may also serve as a hydrophobic nucleus that causes nonspecific aggregation of macromolecules.

IV. Chemical Nature of H-2 and HL-A Antigens

A. Protein Nature

On PAGE, guinea pig transplantation antigen solubilized by sound (see Section III E) gave a homogeneous purified "component 15" of 15,000 mol. wt. No lipid or carbohydrate was detected. Guinea pig strains 2 and 13 displayed a characteristic and reproducible amino acid composition (Reisfeld and Kahan, 1971). The two antigens varied in their content of serine, alanine, valine, leucine, isoleucine, and possibly tyrosine and phenylalanine (Kahan and Reisfeld, 1968a).

Reisfeld and Kahan (1971) reported that

> results strongly suggest that the transplantation antigens isolated from the two inbred, histoincompatible strains of guinea pigs possess allotypic specificities related to protein structure analogous to the polymorphic antigenic determinants found on serum proteins of numerous species. It is reasonable to assume that most of those amino acid differences may have resulted from one-step mutations and that at least some of these amino acids are involved in determining the characteristic immunological properties of the molecules. It is likely that this protein polymorphism reflects the chemical nature of the genetically segregating determinants of transplantation antigens, since these antigens were essentially proteins with no detectable lipid or carbohydrate (at a level of one percent).

When low-intensity sound was used to solubilize HL-A alloantigens from RPMI 1788, the purified materials exhibited no detectable lipid or carbohydrate. There were differences in the amino acid compositions of antigens obtained from cell lines that expressed differences in phenotype (Reisfeld and Kahan, 1971). Purified HL-A alloantigen from RPMI 1788 had an $S_{20,w}$ of 2.35 and a molecular weight of 31,000 daltons (Reisfeld and Kahan, 1972). HL-A antigen oxidized with performic acid had four cysteic acid residues, as shown by the presence of 3.6 carboxymethylcysteine residues by amino acid analysis. Thus the 31,000 mol. wt. antigen seems to be a single polypeptide chain with two intrachain disulfide bridges.

Yamane and Nathenson (1970) purified class II glycoproteins and found them to have a molecular weight of approximately 33,000 in contrast to a molecular weight of 57,000–66,000 for class I glycoproteins. Mann and Nathenson (1969), who made a direct comparison of molecular properties of H-2 and HL-A products, also found that papain treatment produced two glycoprotein classes that differed in size and carried a different series of antigenic specificities. Table XII shows the general chemical compositions for H-2 and HL-A products.

The amino acid compositions of the H-2^b and H-2^d class I fragments differed by approximately 1 mole % in their arginine and glutamic acid contents (Shimada and Nathenson, 1969). Analyses of the class II fragments

Table XII. Chemical Nature of H-2 and HL-A Alloantigens[a]

Alloantigen	Molecular weight	Protein	Neutral carbohydrate	Glucosamine	Sialic acid	Phosphate	Lipid
H-2^b and H-2^d class I	58,000–65,000	80–90%	4%	3–4%	1%	—	—
H-2^b and H-2^d class II	33,000–37,000	70–80%	7%	1% (H-2^d) 4–5% (H-2^b)	1–3%	—	—
RAJI			5–8%		0.95%		
HL-A	50,000	90%		0.5%			
R-4265			6–8%		0.65%	—	—

[a] Data from Nathenson (1970).

revealed a greater divergence between strains as indicated: 4 mole % in serine, 2 mole % in aspartic acid, and from 0.5 to 1.5 mole % in valine, leucine, isoleucine, and tyrosine (Yamane and Nathenson, 1970). The peptide composition of the two class I purified alloantigen fragments was also examined by thin-layer cellulose micromethods (Shimada et al., 1970). Approximately 90% of the resolved peptides produced by cyanogen bromide and trypsin treatments contained identical materials in both H-2^b and H-2^d alloantigens. The H-2^b and H-2^d materials contained three and four identifiable, unique peptides, respectively; 38 peptides were common to both preparations. Nathenson (1970) found the amino acid composition of H-2 and HL-A genotypes in man and mouse to be highly similar.

B. Carbohydrate Content

The carbohydrate composition was studied by using alloantigen preparations that contained radioactively labeled monosaccharides (Muramatsu and Nathenson, 1970). The carbohydrate portion of the glycoprotein, which carried alloantigenic specificities of the H-2^b and the H-2^d genotypes, consisted of two carbohydrate chains each of which contained approximately 12–15 monosaccharides. The pronase-digested glycopeptides from the two strains exhibited identical properties during Sephadex G-50 and DEAE Sephadex A-25 chromatography. At the stage of analysis currently possible, the two genotypes appear to have the same carbohydrate composition. Details of the tentative carbohydrate structural configuration of the H-2 glycoprotein molecule are given by Nathenson and Cullen (1974).

Sanderson *et al.* (1971) strongly emphasized the role of carbohydrate in alloantigenic activity, but little experimental evidence has appeared to indicate the essentiality of carbohydrates for such activity. Removal of all sialic acid, as much as 70% of the galactose, and 20% of the *N*-acetylgalactosamine residues from the papain-treated H-2 antigen had no effect on antigenicity (Muramatsu and Nathenson, 1971). A central role for the protein moiety in determining H-2 antigenic activity is suggested by these findings in conjunction with previous observations on the sensitivity of the alloantigens to protein-denaturing procedures and to selective loss of antigenic activity after specific chemical modification of amino acid groups (Pancake and Nathenson, 1973).

C. β_2-Microglobulin

The 11,000 mol. wt. fragment consistently associated with HL-A was shown to be β_2-M, which, as orginally described by Berggård and Bearn (1968), had about 100 amino acid residues. β_2-M appears to be the invariant or common portion of all 45,000 (approximately 43,000–50,000) mol. wt. HL-A fragments isolated by papain digestion (Nakamuro *et al.*, 1973; Grey *et al.*, 1973). β_2-M is also present in other HL-A active macromolecules of different molecular sizes (65,000, 130,000, 200,000, and 400,000). The 45,000 mol. wt. product can be dissociated with denaturing agents (SDS, urea, and guanidine) to a noncovalently linked 34,000 molecule and to the 11,000 β_2-M entities at a molar ratio of 1:1. β_2-M carries no HL-A specificities or carbohydrate moieties and can be isolated from plasma (Miyakawa *et al.*, 1973), urine (Berggård and Bearn, 1968), and centrifuged tissue culture medium (Tanigaki *et al.*, 1973).

Treatment of human lymphocytes with antiserum to HL-A antigens results in capping of these antigens (Bernoco *et al.*, 1972). Addition of anti-β_2-M antibodies to lymphocytes likewise causes capping of HL-A antigens (Poulik *et al.*, 1973; Solheim and Thorsby, 1974), as well as H-2 antigens (Östberg *et al.*, 1974). β_2-M, the first fragment of the HL-A complex to be sequenced (Fig. 9), reveals a homology of sequence in the constant regions (CH1, CH2, and CH3) of γ_1 heavy chains of immunoglobulin G_1. The greatest homology is seen in the CH3 domain (Cunningham and Berggård, 1974).

Edelman (1970) showed that antibody molecules are composed of a series of compact domains (Fig. 10). Domains in the variable region (VL and VH) mediate antigen-binding functions, whereas those in the C region (CL, CH1, CH2, and CH3) mediate effector functions. Each domain contains about 100 amino acid residues or a single disulfide loop of 60 residues. β_2-M, which appears to be a free Ig domain, contains a

```
1                                        10                                       20
ILE-GLN-ARG-THR-PRO-LYS-ILE-GLN-VAL-TYR-SER-ARG-HIS-PRO-ALA-GLU-ASX-GLY-LYS-SER-


21                                       30                                       40
ASX-PHE-LEU-ASN-CYS-TYR-VAL-SER-GLY-PHE-HIS-PRO-SER-ASP-ILE-GLU-VAL-ASP-LEU-LEU-


41                                       50                                       60
LYS-ASP-GLY-GLU-ARG-ILE-GLX-LYS-VAL-(ASX,HIS,SER,GLX)-LEU-SER-PHE-SER-LYS-ASN-SER-


61                                       70                                       80
TRP-PHE-TYR-LEU-(LEU,TYR,SER)-TYR-THR-GLU-PHE-THR-PRO-THR-GLU-LYS-ASP-GLU-TYR-ALA-


81                                       90                                      100
CYS-ARG-VAL-ASX-HIS-VAL-THR-LEU-SER-GLX-PRO-LYS-ILE-VAL-LYS-TRP-ASP-ARG-ASP-MET
```

Figure 9. Amino acid sequence of β_2-microglobulin. Peterson *et al.* (1972).

single intrachain disulfide loop of 57 amino acid residues similar to the loops of immunoglobulin (constant region).

On their surfaces, cultured lymphocytes have β_2-M, which they actively secrete at a rate of 21 molecules/cell/sec (Hütteroth *et al.*, 1973). Since HL-A antigens are present on the surface of essentially all tissue cells, it would be presumed that β_2-M is present in every instance. On a 45,000 mol. wt. HL-A subunit, β_2-M represents 20–25% of its quaternary structure (Grey *et al.*, 1973).

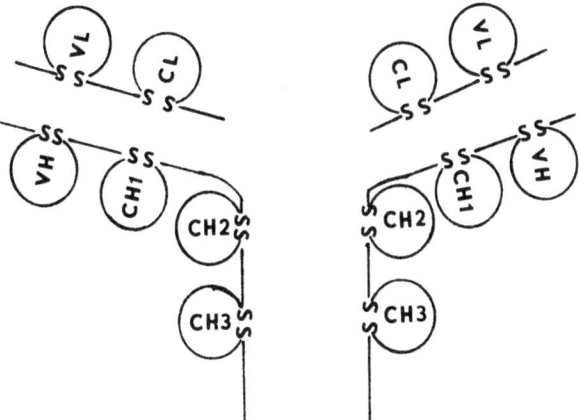

Figure 10. Diagram showing the immunoglobulin domains. The light-chain domains are VL and CL. The heavy-chain domains are VH, CH1, CH2, and CH3. Each domain contains approximately 100 amino acid residues and has a single disulfide loop of some 60 residues.

Although no functions have as yet been attributed to β_2-M, it is of significance that this ubiquitous molecule is found in relation to the cell receptor or recognition molecules. The close resemblance of the H-2 and HL-A subunits (45,000) to IgG heavy chains (50,000), and the strong similarity between these subunits and the 45,000 mol. wt. I gene products (Ia antigens) lead to the speculation that the histocompatibility alloantigen may represent recognition molecules or receptors. This was indicated in the case of I gene products and surface immunoglobulins.

The loci of H-2, I, and Ig regions appear to be interrelated since each, in its own way, participates in immune recognition or in cell–cell recognition or cooperation. Interestingly enough, β_2-M, which is coded by another locus (chromosome 15) and not on chromosome 6, which carries the HL-A region (Goodfellow et al., 1975), may be the link to these three systems. However, β_2-M does not display polymorphism, and it is unlikely to be part of the receptor-specific site of the T lymphocyte or to contribute to the specific determinants of the HL-A antigens.

V. Conclusion

Since the detergent-solubilized alloantigens appear to be of larger molecular size than the papain-digested molecule, it seems reasonable to assume

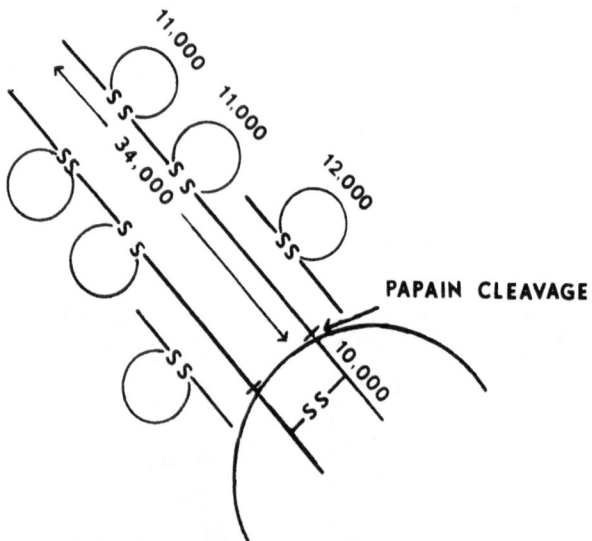

Figure 11. Diagram of an alloantigen molecule on the surface of a cell. Molecular weight of the heavy chain dimer is approximately 88,000. A 10,000 molecular weight hydrophobic region of the heavy chain, which is presumably buried in the membrane, links the dimer by an intrachain disulfide bridge. The location of the 12,000 dalton β_2-M is not known, but it does not appear to play a role in determining specificity at the receptor end.

that the membrane-bound hydrophobic region is cleaved by papain but not by detergent. The heavy chain dimer is probably linked by a disulfide bridge in the hydrophobic region (Fig. 11). The presence of two cysteine groups in the approximately 34,000 mol. wt. moiety indicates the presence of two disulfide loops of about 11,000 mol. wt. each, which represent two domains (Strominger *et al.*, 1974). The position of the noncovalently linked 12,000 mol. wt. β_2-M is not known. This microglobulin lacks polymorphism or alloantigenic activity, displays its greatest homology with the CH3 immunoglobulin domain, and can be shown to be independently associated with the surface membrane. In the mouse, a similar molecule is associated with alloantigens of different specificities (H-2, Ia, *Tla*). For these reasons β_2-M may not be associated with the receptor end of the molecule. Whereas the specific receptor functions and structural aspects of recognition molecules are just now in the process of being clearly delineated, it is probable that HL-A, H-2, Ia, *Tla*, and other alloantigens will have a certain constancy of features and will be similar in molecular configuration at the surface of the cell.

VI. References

Acton, R. T., Letarte-Muirhead, M., and Williams, A. F., unpublished results.

Acton, R. T., Morris, R. J., and Williams, A. F., 1974, *Eur. J. Immunol.* **4**:598.

Allan, D., and Crumpton, M. J., 1970, *Biochem. J.* **120**:133.

Allan, D., and Crumpton, M. J., 1971, *Biochem. J.* **123**:967.

Amos, D. B., 1964, *Prog. Med. Genet.* **3**:106.

Armerding, D., and Katz, D. H., 1974, *J. Exp. Med.* **140**:19.

Armerding, D., and Katz, D. H., 1975, *Fed. Proc.* **34**:1011 (abst.).

Armerding, D., Sachs, D. H., and Katz, D. H., 1974, *J. Exp. Med.* **140**:1717.

Avis, P. J. G., 1972, Pressure homogenization of mammalian cells, in: *Subcellular Components, Preparation, and Fractionation* (G. D. Birnie, ed.), pp. 1–13, University Park Press, Baltimore.

Bach, F. H., 1975, Detection of cell surface alloantigens, in: *The 7th Annual Miami Winter Symposia* (E. E. Smith and D. W. Ribbons, eds.), p. 55, University of Miami, Miami, Fla.

Benacerraf, B., and McDevitt, H. O., 1972, *Science* **175**:273.

Berggård, I., and Bearn, A. G., 1968, *J. Biol. Chem.* **243**:4095.

Bernoco, D., Cullen, S., Scudeller, G., Trinchieri, G., and Ceppellini, R., 1972, HL-A molecules at the cell surface, in: *Histocompatibility Testing* (J. Dausset and J. Colombani, eds.), pp. 527–537, Williams and Wilkins, Baltimore.

Boyse, E. A., Old, L. J., and Stockert, E., 1966, The TL (thymus leukemia) antigen: A review, in: *Immunopathology: IVth International Symposium* (P. Grabar and P. A. Miescher, eds.) pp. 23–40, Grune and Stratton, New York.

Boyse, E. A., Old, L. J., and Stockert, E., 1968, *Proc. Natl. Acad. Sci. U.S.A.* **60**:886.

Boyse, E. A., Flaherty, L., Stockert, E., and Old, L. J., 1972, *Transplantation* **13**:431.

Brown, J. L., Kato, K., Silver, J., and Nathenson, S. G., 1974, *Biochemistry* **13**:3174.

Burton, K., 1956, *Biochem. J.* **62**:315.

Cresswell, P., Turner, M. J., Strominger, J. L., and Sanderson, A. R., 1972, *Fed. Proc.* **31**:737 (abst.).

Cresswell, P., Turner, M. J., and Strominger, J. L., 1973, *Proc. Natl. Acad. Sci. U.S.A.* **70**:1603.

Cullen, S. E., and Nathenson, S. G., 1974, Further characterization of Ia (immune response region associated) antigen molecules, in: *The Immune System: Genes, Receptors, Signals* (E. E. Sercarz, A. R. Williamson, and C. F. Fox, eds.), pp. 191–200, Academic Press, New York.

Cullen, S. E., Schwartz, B. D., and Nathenson, S. G., 1972a, *J. Immunol.* **108**:596.

Cullen, S. E., Schwartz, B. D., Nathenson, S. G., and Cherry, M, 1972b, *Proc. Natl. Acad. Sci. U.S.A.* **69**:1394.

Cunningham, B. A., and Berggård, I., 1974, *Transplant. Rev.* **21**:3.

Dautigny, A., Bernier, I., Colombani, J., and Jolles, P., 1973, *Biochim. Biophys. Acta* **298**:783.

David, C. S., Shreffler, D. C., and Frelinger, J. A., 1973, *Proc. Natl. Acad. Sci. U.S.A.* **70**:2509.

David, C. S., Frelinger, J. A., and Shreffler, D. C., 1975, *Fed. Proc.* **34**:945 (abst.).

Davies, D. A. L., 1969, *Transplantation* **8**:51.

Davies, D. A. L., 1970, Transplantation antigens: Some features of mouse H-2 molecules and their relevance to HL-A in man, in: *Blood and Tissue Antigens* (D. Aminoff, ed.), pp. 101–116, Academic Press, New York.

Davies, D. A. L., Manstone, A. J., Viza, D. C., Colombani, J., and Dausset, J., 1968, *Transplantation* **6**:571.

De Deken-Grensen, M., and De Deken, R. H., 1959, *Biochim. Biophys. Acta* **31**:195.

Demant, P., 1973, *Transplant. Rev.* **15**:162.

Edelman, G. M., 1970, *Biochemistry* **9**:3197.

Eijsvoogel, V. P., 1974, *Prog. Immunol.* **5**:107.

Eijsvoogel, V. P., van Rood, J. J., du Toit, E. D., and Schellenkens, P. Th. A., 1972, *Eur. J. Immunol.* **2**:413.

Eijsvoogel, V. P., Du Bois, R., Melief, C. J. M., Zeylemaker, W. P., Raat Koning, L., and de Groot-Kooy, L., 1973, *Transplant. Proc.* **5**:415.

Goodfellow, P. N., Jones, E. A., van Heyningen, V., Solomon, E., Bobrow, M., Miggiano, V., and Bodmer, W. F., 1975, *Nature (London)* **254**:267.

Green, D. E., Mii, S., and Kohout, P. M., 1955, *J. Biol. Chem.* **217**:551.

Grey, H. M., Kubo, R. T., Colon, S. M., Poulik, M. D., Cresswell, P., Springer, T., Turner, M., and Strominger, J. L., 1973, *J. Exp. Med.* **138**:1608.

Hammerling, G. J., Deak, B. D., Mauve, G., Hammerling, V., and McDevitt, H. O., 1974, *Immunogenetics* **1**:68.

Hartee, E. F., 1972, *Anal. Biochem.* **48**:422.

Hauptfeld, V. D., Klein, D., and Klein, J., 1973, *Science* **181**:167.

Hayman, M. J., and Crumpton, M. J., 1972, *Biochem. Biophys. Res. Commun.* **47**:923.

Hayman, M. J., Skehel, J. J., and Crumpton, M. J., 1973, *FEBS Let.* **29**:185.

Helenius, A., and Simons, K., 1972, *J. Biol. Chem.* **247**:3656.

Helenius, A., and Söderlund, H., 1973, *Biochem. Biophys. Acta* **307**:287.

Hess, M., and Davies, D. A. L., 1974, *Eur. J. Biochem.* **41**:1.

Hunter, M. J., and Commerford, S. L., 1961, *Biochem. Biophys. Acta* **47**:580.

Hütteroth, T. H., Cleve, H., Litwin, S. D., and Poulik, M. D., 1973, *J. Exp. Med.* **137**:838.

Ivanyi, P., 1970, *Contemp. Topics Microbiol.* **53**:1.

Kahan, B. D., 1967 *J. Immunol.* **99**:1121.

Kahan, B. D., and Reisfeld, R. A., 1967, *Proc. Natl. Acad. Sci. U.S.A.* **58**:1430.

Kahan, B. D., and Reisfeld, R. A., 1968a, *J. Immunol.* **101**:237.

Kahan, B. D., and Reisfeld, R. A., 1968b, Progress in the purification of water soluble GP transplantation antigen, in: *Advance in Transplantation* (J. Dausset, J. Hamburger, and G. Mathe, eds.), pp. 295–299, Munksgaard, Copenhagen.

Kahan, B. D., Reisfeld, R. A., Epstein, L. B., and Southworth, J. G., 1967, Biologic activities of water soluble GP transplantation antigen, in: *Histocompatibility Testing 1967* (E. S. Curtoni, P. L. Mattiuz, and R. M. Tosi, eds.), pp. 295–302, Munksgaard, Copenhagen.

Katz, D. H., 1975, The role of products of the histocompatibility gene complex in immune systems, in: *The 7th Annual Miami Winter Symposia* (E. E. Smith and D. W. Ribbons, eds.), pp. 30–32, University of Miami, Miami, Fla.

Katz, D. H., and Benacerraf, B., 1975, *Transplant. Rev.* **22**:175.

Katz, D. H., Hamaoka, T., Dorf, M. E., and Benacerraf, B., 1973, *Proc. Natl. Acad. Sci. U.S.A.* **70**:2624.

Katz, D. H., Dorf, M. E., and Benacerraf, B., 1974, *J. Exp. Med.* **140**:290.

Kissmeyer-Nielsen, F., and Thorsby, E., 1970, *Transplant. Rev.* **4**:70.

Kissmeyer-Nielsen, F., Jørgensen, F., and Lamm, L. U., 1972, *Johns Hopkins Med. J.* **131**:385.

Klein, J., 1972, *Transplantation* **13**:291.

Klein, J., and Park, P. M., 1973, *J. Exp. Med.* **137**:1213.

Klein, J., and Shreffler, D. C., 1971, *Transplant. Rev.* **6**:3.

Klein, J., and Shreffler, D. C., 1972, *J. Exp. Med.* **135**:924.

Klein, J., Hauptfeld, M., and Hauptfeld, V., 1974, *Immunogenetics* **1**:45.

Kochakian, C. D., and Williams, B. R., 1973, *Steroids* **21**:95.

Letarte-Muirhead, M., Acton, R. T., and Williams, A. F., 1974, *Biochem. J.* **143**:51.

Mann, D. L., and Fahey, J. L., 1971, *Annu. Rev. Microbiol.* **25**:679.

Mann, D. L., and Nathenson, S. G., 1969, *Proc. Natl. Acad. Sci. U.S.A.* **64**:1380.

Mann, D. L., Rogentine, G. N., Fahey, J. L., and Nathenson, S., 1969, *J. Immunol.* **103**:282.

Manson, L., Hickey, C., and Palm, J., 1968, H-2 alloantigen content of surface membrane of mouse cells, in: *Biological Properties of the Mammalian Surface Membrane* (L. Manson, ed.), pp. 93–103, Wistar Institute Press, Philadelphia.

McDevitt, H. O., and Benacerraf, B., 1969, *Adv. Immunol.* **11**:31.

McDevitt, H. O., Deak, B. D., Shreffler, D. C., Klein, J., Stimpfling, J. H., and Snell, G. D., 1972, *J. Exp. Med.* **135**:1259.

McDevitt, H. O., Bechtol, K. B., Hammerling, G. J., Lonai, P., and Delovitch, T. L., 1974, *Ir* genes and antigen recognition, in: *The Immune System: Genes, Receptors, Signals* (E. E. Sercarz, A. R. Williamson, and C. F. Fox, eds.), pp. 597–632, Academic Press, New York.

Meunier, J. C., Olsen, R. W., and Changeux, J. P., 1972, *FEBS Let.* **24**:63.

Miller, W. V. (ed.), 1974, Leukocyte and tissue antigens and antibodies, in: *Technical Methods and Procedures*, pp. 225–231, American Association of Blood Banks, J. B. Lippincott, Washington, D. C.

Miyakawa, Y., Tanigaki, N., Yagi, Y., and Pressman, D., 1973, *Immunology* **24**:67.

Muramatsu, T., and Nathenson, S. G., 1970, *Biochem. Biophys. Res. Commun.* **38**:1.

Muramatsu, T., and Nathenson, S. G., 1971, *Fed. Proc.* **30**:2768.

Nakamuro, K., Tanigaki, N., and Pressman, D., 1973, *Proc. Natl. Acad. Sci. U.S.A.* **70**:2863.

Nakamuro, K., Tanigaki, N., Natori, T. and Pressman, D., 1975, *Fed. Proc.* **34**:1016 (abst.).

Nathenson, S. G., 1970, *Annu. Rev. Genet.* **4**:69.

Nathenson, S. G., and Cullen, S. E., 1974, *Biochim. Biophys. Acta* **344**:1.

Neauport-Sautes, C., Lilly, F., Silvestre, D., and Kourilsky, F. M., 1973, *J. Exp. Med.* **137**:511.

Östberg, L., Lindblom, J. B., and Peterson, P. A., 1974, *Nature (London)* **249**:463.

Pancake, S. J., and Nathenson, S. G., 1973, *J. Immunol.* **111**:1086.

Passmore, H. C., and Shreffler, D. C., 1970, *Biochem. Genet.* **4**:351.

Paul, W. E., Shevach, E. M., Ben-Sasson, S. Z., Finkelman, F., and Green, I., 1974, Alloantiserum induced blockade of *Ir* gene product function, in: *The Immune System. Genes, Receptors, Signals* (E. E. Sercarz, A. R. Williamson, and C. F. Fox, eds.), pp. 175–190. Academic Press, New York.

Peterson, P. A., Cunningham, B. A., Berggård, I., and Edelman, G. M., 1972, *Proc. Natl. Acad. Sci. U.S.A.* **69**:1697.

Peterson, P. A., Rask, L., and Lindblom, J. B., 1974, *Proc. Natl. Acad. Sci. U.S.A.* **71**:35.

Poulik, M. D., Bernoco, M., Bernoco, D., and Ceppellini, R., 1973, *Science* **182**:1352.

Rask, L., Lindblom, J. B., and Peterson, P. A., 1974, *Nature (London)* **249**:833.

Reisfeld, R. A., and Kahan, B. D., 1970, *Adv. Immunol.* **12**:117.

Reisfeld, R. A., and Kahan, B. D., 1971, *Transplant. Rev.* **6**:81.

Reisfeld, R. A., and Kahan, B. D., 1972, Human histocompatibility antigens, in: *Contemporary Topics of Immunochemistry* (F. P. Inman, ed.), pp. 51–76, Plenum Press, New York.

Reisfeld, R. A., and Pellegrino, M. A., 1972, Salt extraction of soluble HL-A antigens, in: *Transplantation Antigens: Markers of Biological Individuality* (B. D. Kahan and R. A. Reisfeld, eds.), pp. 259–272, Academic Press, New York.

Reisfeld, R. A., Pellegrino, M. A., and Kahan, B. D., 1971, *Science* **172**:1134.

Sachs, D. H., and Cone, J. L., 1973, *J. Exp. Med.* **138**:1289.

Sanderson, A. R., and Batchelor, J. R., 1968, *Nature (London)* **219**:184.

Sanderson, A. R., and Welsh, K. I., 1972, Purification and structural studies of alloantigen determinants solubilized with papain, in: *Transplantation Antigens: Markers of Biological Individuality* (B. D. Kahan and R. A. Reisfeld, eds.), pp. 273–286, Academic Press, New York.

Sanderson, A. R., Cresswell, P., and Welsh, K. I., 1971, *Nature (London) New Biol.* **230**:8.

Schwartz, B. D., and Nathenson, S. G., 1971a, *Transplant. Proc.* **3**:180.

Schwartz, B. D., and Nathenson, S. G., 1971b, *J. Immunol.* **107**:1363.

Schwartz, B. D., Kato, K., Cullen, S. E., and Nathenson, S. G., 1973a, *Biochemistry* **12**:2157.

Schwartz, B. D., Wickner, S., Rajan, T. V., and Nathenson, S. G., 1973b, *Transplant. Proc.* **5**:439.

Shimada, A., and Nathenson, S. G., 1969, *Biochemistry* **8**:4048.

Shimada, A., Yamane, K., and Nathenson, S. G., 1970, *Proc. Natl. Acad. Sci. U.S.A.* **65**:691.

Shreffler, D. C., 1965, The Ss system of the mouse: A quantitative serum protein difference genetically controlled by the H-2 region, in: *Isoantigens and Cell Interactions* (J. Palm, ed.), pp. 11–19, Wistar Institute Press, Philadelphia.

Shreffler, D. C., 1967, Genetic control of cellular antigens, in *Proceedings of the IIIrd International Conference on Human Genetics* (J. F. Crow and J. V. Neel, eds.), pp. 217–231, Johns Hopkins Press, Baltimore.

Shreffler, D. C., 1974, Genetic time structure of the *H-2* gene complex in cellular selection and regulation, in: *The Immune Response* (G. M. Edelman, ed.), pp. 83–100, Raven Press, New York.

Shreffler, D. C., 1975, Properties and functions of the products of the major histocompatibility complex. General session, American Association of Immunologists Annual Meeting, April 14–18, 1975. Atlantic City, N.J.

Shreffler, D. C., and Klein, J., 1970, *Transplant. Proc.* **2**:5.

Silver, J., and Hood, L., 1974, *Nature (London)* **249**:764.

Snary, D., Goodfellow, P., Hayman, M. J., Bodmer, W. F., and Crumpton, M. J., 1974, *Nature (London)* **247**:457.

Snell, G. D., and Stimpfling, J. H., 1964, Genetics of tissue transplantation, in: *Biology of the Laboratory Mouse* (E. Green, ed.), pp. 457–491, McGraw-Hill, New York.

Solheim, B. G., and Thorsby, E., 1974, *Tissue Antigens* **4**:83.

Springer, T. A., and Strominger, J. L., 1973, *Fed. Proc.* **32**:1018 (abst.).

Srb, A. M., and Owen, R. D., 1953, Linkage, crossing over and chromosome mapping, in: *General Genetics* (G. W. Beadle, R. Emerson, and D. M. Whitaker, eds.), pp. 150–181, Freeman, San Francisco.

Stimpfling, J. H., and Richardson, A., 1965, *Genetics* **51**:831.

Stimpfling, J. H., and Snell, G. D., 1972, Histocompatibility genes and some immunologic problems, in: *Proceedings of the International Symposium on Tissue Transplant* (A. P. Christoffanini and G. Horeckel, eds.), p. 37, University of Chile, Santiago.

Strominger, J. L., Cresswell, P., Grey, H., Humphreys, R. E., Mann, D., McCune, J., Parham, P., Robb, R., Sanderson, A. R., Springer, T. A., Terhorst, C., and Turner, M. J., 1974, *Transplant Rev.* **21**:126.

Tanigaki, N., Katagiri, M., Nakamuro, K., Kreiter, V. P., and Pressman, D., 1973, *Fed. Proc.* **32**:1017.

Taussig, M. J., 1975, Antigen-specific T cell factor in cell cooperation and genetic control of the immune response in: *Symposium: Cellular and Soluble Factors in the Regulation of Lymphocyte Activation,* American Association of Immunologists Annual Meeting, April 14–18, 1975, Atlantic City, N.J.

Taussig, M. J., and Munro, A. J., 1974, *Nature (London)* **251**:63.

Taussig, M. J., Mozes, E., and Isac, R., 1974, *J. Exp. Med.* **140**:301.

Tousler, O., Aronson, N. N., Jr., Dulaney, J. T., and Henderikson, H. J., 1970, *Cell Biol.* **47**:604.

Turner, M. J., Strominger, J. L., and Sanderson, A. R., 1972, *Proc. Natl. Acad. Sci. U.S.A.* **69**:200.

Vitetta, E. S., Klein, J., and Uhr, J. W., 1974, *Immunogenetics* **1**:82.

Wallach, D. F. H., and Kamat, V. B., 1966, *Methods Enzymol.* **8**:164.

Weydert, A., Bernier, I., Colombani, J., and Jolles, P., 1971, *C. R. Acad. Sci. Ser. D* **273**:2006.

Williams, A. F., 1973, *Eur. J. Immunol.* **3**:628.

Wilson, L. A., and Amos, D. B., 1972, *Tissue Antigens* **2**:105.

Yamane, K., and Nathenson, S. G., 1970, *Biochemistry* **9**:1336.

Author Index

Subject Index